# DERMATOLOGY

## Diagnosis and treatment of cutaneous disorders

# DERMATOLOGY

## DIAGNOSIS AND TREATMENT OF CUTANEOUS DISORDERS

---


**Wm. D. STEWART, M.D., F.R.C.P.(C)**

Professor and Chairman, Division of Dermatology,
Department of Medicine, Faculty of Medicine, University of British Columbia;
Head, Division of Dermatology, Department of Medicine, Vancouver General Hospital;
Research Consultant, Shaughnessy Hospital; Consulting Staff, G. F. Strong Rehabilitation Centre; Attending Medical Staff, Cancer Control Agency of British Columbia, Vancouver, British Columbia; Associate Editor, Dialogues in Dermatology, American Academy of Dermatology

**JULIUS L. DANTO, M.D.**

Fellow, American Academy of Dermatology;
Associate Member, Scottsdale Memorial Hospital,
Scottsdale, Arizona

**STUART MADDIN, M.D., F.R.C.P.(C)**

Clinical Associate Professor, Division of Dermatology,
Department of Medicine, Faculty of Medicine,
University of British Columbia;
Active Staff, Vancouver General Hospital,
Vancouver, British Columbia


**FOURTH EDITION**

*with 277 illustrations and 62 color plates*


## The C. V. Mosby Company

Saint Louis 1978

**FOURTH EDITION**



First and second editions published under title: Synopsis of dermatology.
Previous edition copyrighted 1974.

Printed in the United States of America

The C. V. Mosby Company
11830 Westline Industrial Drive, St. Louis, Missouri 63141

**Library of Congress Cataloging in Publication Data**

Stewart, William D
Dermatology.

Bibliography: p.
Includes index.
1. Skin—Diseases. I. Danto, Julius L., joint author. II. Maddin, Stuart, joint author. III. Title.
RL71.S823 1978 616.5 78-12789
ISBN 0-8016-4809-2

TS/U/B 9 8 7 6 5 4 3 2 1

# FOREWORD to first edition

*Synopsis of Dermatology* is not just another textbook. It is an exceptionally complete, accurate, and highly up-to-the-minute presentation of the essentials required for both the recognition and the management of most skin diseases.

The last decades have witnessed the appearance of a number of good, brief textbooks dealing with this specialty. Each of these texts reflects the training, experience, and judgment of its authors. So, like paintings by different artists, each is somewhat different from all the others. I am of the opinion that *Synopsis of Dermatology* is likely to prove, in many respects, the most useful of the newer books.

The book includes short but clear summaries on the embryology, anatomy, and physiology of the human skin; an especially concise and eminently practical presentation of diagnosis by means of regional localizations; and an accurate, up-to-date compilation of the mechanisms and manifestations of cutaneous drug reactions. These are but a few among the many special features that should make this book a front runner for medical students, interns, and residents, as well as for nondermatologists in private practice, who must daily meet and master dermatological problems.

It is only fair to state that my esteem for this text and its three authors is no whit diminished by the fact that I recognize familiar statements and concepts of pathogenesis, as well as practices of therapy, that they and I generated and tested during the years I was privileged to be their preceptor. Nevertheless, I do not believe that I am unduly biased by a teacher's pride when I affirm that I consider *Synopsis of Dermatology* to be one of the most practical and useful didactic texts that have recently come upon the medical scene.

Medicine is rapidly entering an era in which acquisition of knowledge, and especially *communication of knowledge,* is beginning to be accorded the status and attention its importance deserves. I feel sure that all who use this book will recognize the authors' unusual ability to communicate their combined knowledge concerning a category of "organ diseases" which may well constitute about fifteen percent of all medical practice.

*June 12, 1966*

**Marion B. Sulzberger, M.D., F.A.C.P.**
Emeritus Professor of Dermatology, New York University;
Technical Director of Research, Letterman General Hospital,
San Francisco, California

# PREFACE

This is a book on clinical dermatology and does not propose to become a textbook. For this reason, we have shifted the increasing volume of basic science material from its isolated position and prefixed it to the clinical areas where it will be applied, that is, to the disease most relevant to that material. It is true that doing so has the disadvantage of scattering this information throughout the book, but results of investigations indicated that the cluster of information at the beginning of the book in former editions was consulted little, if at all, by the average reader. Thus we hope that the important advances that have been achieved in the past few years will be more easily available to the user in context with the altered function in disease. If there is no area of applicability in the context of this book, the information has been deleted.

There is a great deal more information in this edition than in the third, and even more stringent attention was directed to eliminating unnecessary verbiage. The references used are clarified by a phrase or two, but when this proved too difficult, the reference was eliminated. Illustrations, both in color and in black and white, are more numerous.

Regional diagnosis was so well received that we felt justified in enlarging it while attempting to reduce some of its ambiguity.

Virtually the whole book has been updated, a task that grows significantly each edition and invariably exceeds the time allotted to it. By its completion, however, it has become a more satisfactory achievement, and the reader response makes it a gratifying one.

Mrs. Margaret Anderson has staunchly and inimitably typed, indexed, proofread, copied, edited, criticized, suggested, and, in general, been indispensable to the publication. The staffs of the Biomedical Branch Library at the Vancouver General Hospital, the B.C. Medical Library Service, and the Woodward Medical Library at the University of British Columbia have given freely of their time and skill, for which we are most grateful.

**Wm. D. Stewart**
**Julius L. Danto**
**Stuart Maddin**

# CONTENTS

## COLOR PLATES

PART ONE

# Regional diagnosis

# Introduction

The skin forms a self-replacing, multifunctional, resilient covering for the body that adjusts easily to a remarkable variation in environment, as well as adapting to the needs of the underlying structures that it shelters.

It is a self-contained organ, a semipermeable barrier layer dependent on the vascular, lymphatic, and nerve supply of the body, but carrying out its own unique activities. These include the *production of keratin, sebum, sweat,* and *melanin* (shared with certain other structures) as well as *heat exchange* and *protection.* Similar to some other organs, it performs the specialized functions involved in *perception of sensation, repair of wounds, immunological defense and inflammation, cholesterol synthesis, steroid hormone synthesis, carbohydrate, fat, and protein metabolism.*

## FUNCTIONS OF THE SKIN

The major function of the skin is protective, in the sense of maintenance of the body equilibrium against the disruptive effects of the environment.

1. Protection includes physical protection from (a) trauma, (b) temperature variations, (c) radiations, (d) harmful penetration by both foreign and familiar substances, (e) all concentrations of moisture and humidity, (f) invasion by microorganisms, and (g) damage from macroorganisms. To perform these functions, the skin has a highly integrated, efficient, and complex mechanism of keratinization, in which epidermal cells mature and migrate upward to form the outer compact keratinous stratum corneum (Fig. 1).

2. The skin also maintains itself and repairs its own wounds quickly and efficiently by two distinct epidermal and dermal processes.

3. It produces secretions from its sebaceous and eccrine surface glands that maintain a buffered protective surface film.

4. These glands are the site of an active system of androgen metabolism producing dihydrotestosterone and, perhaps more significant as an active agent, androstenedione.

5. It supports a continually operating chemical factory of carbohydrate, protein, and fat metabolism. Relevant to carbohydrate metabolism, the skin possesses more than half the total amount of glucose contained in the blood. It has not been determined how glucose enters skin cells. The skin is an active site of lipid synthesis. Hair growth represents significant protein synthesis.

6. The skin operates its own delayed hypersensitivity mechanism and develops an immune reaction from simple contact with foreign materials as soon as they have been identified as such.

7. The skin serves, although in a minor way, as an organ of excretion.

8. It also provides an area for irradiation of vitamin D precursors and thus participates in the production of vitamin D.

9. It minimizes loss of internal content and prevents the fluid environment within its confines from leaking out through the barrier.

## HISTORY AND EXAMINATION OF THE PATIENT

### Principles of history taking

A dermatological history simply complements the general medical history and should, in addition to providing the information covered there, emphasize the following points:

1. *Present dermatological illness.* Date and site of first onset, dates of recurrences, apparent cause, course (whether intermittent, seasonal, affected by environmental and occupational factors, other

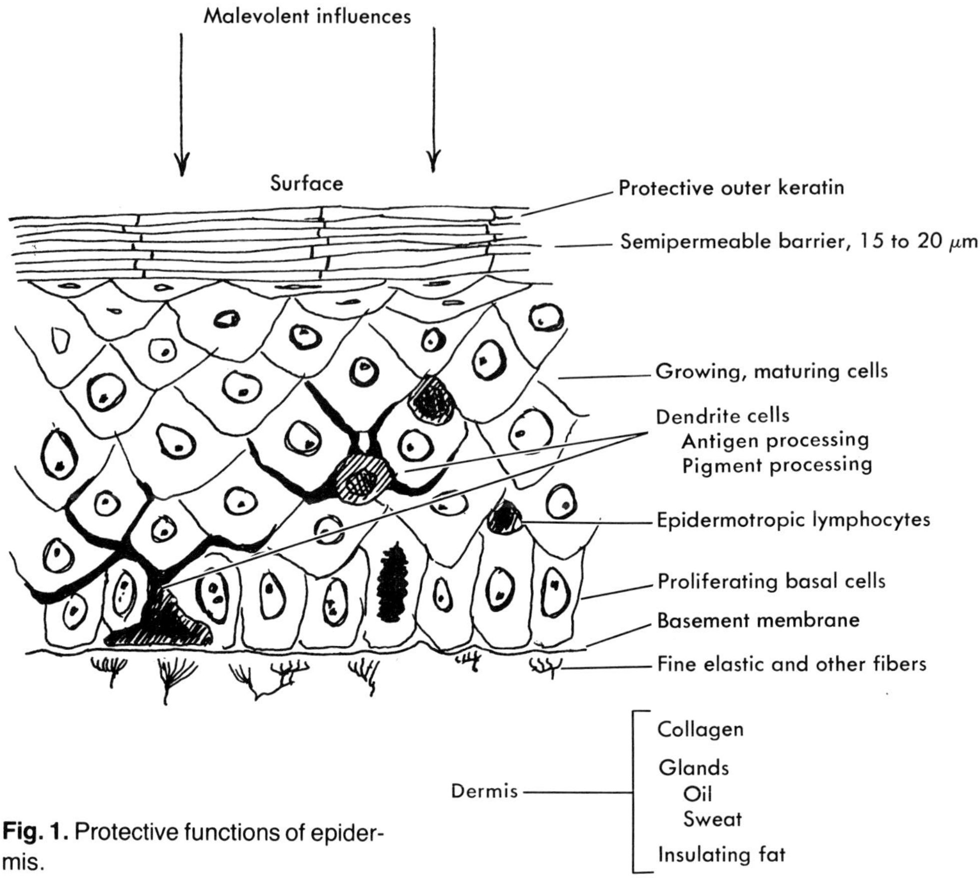


**Fig. 1.** Protective functions of epidermis.

precipitating factors), symptoms, spread of lesions.

2. *Past dermatological illness.* Previous allergic cutaneous reactions, infantile eczema, tolerance of sunlight, metal sensitivity, results of previous patch tests.
3. *General medical background.* History of peptic ulcer, arthritis, heart disease, tuberculosis, asthma, hay fever, current illnesses, recent illnesses.
4. *History of medications.* Important: all current medications prescribed or self-administered, both topical and systemic, must be identified and recorded. Often an old medication rather than a new one is at fault in a drug reaction; previous reactions to medication, proved or suspected. *(Many medications, such as acetylsalicylic acid, cold tablets, antihistamines, or "water pills" are so familiar the patient does not immediately categorize them as medicine.)* This must be gone over at least twice in detail if an unrecognized drug effect is to be elicited.
5. *Family history.* Dermatological disease previously occurring in siblings, parents, predecessors; dermatological disease *currently* occurring in family; allergic genetically related diseases, for example, asthma, hay fever. All known possibly genetically related factors, such as with lupus erythematosus or arthritis.
6. *Travel history.* Recent peregrinations, periods of stay out of country, or being in other parts of country. Contact with other travelers. Exposure to disease.

## Examination of patient

A dermatological examination must be carried out at a suitably comfortable temperature and in a well-lighted room. All skin surfaces should be thoroughly examined and mucous membranes visualized. A systemic approach is advisable so that a routine examination eval-

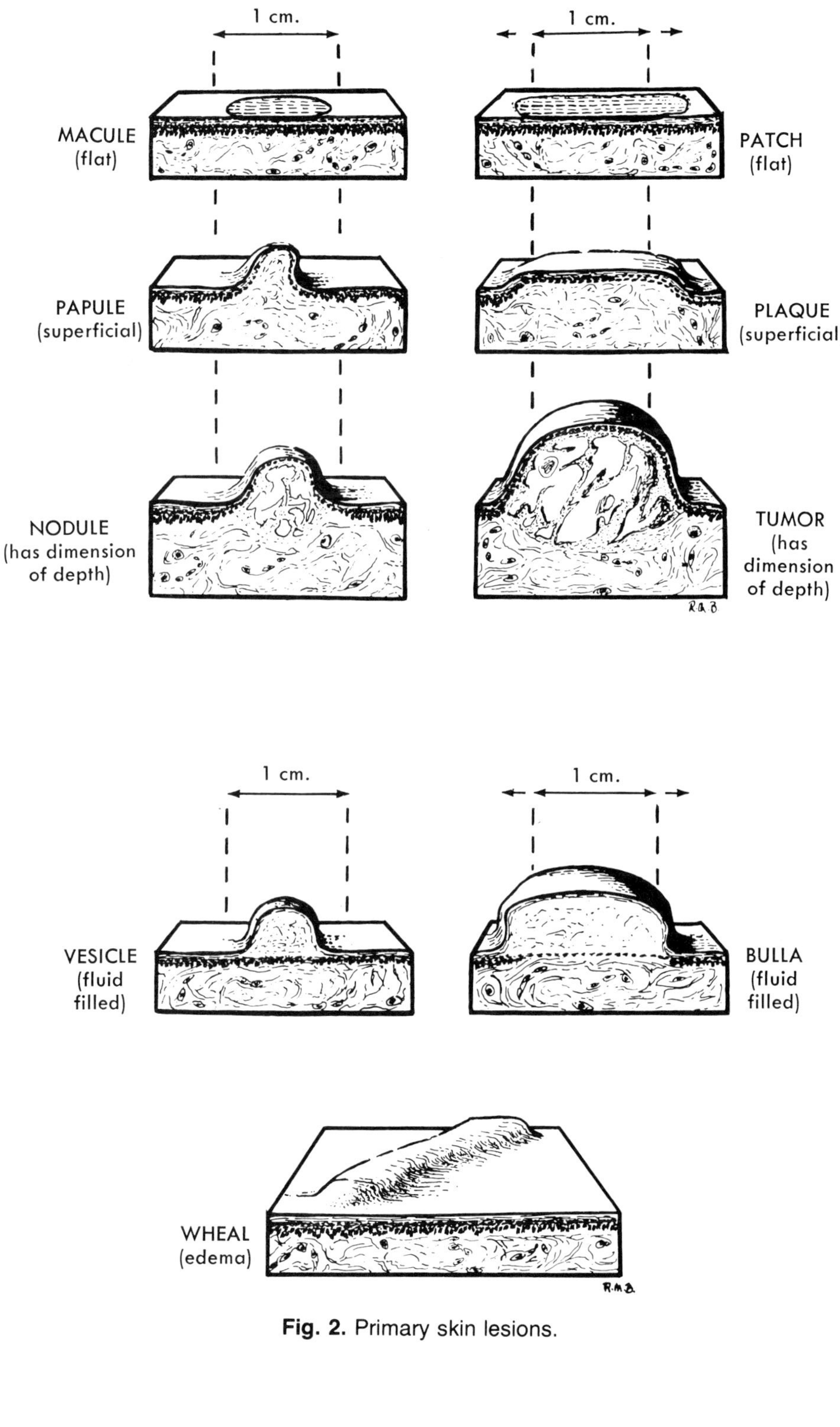


**Fig. 2.** Primary skin lesions.

uates (1) smooth skin, (2) intertriginous skin, (3) hairy areas, (4) mucous membranes, (5) nails, and (6) hair.

One is best advised to determine general patterns of distribution of lesions and then to examine more closely the individually affected areas as to color, scaling, texture, moisture, induration, and definition of borders.

## Cutaneous lesions

Primary cutaneous lesions (Fig. 2) are described in eleven simple terms.

Since there are no agreed-upon definitions of the sizes of cutaneous lesions, and discrepancies exist among authors regarding size and depth of these lesions, we are subscribing to Watt and Jillson's easy-to-remember formula of gradations between these terms*:

### Primary lesions less than 1 cm. in size

**macule** a flat, circumscribed discoloration of the skin or mucous membrane up to 1 cm. in its longest diameter.

**papule** a solid, elevated lesion of the skin or mucous membrane up to 1 cm. in its longest diameter.

**nodule** a solid, elevated lesion of the skin or mucous membrane, with the added dimension of depth in the underlying tissue, but less than 1 cm. in its longest diameter.

**vesicle** a fluid-filled, superficial, elevated lesion of the skin or mucous membrane, less than 1 cm. in diameter.

### Primary lesions greater than 1 cm. in size

**patch** a flat, circumscribed discoloration of the skin or mucous membrane greater than 1 cm. in diameter.

**plaque** a solid, elevated lesion of the skin or mucous membrane greater than 1 cm. in its longest diameter.

**tumor** a solid, elevated lesion of the skin or mucous membrane, with the added dimension of depth in tissue, and greater than 1 cm. in its longest diameter.

**bulla** a fluid-filled, superficial, elevated lesion of the skin or mucous membrane greater than 1 cm. in diameter.

### Primary lesions of varying size

**pustule** a vesicle or bulla containing pus rather than clear fluid.

**wheal** an irregularly shaped, pale to pink, elevated, solid, changing, and transient lesion of the skin or mucous membrane caused by cutaneous edema.

**telangiectasia** a fine, often irregular red line produced by dilatation of a capillary, normally invisible.

*Definitions adapted from Watt, T. L., and Jillson, O. F.: Arch. Derm. **90**:454, 1964.

### Other lesions of varying size

**scar** first red then pale avascular, smooth hyaline wound repair; may be flat, depressed, elevated, or hypertrophic.

**ulcer** loss of tissue from a surface, leaving an uncovered wound.

**sclerosis, sclerotic** indurated, nonpliable.

**scale** a thin flake of surface epithelium separated from the body.

**keratosis, keratotic** thickened, dry, warty, irregular, often pigmented, sharply localized elevation of top layer.

**excoriation** scratch mark.

**eczema** moist, oozing, vesiculation (bubbling up in epidermis).

**crust** dried surface fluid.

**atrophy** *epidermal:* fine, cigarette-paper wrinkling, transparent epidermis; *dermal:* depressed surface, loss of substance, visible blood vessels; *subcutaneous:* more profound loss of substance with no apparent surface structural abnormality.

### Pathological cutaneous processes

Terms used to describe pathological changes in cutaneous disease include the following:

**hyperkeratosis** thickening of the keratin layer of the epidermis. Usually there is an accompanying thickening of the stratum granulosum.

**parakeratosis** incomplete keratinization of the stratum corneum, with retention of nuclei and cellular structure right through the horny layer.

**acanthosis** prolongation of the epidermal rete pegs by hyperplasia of the epidermal cells.

**dyskeratosis** irregular and nonuniform acanthosis with abnormal individual keratinization of cells. They are no longer uniformly placed and spaced. This may be due to malignant changes, but it is seen in some benign disorders.

**vesicle formation** result of edema between epidermal prickle cells that leads to separation of cells and formation of lakes or larger areas of fluid collection. These progress to loculated vesicles that protrude above the surface.

**acantholysis** process by which individual cells lose their tonofilament desmosome attachments, become rounded, and lie in the fluid-filled cavity so formed.

**liquefactive degeneration** change that involves the basal cell layer and denotes edema of the dermoepidermal junction with loss of orientation of the basal cells. There is an inflammatory infiltrate in the area as well.

**desmosome** intracellular structure of epidermal cells of all levels. Bundles of intracytoplasmic filaments loop to attach to the disc surface at sites of contact between adjacent cells. Half desmosomes are at points of intimate contact of basal cells to the basement membrane.

**lysosome** intracytoplasmic membrane-enclosed structure containing a variety of enzymes active in the breakdown of phagocytized material.

CHAPTER 1

# Specific diagnoses by body regions

Brief descriptions of cutaneous diseases as they appear in specific areas of the body are given below. Regional differences are emphasized. Lesions are described by their predominant characteristic, under the following headings: flat lesions, raised (elevated) lesions, depressed (ulcerated) lesions, and loss of hair.

In general, the more common lesions appear first under each heading. The page number after the disease entity refers to the major description of that disease in the book.

## SCALP

### Flat lesions

***Nevus flammeus*** (p. 569). Patches of pink to red, persistent capillary dilatation from birth. On nuchal area in 50% of general population.

***Seborrhea*** (p. 494). Either a noninflammatory, excessive, dry scaling of scalp, "dandruff" (seborrhea sicca), or an excessive oiliness (seborrhea oleosa).

***Seborrheic dermatitis*** (Fig. 1-1, *A*) (p. 494). Diffuse, fine scaling and erythema of scalp. Ordinarily pruritic. May be present as poorly circumscribed patches. Very common.

***Psoriasis*** (p. 462). Early lesions consist of mild patchy scaling only. Later, fully developed red, discrete, or confluent patches possess gray-white heavy scale. May involve entire scalp. No hair loss.

***Atopic dermatitis*** (p. 118). Pruritus, scaling, and dry dermatitis, often with crusting and excoriations. Alopecia produced by long-continued rubbing.

***Seborrheic keratosis*** (p. 508). Early lesion is a flat tan macule.

***Actinic keratosis*** (p. 508). Small, discrete firmly adherent, scaling, reddish macule. Found on bald areas of scalp that have had prolonged exposure to sunlight.

***Nevus*** (p. 523). Discrete, pigmented or nonpigmented macules. Arises at birth or in childhood.

***Primary irritant contact dermatitis*** (p. 430). Erythema and pruritus. May arise from irritating shampoos, permanent waving solutions, and other hair preparations.

***Allergic eczematous contact dermatitis*** (p. 102). Varies from simple erythema in mild cases to severe oozing, exudative dermatitis of scalp, ears, eyelids, forehead, and neck. Common cause: hair dyes.

***Pediculosis capitis*** (p. 336). Associated with pruritus and excoriation of scalp, usually on posterior aspect. Lice found on scalp. Minute gray nits firmly attached to hair shaft. Eyelashes should be examined for nits.

### Raised lesions

***Seborrheic keratosis*** (p. 508). Discrete, soft, rough-surfaced, small brown plaque. Usually in hair-bearing temporal areas.

***Wart (verruca vulgaris)*** (p. 316). Discrete. Ordinarily digitate or filiform.

***Dermatitis herpetiformis*** (p. 140). Persistent, intensely pruritic, crusted vesicopapules.

***Lichen simplex chronicus*** (p. 448). Plaque of lichenification. Sharply localized, very pruritic. Usually suboccipital.

***Zoster*** (p. 303). Unilateral scalp tenderness followed by painful vesicle formation on erythematous base. Early localized lymphadenopathy present.

***Folliculitis*** (p. 244). Discrete, excoriated, crusted, erythematous, perifollicular papules and pustules.

***Acne keloid*** (p. 516). Elevated, smooth,

A

B

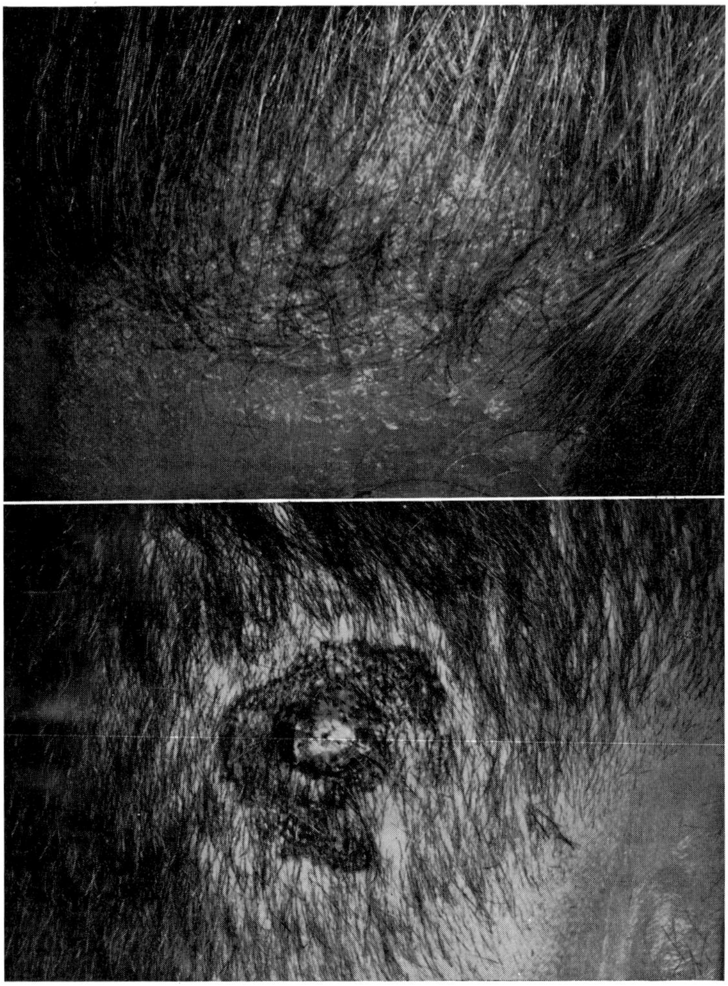

**Fig. 1-1. A,** Seborrheic dermatitis of anterior hairline. **B**, Malignant melanoma of scalp.

firm, pink lesions of posterior aspect of neck, arising from acne lesions.

***Epidermoid cyst and sebaceous cyst (wen)*** (Fig. 1-2) (p. 513). Globular, fluctuant lesions, 1 to 4 cm. in diameter. Rare before puberty. Ordinarily asymptomatic. If infected or irritated, they become painful and enlarged.

***Hemangioma*** (p. 569). Red, soft, rapidly growing tumor of newborn with "strawberry" surface. Asymptomatic.

***Tumors of skin appendages.*** Variety of small nodules, plaques, and cysts on scalp. Frequently present from birth or arising at puberty. Aberrant development of normal components of hair and skin glands. Require microscopic identification as some predispose to recurrence and malignancy.

***Basal cell epithelioma*** (p. 537). Nodular lesion with a distinct rolled border. Tendency toward ulceration in center. Found in frontal aspect or bald areas of scalp. May arise in appendage tumors.

***Squamous cell carcinoma*** (p. 541). May follow actinic keratosis. Indurated and ulcerated nodule demonstrating continued growth.

***Malignant melanoma*** (Fig. 1-1, *B*) (p. 530). Usual origin in pigmented nevus. Malignant transformation accompanied by pigmentary increase, induration, and ulceration. Metastases occur early.

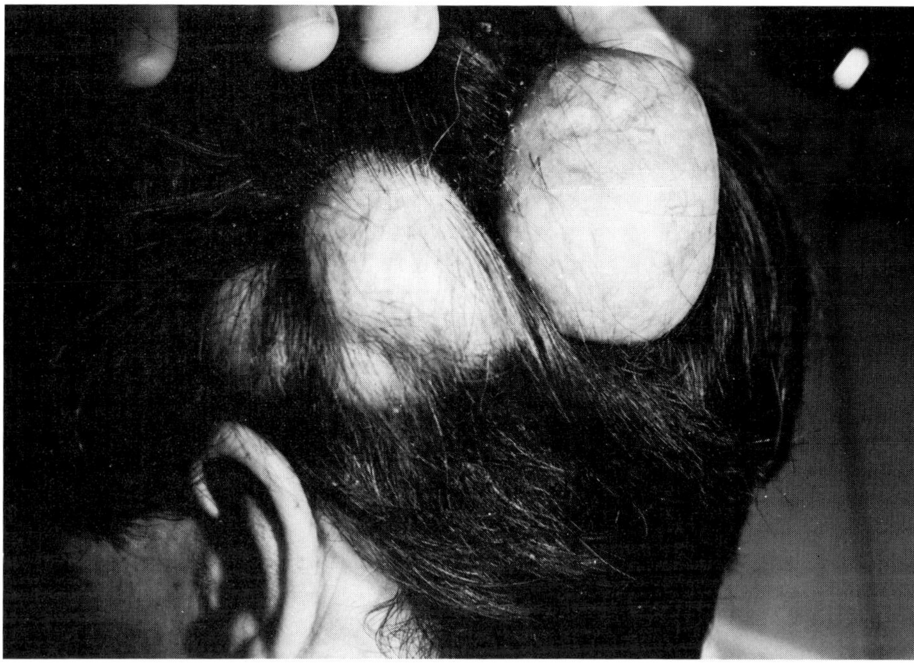

**Fig. 1-2.** Sebaceous cysts. Unusually large, but typical.

***Cylindroma (turban tumor).*** Multiple, smooth, varisized nodules studding scalp. Present from puberty.

***Neurofibroma*** (p. 521). Soft, flaccid, skin-colored pedunculated lesions of neurofibromatosis appear at puberty.

***Dermoid cyst.*** Most are apparent by the third to 5th year, 0.5 to 5 cm., fluctuant, parietal.

***Metastases*** (p. 558). Firm, dome-shaped tumors in an elderly patient's scalp may represent metastases from breast, kidney, or prostate.

## Depressed lesions

***Linear scleroderma (scleroderma en coup de sabre)*** (p. 161). Linear, pale brown lesion, parallel to midline at depth of depressed furrow on scalp and forehead. Atrophy of skin, subcutaneous tissue, and bone may occur. Found in young adults.

### Alopecia (hair loss)—nonscarring

***Physiological male alopecia*** (p. 230). Regression of hair at anterior hairline, above temples, and on vertex. Hereditary.

***Alopecia areata*** (p. 234). Sudden onset of circumscribed, smooth, bald areas. May enlarge and coalesce. Loose, easily removed hairs at periphery of active lesions. Beard may be similarly affected.

***Tinea capitis*** (p. 267). Circular areas of alopecia demonstrating short, broken-off hairs. Type of fungus determines presence or absence of inflammation. Found almost exclusively in children.

***Diffuse alopecia in women*** (p. 230). Asymptomatic, diffuse thinning of scalp hair. No apparent scalp disease. Found from young adulthood on through later life.

***Alopecia caused by chemicals.*** Brittleness and breaking off of hair shafts above skin surface. Excessive exposure to bleaches, waving solutions, and hair straighteners.

***Developmental hair shaft abnormalities*** (p. 233). A variety of malformations of hair shaft, some heritable, some sporadic. Can cause apparent baldness because of fragility and fracture of hairs at or above scalp level. May occur at birth, in childhood, or later.

***Alopecia after pregnancy*** (p. 232). Diffuse postpartum thinning of scalp hair without evi-

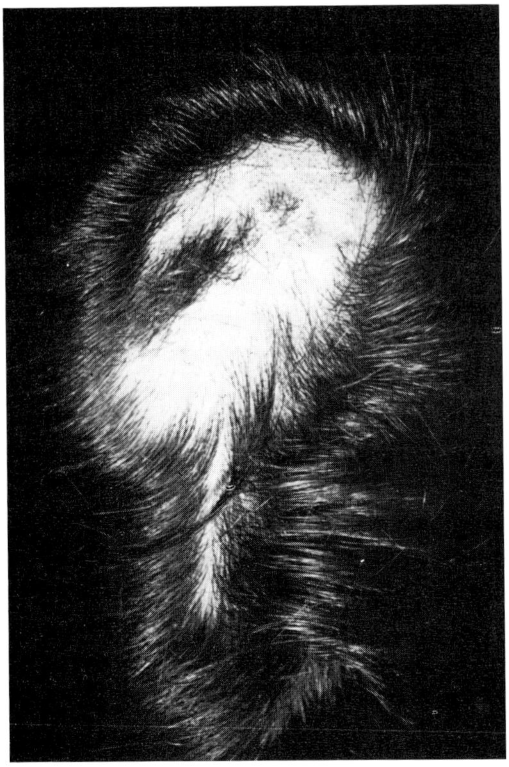

**Fig. 1-3.** Trichotillomania. Appearance can be deceptive in establishing cause of alopecia.

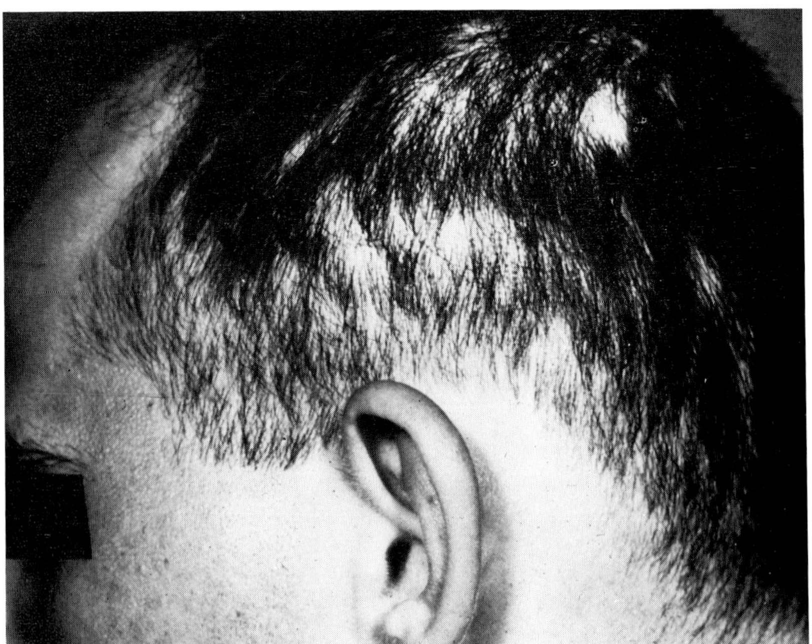

**Fig. 1-4.** Syphilitic alopecia. Moth-eaten appearance.

dence of scalp disorder. May last for several months.

***Alopecia caused by fever*** (p. 232). Diffuse loss of hair on normal-appearing scalp in weeks to months after febrile illness.

***Alopecia caused by drugs*** (p. 232). Cytotoxic drugs, gold, arsenic, and thallium can produce a diffuse loss of scalp hair. Characteristic tapered hair shaft.

***Alopecia caused by endocrine disease*** (p. 232). Pituitary, thyroid, or adrenal disease may produce diffuse hair loss.

***Trichotillomania*** (Fig. 1-3) (p. 478). Incomplete, irregular patches of alopecia caused by tugging of hair by patient.

***Syphilitic alopecia*** (Fig. 1-4) (p. 258). Loss of scalp hair concurrent with mucous patches and generalized skin manifestations. Irregular areas of alopecia that contain some strands of hair. "Moth-eaten" appearance. Serological test for syphilis is positive.

***Alopecia mucinosa.*** Rare. Single or multiple, mildly erythematous, gelatinous papules or plaques devoid of hair. Adults.

## Alopecia (hair loss)—scarring

***Scarring alopecia*** (Fig. 1-5) (p. 235). Scarring proceeds to patchy, permanent loss of hair on scalp.

***Discoid lupus erythematosus*** (p. 235). *Acute:* irregular erythematous, scaling, tender areas that lose hair. *Chronic:* atrophy, depigmentation, and permanent alopecia.

***Bacterial infection*** (p. 240). Pyogenic infections, tuberculosis, and leprosy can produce patchy scarring.

***Tinea*** (p. 267). Some inflammatory and pustular fungal infections can produce scarring.

***Physical injury.*** Mechanical, chemical, radiation, and burns can produce varying amounts of scarring hair loss.

***Lichen planus*** (p. 355). Irregular, scarring follicular lesions in scalp.

***Sarcoidosis*** (p. 488). Scalp lesions. May leave depressed scars despite lack of scarring elsewhere.

***Pseudopelade, folliculitis decalvans*** (p. 236). Idiopathic, patchy forms of alopecia that result in permanent scarring and hair loss.

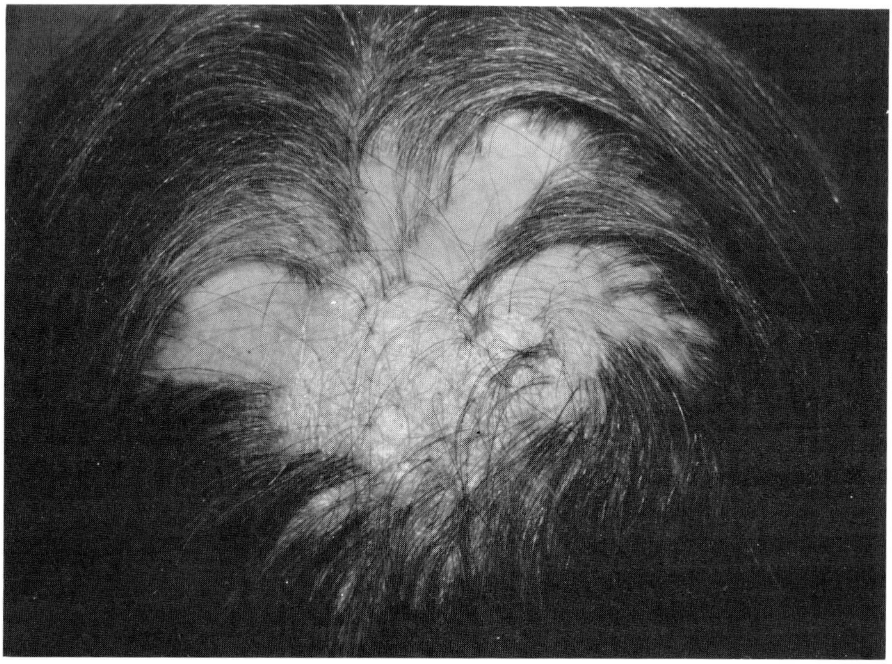

**Fig. 1-5.** Scarring alopecia caused by folliculitis decalvans. Minimal transient initial follicular inflammation.

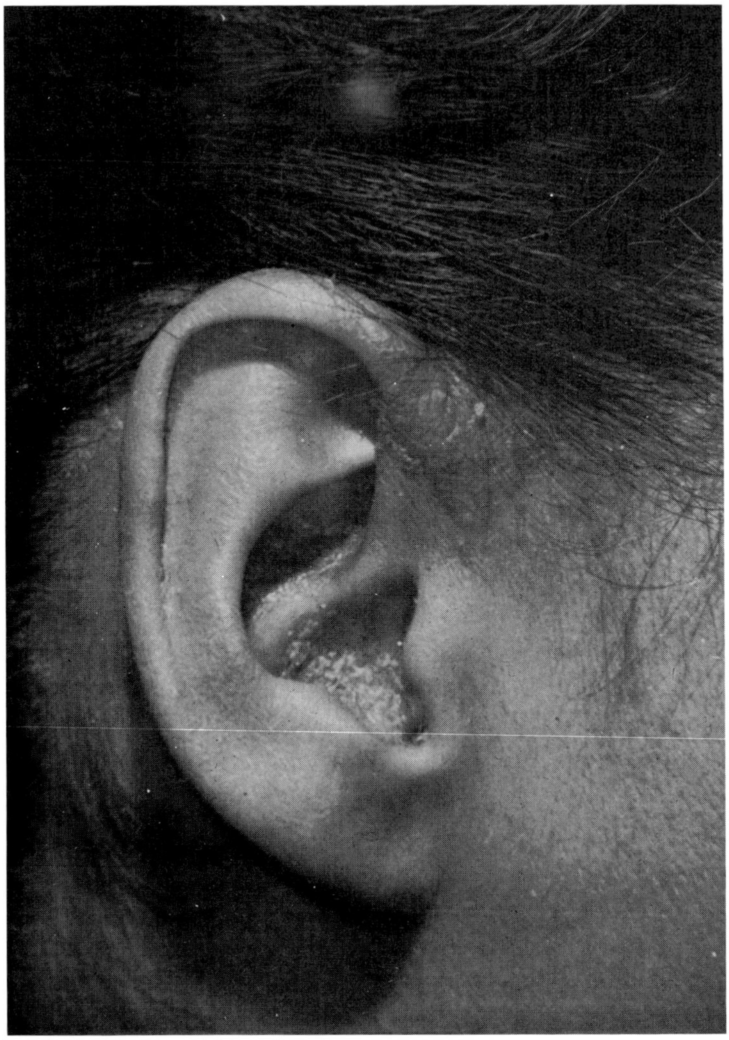

**Fig. 1-6.** Seborrheic dermatitis. Nonadherent, nonscarring, yellow soft scale.

## EXTERNAL EAR

### Flat lesions

***Seborrheic dermatitis*** (p. 494). Pruritus, erythema, fine greasy scale. In postauricular fold, external auditory canal (Fig. 1-6), and periorificial. Becomes moist with irritation.

***Psoriasis*** (p. 462). Red patches with definite silvery scale, periorificial, or shiny erythema in postauricular fold.

***Actinic keratosis*** (p. 508). Poorly defined, reddish, small scaling lesion, usually on sun-exposed helix. Premalignant.

***Atopic dermatitis*** (p. 118). Pruritic, erythematous dermatitis. Often scaly, may be crusted. Diffuse involvement

***Idiopathic otitis externa*** (p. 451). Pruritic, mildly erythematous, and scaling dermatitis of the external auditory canal.

***Allergic eczematous contact dermatitis*** (p. 102). Acute onset of erythema and vesiculation. Common causes: external canal—topical preparations with neomycin; pinna—hair dyes; lobes—metal earrings; posterior folds—spectacle earpieces, hearing aids.

***Dermatoses caused by light*** (p. 360). Minimal to intense inflammation on most prominent areas of ears, and nose and on malar areas. Erythema, plaques, papules, vesicles, or bullae may be present.

***Discoid lupus erythematosus*** (p. 147). Discrete red lesions with hyperkeratotic plugs immediately around orifice of external auditory canal. Ends in atrophic scar.

***Fungal infection*** (p. 270). Rare. Pruritus, scaling, and erythema present in confirmed tinea. Dermatophytes can be cultured.

***Infectious eczematoid dermatitis*** (p. 249). Secondary to purulent process of inner ear. Erythema, with subsequent eczematization and oozing, on area in contact with pus.

***Frostbite.*** Erythema, vesiculation, or ulceration, depending on severity and duration of cold.

### Raised lesions

***Keloid*** (p. 516). Firm, initially erythematous papule. Usually secondary to piercing of earlobe.

***Furuncle*** (p. 245). Painful, tender red swelling in external auditory canal. Becomes pustular, ruptures and suppurates.

***Granuloma pyogenicum*** (p. 522). Soft, rapidly growing, small inflammatory tumor at site of recent earlobe piercing.

***Squamous cell carcinoma*** (p. 541). Indurated, papular lesions that become ulcerated. Steadily enlarging. Usually occurs after scaling actinic keratosis or helix or antihelix. Most common cancer of external ear.

***Bowen's disease*** (p. 545). Velvety, erythematous plaque, slowly but steadily enlarging to progress to invasive squamous cell carcinoma.

***Basal cell epithelioma*** (p. 537). Slowly enlarging translucent papule with ulcerated center and elevated border. Most frequently adjacent to external auditory canal in postauricular region; more rarely, on helix.

***Sebaceous cyst*** (p. 513). Symptomatic, fluctuant tumor on earlobe or postauricular region. If infected, may become red, painful, and tender. Frequently associated with acne.

***Painful nodule of ear (chondrodermatitis)*** (p. 520). Tender nodule on helix of ear involving cartilage. Overlying skin not affected. Usually single.

***Gout.*** Tophi may be seen on antihelix.

***Sarcoidosis*** (p. 488). May cause blue-red, soft swelling symmetrically.

***Leprosy*** (p. 255). Erythematous swelling of lobe may be an early area of involvement.

***Relapsing polychondritis.*** Rare. Cellulitis-like painful ear swelling with distal arthritis, fever, and involvement of cartilage elsewhere. Biopsy diagnosis.

## FACE
### Flat lesions

***Freckle (ephelis)*** (p. 415). Discrete tan-brown macule that waxes and wanes seasonally because of sun exposure. Fair-complexioned children.

***Juvenile lentigo*** (p. 416). Discrete brown macule that does not vary in intensity with sun exposure.

***Senile lentigo*** (Fig. 1-7) (p. 416). Discrete, benign, irregular scaling, gray-brown macule on exposed actinic skin of older patient. Benign.

***Seborrheic keratosis*** (p. 508). Starts in adult life as flat, irregularly-shaped, tan patch, slowly darkens and develops typical thickening to verrucous surface.

***Telangiectasia*** (p. 273). Multiple, branching, linear, capillary dilatations. Occurs after actinic damage, particularly over bony prominences in fair individuals. Hereditary form (Rendu-Osler-Weber disease), small, almost punctate lesions of face and fingers with mucous membrane involvement. Also, rectangular "mats" of telangiectasia seen in scleroderma.

***Nevus araneus (spider nevus)*** (p. 572). Pinhead-sized arteriole with radiating branches that blanches on pressure.

***Nevus flammeus*** (p. 569). Irregularly shaped, reddish purple stain. Present from birth. May be very small or involve half of face. Surface may slowly become roughened and nodular.

***Seborrheic dermatitis*** (p. 494). Fine scaling and erythema of nasolabial folds, free edges of eyelids, temples, and forehead adjacent to hairline.

***Atopic dermatitis*** (p. 118). Dryness, fine

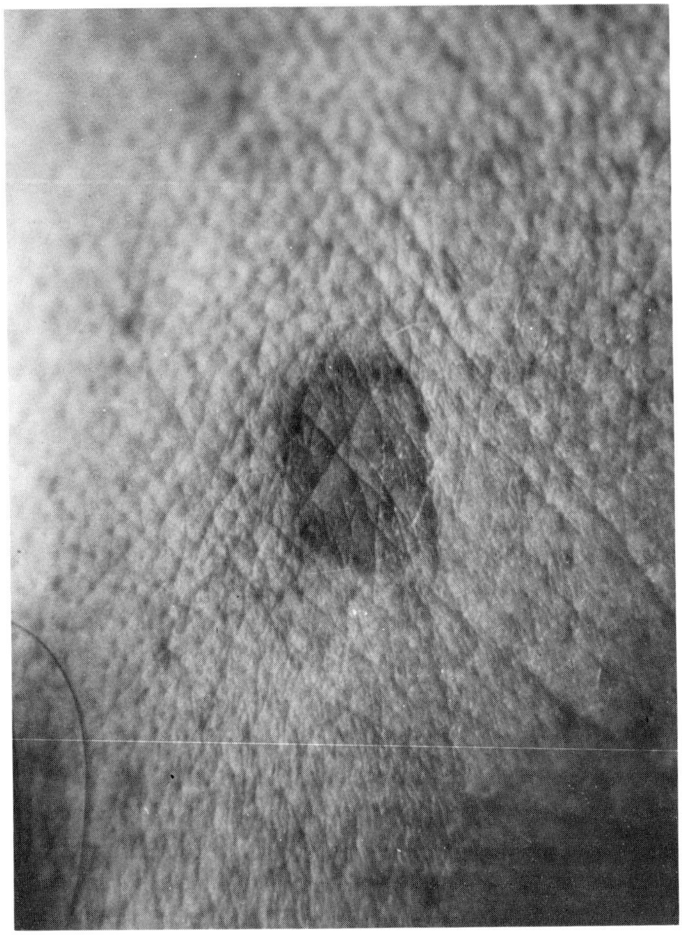

**Fig. 1-7.** Senile lentigo. On dorsum of hand, a common site.

scaling, mild erythema, excoriations. On forehead and cheeks. Pruritic.

***Pityriasis alba (dartre volante).*** Pink hypopigmented, finely scaling patches on cheeks. Found in children. Self-limited, recurrent.

***Allergic eczematous contact dermatitis*** (p. 102). Mild erythema to weeping dermatitis or dry, scaling lesion in more chronic phase. Pruritic. Common causes: neomycin, preservatives in topical medications and perfumes, emulsifying agents in face creams and cosmetics.

***Actinic skin*** (p. 360). Atrophic, dry, finely wrinkled, scaling skin resulting from prolonged exposure to sunlight. Areas of depigmentation, hyperpigmentation, and telangiectasia.

***Actinic keratosis*** (Plate 1) (p. 508). Flat, skin-colored, scaling, small lesion on sun-exposed skin. Often easier to feel than to see. Premalignant.

***Chloasma*** (p. 417). Mottled brown hyperpigmentation. "Mask of pregnancy." Forehead, malar prominences, or moustache area.

***Junction nevus*** (p. 523). Flat, tan to dark brown, asymptomatic macule or patch. May arise in infancy or appear later.

***Allergic photocontact dermatitis*** (p. 111). Same as above, but needs light exposure plus contactant to produce it. Common causes: antiseptics in soaps and cosmetics, ragweed pollen, and phenothiazine.

***Psoriasis*** (p. 462). Red patches with mini-

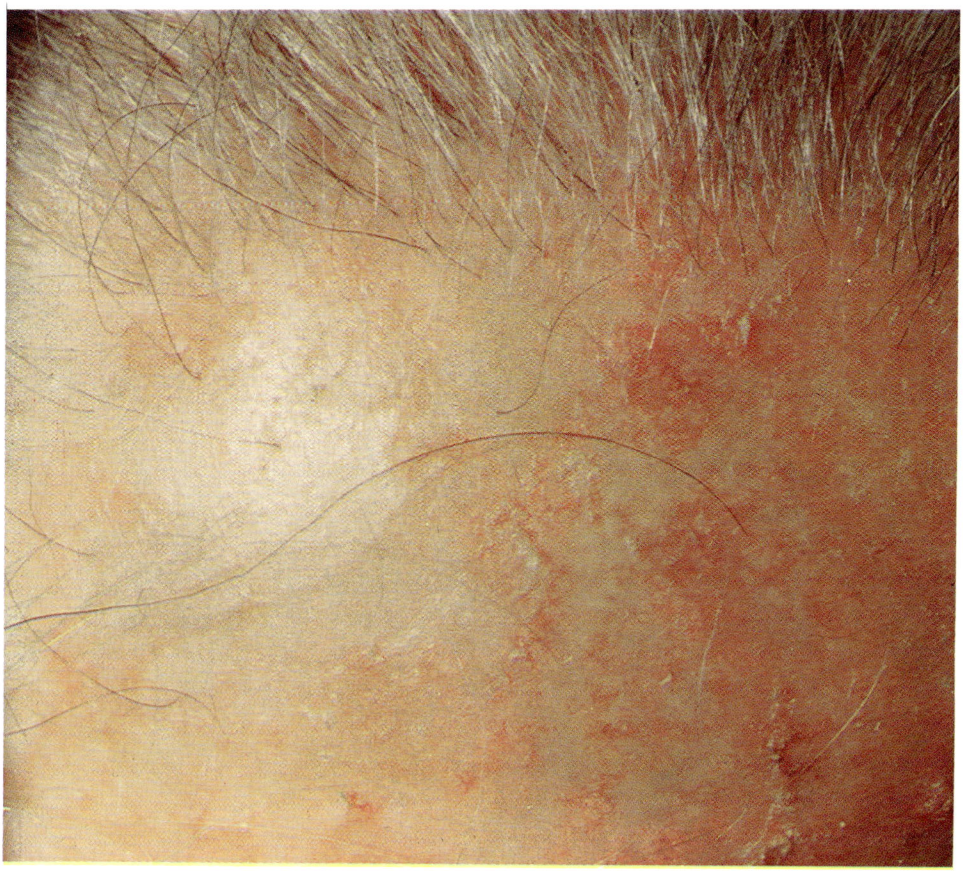

**Plate 1**

Actinic keratosis. Extensive involvement of the forehead.

mal scale. On eyebrows, paranasal and nasolabial areas, and anterior hairline.

***Rosacea*** (Fig. 1-8) (p. 92). Areas of erythema of forehead, nose, malar prominences, and chin. Accompanied by papules and pustules. Telangiectasia is common. Excessive oiliness.

***Polymorphous light eruption*** (p. 363). Several forms. May be macular; papular, plaquelike, or vesicular; transient or persistent. Sun-exposed areas. Can occur through window glass. Appearance delayed after exposure.

***Fungal infection*** (p. 265). Mildly erythematous, circumscribed, scaling lesion, particularly on periorbital area in children, forehead in adults. Scrapings of scales give positive culture.

***Photosensitivity*** (p. 362). Diffuse erythema and pigmentation of face, sides of neck, V of chest, and dorsa of hands. Photosensitizing agent may be external or ingested.

***Discoid lupus erythematosus*** (Fig. 1-9) (p. 147). Erythematous, well-demarcated, scaling lesions leading to atrophic depigmented scars. On malar areas and bridge of nose. Usually sun sensitive.

***Erysipelas*** (p. 247). Tender, well-demarcated, irregular, red unilateral, edematous, acute, spreading lesions.

***Leprosy*** (p. 255). Red-brown shiny macules poorly defined hypopigmented, slightly scaly patches.

***Malignant lentigo*** (p. 530). Mottled, irregularly enlarging area of tan pigmentation.

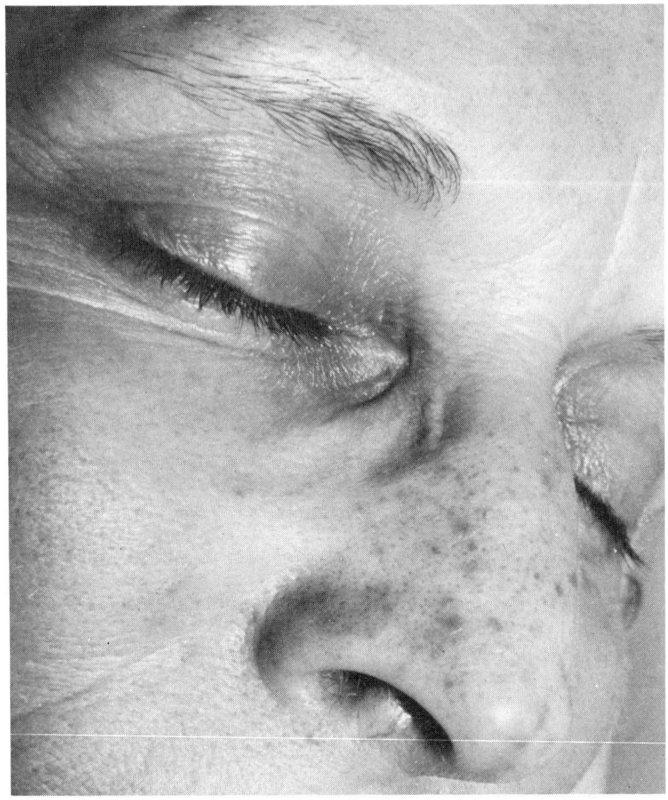

**Fig. 1-8.** Early rosacea affecting nose only. Papules predominate.

May slowly evolve into a malignant melanoma. First sign may be nodule formation. Occurs in elderly patients.

***Drug eruption*** (p. 199). Photosensitizing drugs (for example, chlorpromazine hydrochloride) will produce a red-brown facial pigmentation on sun exposure.

***Porphyria*** (p. 371). Erythema or vesicles and bullae of face or back of neck occurring after trauma or sun exposure. Chronic cases have hyperpigmentation, hirsutism, and eye suffusion as well. Skin easily damaged by minor trauma.

***Sarcoidosis*** (p. 488). Asymptomatic, pigmented, flat, reddish brown annular lesion. Chiefly on forehead and temples. May scar.

***Xeroderma pigmentosum*** (p. 368). Atrophic, irregularly pigmented skin. Increasingly apparent freckles and keratoses leading to malignancies from sun exposure. First found in children.

***Vitiligo*** (p. 422). Sharply demarcated white patch completely devoid of pigment. Appears first around eyes and mouth.

## Raised lesions

***Senile sebaceous hyperplasia*** (p. 516). Minute, pale yellow, circumscribed, flat-topped papules on forehead and nose of elderly individuals.

***Acne vulgaris*** (p. 79). Comedones, papules, pustules, cysts, and scars. Found in some adults as well as in teen-agers.

***Perioral dermatitis*** (p. 410). Erythematous patches, as well as pinhead-sized papules, on chin, nasolabial folds, and periorbital area. Found in women.

***Wart (verruca)*** (p. 316). Multiple, flat-topped, fawn-colored, slightly raised lesions or small projections.

***Nevus*** (p. 523). "Mole." May be skin colored or pigmented. Most common form is dome shaped and often hair bearing.

***Seborrheic keratosis*** (p. 508). Slow-grow-

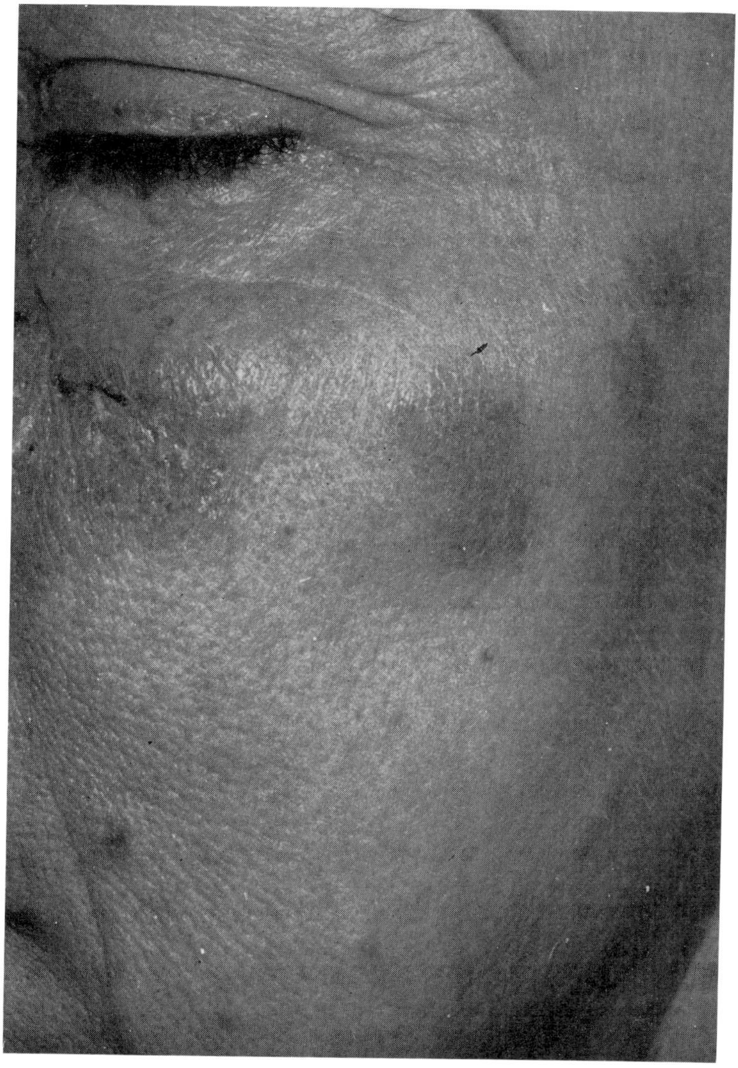

**Fig. 1-9.** Discoid lupus erythematosus. Lesions of recent origin.

ing warty lesion, skin-colored to black. Begins as flat brown patch. Appears to be "stuck on" normal skin.

***Milium*** (p. 513). Minute, globular, 1 to 2 mm. white epithelial cyst, usually multiple. Most often infraorbital.

***Folliculitis*** (p. 244). Discrete, erythematous, follicular papules and pustules of bearded area. Often attributed to "ingrown hair."

***Herpes simplex*** (p. 295). Cluster of minute vesicles on erythematous base that progress to crusting. Early local lymphadenopathy. May be anywhere on face.

***Zoster*** (p. 303). Unilateral, tender paresthesia on area supplied by one branch of trigeminal nerve. Progresses through erythema, vesicles, crusts, and scars.

***Urticaria*** (p. 113). Localized, pruritic, discrete wheals that last for minutes to hours and disappear. May affect face with massive swelling (angioneurotic edema) involving lips, buccal mucosa, tongue.

***Impetigo contagiosa*** (p. 242). Rapidly spreading, loosely adherent yellow crusts on erythematous base.

***Furunculosis, folliculitis*** (p. 244). Pustular, inflamed, indurated lesions of bearded area in males or elsewhere. Usually staphylococcal.

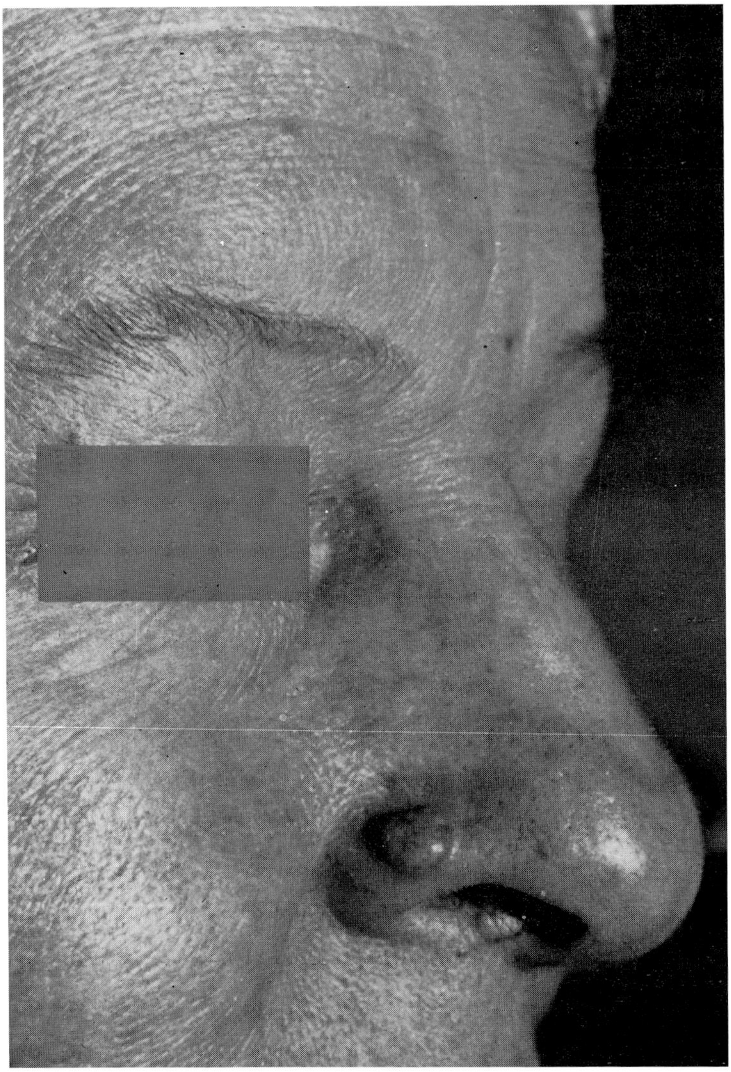

**Fig. 1-10.** Basal cell epithelioma of nose.

***Molluscum contagiosum*** (p. 311). One or more small, waxy, umbilicated, globular lesions. Usually found in children.

***Basal cell epithelioma*** (Fig. 1-10) (p. 537). Slowly enlarging, translucent papule that ulcerates, exhibiting raised, pearly border. Telangiectatic vessels on surface. Most often on upper half of face. Invasion of cartilaginous and bony structures can occur.

***Granuloma pyogenicum*** (Fig. 1-11) (p. 522). Smooth, moist, small red tumor. Grows rapidly at site of minor trauma, usually cheeks.

***Cutaneous horn*** (p. 512). Localized hyperkeratotic lesion producing a horny projection. Base may show changes of actinic keratosis or squamous cell carcinoma.

***Blue nevus*** (p. 528). Blue, dome-shaped or flat lesion. May be present at birth.

***Dermatosis papulosa nigra.*** Common in blacks. Smooth, skin-colored papules from adolescence onward. On malar areas.

***Trichoepithelioma*** (p. 515). Multiple, small, skin-colored papules clustered around eyes, nose, and upper lip. Dominant inheritance. Appears at puberty.

***Adenoma sebaceum (Pringle's disease)*** (p. 515). Small, multiple, yellow-tinted papules with telangiectasia. Occurs from childhood

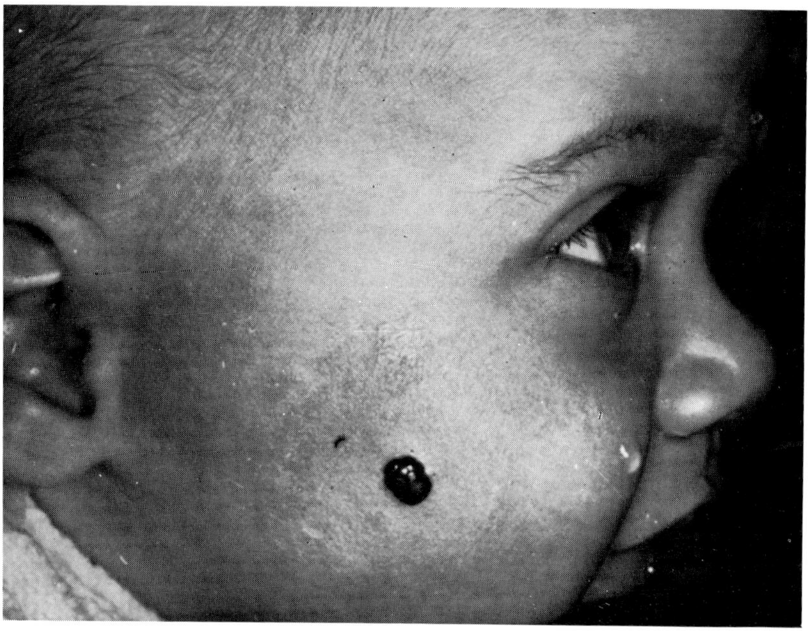

**Fig. 1-11.** Granuloma pyogenicum. This lesion has been darkened by hemorrhage into it.

through later life. On paranasal area and cheeks. Epilepsy and mental retardation possible.

***Granuloma annulare*** (p. 167). Single or multiple annular lesions with papular borders.

***Lymphocytoma cutis.*** Papular plaque or nodular, benign infiltrate. Blue-red, soft, asymptomatic.

***Sarcoidosis*** (p. 488). Red-brown plaque or nodule, or may consist of multiple minute papules 1 to 5 mm. May be yellow-brown-red tumor, paranasal to periorbital. Rarely affects nose, cheeks, ears with large soft blue-red swellings. Atypical in blacks.

***Leishmaniasis.*** A small facial papule. Enlarges slowly. Ulcerates, crusts, and heals with scarring over a long period. Recurrent forms exist.

***Lupus vulgaris*** (p. 253). Soft yellow-brown papules that become plaques with atrophic centers.

***Strawberry hemangioma*** (p. 569). Red, elevated, varisized, soft tumor, with pitted and lobulated surface. Present on face from birth or very shortly thereafter. Rapid enlargement, then resolution.

***Keratoacanthoma*** (p. 512). Rapidly enlarging, red to skin-colored lesion that resembles squamous cell carcinoma. Central crust, plug, or umbilication. Papule, nodule, or tumor. Often paranasal.

***Squamous cell carcinoma*** (p. 541). Steadily enlarging, ulcerated nodule that develops from actinic keratosis. Occasionally on normal-appearing skin. Frequency of occurrence is in cheeks, nose, and then upper lip. Metastasis to cervical nodes is slow. Preauricular nodes first involved.

***Bromoderma, iododerma.*** Pustular, acnelike lesions that may be bullous, or become crusted, heaped up.

***Actinomycosis*** (p. 288). Induration, nodules, sinus tracts, and granular purulent discharge in mandibular area. Found in country dwellers.

***North American blastomycosis*** (p. 290). Ulcerating nodules that progress to verrucous lesions.

***Lymphoma, mycosis fungoides*** (p. 555). Indurated, firm, red papules that enlarge to plaques and nodules. Asymptomatic.

### Depressed or atrophic lesions

***Compulsive excoriations*** (p. 477). Caused by fingernail picking and digging of acne and other lesions. Produces crateriform scars.

### Hair loss

***Alopecia areata*** (p. 234). One or more well-circumscribed, smooth, hairless patches on bearded area. May be depigmented as well.

## EYELIDS

### Flat lesions

***Seborrheic dermatitis*** (p. 494). Crusting, sealing, and redness of upper and lower eyelids, with characteristic reddened margin (blepharitis). Eyebrows and scalp scaling.

***Hemangioma*** (p. 569). Usually flat, transient, and fading. Found in infants at birth; disappears in weeks.

***Allergic eczematous contact dermatitis*** (p. 102). May be acute, edematous dermatitis with vesicles and erythema, but is usually dry, scaling, and pruritic. Common causes: fingernail polish or hardener, hair dyes, hand lotion, and medicated and cosmetic creams applied to eyelids. (See Plate 9, p. 103.)

***Atopic dermatitis*** (p. 118). Pruritic, nonerythematous lichenification of upper eyelids.

***Dermatomyositis*** (p. 155). Swelling of periorbital tissue with very characteristic purplish (heliotrope) tint to eyelids. Signs of muscle tenderness and weakness may not be immediately apparent, but follow shortly. (See Plate 16, p. 156.) Found in children and adults.

### Raised lesions

***Urticaria*** (p. 113). "Hives" or common urticaria. Often affects loose tissues of eyelids first, causing profound edema. Must be differentiated from true edema of soft periorbital tissues associated with renal, cardiovascular, or collagen disease.

***Molluscum contagiosum*** (p. 311). Skin-colored, umbilicated papule less than 1 cm. in diameter. Viral infection.

***Milium*** (p. 513). Asymptomatic, white, pinhead-sized papule on inferior periorbital surface, sometimes on eyelids.

***Stye (hordeolum).*** Inflammation from obstruction and subsequent infection of sebaceous gland of lid.

***Pediculosis*** (p. 336). Crusting of eyelids associated with blepharitis caused by infestation by pubic lice. Nits will be found attached to eyelashes as small gray-white swellings of hair shaft. Pubic area is involved first.

***Xanthelasma*** (p. 382). Yellow papules or plaques on medial upper and lower eyelids. Asymptomatic, chronic, and associated with hypercholesterolemia and atherosclerotic vascular disease in significant number of patients. May be familial.

***Perioral dermatitis*** (p. 410). Papules may affect eyelids as well as perioral area.

***Basal cell epithelioma*** (p. 437). Papule or nodule with distinct rolled border, often on inner canthus. Extends laterally in all directions beneath epidermis. Can involve more area than apparent on first examination. (See Fig. 35-4, p. 538.)

***Syringoma.*** Composed of multiple, small, soft, yellow-tinted papules. Found in women from puberty through later life. Infraorbital.

***Amyloidosis*** (p. 173). Discrete purpuric lesions of periorbital areas.

### Hair loss

***Alopecia areata*** (p. 234). Patchy or complete hair loss that may involve only one or both eyelashes or eyebrows.

***Atopic dermatitis*** (p. 118). Continued rubbing of these areas because of pruritus can result in partial or complete loss of eyebrows.

***Myxedema*** (p. 175). Pale, boggy infiltration associated with some loss of lateral third of eyebrows. Skin generally becomes dry; scalp hair, sparse and coarse.

## LIPS

### Flat lesions

***Primary irritation cheilitis*** (p. 430). Caused by licking and biting of lip, resulting in scaling, erythema, and fissuring. May be present as circumoral dryness and erythema with normal-appearing lips.

***Actinic cheilitis*** (p. 361). Diffuse, pale, dry scaling with thinning and fragility that lead to fissuring. Caused by sunlight.

***Allergic contact cheilitis.*** Dry, scaling, chronic fissuring. Common causes: perfume, dye or oil in lipstick, sunscreens, and topical medications.

***Candidosis.*** *Perlèche (angular cheilitis)* (p. 390): moist, erythematous, angular fissures leading away from corners of mouth. Results from moisture accumulating where *Candida albicans* appears as secondary invader. Found in older patients and especially those with dentures and in association with denture stomatitis. Vitamin B deficiency can produce similar crusted and inflamed augular fissures. *Hyperplastic cheilitis* (p. 285): chronic, thickened lips with persistent fissures and erythema. Responds to nystatin ointment.

***Leukoplakia*** (p. 394). White, thickened plaque resulting from chronic irritation. Premalignant. May eventuate into squamous cell carcinoma.

***Lichen planus*** (p. 355). Papules or small plaques, erythema or crusted surface. Tendency to fissure. Lower lip.

***Discoid lupus erythematosus*** (p. 147). Painful, localized area of erythema with heavy scaling and fissuring. Lower lip.

***Angioma.*** Occurs on lips in form of soft, blue venous lake.

***Telangiectasia*** (p. 573). Punctate red macules characterize Osler's essential hereditary hemorrhagic telangiectasia. May bleed.

***Nevus*** (p. 523). Macular, pigmented lesions of junction nevus type. Not uncommon on lips.

***Ephelis (freckle)*** (p. 415). Brown macule. Appears infrequently on exposed surfaces of lips.

***Peutz-Jeghers syndrome.*** Multiple tan to black freckles of lips, peribuccal area, fingers, and toes. Associated with multiple polyps of small intestine. Appears at birth or shortly thereafter (Fig. 1-12).

## Raised lesions

***Herpes simplex*** (p. 295). Localized area of irritation at vermilion border. Develops cluster of tiny vesicles that progress to crusting. Tender submental adenopathy. (See Plate 30, p. 296.)

***Erythema multiforme*** (p. 312). Affects lips severely in children (Stevens-Johnson syndrome). Vesicles and painful erosions. Systemic symptoms. Less severe lesions in more common adult forms.

***Urticaria (angioneurotic edema)*** (p. 113). Acute edema of lips, eyelids, tongue, and larynx. May be transient and recurring.

***Mucous retention cyst*** (p. 396). Fluctuant,

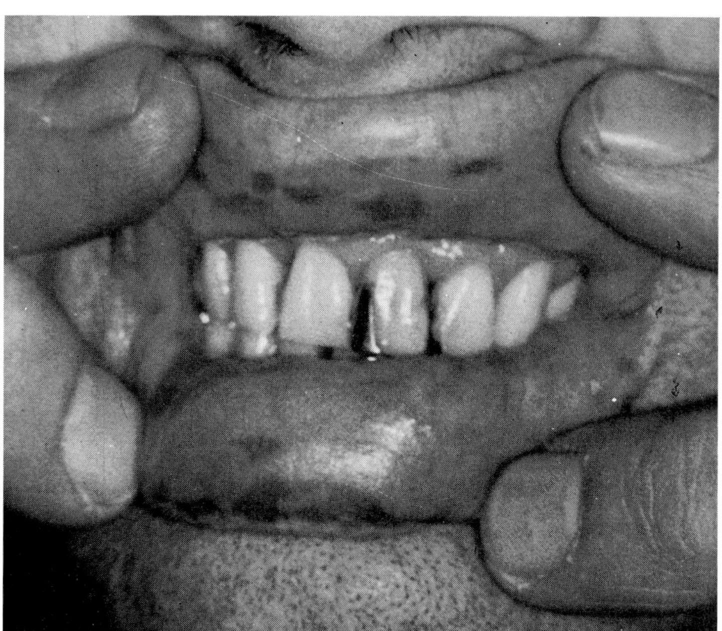

**Fig. 1-12.** Peutz-Jeghers pigmentation.

soft, translucent tumor. Enlarges rapidly and contains mucinous fluid. Appears on inner aspect of lower lip. Asymptomatic.

***Lymphedema.*** Persistent swelling attributable to lymph channel obstruction after recurrent streptococcal infection of area.

***Wart (verruca)*** (p. 316). Pinhead-sized, flat, skin-colored papules or elongated filiform warts. Lips and mucocutaneous junction not uncommon sites.

***Papilloma*** (p. 516). Benign overgrowth of squamous epithelium that possesses multiple, small, papillary projections. Color varies from pink to white.

***Fordyce's disease.*** Discrete yellow papules along inner aspect of lips, 1 to 2 mm. in diameter. These are ectopic sebaceous glands, asymptomatic, with no clinical significance.

***Pyogenic granuloma*** (p. 522). Rapidly growing, red-blue, smooth, globular papule, often at site of minor trauma.

***Syphilitic chancre*** (p. 258). Painless, indurated ulcer associated with regional lymphadenopathy. *Split papule* at corner of mouth, with one half on each lip, is characteristic of stage occurring after disappearance of chancre, 2 to 6 months after exposure. Associated with *mucous patches* of buccal mucosa and tongue and generalized cutaneous manifestations.

***Squamous cell carcinoma*** (p. 541). May begin as a plaque of leukoplakia, a firm red induration, a persistent fissure, an ulcer, or a warty growth. Aggressive behavior. Commonest site of oral carcinoma is on lower lip, where metastasis is to submaxillary lymph nodes. Carcinoma of upper lip metastasizes to preauricular nodes, then to cervical chain. (See Plate 55, p. 541.)

***Keratoacanthoma*** (p. 512). Rapidly growing, indurated lesion with central crater. Involves lip and adjacent skin. Biopsy should take total lesion for correct diagnosis.

## ORAL CAVITY AND TONGUE

### Flat lesions

***Denture stomatitis.*** Pain, irritation, and disturbed salivation result from this. Inflammation beneath dentures. May be attributed to direct trauma. Often associated with candidosis and, with chronicity, becomes atrophic.

***Geographic tongue.*** Asymptomatic, irregular, smooth, depressed, erythematous areas on dorsum of tongue caused by loss of filiform papillae (Fig. 1-13). May be recurrent and migratory, with constantly changing patterns.

***Black hairy tongue.*** Dark brown to black discoloration with or without hypertrophy of filiform papillae. Caused by pigment-producing bacteria.

***Glossodynia.*** Subjective complaint of persistent sensation of tongue with no objective findings. Most frequently found in women past middle age.

***Koplik's spots.*** Multiple irregular spots with bluish white centers along the bite line with palatal pharyngeal erythema. Precedes measles rash. Buccal mucosa involved.

***Chronic gingivitis.*** Virtually universal. Varies from minimally inflamed gingival interdental papillae to swollen, red, tender, shiny gingival margins throughout the mouth. Caused by accumulation of calcareous accretions, plaque, and food impaction.

***Median rhomboid glossitis.*** Red depressed area on midpoint of dorsum of tongue with absent papillae and irregular, smooth, lobulated elevations. Developmental abnormality. Some cases caused by *candida*. Often adult males.

***Candidosis (candidiasis, moniliasis)*** (p. 280). Multiple oral manifestations.

***Thrush*** (p. 284). Creamy white patches, with friable, reddened, underlying surface on buccal mucosa and tongue. Usually found in infants and young children, from 1 week after birth. Smears and culture of white patches demonstrate *Candida albicans*.

***Chronic hyperplastic candidosis*** (p. 285). White, firm, lobulated, adherent plaques on erythematous base. Affects buccal mucosa, retrocommissural area, dorsum tongue, and posterior palate. (See denture stomatitis, p. 390.)

***Herpetic gingivostomatitis*** (p. 388). Fiery red, swollen gingiva, mucosal vesicles. May have exudate accompanied by fever, malaise,

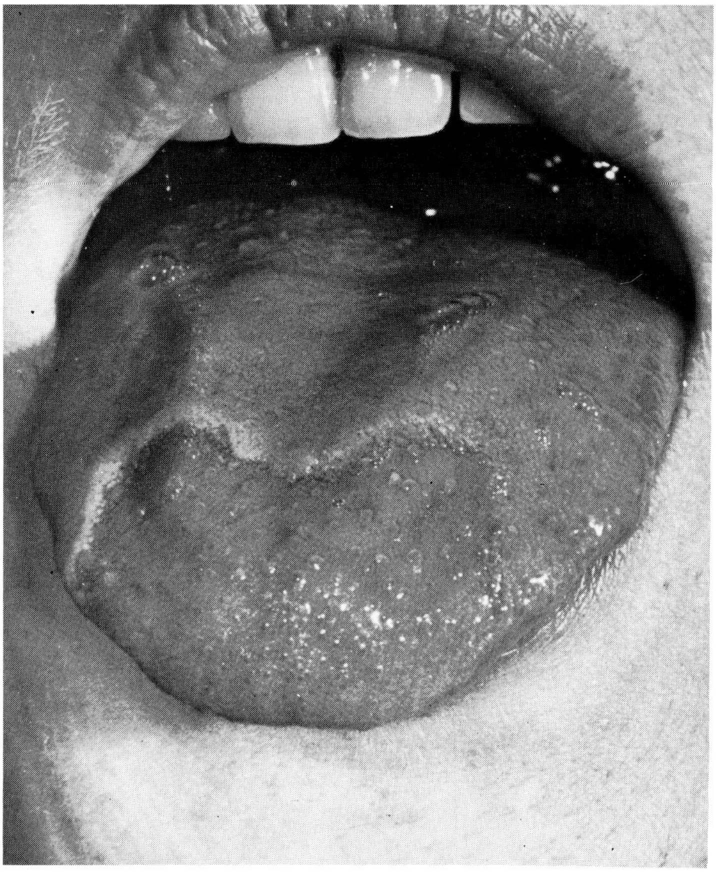

**Fig. 1-13.** Geographic tongue.

and lymphadenopathy. Chiefly children 2 to 4 years of age. Fairly common.

***Hemangioma*** (p. 569). Capillary, strawberry, or cavernous types appear here as elsewhere. Found in children.

***Allergic contact stomatitis.*** Rare. Well defined erythema and inflammation of mucosa at site of direct contact with material producing dermatitis. Bullae may be present. In chronic cases, hyperplasia with polypoid lesions gradually appears. Common causes: ingredients in lozenges and cough drops, flavoring agents, mouthwashes, and dentifrices.

***Drug eruption (stomatitis caused by systemic drugs).*** Erythema, bullae, gingivitis, or painful erosions may be present. Lichenoid drug eruptions can produce lacy, gray, lichen planus–like patterns on the buccal mucosa.

***Fordyce's disease.*** Multiple, minute, white-yellow papules on anterior mucosal surface. Heterotopic sebaceous glands.

***Smooth tongue.*** Red, shiny surface attributable to atrophy of papillae on dorsum of tongue. May be indicative of pernicious or iron-deficiency anemia, sprue, pellagra, or vitamin B complex deficiency. In severe anemia, tongue may be significantly reduced in size.

***Scarlet fever.*** Reddened, edematous oropharynx and tongue, often with yellow exudate. Followed within 3 days by diffuse erythema.

***Diphtheria.*** Patchy, tenacious, gray-white membrane covering erythematous lesions of oropharynx. May extend to uvula and buccal mucosa.

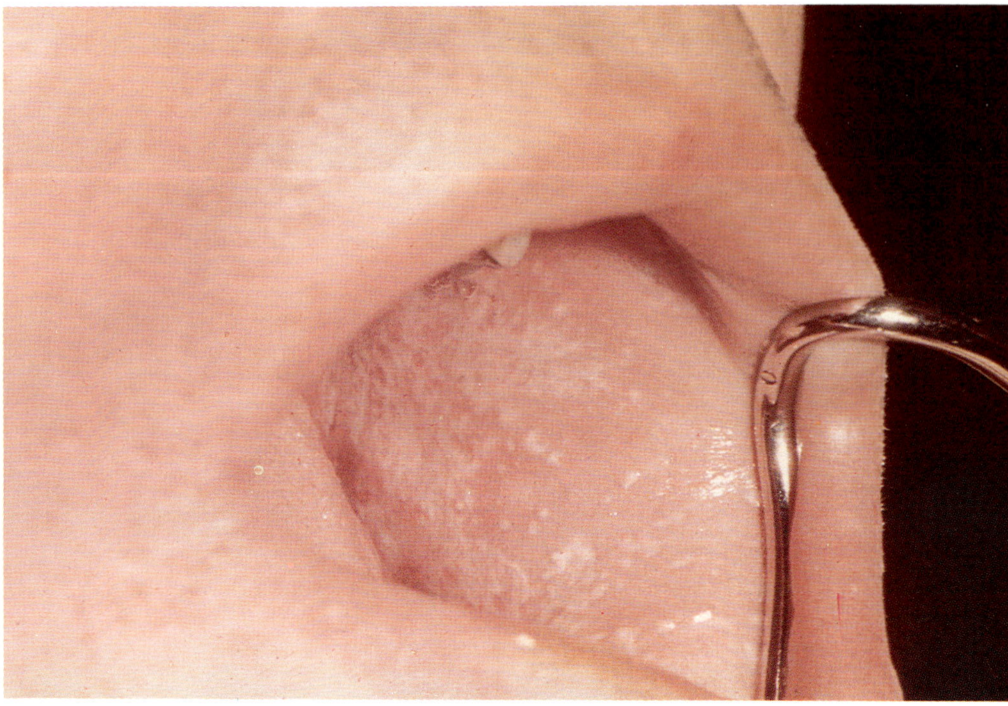

**Plate 2**

Lichen planus. Pathognomonic lacy gray appearance.

***Scurvy.*** Hyperplastic gingival swelling with ulceration and hemorrhage.

***Pellagra.*** Patchy atrophy of lingual papillae, with strongly reddened tongue. Ulcerations often present.

***Lichen planus*** (Plate 2) (p. 355). On buccal mucosa, an asymptomatic, white, lacy reticulation. On tongue, a milky white patch, papule, or erosion. An acute inflammation may occur, and residual persistent ulcerations that are potentially premalignant appear.

***Bullous diseases*** (p. 127). Bullae on tongue and buccal mucosa that quickly rupture, leaving tender, denuded surfaces. Produced by erythema multiforme bullosum, pemphigus, epidermolysis bullosa, drug reactions, lichen planus, pemphigoid, and benign mucous membrane pemphigoid.

***Leukoplakia*** (p. 394). Varies from thin, faintly white patches on thick adherent plaques. Some are speckled white on red. Most common locations are buccal mucosae, commissures, alveolar ridge, tongue. Biopsy and microscopic examination required. Premalignant.

***Syphilitic mucous patches*** (p. 261). Red, macular, or papular lesions progressing to ulceration covered by gray membrane. Tongue. Appear 2 months to 1 year after chancre. Serological tests are positive. *Highly infectious.* Syphilitic glossitis with mucosal atrophy and "bald tongue" may be present at this stage.

***Melanin pigmentation.*** Poorly defined, brown pigment deposition. Common on gingiva and inner surface of lips in blacks and other darkskinned persons. Antimalarial drugs can cause palatal melanosis.

***Nevus*** (p. 523). In oral cavity and tongue, nevi are usually pigmented. May be flat or elevated. Junctional, intradermal, compound or blue. Palate, gingiva, or buccal mucosa. Usually less than 1 cm.

***Metallic pigmentation.*** Bismuth, mercury, lead, silver, and gold can produce metallic pigmentation along gingivae after systemic absorption, ingestion, or local use, particularly with poor oral hygiene. Bismuth, mercury, and gold may also produce erosive lesions on oral mucosa.

***Addison's disease*** (p. 419). Freckles and blotchy brown pigmentation of buccal mucosa and lips.

## Raised lesions

***Denture granuloma.*** Soft, tender, red tumor at site of irritation by dentures. May be discrete or multiple. May be diffuse as in papillary hyperplasia of palate.

***Coated tongue.*** Not significant. Retention of papillary hypertrophy and epithelial debris on tongue surface.

***Nicotine stomatitis.*** Papular, verrucous gray alteration over vault of hard palate, often with central red puncta at site of multiple gland orifices. Asymptomatic. Found chiefly in pipesmokers.

***Papillitis.*** Enlarged, erythematous papillae. Usually on top of anterior tongue margins because of rubbing, local irritants, smoking, hot foods, and the like.

***Torus palatinus.*** Very common, bony excrescence on midline of hard palate. Developmental.

***Dental abscesses.*** Painful, fluctuant lesions on gingiva or palate, or a diffuse local cellulitis.

***Mucous cyst (mucocele)*** (p. 396). Soft, painless, fluctuant, with characteristic blue cast. On lower lip, or floor of mouth on one side. May be superficial or deep. Common.

***Dental cyst.*** A variety of cysts may arise from tooth structures and present as noninflamed fluctuant swellings. Common.

***Gingival cyst.*** Small white, 1 to 3 mm. cysts on alveolar mucosa of infants and newborns. Very common. Disappear spontaneously.

***Wart (verruca)*** (p. 316). Common, grainy-surfaced warts occur here as elsewhere, chiefly on tongue or inner gingival surface. Condylomata acuminata also occur in mouth.

***Fibroma.*** Pink to red, firm fibrous bilateral or single tumors anywhere in oral mucosa, including tongue. Common.

***Giant cell granuloma.*** Soft, blue-red swelling near teeth on alveolar ridge. Rapid growth. May ulcerate. Strong tendency to recurrence. Benign.

***Hypertrophic gingivitis.*** Diffuse enlargement of gingiva caused by the following: *Pregnancy*—maximum eighth month, fiery red, swollen, tends to bleed; up to 100%. *Drugs*—firm, pale, resilient, nonfragile; up to 60%. *Leukemia*—shiny, edematous, pale; may be massive; bleeds; can also be hereditary.

***Pyogenic granuloma*** (p. 522). Bright red, smooth, dome-shaped, rapid-growing small tumor of gingiva, less often on tongue, lip, or oral mucosa.

***Pregnancy granuloma.*** Occurs along gingival margin in pregnancy.

***Papilloma.*** Pedunculated, white or gray, cauliflower-like. Small. Benign.

***Squamous cell carcinoma*** (p. 541). Painless nodule, ulcer, or induration. May evolve from plaque of leukoplakia on tongue or mucosa. *The tongue follows lower lip as second most common site of oral squamous cell carcinoma.* Usually on lateral border or ventral surface. Metastasis occurs early in deep lymph nodes on floor of mouth.

***Malignant melanoma*** (p. 530). Rare, painless, soft, brown to black tumor. May be nonpigmented. May or may not arise on pre-existing nevus. Gingiva, palate, and lips. Very prone to metastasize regionally and distantly.

***Hereditary hemorrhagic telangiectasia*** (p. 574). Punctate, deep red papules that bleed frequently. Also found on lips, conjunctiva, face, and in many viscera.

***White sponge nevus.*** Thick, white, spongy lesions in buccal mucosa. May involve all or part of oral mucosa. Congenital. Benign.

***Lipoma*** (p. 519). Yellow or pink, pedunculated soft tumor on floor of mouth, gingiva, tongue, or oral mucosa.

***Lymphangioma.*** Pale pink, diffuse swellings that superficially demonstrates small clear lymph vesicles. May involve tongue, lips, or mucous membrane.

***Angioneurotic edema*** (p. 113). Immediate, allergic, urticarial reaction causing noticeable swelling of lips, tongue, perioral tussues, and pharynx. Causative agent is usually a food or drug.

***Macroglossia.*** Enlargement of tongue. Occurs in primary amyloidosis and hypothyroidism. Asymmetrical in neurofibromatosis.

### Depressed lesions

***Aphthous ulcers*** (p. 387). Tender, painful, pinhead- to pea-sized, gray, denuded areas surrounded by erythema on vestibule, buccal mucosa, or ventral surface of tongue. Lesions last 1 to 2 weeks, disappear, and recur.

***Ulcer.*** Large ulcers may occur from trauma, radiation, anticancer drugs, drug reactions, systemic disease, malignancy, lupus erythematosus, lichen planus, erythema multiforme, and bullous diseases.

***Scrotal tongue.*** Deep and shallow fissuring of tongue. Nonconsequential defect. Congenital or acquired.

***Vincent's infection (acute necrotizing gingivitis)*** (p. 388). Painful areas of inflammation and necrosis of gingival papillae between teeth. Spreads along gingival margin. Associated with tender cervical lymphadenopathy and fetid odor. Transmissable.

***Syphilis*** (p. 258). *Chancre:* painful ulcer that appears at site of inoculation after 2 to 6 weeks and subsides in 2 to 5 weeks. Noticeable local lymphadenopathy. Dark-field examination is not sufficient to make diagnosis because of similarity between oral spirochetes and *Treponema pallidum.* Serological test for syphilis may still be negative in early phases of chancre. *Gumma:* may occur on palate, with perforation; on tongue, with fibrosis.

***Behçet's syndrome.*** Recurrent, small, painful, irregular ulcers of lips and buccal mucosa. Associated with similar lesions on genitalia, uveitis, vasculitis, and arthritis. Multiple organ disease.

## NECK

### Flat lesions

***Allergic eczematous contact dermatitis*** (p. 102). Erythema that may have papules or vesicles. Common causes: necklace-clasp posteriorly, necklaces, chains, textile finished in collars, pendants anteriorly, nail polish at sides of neck.

***Berloque dermatitis*** (p. 419). Brown pigmentation in trickle pattern on sides of neck caused by perfume and sunlight.

***Poikiloderma of Civatte*** (p. 419). Telangiectasia and hyperpigmentation of sun-exposed sides and anterior neck in rows. Anterior-chin shaded area spared. Very common in women.

***Photosensitivity*** (p. 362). Diffuse erythema and pigmentation of exposed parts of neck and V of chest. Associated with ingested or applied photosensitizing agent.

***Actinic keratosis*** (p. 548). Localized scaling and erythematous lesions on anterior sun-exposed V of neck.

***Tinea versicolor*** (p. 278). Hypopigmented and hyperpigmented finely scaling, irregular patches on sides and posterior aspect. Extend up to mandible and to hairline.

***Hailey-Hailey pemphigus*** (p. 133). Sharply bordered erythematous, moist patches at base of neck bilaterally. Surface is fissured.

***Pseudoxanthoma elasticum*** (p. 169). Pale yellow, soft, velvety macular and papular alteration in skin along sides of neck at base. Papules coalesce to become plaques. Other flexures involved.

***Pellagra*** (p. 368). Erythema, scaling in sharply defined "necklace of Casal" outlined by hyperpigmentation in sun-exposed anterior V of neck.

### Raised lesions

***Lichen simplex chronicus*** (p. 448). Lichenified, pruritic hyperpigmented plaque at base of sides of neck or posteriorly. May be bilateral. Orientals predisposed.

***Acrochordon (skin tags)*** (p. 516). Tiny skin-colored papillomas on sides and front of neck. Heritable. Women.

***Epithelial nevus.*** Yellow-brown, velvety plaque, to side of midline anteriorly from birth.

***Keloid*** (p. 516). Firm, small, smooth, pale, globular lesions in suboccipital hairy region at site of folliculitis or acne lesions.

***Cyst.*** *Branchial cleft remnant:* At site of cervical fistulae at anterior border of sternocleidomastoids from childhood to early adult life. *Thyroglossal duct remnant:* From submental area to suprasternal notch. Moves with hyoid bone in swallowing.

## FOREARM AND DORSUM OF HAND
### Flat lesions

***Seborrheic keratosis*** (p. 508). Brown, macular lesions that become roughened and appear "stuck on" normal skin. Seen chiefly in those past middle age.

***Lentigo*** (p. 416). Persistent, macular, tan lesions. Seen at all ages. May be scaling and roughened in older persons (senile lentigo). No malignant potential.

***Pigmented nevus*** (p. 523). Tan to black, flat or slightly elevated, discrete lesion. Present since childhood.

***Blue nevus*** (p. 528). Striking blue color to flat, discrete lesions. Present from birth.

***Actinic keratosis*** (p. 508). Scaling, discrete, reddish macular lesion on dorsum of hand and on areas exposed to sunlight. May become heaped up and hard. Premalignant.

***Senile purpura*** (p. 481). Large, irregular ecchymoses of dorsa of wrists and hands in elderly patients. Asymptomatic.

***Primary irritant contact dermatitis*** (p. 430). Erythema, dryness, scaling, sometimes with interfinger involvement. Affects dorsum of hand, fingers, and wrist flexures.

***Allergic eczematous contact dermatitis*** (p. 102). Erythema and scaling of dorsum of hand and fingers, particularly over knuckles. Occurs in reactions to rubber gloves.

***Atopic dermatitis*** (p. 118). Pruritus, scaling, and excoriations of hand, fingers, and wrist flexures that progress to lichenification and fissuring. Often in children and young adults. Hands may show only manifestations of this disease. Antecubital fossae involved as part of flexural distribution of this disorder in older children and young adults. Lichenified, excoriated, pruritic.

***Lichen simplex chronicus*** (p. 448). Localized, well-demarcated patch of hyperpigmentation and lichenification. Pruritic, unilateral. Persistent on forearm and dorsum of hand. (See Plate 45, p. 458.)

***Nummular eczema*** (p. 435). Coin-shaped, erythematous lesions with moist surface. May be crusted. On dorsa of hands and on extensor surfaces of forearms and legs.

***Photosensitivity dermatitis*** (p. 199). Diffuse erythema of dorsa of hands caused by contact with photosensitizing chemical or ingestion of photosensitizing drug. Vesicles or bullae may occur. Hyperpigmentation usually follows.

***Erythema multiforme*** (p. 202). Distinctive, circular, erythematous, and edematous lesions with depressed center ("target" or iris lesions). May become bullous. Begin distally and spread proximally. (See Plate 23, p. 213.)

***Vitiligo*** (p. 422). Circumscribed area of complete depigmentation. Symmetrical. May demonstrate glove distribution.

***Fungal infection*** (p. 265). Dry, pruritic crescentic patches of scaling, erythematous dermatitis. Peripheral vesicles. Dorsa of hands.

***Syphilis*** (p. 258). Nonpruritic erythematous macules or papules on palms and soles concurrent with generalized eruption. Serological test for syphilis positive at this stage.

***Polymorphous light eruption*** (p. 363). Scaling and erythema, papules, or vesicle and bulla formation. Begins hours to a day or more after sun exposure.

***Porphyria*** (p. 371). Sun-sensitive hands with fragile, easily damaged epidermis. Heals with hyperpigmented scars. Sun may cause vesicles or bullae.

***Fixed drug eruption*** (p. 199). Red-brown round lesion with shading of colors. May develop bullae. Recurrent.

***Acrocyanosis*** (p. 574). Bluish discoloration of fingers, with aching on cold exposure and dependency. Found in women.

***Raynaud's disease*** (p. 584). Complete, sharply limited finger pallor, followed by cyanosis and rubor. Leads to fingertip ulcers.

***Scleroderma*** (p. 158). Skin of distal phalanges becomes hardened, atrophic, and bound down. Fingers slowly acquire fixed, clawlike position with areas of atrophy, hyperpigmentation, and depigmentation. Small terminal ulcers on digits. Raynaud's phenomenon present.

***Systemic lupus erythematosus*** (p. 151). Erythema and telangiectasia over phalangeal joints, base of fingernails, and elbows. Fingertips erythematous and tender. Small purpuric lesions.

***Dermatomyositis*** (p. 155). Telangiectatic and erythematous patches extensor aspect of joints, fingers, and elbows.

### Raised lesions

***Wart (verruca)*** (p. 316). Small, slightly elevated, flat, fawn-colored freckle-like lesions on dorsum of hand (verruca juvenilis) or hyperkeratotic, rough-surfaced papules with central puncta (verruca vulgaris) anywhere on hand.

***Paronychia*** (p. 403). Tender, red, sometimes purulent swelling at base of nail in persons doing "wet work."

***Scabies*** (p. 325). Vesicles and papules in interfinger webs, wrist flexures, and elbows. Acute and recent onset. Infectious. Pruritic.

***Granuloma annulare*** (p. 167). One or more red to skin-colored papules that enlarge slowly to form circular lesion with depressed center. Peripheral extension of raised borders. On dorsa of hands and fingers. Asymptomatic.

***Lichen planus*** (p. 355). Pruritic, discrete, shiny, flat-topped, polyangular reddish papules on dorsa of hands and flexor surfaces of wrists.

***Dermatitis herpetiformis*** (p. 140). Extremely pruritic grouped vesicles that are excoriated as they appear, distal to elbow. Chronic lesions, hyperkeratotic, hyperpigmented.

***Granuloma pyogenicum*** (p. 522). Rapidly growing, small, smooth, brightly erythematous tumor composed of granulation tissue. Often arises at site of minor trauma.

***Knuckle pads.*** Asymptomatic, hyperkeratotic papules over interphalangeal joints. Inherited as a Mendelian dominant. May be associated with Dupuytren's contracture.

***Myxoid cyst (ganglion)*** (p. 519). Noninflammatory, fluctuant, asymptomatic, small swelling of dorsum of distal phalanx, adjacent to nail fold or dorsum of hand. Contains clear, jellied fluid.

***Sweat retention (dyshidrosis)*** (p. 505). Discrete, small, skin-colored vesicles with erythematous halo on dorsa of hands and sides of fingers. This eruption is strongly pruritic. Often follows an inflammatory dermatosis.

***Glomus tumor*** (p. 522). Sharp, lancinating pain that arises from this minute vascular tumor is an identifying feature. Often found under a fingernail.

***Arsenical keratoses*** (p. 559). Affect dorsa fingers and knuckles with localized conical, hard, keratotic lesions less than 0.5 cm. Palms and soles also involved.

***Squamous cell carcinoma*** (p. 541). Arises in rough, thickened skin with multiple keratoses, from sun or other factors. Induration occurs, followed by hyperkeratosis, erythema, tenderness, and then ulceration. Slow growing and slow to metastasize. If it arises again in normal skin, it will spread faster.

***Basal cell epithelioma*** (p. 537). Less common than squamous cell in this site. Smooth, localized, with rolled edge and pearly appearance. Ulcerates.

***Fish tank, swimming pool granuloma.*** Red-brown papular crusted lesions on hand or fingers after abrasion in aquarium or pool. May ulcerate superficially. Usually single. May present linear sporotrichoid spread.

***North American blastomycosis*** (p. 290). Papule or nodule that ulcerates and forms persistent, nonhealing verrucous plaque on dorsum of hand or forearm. Associated lymphadenopathy and lymphangitis.

***Sporotrichosis*** (p. 289). Papules and nodules arise and develop slowly. Occurring over hand and arm. Tend to follow lymph channels in linear fashion. Eventually ulcerate.

***Milker's nodules*** (p. 312). Discrete erythematous papules on hands or wrists. Become pigmented. Self-limited. Contracted from cow.

***Erysipeloid.*** Blue-red nodules at areas of trauma on hands. From contact with fish.

### Ulcerations

***Anthrax, diphtheria, tularemia.*** Distinctive ulcerations on finger or hand, with regional adenopathy.

## PALMS AND SOLES

### Flat lesions

***Contact dermatitis*** (p. 102). The following two clinical entities are so similar in appearance that it is often impossible to distinguish one from the other. Both may begin with vesicles and redness. Patch testing may be definitive. *Primary irritant contact dermatitis* (p. 431): one of most common dermatoses encountered anywhere. Dryness, scaling, and

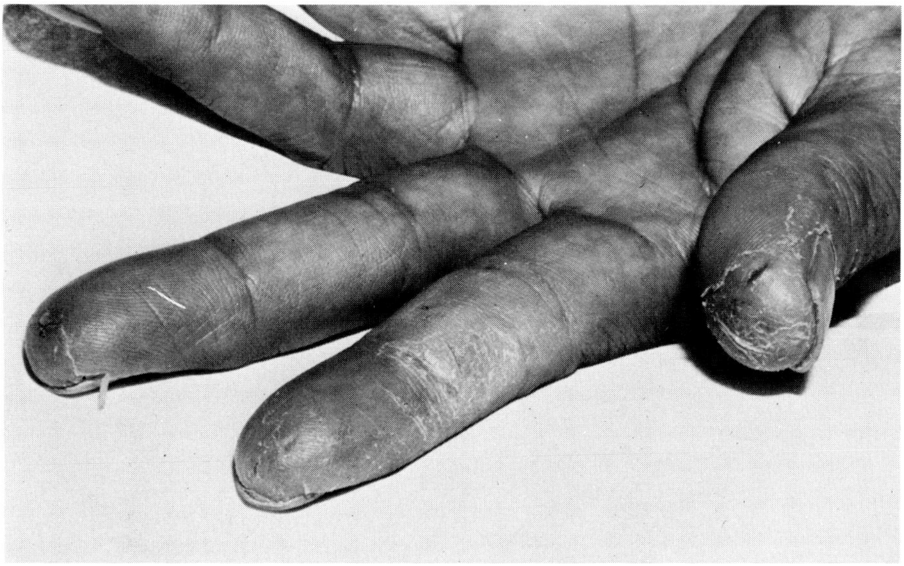

**Fig. 1-14.** Allergic contact dermatitis of a dentist's fingers from local anesthetic. Proved by patch testing.

erythema of palms with fissuring in long-standing cases. Most common in women as "housewife's eczema." Often begins beneath rings. *Allergic contact dermatitis* (Fig. 1-14): pruritus, erythema, and vesiculation, followed by scaling, fissuring, and lichenification in long-standing cases. May mimic other dermatoses. Causes: rubber components, leather, metals, dyes, antibiotics, lanolin, and plant chemicals. Solid substances produce erythema strictly at site of contact with sensitizing agent, whereas liquids tend to produce interfinger irritations. Both types of contact dermatitis are unusual on soles.

***Psoriasis*** (p. 462). May affect palms and soles in three ways: (1) Discrete hyperkeratotic areas that slowly enlarge and fissure as they thicken. (2) Characteristic scaling, red, psoriatic lesions. (3) Vesicular or pustular involvement, with multiple tender, painful 1 to 3 mm lesions that either harden to a yellow, inactive residual and peel, or lead to a phase of fissuring and bleeding.

***Tinea*** (p. 276). Diffuse erythema with fine dry scale, or vesicopustules similar to psoriasis. Erythematous patch with peripheral vesicles likely to be fungus. Scrapings will show hyphae.

***Pompholyx.*** Groups of vesicles appear suddenly, over palms, along fingers, and sometimes on soles. Become pruritic and tender and then subside synchronously over 1 to 3 weeks. The skin peels. Recurrences are the rule. May become secondarily infected.

***Atopic dermatitis*** (p. 118). Painful, mildly erythematous, dry scaling and fissuring of sole, particularly toes and ball of foot. In children in winter, "winter feet." Palms easily irritated by strong cleansers, frequent washing.

***Pitted keratolysis*** (Fig. 1-15) (p. 250). Punched-out, asymptomatic shallow craters of soles on weight-bearing areas.

***Keratosis palmaris et plantaris*** (p. 352). Diffuse, hyperkeratosis of palms and soles accompanied by cracking and fissuring. Lifelong, from infancy. Hereditary. Often hyperhidrotic. NOTE: Palmar and plantar keratosis may be local, punctate or diffuse, isolated, or part of a generalized cutaneous disorder. It may be an inherited defect sui generis, or of chemical origin.

***Lichen planus*** (p. 355). Hyperkeratotic papules extending to periphery of palms and soles from adjacent wrists. Also, acute erythematous, painful, diffuse thickening of palms and soles.

***Syphilis*** (p. 258). Nonpruritic erythema-

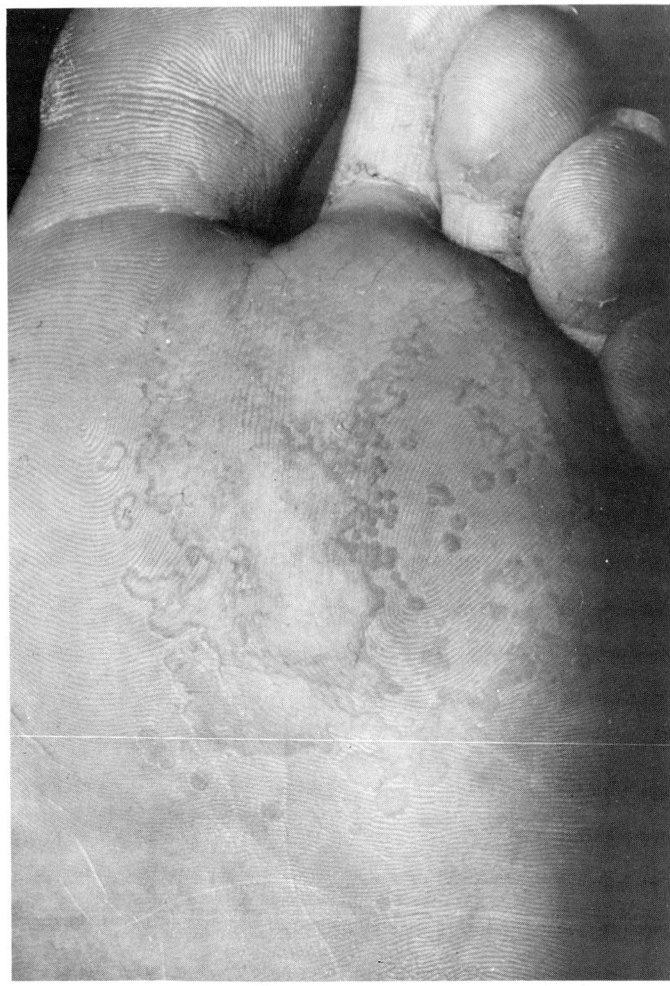

**Fig. 1-15.** Pitted keratolysis. Note geographic areas of keratin dissolved in the inflammatory process.

tous macules or papules on palms and soles concurrent with generalized eruption. Serological test for syphilis positive at this stage.

***Erythromelalgia (erythermalgia)*** (p. 575). Burning discomfort on soles of feet, often without visible changes. Associated with increased environmental temperature.

***Pyoderma*** (p. 248). Painful, erosive, moist lesions, often first seen at base of toes, with peripheral spread. May be staphylococcal, streptococcal, pseudomonas, or other.

## Raised lesions

***Wart (verruca)*** (Fig. 1-16) (p. 316). As elsewhere is keratotic and discrete with black dots of thrombosed capillaries for identification. Lines of epidermal ridges separate to go around warts.

***Punctate keratoderma*** (p. 253). Some forms of keratosis palmaris et plantaris are spotty and consist of individual keratotic lesions. Many inflammatory. Arsenical keratoses to be ruled out.

***Callus*** (p. 254). Tender; hyperkeratosis on weight-bearing areas.

***Reiter's disease (keratoderma blennorrhagicum)*** (p. 469). Lesions are sharply bordered, erythematous, and heavily crusted and may be pustular. Pustules give way to hard conical yellow-brown keratotic lesions. Association

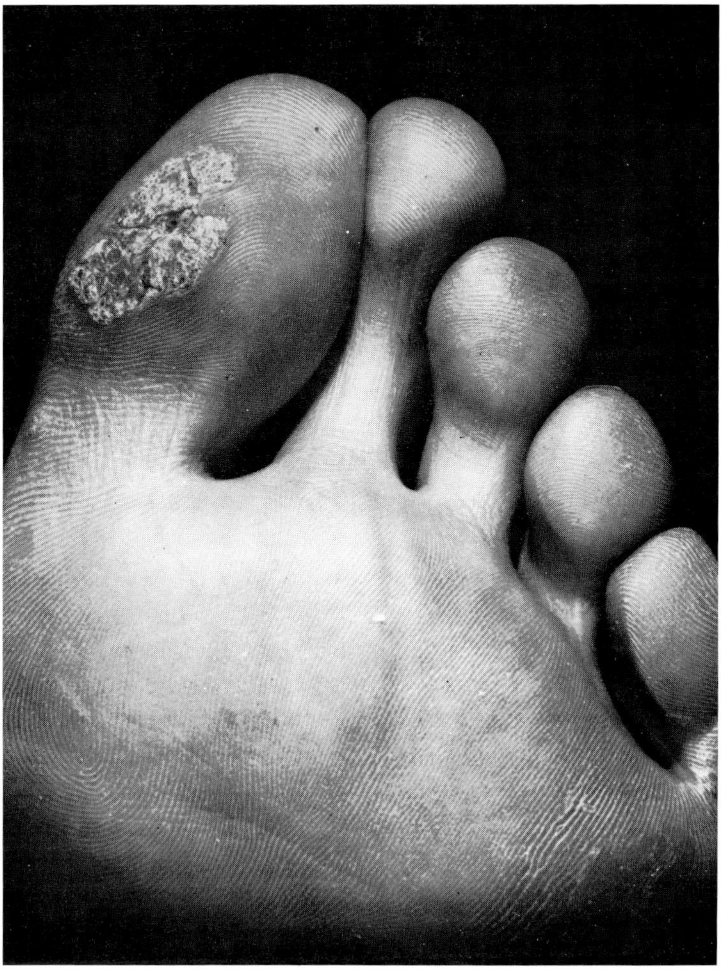

**Fig. 1-16.** Plantar wart.

with penile lesions, arthritis, and conjunctivitis.

***Keratoderma climactericum.*** Punctate hyperkeratoses. Increase slowly to confluency, around periphery of weight-bearing and frictional areas. Fissuring and uncomfortable. Women 35 to 65 years of age.

## TORSO
### Flat lesions

***Freckle*** (p. 415). Tan, small or large, irregular macule that appears with sun exposure, fades with avoidance. Axillary freckling indicates neurofibromatosis.

***Lentigo*** (p. 416). Tan, 1 to 5 mm. macule. No change with seasons or sun. Increased numbers in leopard syndrome and with some congenital syndromes.

***Pigmented nevus*** (p. 523). Flat, tan to black, irregularly shaped, multiple macules. 1 to 10 mm. Appear at birth, during adolescence, during pregnancy. May disappear as well.

*Special forms*

ITO'S NEVUS. Large. Shoulder and arm. From birth.

BECKER'S NEVUS. Light tan, mildly hairy. Shoulder area. Appears in male teenagers.

HALO NEVUS (p. 524). Depigmented halo appearing around pigmented nevus. Eventually results in disappearance of "mole."

MONGOLIAN SPOT (p. 528). Dusky blue macular lesions commonly found in sacral region in newborn Oriental infants. Disappears during childhood.

***Café-au-lait patch*** (p. 416). Light tan, smooth, irregular patches from birth. Six or more larger than 1.5 cm. indicate neurofibromatosis.

***Postinflammatory hyperpigmentation*** (p. 419). Patches of hyperpigmented skin appear at sites of previous inflammation and may last for weeks to months. Lichen planus, bullous dermatoses, pityriasis rosea, and fixed drug eruptions may produce these changes.

***Seborrheic keratosis*** (p. 508). Begin as flat, tan, irregular-shaped macule that progresses to typical lesion (see raised lesions).

***Psoriasis*** (p. 462). Dull red, large, irregular-shaped patches and plaques with thick, prominent, silvery scale, many similar small lesions, or diffuse scaling and erythema involving large portions of body surface.

***Seborrheic dermatitis*** (p. 494). Irregularly shaped, poorly defined, erythematous patches on presternal, interscapular and umbilical areas, possessing fine, slightly greasy scale.

***Pityriasis rosea*** (p. 426). Red, scaling, oval macular lesions whose long axes follow lines of cleavage of skin. Initial lesion (herald patch) occurs before others in a pathognomonic pattern. (See Plate 7, p. 54.)

***Tinea versicolor*** (p. 278). Discrete, confluent, fawn-colored to brown, slightly scaling lesions of irregular shape. Spreads slowly. Sunlight produces characteristic combination of hyperpigmentation and hypopigmentation. Actual lesions pale in summer, tan in winter. Upper half of torso.

***Allergic eczematous contact dermatitis*** (p. 102). Acute, pruritic inflammation ranging from erythema to vesiculation. Common causes: metal fasteners, rubber waist bands, dyes, formaldehyde in textile finishes of slips and shirts, perfumes, and certain sunscreens. Perspiration leaches these chemicals from clothing.

***Atopic dermatitis*** (p. 118). Pruritic, scaling, erythematous inflammation. Lichenification of upper back, chest, and waist. Chronic. Skin generally dry. (See Plate 13, p. 123).

***Vitiligo*** (p. 422). Irregular, completely depigmented areas. May gradually enlarge. Texture of skin surface not altered. Symmetric distribution, often axillary.

***Tinea corporis*** (p. 270). Multiple, round, red, scaling, macular lesions with fine, vesicular border. Found chiefly in preadolescents after exposure to kittens.

***Scabies*** (p. 325). Pruritic, excoriated, vesicopapules on anterior and posterior axillary folds, waist, and areolae of nipples in women. Can see burrows on careful examination.

***Discoid lupus erythematosus*** (p. 147). Sharply bordered, nonpruritic, dull red, scaling lesions of upper midback, neck and V of chest that produce scarring.

***Candidosis (moniliasis)*** (p. 280). Patches of diffuse, moist erythema with flaccid pustules on periphery. Found on submammary areas, extending to inferior aspect of breast.

***Drug eruption*** (p. 199). Commonest site. May be macular, morbilliform, papular, bullous, urticarial, purpuric, or pustular.

***Bowen's disease*** (p. 545). Discrete, dusky red patch. Enlarges very slowly and persistently. Biopsy necessary to establish diagnosis. Asymptomatic.

***Superficial basal cell epithelioma*** (p. 537). May be clinically indistinguishable from Bowen's disease, but may have recognizable threadlike round border. Psoriasiform appearance (Plate 4, p. 35).

***Erythema marginatum.*** Slightly elevated rings and polycyclic patterns of erythema. Recurrent, asymptomatic.

***Progressive systemic scleroderma*** (p. 158). Tight, shiny skin with reduced flexibility. Leads to restriction of chest motion.

***Urticaria pigmentosa*** (p. 562). *Childhood:* multiple, up to several centimeters, oval, brown maculopapular lesions become reddened and elevated when rubbed. Can blister in infancy (Fig. 1-17). *Adult:* small, macular, generalized, telangiectatic lesions.

***Tuberous sclerosis*** (p. 515). Multiple depigmented white angular or leaf-shaped macules, 1 to 3 cm. long. Occur on the trunk or

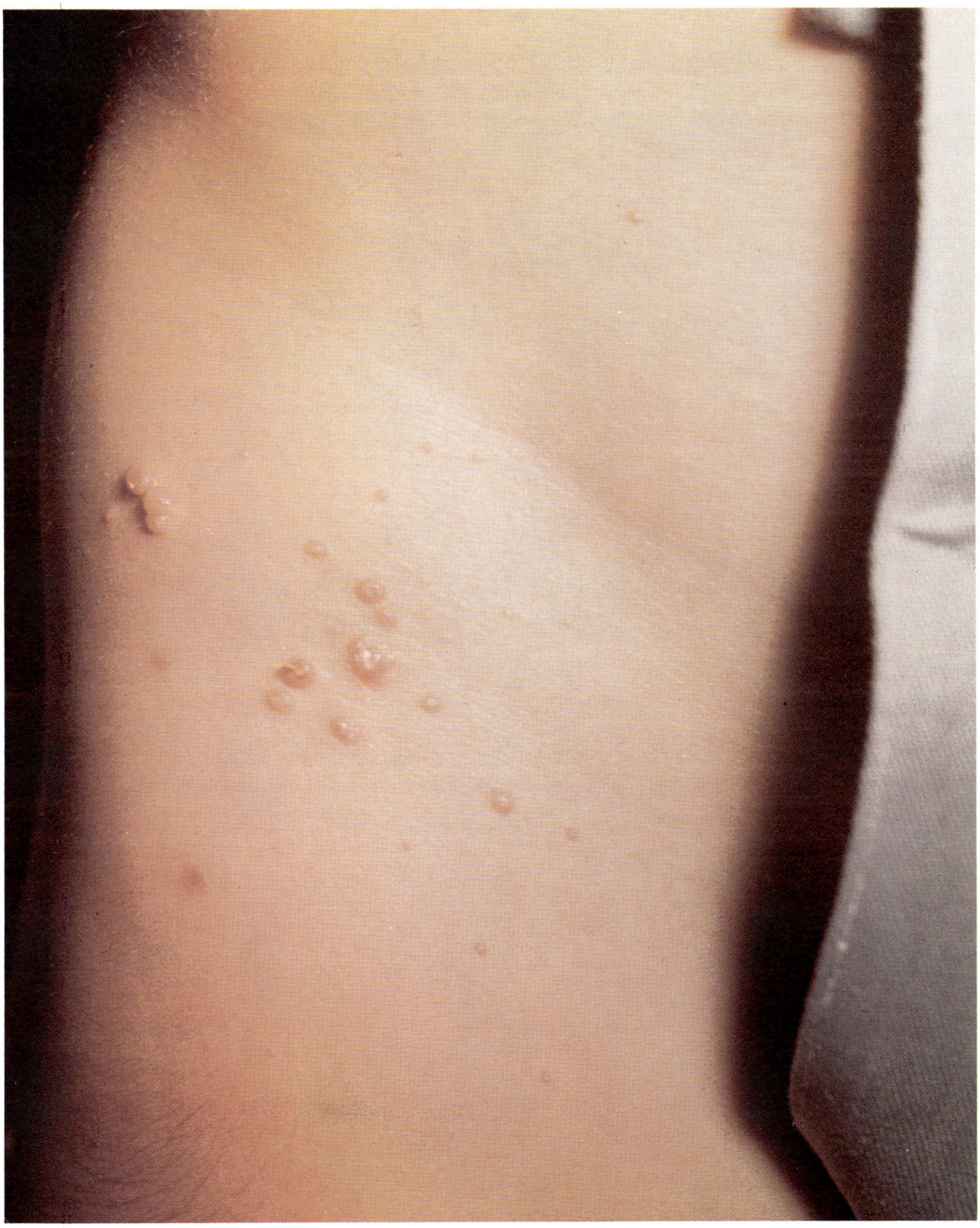

**Plate 3**

Molluscum contagiosum. Waxy pink globules with umbilicated centers.

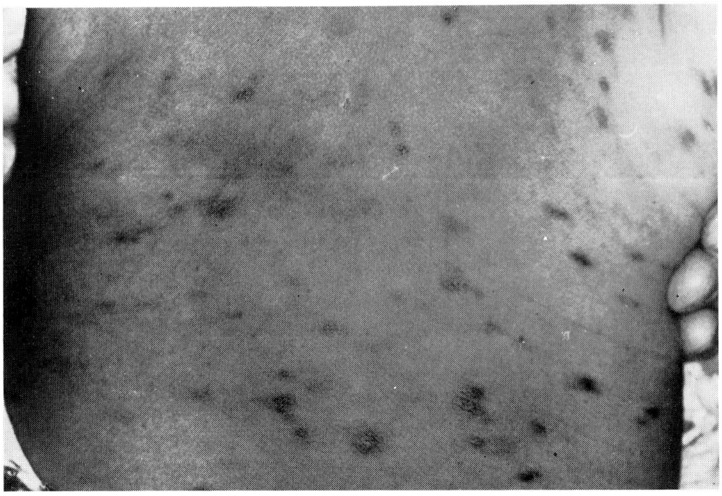

**Fig. 1-17.** Urticaria pigmentosa.

buttocks in most patients with tuberous sclerosis.

***Malignant lentigo*** (p. 530). Begins as small, mottled light brown, irregular macule on upper torso. Very slowly extends peripherally with increasing disparity of colors. Eventually produces a nodular surface, which may ulcerate. Slow to metastasize.

***Superficial spreading melanoma*** (p. 532). Begins in upper torso, on back, with enlarging lesion. Displays irregular coloring. Black, brown, pink, blue and white may be present.

## Raised lesions

***Acne vulgaris*** (p. 79). Comedones, papules, pustules, and cysts on back, midchest, shoulders, and upper arms. May occur on buttocks. Larger lesions produce scars and keloids. Skin is likely to be oily.

***Pigmented nevus*** (p. 523). Multiple, brown to black lesions, slightly raised or dome shaped. Varying in size from 1 to 10 mm. May be hairy.

***Giant hairy nevus, bathing suit nevus*** (p. 526). Present from birth. Often very large, covering extensive parts of skin surface. However, may be any size. Usually dark brown, raised, rugose. Incidence of melanoma significant.

***Seborrheic keratosis*** (p. 508). Tan to dark brown, warty, greasy, roughened soft tumor. May be pruritic.

***Acrochordon (skin tag)*** (p. 516). Tiny, asymptomatic, noninflamed outpouchings of subepidermal connective tissue about neck, upper chest, and upper back.

***Senile angioma (cherry angioma, Campbell de Morgan spot*** (p. 572). Pinhead-sized, bloodred, asymptomatic vascular papule 1 to 3 mm in diameter. Found in most adults after middle age. No clinical significance.

***Molluscum contagiosum*** (p. 311). Multiple, small, discrete, waxy globules with central depression. Usually found in children (Plate 3, p. 33).

***Keloid, or hypertrophic scar*** (p. 516). Firm plaque. Pink to skin colored. Pruritic early. Older lesions white. Anterior presternal area in children and young adults. Prevalent in darkskinned races (Fig. 1-18).

***Sebaceous cyst*** (p. 513). Fluctuant, skin-colored globular tumor, 0.5 to 3 cm. or more in diameter. Asymptomatic. Acne or seborrhea usually present.

***Lipoma*** (p. 519). Soft, poorly defined, compressible fatty tumor. Asymptomatic and essentially unchanging.

***Urticaria*** (p. 113). Pale, pruritic wheals on an erythematous background, with bizarre

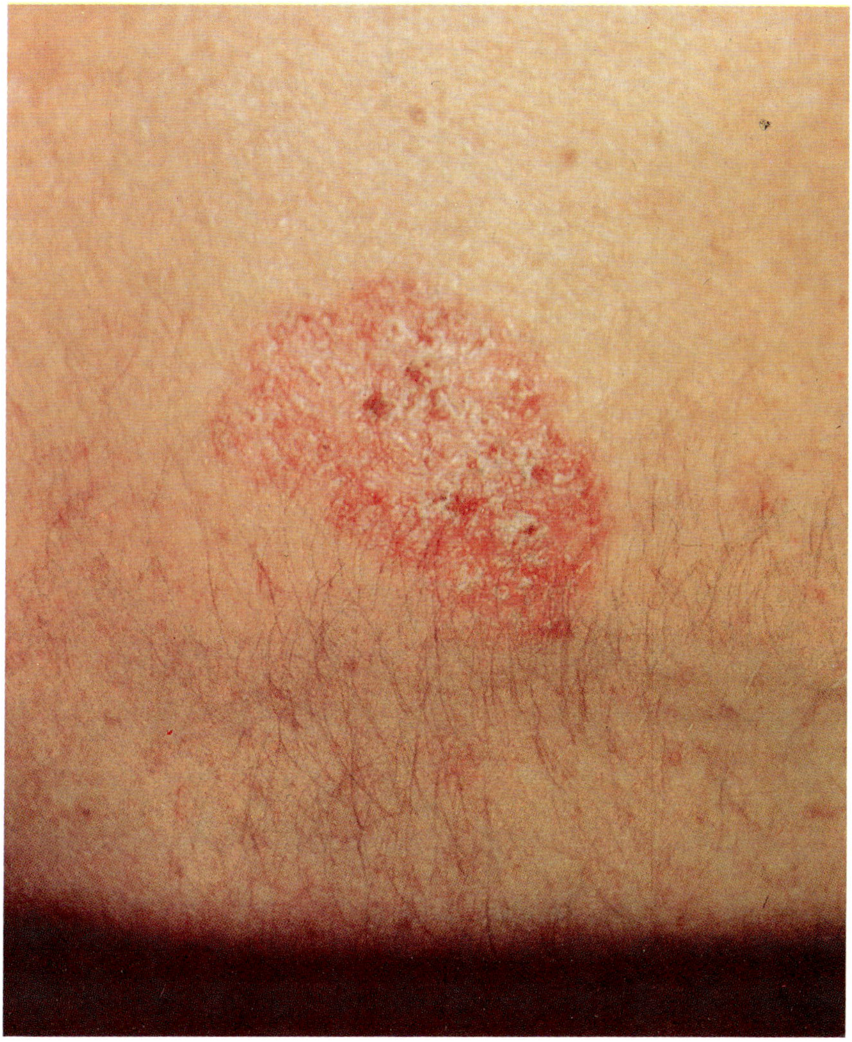

**Plate 4**

Superficial basal cell epithelioma. Characterized by slow, persistent enlargement.

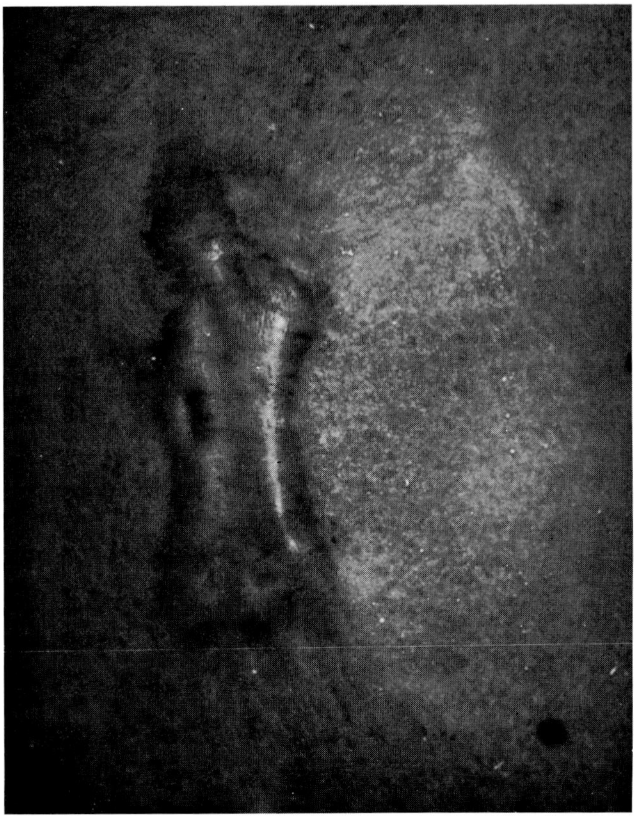

**Fig. 1-18.** Keloid, presternal area.

A

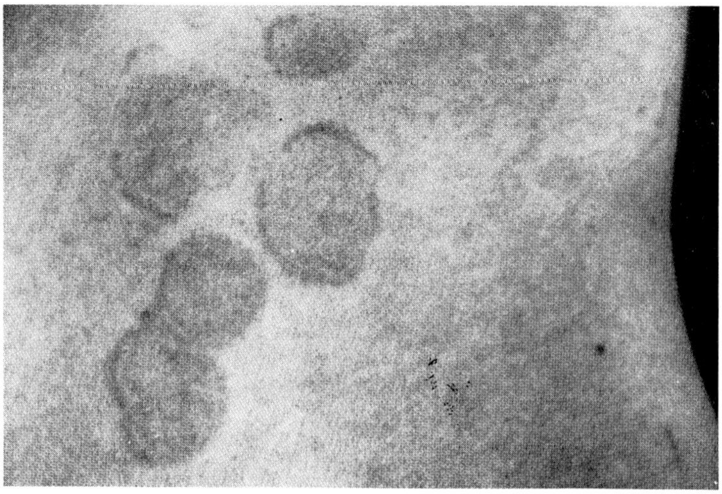

**Fig. 1-19. A,** Urticaria. Transience of individual lesions is the hallmark.

sizes and shapes (Fig. 1-19, *A*). Lesions are transient, clearing from one site after several hours, only to appear in other areas.

***Dermographism*** (p. 115). Wheals appear on stroking, scratching, or pressure.

***Pediculosis corporis*** (p. 336). Papules and long, deep, linear excoriations from infestation with body lice. Associated with poor hygiene.

***Varicella*** (p. 302). Initially clear vesicles on erythematous base in varying stages. First on face and back. Spreads outward. Found in children.

***Vaccinia*** (p. 309). Pustules occurring after vaccination 1 week previously. Grave in atopic patients.

***Herpes simplex*** (p. 295). Initial clustered vesicles, progressing on to crusting. Recurrent lesion of buttock.

***Zoster*** (p. 303). Vesicular, crusting eruption occurring after unilateral, segmental, neural distribution (Fig. 1-19, *B*). Preceding prodromal pain. May be followed by postherpetic neuralgia.

***Erythema multiforme*** (p. 212). Papules, vesicles, and bullae with characteristic "bull's-eye" form, having a pale periphery and darker, fluid-filled center.

***Lichen planus*** (p. 355). Very pruritic, discrete, flat-topped, angular, violaceous papules. Eruption over thorax may be diffuse, maculopapular, and less specific.

***Dermatitis herpetiformis*** (p. 140). Intensely pruritic. Macules, papules, vesicles, and bullae may all be present, but usually clusters of excoriated vesicles. Residual hyperpigmentation. Found in interscapular, sacral areas (Fig. 1-20).

***Pemphigus*** (p. 133). Bullous lesions that rupture easily, leaving a red, denuded surface. Epidermis is found to be quite fragile and easily separated from dermis. Patient has systemic toxic symptoms.

***Variola*** (p. 307). Patient ill. Vesicles becoming pustules. All same stage of development. First on face and extremities.

***Sweat retention (miliaria)*** (p. 505). Pruritic, discrete, erythematous papules and vesicles. May follow an episode of cutaneous inflammation or excessive perspiration in predisposed individual.

***Dermatofibroma*** (p. 516). Small, reddish brown tumor. Sometimes has yellow cast. Firm, dome shaped. Less than 1 cm. in diameter, discrete, stationary, asymptomatic.

***Parapsoriasis.*** *Acute:* small vesiculopapules and crusting lesions scattered over torso and extremities. Lesions in various stages. *Chronic (en plaque):* erythematous, large, scaling plaques on thorax, thighs, buttocks.

***Xanthomatosis*** (p. 378). Multiple, papular or nodular, yellow-brown–toned lesions extending over buttocks. Associated with lesions on extensor surfaces elsewhere.

B

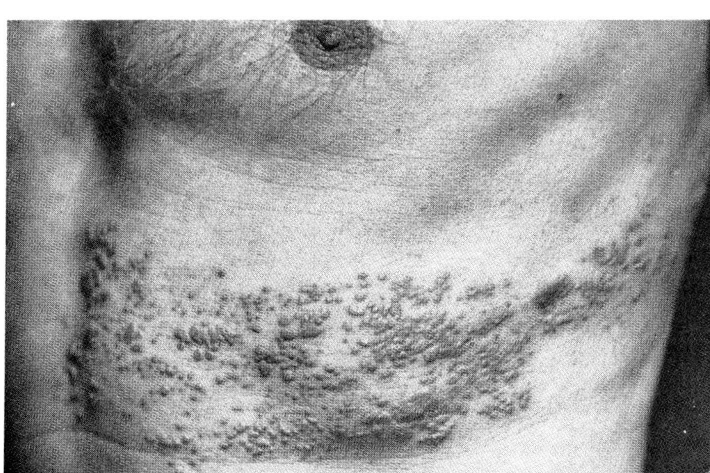

**Fig. 1-19, cont'd. B,** Zoster. Note abrupt cessation at midline.

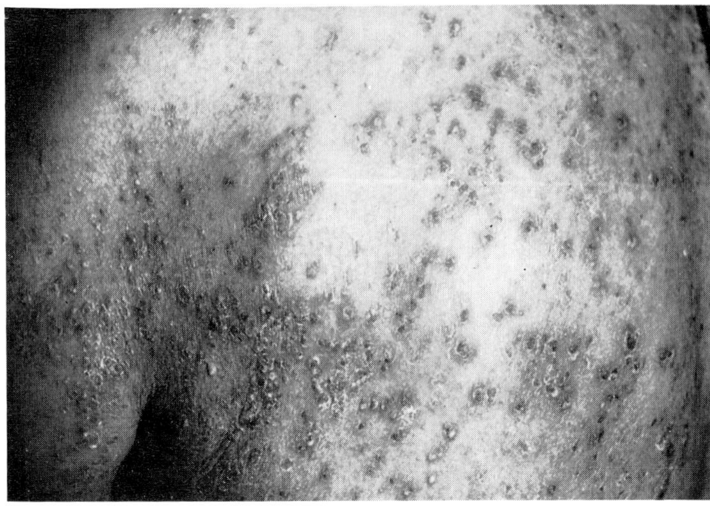

**Fig. 1-20.** Dermatitis herpetiformis.

***Neurofibromatosis (von Recklinghausen's disease)*** (p. 521). Multiple, soft, varisized, compressible, pedunculated tumors seen after puberty. Also, large, light brown macules (café-au-lait spots) present from birth.

***Keratosis follicularis (Darier's disease)*** (p. 351). Hereditary. Dirty brown, greasy follicular papules. May enlarge and coalesce to form large verrucous growths on midback and chest. Extend onto neck. Usually childhood onset.

***Malignant melanoma*** (p. 530). *Superficial spreading melanoma:* elevated plaque on upper torso with rapid extension and black-brown, rose, white, color variation. *Nodular melanoma:* tan to black, enlarging and darkening nodule. Back is most frequent site in males in Australia. May arise from preexisting pigmented nevus.

***Superficial basal cell carcinoma*** (p. 537). Skin-colored, flat papules extending slowly peripherally. Minute rolled border. Multiple (Plate 4, p. 35).

***Mycosis fungoides*** (p. 555). Well-demarcated erythema in early stages. Slowly evolves over years into discrete plaques and ulcerated tumors. (see Plate 60, p. 556.)

***Pseudoxanthoma elasticum*** (p. 169). Degenerative hereditary involvement of sides of neck and supraclavicular areas. Minute yellow papules in background of ruddy telangiectasia. Skin becomes redundant. Childhood onset.

***Actinomycosis*** (p. 288). Woody induration of affected thoracic area. Frequent in sinus tract to thoracic cavity.

***North American blastomycosis*** (p. 290). Arising from pulmonary focus. Present on skin of lateral thorax as papule or pustule with slow peripheral extension.

***Scleredema adultorum.*** Acute onset of progressive "solid edema" of neck, back, and thorax.

## Depressed or ulcerated lesions

***Localized scleroderma (morphea)*** (p. 161). Indurated, mildly erythematous, initially hyperpigmented patch or patches that slowly give way to atrophy or pallor. Present on front and sides of thorax and abdomen. (See Plate 17, p. 162).

***Lichen sclerosus et atrophicus*** (p. 164). Depigmented, pale, atrophic patches on normal skin, with small, flat, peripheral papules. Initial inflammatory phase usual. On upper back and shoulders.

***Macular atrophy.*** Pale oval lesions, 1 to 2 cm. in diameter. Single or multiple, covered by thin, slightly bulging atrophic skin. May or may not be inflamed.

## FEMALE BREAST

### Flat lesions

***Striae*** (p. 204). Appear late in puberty after secondary sexual characteristics as jagged linear bands. First red-blue, soon become white and inconspicuous. Depressed, asymptomatic may appear with pregnancy or after use of topical fluorinated glucocorticoids.

***Scabies*** (p. 325). Crusting, vesicular, intensely pruritic dermatitis of nipples and areolae of mature females.

***Allergic eczematous contact dermatitis*** (p. 102). Well-defined erythema in mild cases and vesiculation in more severe cases. Common causes: Nickel bra fasteners, rubber and associated chemicals, or, less commonly, clothing finishes and black dyes, and synthetic materials.

***Intertrigo*** (p. 282). Red, moist patches or erosions with well-demarcated borders beneath breast. Frequently *Candida* present. Warmth and moisture predispose.

***Eczema.*** Moist, vesicular dermatitis of areola and nipple of young adult females. Idiopathic. Not uncommon. May be unilateral or bilateral. Chief significance lies in Paget's disease (see below).

***Paget's disease of the nipple.*** Moist, slightly crusted dermatitis of nipple and areola. Usually unilateral. Manifestation of a deeper intraductal mammary malignancy. Can easily be mistaken for benign lesion. *Biopsy essential.* (See previous discussion of eczema.)

***Syphilitic chancre*** (p. 258). Small, red macule that goes on to erode with formation of very superficial clean ulcer. Painless, round, but indurated. 1 to 2 cm. Regional lymphadenopathy.

### Raised lesions

***Seborrheic keratosis*** (p. 508). Skin-colored to brown or even black, warty growths "stuck onto" the skin chiefly in inframammary areas of middle-aged women. Often itchy.

***Fox-Fordyce disease.*** Intensely pruritic, small, flesh-colored papules closely studded over areolae of postpubertal females. Occasionally in prepubertal males.

***Metastatic carcinoma*** (p. 558). Most common site of metastatic carcinoma of the skin. Usually from breast malignancy. Painless 1- to 3-cm. skin-colored nodules that go on to ulcerate. Usually freely movable.

## AXILLARY-INGUINAL

### Flat lesions

***Intertrigo*** (p. 282). Moist, tender patches of erythema starting from depth of flexures. Often irritant origin. From heat, perspiration.

***Tinea cruris*** (p. 272). Males. Most common inguinal dermatitis. Red-brown, scaling, crescentic lesion extending down thigh from inguinal fold. Pruritic. Border active, vesicular. Often extends to perianal area. Scrapings essential.

***Psoriasis*** (p. 462). Characteristic dull red macule with thick white scale, or a glistening erythematous patch. May be entirely intertriginous (psoriasis inversa).

***Seborrheic dermatitis*** (p. 508). Localized, moist, erythematous patch.

***Candidosis (moniliasis)*** (p. 280). Sharply demarcated, shiny, erythematous patch with peripheral satellites of flaccid pustules. Inguinal form more common.

***Allergic eczematous contact dermatitis*** (p. 102). Erythema, progressing to pruritic, localized, moist dermatitis. When causative allergen is in clothing, dress shields, dyes, or textiles, dermatitis is limited to periphery of axilla, leaving apex uninvolved. When causative allergen is an antiperspirant or deodorant, vault and apex are affected, with the periphery being spared.

***Erythrasma*** (p. 250). Asymptomatic, reddish brown patches covered by fine superficial scale. Fluoresces red under Wood's light.

***Diaper dermatitis*** (p. 178). May be moist or scaling, discrete or diffuse, clean or purulent. Flexural, depending on cause.

***Vitiligo*** (p. 422). Completely depigmented, symmetrical patches, asymptomatic with sharp borders. May appear in flexures first.

***Freckle*** (p. 415). Multiple, small brown to black freckles in axilla are pathognomonic of neurofibromatosis.

### Raised lesions

***Venereal inguinal lymphadenopathy.*** Aside from general causes of lymphadenopathy that apply to all nodes, inguinal lymph gland enlargement may be attributable to *pyogenic anogenital infection, herpetic balanitis* or *vulvovaginitis*, or *primary syphilis* (50% of cases) in association with a chancre. *Chancroid:* lymphadenopathy develops and then may ulcerate after the appearance of a genital lesion 5 to 20 mm. in size. Sinus tracts may occur. *Granuloma inguinale:* destructive groin lesions develop and then ulcerate and enlarge, not always in association with a genital lesion. *Lymphogranuloma venereum:* inguinal dermatitis, swelling, and sinuses occur after genital lesion. May go on to extensive lymphatic damage with matted glands above and below inguinal ligament.

***Acrochordon (skin tag)*** (p. 516). Small, pedunculated, skin-colored connective tissue growth. Most common in axilla but occasionally in groin.

***Furuncle*** (p. 245). Tender, red, nodular lesion that becomes fluctuant and suppurates.

***Warts*** (p. 316). Row of common warts may occur along groin fold in moisture and warmth.

***Lichen planus*** (p. 355). Flexural areas may be affected with few characteristic lesions elsewhere. Color is typically deep red-purple.

***Hidradenitis suppurativa*** (p. 90). One or more tender, erythematous nodules that suppurate and may form sinus tracts. Tends to heal with scar formation and to recur. Deeper, more extensive, and more persistent than furunculosis (Fig. 3-9, p. 91). May extend to perineum.

***Pemphigus vegetans*** (p. 134). Large, flaccid bullous lesions. Moist erosions on which papillomatous or verrucous masses may subsequently arise.

***Pemphigoid*** (p. 137). Tense, clear pruritic blisters in elderly patients, particularly female. Extend down thighs, legs, and elsewhere.

***Pseudoxanthoma elasticum*** (p. 169). Yellow papules in the darkened, loose redundant skin of axilla or groin.

***Fox-Fordyce disease.*** Small, closely set axillary papules, with a yellow cast. Exceptionally pruritic. Chiefly found in adult women at or shortly after puberty.

***Pediculosis*** (p. 336). Infestation with pubic lice. Close examination reveals gray nits on hair shafts. Pubic involvement present first, then axillary. Pruritic, erythematous.

***Trichomycosis axillaris.*** Small nodules or concretions on hair shafts. May be yellow or black. Fungal or bacterial origin. Asymptomatic. Axillary only.

***Acanthosis nigricans*** (p. 421). Velvety or verrucous brown to black hyperpigmentation of axillae. (See Fig. 24-4, p. 420).

## FEMALE GENITALIA

### Flat lesions

***Pruritus vulvae*** (p. 447). Diffuse labial lichenification, either moist or dry. There may be secondary erythema and edema, excoriations, and even infection.

***Psoriasis*** (p. 462). Rather diffuse erythema ordinarily with minimal, but characteristic scaling. Extends along perineum or vulva and over mons pubis. Pruritic.

***Seborrheic dermatitis*** (p. 494). Pruritic, intertriginous, scaling, and erythematous lesions chiefly affecting hair-bearing pubic region and extending to labia majora and perineum.

***Erythrasma*** (p. 250). Well-defined brown fine scaling patches in intergluteal or genitofemoral area. Fluoresces red under Wood's light.

***Candidosis (moniliasis)*** (p. 280). Creamy white patches on reddened base in vagina. Lumpy white discharge. Pruritic.

***Trichomoniasis.*** *Trichomonas vaginalis* produces foamy, vaginal discharge. Vulva reddened, itchy, with fiery red burning granular vaginal mucosa, sometimes petechial. Diagnosis by culture or direct examination of discharge.

***Contact dermatitis*** (p. 102). Various stages of inflammation, from mild erythema to severe weeping and vesiculation. May be (1) *primary irritant:* caused by soaps and excessive cleaning, incontinence, deodorant sprays, and disinfectants, or (2) *allergic:* caused by preservatives and ingredients of topical medications, synthetic rubber in contraceptives, textile dyes in underclothing, nail polish, personal hygiene products, and the like.

***Leukoplakia*** (p. 394). Premalignant lesion. Thickened white plaque on mucous membranes of vagina or labia. Distinct induration not seen in lichen sclerosus et atrophicus. May develop in area of primary atrophy or lichen sclerosus et atrophicus. Must be examined for dysplasia.

***Herpes simplex*** (p. 295). Group of small vesicles on erythematous base that rupture. May be very small area, recurrent. Initial episode, severe and extensive with systemic symptoms. Cutaneous genital lesion may accompany cervical infection.

***Bowen's disease*** (p. 245). Red, slightly scaling or velvety patch on labia that persists. Biopsy.

### Raised lesions

***Condylomata acuminata*** (p. 319) Gray-pink, soft papules on introitus, vaginal mucosa, and around anus. May affect cervix.

***Lichen planus*** (p. 355). Flat-topped papules that become confluent. Extremely pruritic. Mucous membrane of vagina or labia minora may show lacy, gray, linear lesions.

***Lichen simplex chronicus*** (p. 448). Very pruritic, well-circumscribed, lichenified plaque. White on mucosal surfaces, pigmented on skin. On labia or perineum. Usually unilateral (See Plate 45, p. 458).

***Epidermal cyst.*** Labia and around clitoris. May become inflamed.

***Pediculosis pubis*** (p. 336). Pruritic, discrete, excoriated pubic papules. Lice may be found at base of hair. Occasionally bluish macules found over lower abdomen.

***Urethral caruncle.*** Bright red, fleshy, often painful lump. Most often in postmenopausal women. Benign.

***Carcinoma*** (p. 541). Begins as lump or ulcer, or simply bleeding, in any vulvar area, but most often in labia. Can arise on patch of leukoplakia.

***Melanoma.*** (p. 530). Unusual. Mostly pigmented and central, but amelanotic lesion can occur.

***Extramammary Paget's disease*** (p. 549). Well-defined, painful or itching reddish plaque. Labia majora. May extend to inguinal fold. Rare.

### Ulcerated or atrophic lesions

***Senile atrophy.*** Postmenopausal women may develop thinning and depigmentation of vulvar areas, without stenosis. Often pruritic.

***Lichen sclerosus et atrophicus*** (p. 164). White patches and papules on and around vulva, extending in figure eight pattern to perianal area. Later, atrophy with stenosis of orifice and thin, wrinkled depigmented skin. Leukoplakia rarely occurs in this disease, but biopsy must be done to rule out dysplasia. Chiefly premenarche or postmenopause. (See Plate 18, p. 165).

***Primary atrophy.*** Soreness, dyspareunia, dysuria with redness, sclerosing and flattening of labia minora, and vestibule. Finally, white, atrophic. Postmenopausal.

***Chancre (syphilis)*** (p. 258). Red, flat erosion that ulcerates with surrounding induration. Labia minora, clitoris, urethra, or posterior commissure. Often unapparent.

***Chancroid*** (Fig. 1-21, p. 42). Painful papule within introitus that ulcerates and develops ragged edges and satellite ulcers. Inguinal nodes enlarge and may ulcerate.

***Gonorrhea*** (p. 251). Few signs. Urethritis with infection and swelling of paraurethral Skene's glands (analog of prostate) and labial Bartholin's glands. Cervix and rectum inflamed. Culture must be taken from rectum, cervix, and urethra.

## MALE GENITALIA
### Flat lesions

***Primary irritant dermatitis (acute balanitis).*** Erythema of glans and prepuce. Often moist. May be vesicular. Overzealous cleansing, antiseptics, or poor hygiene are frequent causes. Any age.

***Allergic eczematous contact dermatitis.*** Pruritus and erythema. Often weeping and vesiculation. Entire glans, shaft, and scrotum may be involved. Most common causes are topical applications, rubber condoms, and plant (poison ivy) contact through fingers.

***Candidosis (moniliasis)*** (p. 280). Patchy erythema of glans. Most often transient after intercourse because of candidal contact. May be stubborn in diabetic person.

***Circinate balanitis.*** Red, moist erosions of glans with crescentic, polycyclic edges that move and change slowly. May be crusted. Accompanies Reiter's disease.

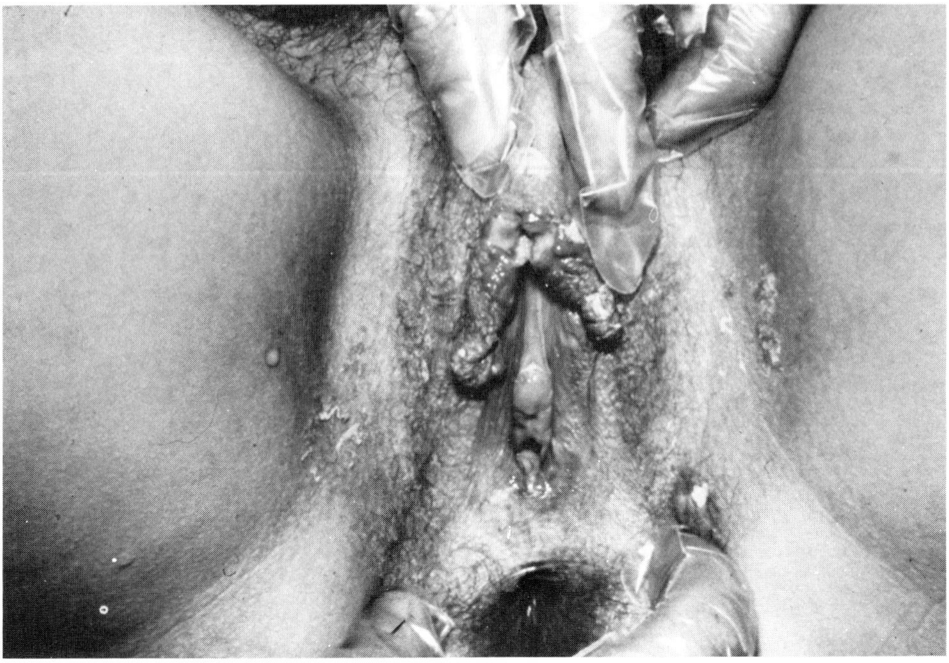

**Fig. 1-21.** Chancroid. Multiple superficial satellite ulcers on labia and bordering introitus. (Courtesy Dr. Allan R. Ronald, Winnipeg, Manitoba.)

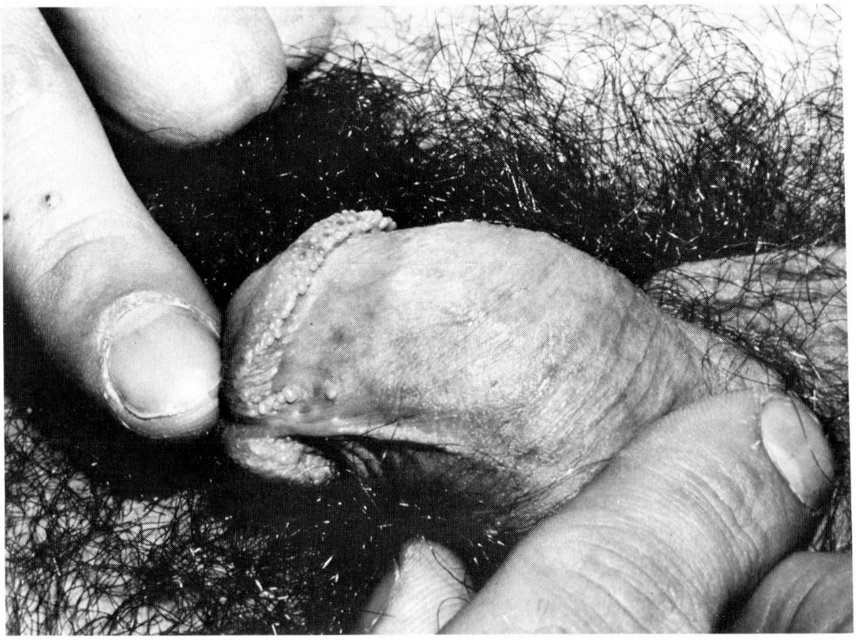

**Fig. 1-22.** Pearly penile papules. An accentuation of normal anatomy.

***Acute infective balanitis*** (p. 392). Bright red, exudative inflammation of glans and prepuce with yellow, creamy exudate. May become edematous and phimosis is a danger. Mixed bacterial origin.

***Seborrheic dermatitis*** (p. 494). Diffuse erythema and scaling in hair-bearing pubic region. Extends onto base of shaft and scrotum. Erythematous macular lesion or diffuse erythema on glans.

***Tinea cruris*** (p. 272). Scaling and erythema, fine, vesicular border. Scrotum and perineum. (see Plate 28, p. 273).

***Pediculosis pubis*** (p. 336). Strong pruritus of pubic region and, secondarily, of scrotum. Excoriated discrete papules. Active lice seen. Red dust may be present on skin.

***Chronic circumscribed balanitis (Zoon)*** (p. 392). Deep red, shiny patches with sharply demarcated border in adult males. Biopsy.

***Erythroplasia of Queyrat (Bowen's disease)*** (p. 546). Red, velvety, sharply bordered plaque on glans. Slow to enlarge. May be present for long periods without extension. Eventually invades. Asymptomatic.

***Nevus*** (p. 523). Ordinarily of pigmented junctional type.

## Raised lesions

***Pearly penile papules.*** Because of frequent anxiety over these normal structures on coronal sulcus, it seems helpful to include a picture (Fig. 1-22).

***Wart (verruca accuminata)*** (p. 319). Soft, pink to gray papillomas form small cauliflower-like growths. Mostly in coronal sulcus.

***Scabies*** (p. 325). Characteristic burrows and pruritic, excoriated papules, 2 to 3 mm., on shaft or glans of penis.

***Herpes simplex*** (p. 295). Prodromal itching or burning is followed by grouped vesicles on erythematous base. Vesicles rupture, leaving denuded, tender red area for 1 to 2 weeks. Recurrent. Shaft or glans.

***Angiokeratoma*** (p. 522). Blue papules of venous dilatations of scrotum in elderly men. Capped by hyperkeratotic epidermis.

***Lichen planus*** (p. 355). Discrete, polyangular, confluent small, flat-topped, reddish papules on shaft or glans. May have annular configuration.

***Syphilis*** (p. 258). Condylomata lata may occur in coronal sulcus as flat moist papules. Serological test for syphilis positive at this stage.

***Bullous eruptions*** (p. 127). Vesicles and bullae of glans on erythematous base. Erythema multiforme, pemphigus, pemphigoid, and drug eruptions may be cause. (See Plate 20, p. 194.)

***Fixed drug eruption*** (p. 199). Red-brown, recurrent or persistent, sharp, round lesion usually on glans. May blister and will hyperpigment.

## Ulcerations and atrophies

***Syphilitic chancre*** (p. 258). Painless, indurated ulcer. Usually present on glans or corona of penis. Always associated with regional inguinal adenopathy. Serological test for syphilis may not be positive in early stages of chancre.

***Balanitis xerotica obliterans (lichen sclerosus et atrophicus)*** (p. 166). Atrophic. Depressed gray-white lesions on glans in adults. May lead to stenosis of urethral orifice.

***Chancroid.*** Tender and painful, red, shallow ragged-edged ulcer on preputial fold, glans, or shaft. May be multiple. Nonindurated.

***Granuloma venereum.*** Painless papules or vesicles that erode to become velvety, granulomatous. Extend to adjacent area. Scars.

***Squamous cell carcinoma*** (p. 541). Chronic, indurated nodule on penile shaft that tends to ulcerate and bleed. At junction of glans and prepuce, moisture produces softened, friable granulomatous-appearing lesion that bleeds easily. Metastasizes early. May follow leukoplakia. Rarely found in males circumcised early. Scrotal carcinoma may be related to occupation and is characterized by noduloulcerative lesion.

# PERIANAL AREA

## Flat lesions

***Pruritus ani*** (p. 443). Lichenification, often mild erythema, hyperpigmentation, mac-

A

B

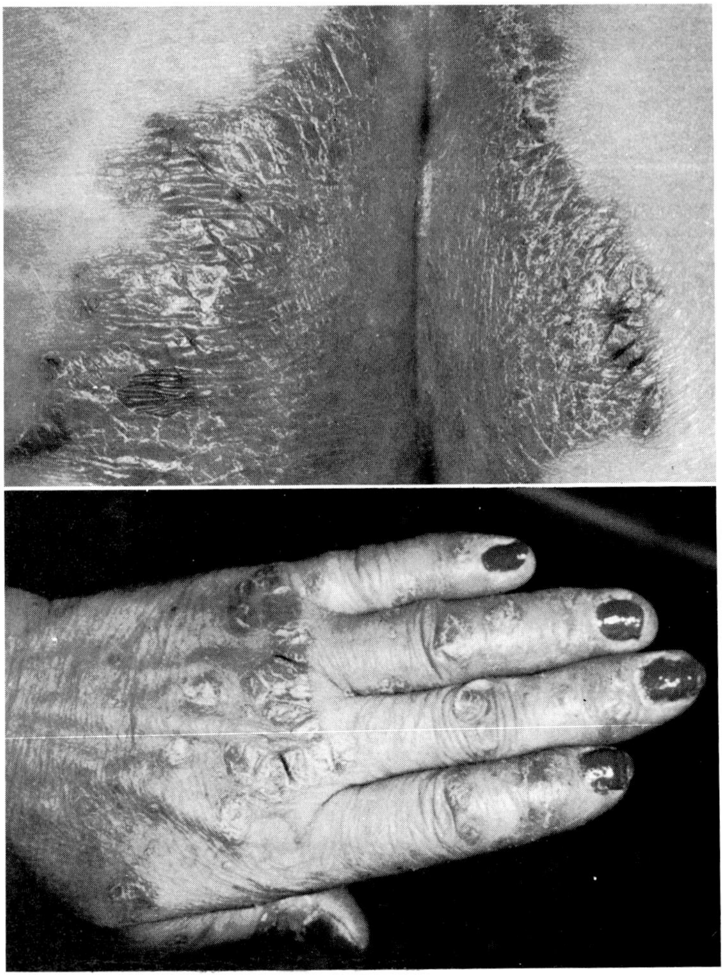

**Fig. 1-23. A,** Psoriasis of gluteal fold. **B**, Psoriasis of hand.

eration, excoriations and perhaps moisture. Produced by variety of underlying diseases.

***Psoriasis*** (p. 462). One of areas most frequently involved by psoriasis. Glistening, erythematous patch with a fissure in depth of gluteal cleft (Fig. 1-23, *A*).

***Seborrheic dermatitis*** (p. 494). Pruritic, scaling, erythematous dermatitis. Also affects pubic area in women, and scrotum and inner thigh in men.

***Primary irritant dermatitis*** (p. 430). Diffuse, pruritic erythema of perianal area. Acute cases moist and weeping. Chronic cases thickened, dry, fissured, hyperpigmented, and lichenified. Caused by excessive use of hot water, soap, disinfectants, and assorted irritants.

***Intertrigo*** (p. 282). Pruritic, macerated, erythematous dermatitis of gluteal walls, perineum, and inguinal folds. Associated with heat, moisture, friction, obesity.

***Candidosis (moniliasis)*** (p. 280). Moist, shiny erythema with flaccid, peripheral, pustular lesions on perineum and gluteal fold walls.

***Allergic eczematous contact dermatitis*** (p. 102). Dry, scaling, erythematous inflammation of perianal area is mildest form. When severe, is moist and intensely pruritic, and extends onto gluteal walls and perineum.

Chronic lesions are dry, thickened, and lichenified with fissures and hyperpigmentation. Causes: anesthetic ointments, suppositories, preservatives in topical medications, and toilet tissues. (See Plate 44, p. 444.)

***Fungal infection*** (p. 270). Localized, scaling, erythematous, pruritic patch. Active vesicular border. May extend to perineum, inguinal folds, inner surface of thighs. Scrapings and identification of fungus are essential.

***Gonorrheal proctitis.*** Acute, painful, irritating anal and perianal process. May be fissures. Painful defecation.

***Chancre, syphilitic*** (p. 258). Ulcerated lesion. Anal chancre often misdiagnosed. Can masquerade as hemorrhoids or fissure in ano. May be in anal canal.

***Anal fissure.*** Sharp pain on defecation. Rarely pruritic.

***Squamous cell carcinoma*** (p. 541). Patch of velvety, erythematous inflammation (Bowen's disease) or an indurated nodule or ulcer on anal margin or mucosa. Prone to metastasize.

***Extramammary Paget's disease*** (p. 549). Pruritic, persistent, spreading, vesicular, erythematous involvement of perianal, perivulvar, or scrotal area, with characteristically well-demarcated advancing border. Association with underlying adenocarcinoma.

***Acanthosis nigricans*** (p. 421). Pigmented, verrucous involvement of perineum.

## Raised lesions

***Condylomata acuminata*** (p. 319). Pale pink, soft papillomas on margin of rectal mucosa. Often in children. May enlarge and coalesce. Single giant type sometimes seen.

***Lichen simplex chronicus*** (p. 448). Lichenified, isolated, very pruritic plaque. Usually unilateral.

***Condylomata, syphilitic*** (p. 261). Flat, moist, broad-based papules. Secondary stage. VDRL test positive.

***Hidradenitis suppurativa*** (p. 97). Deep-seated, purulent nodules and abscesses. Sometimes with sinus tract formation in perianal skin. Gluteal fold, or buttocks.

***Pilonidal cyst.*** Upper portion of gluteal fold. Cyst at site of depression or "dimple." May become infected, with sinus tracts and abscesses.

***Melanoma*** (p. 530). Pigmented or nonpigmented, cutaneous, perianal papule or nodule that enlarges or becomes ulcerated. Rapid growth and spread.

***Lymphogranuloma venereum and granuloma inguinale.*** Papular, verrucous, heaped-up and scarring, inflammatory lesions of perineal, perianal, and genital areas.

## LEGS AND DORSUM OF FEET

### Flat lesions

***Psoriasis*** (Fig. 1-23, *B*) (p. 462). Heavily scaling plaques on knees. Earliest lesions of thighs may resemble folliculitis. Patches and plaques with less scaling may appear on legs, or dorsa of feet, hands, fingers, or toes.

***Hypostatic dermatitis*** (Fig. 1-24) (p. 585). At first, minute petechiae in clusters. Become confluent and spread into distinct erythema with scaling. Finally, diffuse reddening and brown with woody induration. Venous varicosities present.

***Interdigital intertrigo.*** Maceration, erythema, weeping, itching, and burning between toes resembling fungal infection, but caused by heat, sweat, or occlusive footwear. Not uncommon in children.

***Erythrasma*** (p. 250). Macerated or scaling lesions of intertoe webs. Red fluorescence under Wood's light.

***Senile pruritus*** (p. 454). Subjective complaint. Associated with scaling and dry skin. Chiefly in elderly males.

***Ichthyosis*** (Fig. 1-25) (p. 344). One of several congenital disorders producing dryness and plate-like scaling of skin. Most apparent in leg area. May show considerable hyperpigmentation.

***Atopic dermatitis*** (p. 118). In infants and children, an excoriated, erythematous, dry dermatitis, or excoriated, small plaques. In older age group, a pruritic, papular, or lichenified eruption. Toes often pruritic.

***Common bacterial infections*** (Fig. 1-26) (p. 242). *Impetigo:* Verrucous, gray scabs. Yellow honey crusting over erythema. Bullous in children. *Ecthyma:* Sanguinous, adherent crust over ulcer. *Pustular folliculitis:* Pustular

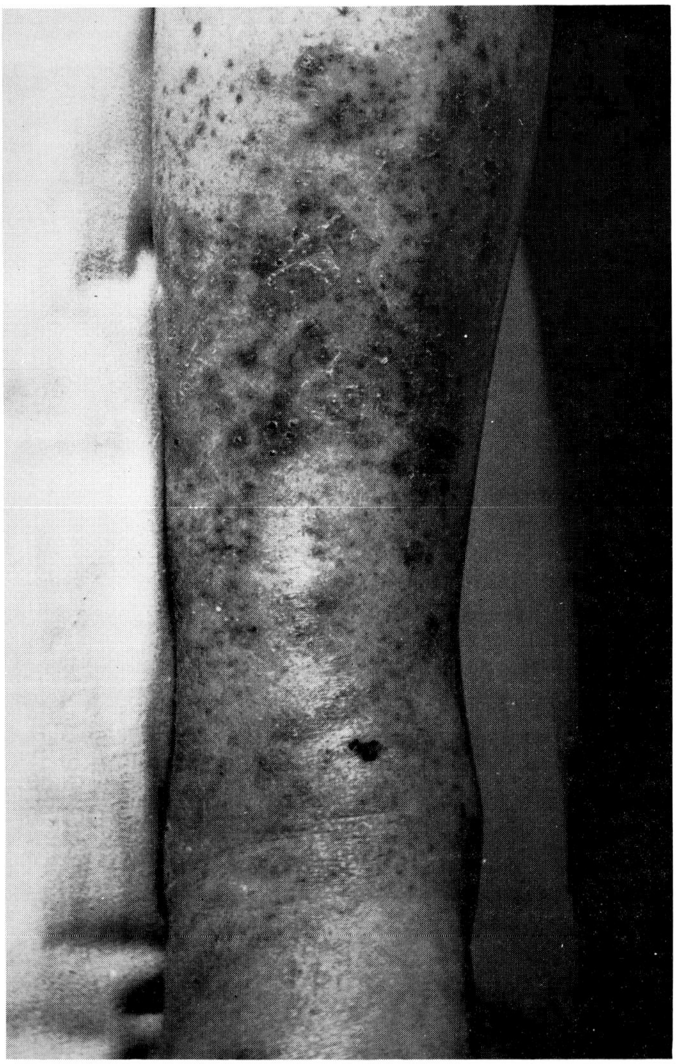

Fig. 1-24. Hypostatic dermatitis.

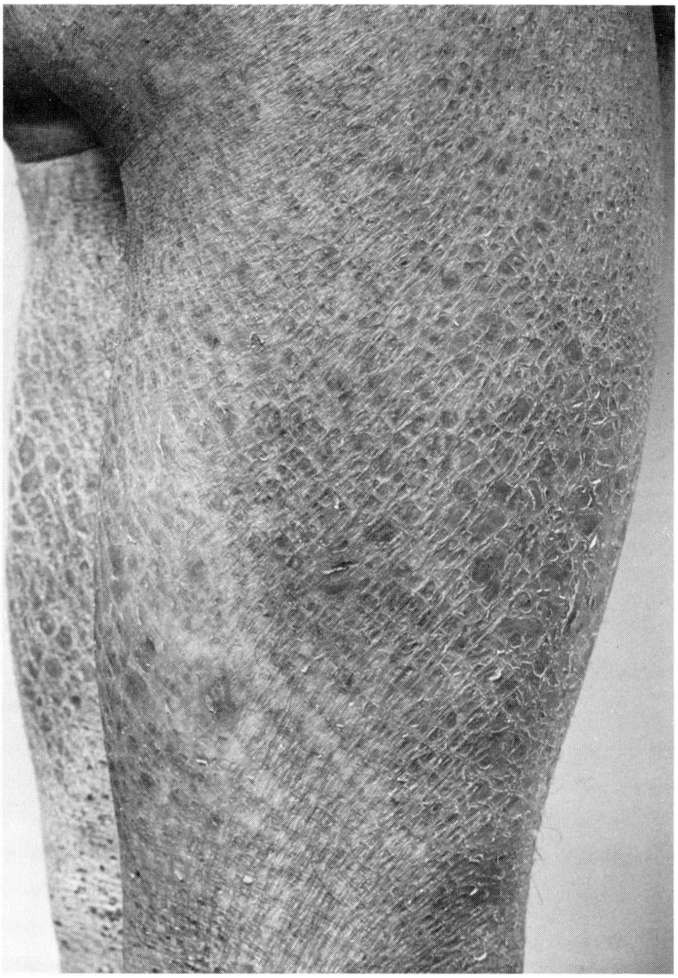

**Fig. 1-25.** Thighs of male with sex-linked recessive ichthyosis.

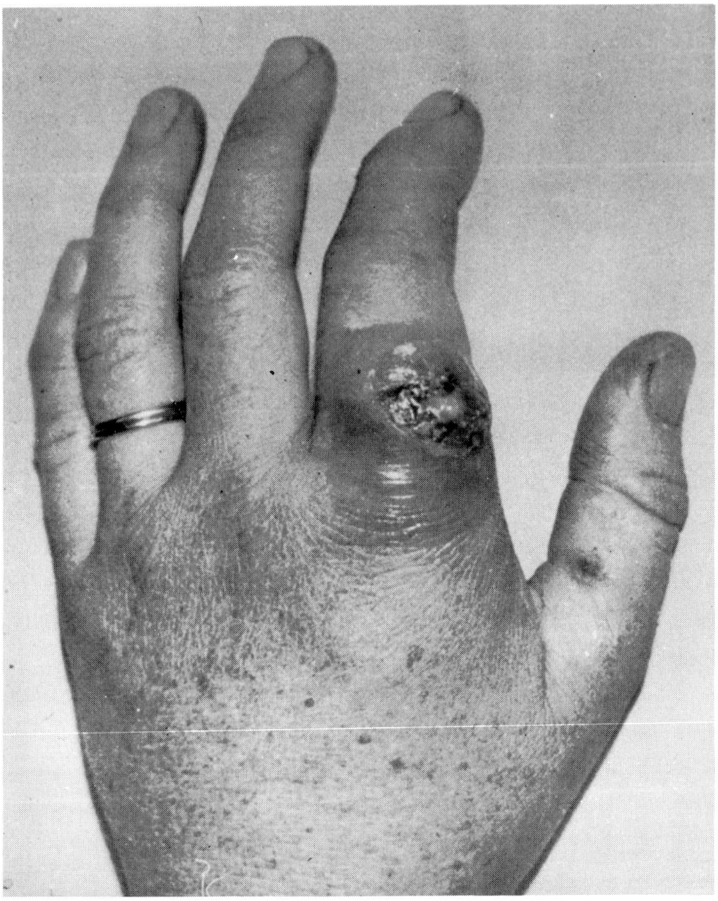

**Fig. 1-26.** Staphylococcal infection of finger. Pyoderma.

lesion, hairy legs. *Erysipelas:* Sharp-bordered, red, indurated edema with systemic signs. Fever. *Pyoderma:* Crusted, indurated, discrete, posttraumatic lesions. May contain *Pseudomonas* and *Proteus.*

***Fungal infection (superficial)*** (p. 270). Pruritic, circular lesions with red, finely scaling center and unobtrusive vesicular border on *legs.* Scrapings. On *feet,* intertoe scaling, fissuring, and maceration can spread to dorsum. Crescentic lesions, active vesicular border. Chronic, hyperkeratotic dermatitis with *sides of feet* affected by thickening, redness, and scaling. May be unilateral.

***Allergic eczematous contact dermatitis*** (p. 102). Ranges from erythema to oozing dermatitis. Causes: *thighs*—sensitizing material (keys, matches) in pockets, elastic in underwear; *inner thighs*—formalin in permanent-press fabrics or clothing dye or finish; *legs*—ingredients in topical medications for hypostatic dermatitis; *popliteals*—rubber boots, stockings, panty hose dyes and finishes; *feet*—leather, metal buckles, chromium, textile dyes (Fig. 1-27).

***Erythema ab igne.*** Reticulated network of red-brown lines around calves, in areas chronically exposed to heat.

***Livedo reticularis*** (p. 574). Purplish, permanent reticulated mottling of thighs, legs, and feet, particularly apparent in cold. May be associated with discomfort and even ulceration. Women.

***Drug eruption*** (p. 183). Carbromal sensi-

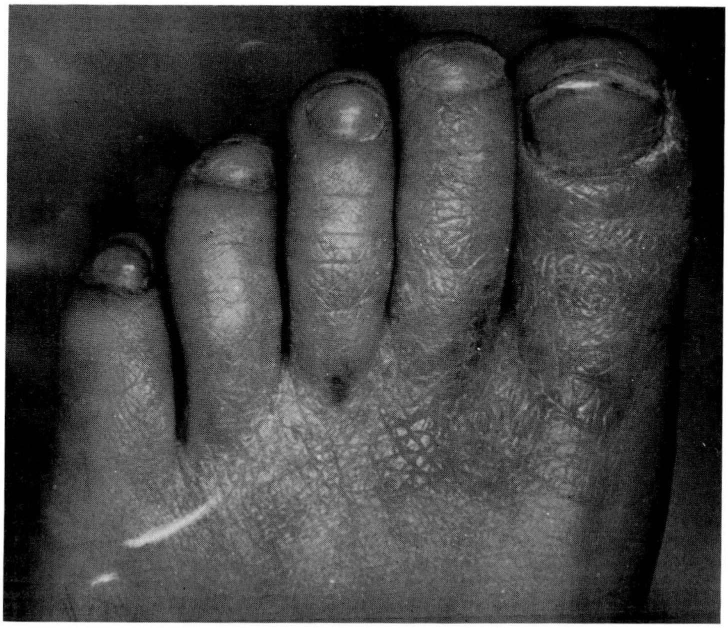

**Fig. 1-27.** Contact dermatitis caused by shoe dye. Erythema, scaling papules, and pruritus over first and second toes and dorsum of foot.

tivity produces specific, purpuric, "cayenne pepper" dermatitis, beginning in ankles and extending proximally. Pruritic.

***Purpura*** (p. 481). Legs may be area first and most affected by many purpuras because of orthostatic element. Hematological, vascular, collagen, infectious, and allergic diseases may be causative.

***Pigmented purpuric dermatosis*** (p. 483). Patches or papules of clusters of petechiae that persist. Extend slowly. May be pruritic. Four types. Capillary vasculitis.

***Hand, foot, and mouth disease*** (p. 322). Transient vesicles with red areolae on dorsum of fingers and toes around nails, palms, and soles, concomitant with a stomatitis.

## Raised lesions

***Clavus (corn)*** (p. 354). Tender, hard, hyperkeratotic lesion in shape of an inverted pyramid. On dorsa of most women's fifth and other phalangeal joints. Also, soft, macerated hyperkeratosis between toes, characteristically fourth interspace. Caused by shoes.

***Granuloma annulare*** (p. 167). One or more skin-colored to reddish papules. Enlarge peripherally to develop depressed center and form ringed lesion. On dorsum of foot.

***Folliculitis*** (p. 244). Discrete, erythematous, follicular papules and pustules on anterior thighs. Oils and greases often the cause. "Hand wiping" at work.

***Dermatofibromas*** (p. 516). Common, discrete, firm, skin-colored to brown, subcutaneous pea-sized nodule. Unchanging in appearance.

***Insect bites*** (p. 332). Discrete, pruritic papules that become urticarial, vesicular, and bullous. Most often around ankles from fleas that jump and bite, then leave. Children.

***Lichen planus*** (Plate 5) (p. 355). Pruritic, discrete, confluent, reddish purple papules below malleoli. May progress on shins to form heaped-up hypertrophic plaques. Papular polyangular lesions elsewhere.

***Keratosis pilaris*** (p. 349). Follicular, conical, hyperkeratotic papules of lateral thighs and arms. Most prominent at puberty and in teens. Hereditary.

***Hyperkeratotic lesions of legs and feet.***

1. *Actinic keratoses.* Conical and inflamed,

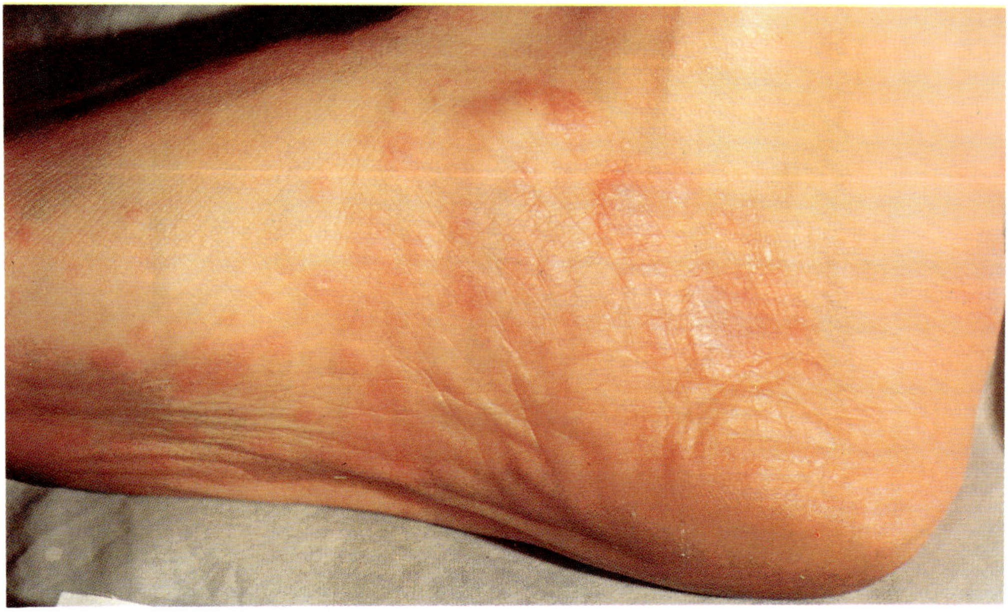

**Plate 5**

Lichen planus. Note polyangular papules.

tender hyperkeratoses in areas of actinic damage. Bleed on removal.

2. *Stucco keratoses.* Uniform white superficial 1 to 3 mm. hyperkeratoses of lower one third of legs, and feet.

3. *Disseminated superficial actinic porokeratosis.* Follicular keratotic papules progress to small annular lesions in sun-exposed areas. Fade in winter.

4. *Arsenical keratoses.* Small hyperkeratotic lesions on legs, feet, palms, and soles.

***Thrombophlebitis.*** Tender, painful, inflamed tumor of leg. Usually unilateral. Associated with dependent edema. Linear, firm cords may be palpable. May be superficial, migrating, or deep.

***Lichen simplex chronicus*** (p. 448). Localized, pruritic lichenified lesions with sharp borders. Ankle, leg, or foot. Unilateral.

***Blue nevus*** (p. 528). Sharply demarcated, blue-black, circular papule or nodule present since birth.

***Cutaneous vasculitis*** (p. 576). Multiple, circumscribed, red papules or nodules, petechiae, ecchymoses, vesicles, bullae, ulcers. Tender and occurring in crops. Hemorrhage is always present. May be extensive.

***Pyoderma gangrenosum.*** Papule or pustule arising with blue-red areola, ulcerates and persists as ragged-edged, shallow erosion or ulcer with cobblestone base. Thighs, legs.

***Erythema nodosum*** (p. 218). Symmetrical, discrete, painful, tender, red nodules on shins. 4 to 6 weeks each.

***Xanthoma tuberosum*** (p. 378). Brown to yellow papules. Enlarge and coalesce to form larger, red-brown to yellow nodules on knees, ankles, and tendons.

***Bullous lesions in unconscious patients*** (p. 145). Dusky plaques, tense vesicles, or large, tense, clear bullae surrounded by a narrow rim of erythema. On pressure areas or traumatized sites. Arise in comatose patients. Most often found on legs.

***Swimming pool granuloma.*** Brown-red papules or plaques, crusted and scaling. Localized area of previous abrasion from swimming pool, or aquarium. Dorsa of feet, knees.

***Glomus tumor*** (p. 522). Minute, blue-red lesion often on nail plate. Intense pain on pressure.

***Gout.*** Very painful, intermittent, red swelling over small joints. White chalky exudate from ulcerating pale papules.

***Malignant melanoma*** (p. 530). Darkly pigmented macule, papule, or ulcer. Rarely nonpigmented, when it can be mistaken for wart or foreign body.

***Larva migrans (creeping eruption)*** (p. 439). Irregularly shaped, weaving, looped line that is red, vesicular, and very pruritic on sole, dorsum, and sides of foot. Found in warm climates.

***Epidermolysis bullosa*** (p. 142). Bullous lesions on friction areas. May first appear in infancy or be delayed until severe trauma later in life produces them.

***Kaposi's hemorrhagic sarcoma.*** Blue-purple papules and nodules of firm consistency emerging through a collarette of epidermal tissue. Legs, feet, ankles (Plate 58, p. 550).

***Keratoacanthoma*** (p. 512). Closely mimics appearance of squamous cell carcinoma. Dome-shaped, rapidly growing lesion with central crater. Legs.

***Squamous cell carcinoma*** (p. 541). Firm, enlarged nodule that develops persistent, depressed ulceration. Does not metastasize rapidly. Progresses by local extension at first.

***Melanoma*** (p. 530). Brown to black macule, papule, nodule, or ulcer. Regional lymphadenopathy may occur early. Legs most common site in women.

***Sporotrichosis*** (p. 289). Erythematous, ulcerating, pustular nodules along course of lymphatic channels.

***North American blastomycosis*** (p. 290). Verrucous nodular lesion that ulcerates, pigments, and scars. Surface demonstrates minute abcesses.

***Coccidioidomycosis*** (p. 289). Erosive, ulcerated, warty, or vegetating granuloma. Often secondarily infect.

***Erythema induratum*** (p. 255). Relatively painless reddish blue nodules that ulcerate. Found chiefly on calves. May be early lesion in sarcoidosis.

***Weber-Christian panniculitis*** (p. 218). Tender nodules and plaques that leave depressed, pigmented lesions. On thighs in adult women.

***Pretibial myxedema*** (p. 175). Large skin-colored plaques and nodules on shins. Prominent follicles. Asymptomatic.

***Cutaneous amyloidosis*** (p. 173). Intensely pruritic, pale waxy to brown, closely set papules on shins in ripple pattern.

***Periarteritis nodosa*** (p. 581). Discrete, painful, tender red nodules.

### Ulcers and atrophies

***Atrophie blanche.*** Tender petechiae on dorsum of foot or lower one third of leg. Progress to white patches and telangiectasia with shallow scars. One third ulcerate with slow healing. Varicose veins associated.

***Hypostatic ulcer*** (p. 585). Punched-out slowly healing ulcer on medial malleolar surface. Relatively painless. Varicose veins, pigmentation, and hypostatic dermatitis also present.

***Leg ulcer (other than hypostatic ulcer)*** (p. 585). Many causes.

***Diabetic dermopathy.*** Localized tan to brown, slightly depressed, asymptomatic lesions on anterior shin bilaterally. Diabetes present.

***Necrobiosis lipoidica (diabeticorum)*** (p. 169). Red-brown-yellow atrophic patches with erythematous halo and telangiectasia (Plate 6, p. 52). In later stages, epidermis becomes translucent. Shins.

## NAILS
### Color changes

***Opacity.*** Nails become dull yellow with invasion by fungal elements.

***Gray-black nail.*** Gray-black, discolored areas with roughened, distorted surface occur with *Candida* infection. Often at lateral or proximal edges of nails.

***Brown nail.*** Potassium permanganate soaks, tobacco, hair dyes, medications (resorcin) and the like, as well as some fungal and yeast nail infections, cause browning of nail.

***Brown or black longitudinal streaks.*** Pigmented mole or melanoma of nail fold affecting matrix. Multiple streaks common with dark skin. Malnutrition also a cause. Addison's disease.

***Blue-green, gray-green nail.*** May result

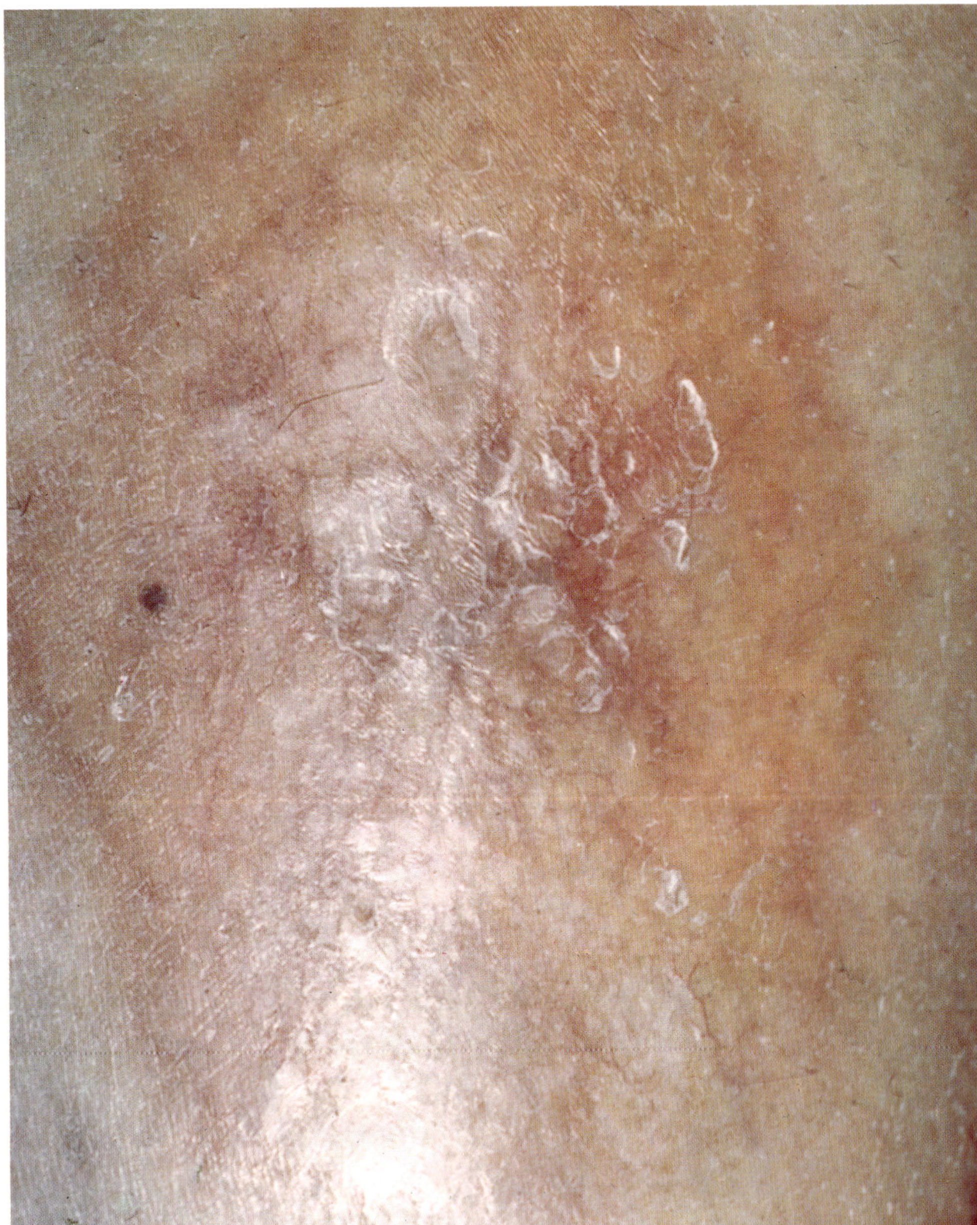

**Plate 6**

Necrobiosis lipoidica. Note telangiectasia and yellow color in this pretibial lesion.

from pyocyanin pigment in *Pseudomonas* infection.

***Orange or yellow nail.*** Some red nail polish will stain nail tissue orange.

***Leukonychia.*** Asymptomatic "white spot" or chalk streak in nail caused by incomplete keratinization. Can occur from trauma.

***White nail.*** Diffuse whiteness occurs in ground glass effect from cirrhosis of liver. Chronic renal disease produces white nails with distal pink zone. Nail bed pallor. Onycholysis.

***Hemorrhages.*** Minute, discrete lesions may indicate subacute bacterial endocarditis or other systemic conditions producing embolic phenomena. Trauma. Also occasionally idiopathic psoriasis, dermatitis, fungus.

***Yellow nail syndrome.*** (p. 403). Acquired discoloration of all nails with thickening and curvature of plate. (See Plate 40, p. 404.)

***Nail bands.*** Single and double white bands, pink bands, blue and red lunulae (p. 405).

***Color change from drugs.*** Atabrine, chloroquine—blue. Phenolphthalein—blue lunulae. Tetracycline—yellow.

***Brittleness.*** Breaking off from free edge of nail can occur from frequent immersion in soapy water, and in iron deficiency. Ichthyosis.

***Splitting or peeling.*** Often a sequel of repetitious exposure to wet work and multiple forms of minor trauma.

## Structural changes

***Destruction.*** Softening, erosion, fragmentation, dystrophy, and crumbling of distal portion of nail or piling up of hyperkeratotic tissue beneath distal half, is not uncommon and may be caused by psoriasis or by fungal infection of nail.

***Transverse ridging*** (p. 405). Chronic, inflammation (for example, atopic dermatitis, primary irritant dermatitis) may cause multiple ridging and distortion of nail when paronychial tissue is affected. Single ridges (Beau's lines) associated with systemic febrile infection, childbirth, trauma, and alopecia. Can be severe enough to shed nails.

***Pitting of nails*** (p. 407). Most often observed with psoriasis, but also with onychomycosis, allergic contact dermatitis, and alopecia areata. Idiopathic.

***Thickened nail.*** From chronic pressure of ill-fitting shoes or other trauma, onycholysis, or vascular stasis or insufficiency.

***Onycholysis*** (p. 405). Partial separation of nail from nail bed. May arise from trauma to ends of fingernails and from too vigorous use of nail file. Sometimes associated with psoriasis, bullous dermatoses, maceration, fungus, and local infection. Also idiopathic.

***Koilonychia (spoon nail)*** (p. 405). Iron-deficiency anemia, exposure to strong cleansers and alkalis, and hereditary factors cause thin concave nail.

***Clubbing (hippocratic nail)*** (p. 405). Broad convex nail that occurs on all fingers and toes. May be inherited, congenital, or associated with chronic pulmonary disease, carcinoma of lung, and congenital heart disease, or other systemic disease. Also, may have no identifiable cause in healthy individuals.

***Thinning or longitudinal ridging.*** Occurs normally with age, lichen planus, anemias, ischemia (Raynaud's disease), tumor, cyst of nail-fold area, median canal dystrophy.

***Shedding.*** Periodic shedding disorder, posttraumatic, onycholysis, severe illness. With residual scarring: lichen planus, bullous eruptions, congenital ectodermal defect, trauma, radiation, pterygium, ischemia.

## Adjacent tissue changes

***Ingrown nail*** (p. 405). Result of pressure from ill-fitting shoe, improper cutting of toenail, or, sometimes, exaggerated lateral curvature of nail. Free distal corner of nail cuts into skin that obstructs its growth.

***Inflammation of nail fold.*** With red, tender, edematous tissue, and purulent discharge; *acute paronychia* may be bacterial in origin. *Chronic paronychia* usually is result of excessive or prolonged exposure to water.

***Pterygium.*** Congenital ectodermal defect, impaired circulation, lichen planus. Idiopathic.

## Raised lesions

***Subungual exostosis*** (p. 520). Hard, bony tumor of toenail bed that forces nail upward.

Usually no pain or tenderness involved.

***Malignant melanoma*** (p. 530). Most notable form is pigmented tumor or "whitlow." Causes swelling of distal phalanx under nail, with pain and tenderness.

***Glomus tumor*** (p. 522). Red, punctate discoloration of nail bed that may demonstrate lancinating, spontaneous pain, or pain on pressure.

## GENERALIZED ERUPTIONS

### Flat lesions

***Psoriasis*** (p. 462). Deep red, sharply bordered, irregular symmetrical macules and plaques with thick scale. However, problems in diagnosis arise when skin is universally involved, scaling, and red.

***Seborrheic dermatitis*** (p. 494). Erythematous, pruritic dermatitis of scalp, central face, midsternal area, navel, and perianal region, with fine, yellow, greasy scale. When generalized, can be acute, pruritic, chronic, or asymptomatic. In infants, generalization can occur rapidly. Often infected.

***Pityriasis rosea*** (p. 426). Initial herald patch followed by generalized outbreak of discrete, light red, parallel oval lesions with very fine scale (Plate 7). May become universal.

***Atopic dermatitis*** (p. 118). Erythematous and lichenified lesions appear first in flexures. When generalized, all areas are pruritic, dry, thickened, and scaling. Areas may be reddened but not intensely so. Excoriated.

***Drug eruption*** (p. 183). May take variety of forms. Most frequent are maculopapular and morbilliform types. Patients with infectious mononucleosis are particularly prone to develop these eruptions when taking ampicillin.

***Erythema multiforme*** (p. 212). Circular wheal-like lesions. Many with depressed darker center of typical "target" appearance are usually present somewhere. Begins distally. Spreads centripetally. May become bullous.

***Exfoliative dermatitis*** (p. 222). Generalized erythema and extreme scaling. Nails and hair may be shed. Characteristic chilling sensation

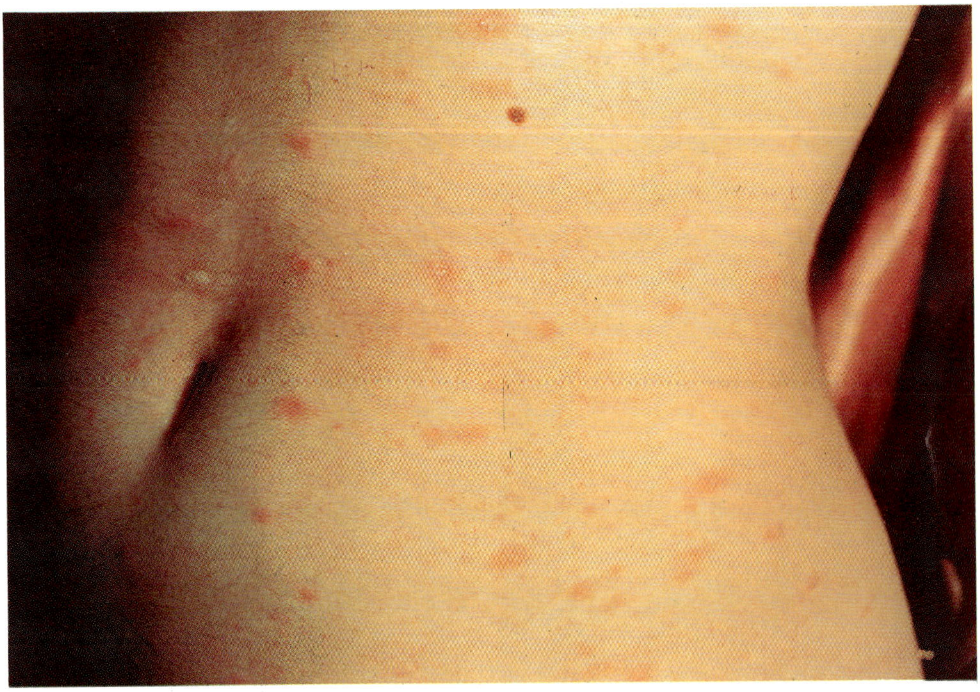

**Plate 7**

Pityriasis rosea. Oval, parallel, light pink lesions with fine scale.

associated. Generalized lymphadenopathy almost always present.

***Syphilis (secondary)*** (p. 261). Oval, discrete macules or papules. Palms, soles, and mucous membranes involved. Malaise, myalgia, and low-grade fever with generalized lymphadenopathy. Serological test for syphilis positive.

***Rubella, rubeola, and roseola infantum*** (p. 314). Spreading outward, erythematous, discrete macular lesions, associated with fever. Usually occur in children.

***Viral exanthems*** (p. 322). Measles-like eruptions resulting from infection by coxsackievirus, echovirus, and other enteroviruses.

***Infectious mononucleosis.*** Morbilliform eruptions in some cases. Some urticarial reactions. Serological test for syphilis may be positive in a small percent.

***Scarlet fever.*** Diffuse, erythematous, confluent, blanching dermatitis with circumoral pallor and desquamation. One day to 1 week after fever and streptococcal sore throat.

***Meningococcemia.*** Rapidly spreading, red, macular lesions becoming quickly purpuric. Individual lesions enlarge peripherally. Found in seriously ill patient, often a child. Signs of meningeal irritation.

***Mucocutaneous lymph node syndrome.*** Children. Acute process with cervical adenopathy. Edema of hands and feet, followed by exanthem, spreading from fingertips proximally.

***Rickettsial eruptions.*** Chiefly thoracic, erythematous, macular lesions becoming purpuric and associated with fever. *Epidemic* or *endemic typhus* and *Rocky Mountain spotted fever*. *Rickettsialpox* becomes generalized and vesicular following an individual discrete lesion occurring at site of mite bite.

***Pityriasis rubra pilaris*** (p. 351). Universal fine scale on an erythematous base, with follicular prominences on dorsum of hands and fingers. Islands of normal skin.

***Histiocytosis X*** (p. 384). Crusting, erythematous, and petechial lesions. Resemble very severe seborrheic dermatitis, often with similar scaling. On thorax, face, scalp, and buttocks. Xanthomatous lesions may be present. Found in early childhood.

***Toxic epidermal necrolysis*** (p. 144). Diffuse erythema with advancing firm border, becoming generalized. Epidermis softens, slips, and detaches in large sheets. Flaccid fluid-filled bullae may form. Patient febrile and toxic. Found in children and adults.

***Urticaria pigmentosa*** (p. 562). Tan to brown pigmented lesions. Generalized, may become universal with skin thickening, redness, and episodes of flushing. *Adult form:* telangiectactic, pigmented patches everywhere but palms, soles, and mucous membranes. Erythema may be present.

## Pigmented lesions

***Addison's disease*** (p. 419). Diffuse pigmentation, accentuated in exposed areas. Flexures, creases, and buccal mucous membrane have localized pigmentation.

***Hyperthyroidism.*** Diffuse pigmentation. May have accentuation of exposed areas, particularly eyelids.

***Lymphomas*** (p. 554). Hodgkin's disease, particularly, produces dusky, generalized pigmentation with areas of more intense color. Notable in zones of pruritus. Possibly secondary to rubbing and scratching.

***Scleroderma*** (p. 158). Generalized tan pigmentation sometimes seen in areas otherwise uninvolved with the disease. Sclerodermatous areas also show hypopigmentation.

***Uremia.*** Advanced renal failure is often associated with yellow-brown, diffuse pigmentation. Most noticeable on exposed areas. Chiefly in long-standing renal failure.

***Hemochromatosis*** (p. 420). Bronze pigmentation. Accentuated on exposed skin. Definitely generalized. Almost universally present in this disorder.

***Ichthyosis*** (p. 344). Fine or coarse, dry scales with tendency to tan pigmentation, some pruritus. Has distribution pattern dependent on type of genetic inheritance. Some forms deeply pigmented.

***Malabsorption syndrome.*** Associated with irregular mild pigmentation in patches. Frequently occurring after erythematous scaling, nonspecific dermatitis. May be generalized and diffuse. Variable association with pruritus, ichthyosis, and follicular hyperkeratosis.

***Arsenical pigmentation.*** Diffuse, dusky involvement of trunk and less noticeable on extremities, with paler "raindrops on a dusty road" appearance. May result from prolonged arsenic ingestion.

***Poikiloderma atrophicans vasculare.*** Hyperpigmentation, hypopigmentation, and telangiectasia with atrophic epidermis. Symmetrical patchy local or general, universal and permanent.

## Raised lesions

***Scabies*** (p. 325). Punctate lesions, linear burrows, and excoriated papules. Extreme pruritus involves entire cutaneous surface.

***Urticaria*** (p. 113). Migratory and pruritic wheals may involve entire skin surface with irregular and changing lesions. All are transient.

***Generalized vesicular eruptions*** (p. 303). Varicella, variola, disseminated herpes zoster, vaccinia, and Kaposi's varicelliform eruption are infections that produce generalized vesicular eruptions.

***Dermatitis herpetiformis*** (p. 140). Chronic, intensely pruritic dermatitis of grouped vesicles, macules, papules, and occasionally bullae. Lesions heal with hyperpigmentation. Excoriations prominent early.

***Lichen planus*** (p. 355). Distinctively flat-topped, pruritic, red-violet, angular papules usually present on wrists, although remainder of skin involvement may be simply erythematous. Lacy, gray mouth lesions.

***Parapsoriasis.*** *Acute* form consists of vesicles and small necrotic papules. Self-limited. Found in young adults. *Chronic* form consists of larger, multiple, discrete, slightly elevated asymptomatic lesions with scaling surfaces.

***Neurofibromatosis*** (p. 521). Large, scattered café-au-lait spots with multiple, flaccid, pedunculated, and sessile tumors.

***Pemphigus*** (p. 133). May be characterized by generalized bulla formation, or erosive lesions that develop vegetations. Buccal mucosa membrane involved early.

***Bullous pemphigoid*** (p. 137). Shows large, tense, clear bullae with predilection for groins, thighs, and flexures of elderly. Chronic. Mucous membranes not involved.

***Bullous erythema multiforme*** (p. 212). Bullae develop in centre of target lesions in severe cases. Many follow herpes simplex.

***Mycosis fungoides*** (p. 555). Has three distinct stages: eczematous, plaque, and tumor. Evolves over prolonged period, often many years.

PART TWO

# Clinical dermatology

CHAPTER 2

# Dermatological therapeutics and techniques

## Dermatological therapeutics

### TOPICAL THERAPY

#### Wet dressings

Wet dressings are used in acute, oozing dermatoses. Their action is drying, anti-inflammatory, and antipruritic. These compresses should be applied with soft cloths, such as freshly laundered handkerchiefs, diapers, sheeting, or pillowcase material—preferably not gauze squares, which are hard to handle and deteriorate quickly. Sterility is not essential, but cleanliness is.

A dressing should be thoroughly soaked with the solution and applied directly to the lesions. It is left on for 10- to 15-minute periods and allowed to air dry. No rubbing or blotting with towels. Usually, additional compresses are applied at 2- to 3-hour intervals. *They are kept at room temperature.* Types of dressings include the following:

1. Cool tap water.
2. Physiological saline solution, 2 teaspoonfuls of salt per quart of water.
3. Aluminum acetate solution, or Burow's solution. This is probably the most widely prescribed compress in current dermatological therapy. It has a mild antibacterial and drying action. The most practical method is the use of prepared powders or tablets, such as Domeboro or Buro-Sol, 1 packet of powder or 1 tablet to a pint of cool tap water.
4. Potassium permanganate compresses. One 5-grain tablet to 3 quarts of water makes a 1:10,000 solution, suitable for compresses. *This is a staining solution* and leaves its traces on skin, clothes, and containers, including bathtubs. It is antifungal and mildly antibacterial.

#### Balneotherapy

For widely disseminated lesions, baths are sometimes the most practical method of therapy. They serve the same function as wet compresses, that is, providing cooling, antipruritic, antiflammatory, and cleansing actions. The tub should be close to half full, which requires an average of 20 gallons of water. The water should be tepid and not allowed to cool excessively. The duration usually is short—10 to 15 minutes. Drying is by blotting with a soft towel in a warm room so that no great temperature fluctuations are encountered. Light, loose clothing should be worn after the bath, or the patient should go directly to bed.

***Colloid baths.*** An oatmeal bath consists of 1 cupful of Aveeno or plain oatmeal in a cloth bag placed in tub water or used directly on the skin. The effect is both antipruritic and drying. Aveeno Oilated is antipruritic, nondrying, and somewhat lubricating.

A cornstarch bath consists of 2 cupfuls of Linit starch or plain edible starch to a quart of water, to make a paste; then the mixture is added to bath water. This agent is antipruritic and quite drying.

***Tar baths.*** Commercial tar bath solutions (1 to 2 teaspoonfuls) added to the bath water, liquor carbonis detergens (1 oz.), or other similar tar bath preparations are antipruritic and nondrying. These preparations are employed for chronic pruritic dermatoses. No soap should be added.

***Bath oils.*** For pruritic and dry skin diseases a commercially available bath oil may be added to the bath with benefit. These are formulated to have a rapid dispersant action in water, resulting in a homogeneous distribution in the bath. Its effect rarely lasts more than a few hours. A similar effect can be obtained if a lubricating agent, such as Dermabase, is applied to the moist skin after the bath.

Alpha-Keri, an oil-soluble lanolin fraction in a form of mineral oil, seems to provide good lubricating effect. Also available are Aveeno Oilated, Domol, Lubath, Jeri-bath, and other preparations. A similar effect can be obtained if a lubricating agent is applied to the moist skin after the bath.

## Lotions

Lotions are liquid vehicles for carrying medications. They may be *lubricating*, *cooling*, *antipruritic*, or *drying*, and they require frequent application. Ordinarily they are not washed off between applications. For enhanced antipruritic effect, 0.5% menthol and 0.25% phenol may be added to these lotions.

1. Calamine lotion, U.S.P., B.P., drying
2. Alcoholic shake lotion

| | |
|---|---|
| Zinc oxide | 15 mg. |
| Talc | 15 mg. |
| Glycerin | 10 ml. |
| Isopropyl alcohol | 40 ml. |
| Water | 40 ml. |

Skin coloring may be added. The lotion is best applied with a paintbrush, although fingers are satisfactory. The effect is drying.

3. Emollient lotion

| | |
|---|---|
| Dermabase | 2 oz. |
| Water | q.s. ad 8 oz. |

Bland, lubricating lotion

4. Antiperspirant lotion

| | |
|---|---|
| Aluminum chlorhydroxide complex | 15% |
| Glycerin | 5% |
| Alcohol | 40% |
| Water | q.s. ad 100 mg. |

5. Glutaraldehyde lotion

| | |
|---|---|
| Glutaraldehyde | 3% to 10% |
| Water | q.s. ad 100 mg. |

Drying, antiperspirant, antifungal. (Above 5% may cause browning of skin.)

***Amounts required.*** Schlagel determined through a series of careful experiments that lotions and ointments are used in equivalent weights on application. Twelve to 26 Gm. were used to cover the entire skin surface of an average-sized male when applied sparingly under controlled conditions. When uncontrolled or "ad lib" instructions were issued, the variation ranged from 7 to 115 Gm.

The amounts required by trained operators to cover specific areas with a thin layer are as follows:

| | |
|---|---|
| Head, excluding hair | 1.2 Gm. |
| Trunk | 5 Gm. |
| One arm | 2 Gm. |
| One leg | 4 Gm. |
| Anogenital area | 1.5 Gm. |

## Ointments and creams

Ointments are used for *lubrication*, as vehicles for active medications, and for *protection*. Arbitrarily, ointments generally are greasy or oily bases, whereas creams are lighter, are usually water-washable substances, and will rub into the skin without leaving an easily demonstrable film.

*White* or *yellow petrolatum*, *hydrophilic petrolatum*, U.S.P., and *anhydrous lanolin* are bland and protective, if somewhat occlusive. They are not to be used in areas where heat dissipation is advisable. *Mineral oil* is a liquid form of a similar nature and can be heavy or light.

*Lanolin*, *Eucerin*, and *Qualatum* are so-called water-in-oil bases that are lighter and less occlusive than petrolatum, but are not easily water washable.

*Hydrophilic ointment*, paradoxically named, is a water-washable cream. *Unibase*, *Emulsion base*, and *Dermabase* are similar bases and are easily applied, light creams. *Glaxal base* is well accepted by patients.

## Gels

Gels are a form of ointment with propylene glycol and carboxypolymethylene that are clear and nongreasy on application, despite a viscous appearance. They are thixotropic, becoming thinner with rubbing or movement. Some sting on application. They may be used on hairy areas, a usage that is a distinct advantage.

## Pastes

Pastes are stiff vehicles made up of powder in ointments. They are *porous* and *less occlu-*

*sive* than ointments and can be used as *protectives*, even on weeping surfaces. Pastes are often hard to remove. They are applied most easily with tongue depressors to "butter" them on.

| | | |
|---|---|---|
| 1. | Zinc oxide | 25% |
| | Starch | 25% |
| | White petrolatum | q.s. ad 100 mg. |
| | Protective. | |

## Powders

Generally used in moist locations, between toes, and in intertriginous areas, powders are *absorbent* and may have antifungal and antibacterial agents added. They should be dispensed with a shaker top.

1. Unscented talc, drying
2. Zinc oxide, drying
3. Cicatrin powder (neomycin-bacitracin) (Calmic) antibacterial
4. Zeasorb powder, antiseptic, absorbent
5. Nystatin (Mycostatin) dusting powder, anticandidal
6. Menthol 2%
   Phenol 1%
   Talc q.s. ad 100 mg.
   Antipruritic.
7. Tolnaftate powder, antifungal

## Occlusive dressings

Thin, transparent, pliable plastic films used as occlusive dressings produce an intensification of the effect of topically applied medications. By producing moisture retention, nonevaporation of the vehicle, and maceration of the epidermis, an increased penetration of certain medications result. Glucocorticoids for inflammatory disorders, salicyclic acid for calluses, and cantharidin and salicyclic acid for warts are all made more useful by their application under occlusive dressings. Dangers of this addition to topical therapy include bacterial and candidal infection, sweat retention, folliculitis, and increased incidence of side effects of the medication used.

## Shampoos

Liquid soaps are more satisfactory for cleansing hair, since they impart more gloss than soaps in bar form.

*Selenium sulfide suspension* is an effective antiseborrheic shampoo, but it produces scalp oiliness in many individuals. It does eliminate dry scaling and dandruff.

*Betadine shampoo* is a good antibacterial cleanser, especially for patients with scalp folliculitis.

*Zinc pyrithione* in a concentration of 2% has recently been introduced and has been found to be an effective antiseborrheic agent when incorporated in shampoos or hair dressings.

*Tincture of green soap* shampoo, an alcoholic solution of soft soap, is quite drying and is a good cleanser. Liquor carbonis detergens, 5%, may be added to make a *tar shampoo* of satisfactory quality for scaling scalp conditions.

*Triethanolamine sulfate*, 40% in water, makes a bland shampoo to which medications can be added.

*Coconut oil shampoo* is a nondetergent vegetable oil shampoo that provides good cleansing action.

## Soaps

As a rule of thumb, the common soaps are the least likely to cause irritation. Some strongly perfumed soaps, as have been popular recently, do seem to produce untoward irritation. Despite patient doubts, however, it is unusual for soap to cause skin problems, other than a very mild and transient tight feeling. The value of soaps vastly outweighs any problems they may have been responsible for.

Soaps to which bacteriostatic agents are added may be satisfactory in reducing the bacterial flora of the cutaneous surface. Soaps containing hexachlorophene, such as pHisoHex, are of this type. These may be helpful in a family with staphylococcal or other cutaneous bacterial disease. However, hexachlorophene has been limited to prescription use and is banned for use on infants in Canada, since evidence was obtained of possible neurological effects from daily application on infants. Povidone-iodine or chlorhexidene cleansers are useful substitutes when hexachlorophene is contraindicated.

*Emulsifying ointment B.P.* provides a very satisfactory soap substitute for individuals with dry, sensitive skin.

## Sunscreening agents

Certain chemicals applied to the skin have the capacity to absorb specific wavelengths of light from the sun and thus protect the cutaneous surface. This ability has especial value in cases of *photosensitive dermatoses, chloasma, vitiligo, actinic skin, polymorphous light eruptions, porphyria,* and so forth, in which light plays an important causative part in the dermatosis.

There are also certain opaque chemicals that act to block light by virtue of their opacity. They are often the most efficient but are less acceptable cosmetically than the light absorbers, since they can be easily seen.

So-called suntanning agents, which are proclaimed to retard burning and enhance tanning, probably do retard some burning, but probably also retard tanning. Mineral oil, creams, and ointments do not offer protection against sunburn.

Sunscreening agents are applied to light-exposed areas and are effective for perhaps 3 to 4 hours, depending on the thickness of the material applied, the amount of rubbing, perspiration, or water immersion. Wet skin burns and also tans much more quickly than dry skin does.

### Opaque agents

1. Titanium dioxide 5% to 7%
   Hydrophilic ointment q.s.
2. Doak Solar Cream; A-Fil ointment.
3. Covermark, an opaque covering makeup blended to the skin color that can be obtained in a waterproof form.
4. Dihydroxyacetone, a clear liquid that colors the skin, blocks long wavelengths only partially, and must be used daily (does not protect against sunburn).

### Light-absorbing agents

#### *Sunburn range*

1. Para-aminobenzoic acid 5%
   Alcohol q.s.
   Absorbs light in the sunburn region from 250 to 310 nm. (Presun, Pabanol, PABA gel).
   Many esters of PABA have been incorporated into other products (Eclipse, Pabafilm).
2. Neo A-Fil ointment, with digalloyl trioleate being the light absorber, again in the sunburn range.

#### *Sunburn and longer range*

3. Benzophenone derivatives, sulisobenzone (Uval, Solbar, and others) and oxybenzone, in mineral oil or in water-washable bases, which screen light in a wider range than the first two agents listed; may be irritating on application to sensitive skin.
4. Red Vet Pet (RVP), a petrolatum that is rather greasy, but screens light in the longer wavelengths; more suitable for patients with porphyria who have trouble from this part of the light spectrum; in addition, RVPaque incorporates an opaque component, zinc oxide. RVPlus also contains titanium.
5. Dihydroacetone 3%
   Naphthoquinone 0.25%
   Alcohol-water vehicle
   Applied nightly, will provide long and some shorter wave ultraviolet-light protection. Stains skin.
6. MacLeod and Frain-Bell long- and short-wave protective cream:

| | |
|---|---|
| Titanium dioxide | 20% |
| Zinc oxide | 6% |
| Kaolin | 2% |
| Red ferric oxide | 1% |
| Mexenone (Uvistat) | 4% |
| Cream to | 100% |

   Apply prior to sun exposure.

#### *Systemic (oral)*

7. Betacarotene (Solatene) is now available for general use in the United States, although still restricted in Canada. It is effective in blocking the effects of long wave ultraviolet light in individuals with a serum level of 600 mg./ml. or an adequate deposition in the skin. It is essentially nontoxic although it stains the skin orange. It is not effective against shorter wave sunburn-range ultraviolet light. Dose: 30 mg. capsules, t.i.d.

## Topical antibacterial agents

### Antiseptics

It is difficult to assess the efficacy of topical antibacterial agents except by their clinical effectiveness. Their chief uses are the following:

1. To treat carriers of pathogenic microorganisms (for example, nose, scalp, anogenital or flexural areas)
2. To reduce the skin overall bacterial count in a patient with recurrent clinical infections (for example, atopics)
3. To reduce skin bacterial count in a patient at risk of developing an infection (such as in surgery, immunosuppression, and diabetes)

Some potent antibacterial agents are too irritating to be used. Effective topical antiseptic agents that are not harmful to infected or abraded skin include the following:

1. Chlorhexidine (Hibitane), available as solution or cleanser
2. Povidone-iodine (Betadine), available as spray, solution, shampoo, or cleanser
3. Hexachlorophene, available as solution, powder, or cleanser *(not to be used on infants or children)*
4. Alcohol 70%, for temporary effect only, but has increased antiseptic effect when used in addition to the above

## Antibiotics

Not all antibiotics should be used as topical agents. Pencicillin and sulfa drugs are too sensitizing for this purpose. Once an allergy is produced by a medication, that medication can no longer be used systemically. Some do not produce sensitization often. Erythromycin has a very low incidence of sensitization topically.

The following topical antibiotic agents are particularly useful in recurrent cutaneous infections caused by gram-negative organisms and staphylococci. If there is culture evidence of a nasal carrier state, it is wise to use these agents inside the nostrils three times daily to eliminate any possible infection harbored there. Persistent nasal crusting is a clue to the existence of such an infection. It is important to note here that normal dryness of the skin surface provides an unfriendly environment for bacteria, whereas moisture and maceration encourage their growth. Production of dryness in an infected area may be more useful in antibacterial effect than the use of a topical antibiotic. Other carrier areas are the hairy scalp and the perineum.

***Neomycin.*** Neomycin is used in 0.5% to 1% concentration, but it must be formulated with care because some vehicles are incompatible with its use. It is active against both gram-positive and gram-negative organisms. Reports indicate that most cases of sensitivity are caused by its use in an ointment base. Cross sensitivity may be present to streptomycin and kanamycin.

***Bacitracin.*** Bacitracin is active against gram-positive bacteria and rarely produces sensitivity.

***Polymyxin B.*** Polymyxin B is active against gram-negative bacteria, including *Pseudomonas*.

***Chloramphenicol.*** Because chloramphenicol is now rarely used systemically, it is more justifiable to use it topically. It rarely produces sensitivity and is used in cream or lotion in 1% to 3% concentration.

***Silver sulfadiazine (Silvadene).*** This is now generally used in prophylactic application to prevent and to treat infections in burn patients. It is not so widely used in chronic or chronic, recurrent infections in dermatologic patients to our knowledge.

***Gentamicin.*** Available in cream or ointment form, gentamicin is effective against gram-negative and gram-positive bacteria and *Proteus* species.

As a result of the topical use of gentamicin, resistant strains are being reported in various parts of the world. It remains as one of our most important systemic antimicrobial agents against serious infections. *Gentamicin should be used topically only in restricted circumstances, such as the prophylaxis of burn cases, where it may be as important to the patient as in systemic infection. Its widespread use is resulting now in more and more resistant* Pseudomonas *and* Proteus *strains.*

### REFERENCES


Anderson, V.: Over the counter topical antibiotic products. Data on safety and efficacy, Int. J. Dermatol. **15**(suppl. 2):3, 1976.

**An in-depth review of all available information.**

Fusaro, R. M., and Johnson, T. A.: Protection against long-wave ultraviolet light with topical dihydroxyacetone, Dermatologica **159**:346, 1975.

**0.25% lawsone added to 3% DHA in alcohol-water vehicle gives immediate protection over a wide spectrum of UVL.**

Keys, T. F., and Washington, J. A.: Gentamycin resistant *Pseudomonas aeruginosa*. Mayo Clinic experience. Mayo Clinic Proc. **52**:797, 1977.

**Of growing importance in larger medical centres.**

Macleod, T. M., and Frain-Bell, W.: A study of chemical light screening agents, Br. J. Dermatol. **92**:417, 1975.

**A confirmation of the effectiveness of 5% PABA plus ester against sunburn.**

Mathews-Roth, M. M., Pathak, M. A., Fitzpatrick, T. B., et al.: Beta-carotene therapy for erythropoietic protoporphyria and other photosensitivity diseases, Arch. Dermatol. **113**:1229, 1977.
**A significant benefit to selected groups of patients. One third of polymorphous light eruptions were helped.**

Schlagel, C. A., and Sanborn, E. C.: The weights of topical preparations required for total and partial body inunction, J. Invest. Dermatol. **42**:253, 1964.
**A significant difference in amounts used between "ad lib" use and trained applicators.**

## GLUCOCORTICOID AGENTS

### Topical therapy

Topical glucocorticoids are by far the most widely used therapeutic agents in dermatology today. Their chief effect is a profound local anti-inflammatory action. The anti-inflammatory effect is palliative, and the medication must be repeated until the disease undergoes a remission or until the causative agent has been eliminated. Under such circumstances these medications approach the ideal therapeutic agent for the following reasons:

1. They are applied directly to the area requiring their effect. Other tissues are affected minimally, if at all.
2. They have minor side effects when used in proper concentrations and circumstances.
3. A profound anti-inflammatory effect is exerted locally by a small concentration of medication.
4. They can be applied for prolonged intervals with continuing effectiveness.
5. Effective concentrations can be attained at essentially low cost.
6. They are essentially free of sensitizing properties.

### Cellular effects

After skin penetration, the glucocorticoid probably loses its highly branched side chain that helped it pass the lipid protein barrier, and is absorbed into the target cell. Here, after combining in the nucleus with receptor proteins, it binds with the chromatin of the regulatory gene and the cell's activities undergo a change. It now produces proteins that restore, rebuild, modulate, or carry on other anti-inflammatory activities, depending on the type of cell affected. It also stabilizes lysosomal membranes so that damaging enzymes cease to be released. Prostaglandin inflammatory activity is reduced, and there may be salutory effects on cAMP as well. The inflammation-producing activities of committed lymphocytes are curbed by steroids, which will destroy lymphocytes in high enough concentrations (Voorhees).

Cortisone is not effective topically. Hydrocortisone is effective topically at 1% concentration. The original hydrocortisone molecule has had innumerable effective chemical substitutions with as many molecules and side chains in the past 20 years. The areas of alteration of the molecule are diagrammed in Fig. 2-1, and the resulting available steroids for topical use are presented in Fig. 2-2. These alterations, most of which involve a fluorine group, produce an incredible increase in potency and effectiveness. This is achieved either by increasing the intrinsic activity of the compound at its site of action, by increasing the compound's ability to penetrate the skin, or by making a compound that takes longer to metabolize to its inactive components so that it has a longer duration of action.

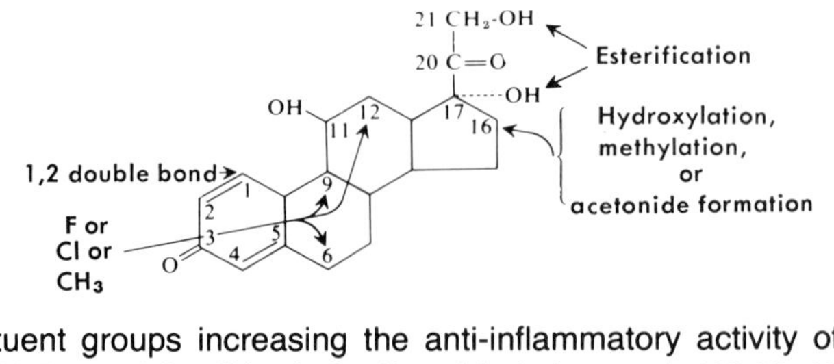


**Fig. 2-1.** Substituent groups increasing the anti-inflammatory activity of hydrocortisone. (From Stewart, W. D., and Runikis, J. O.: Can. Med. Assoc. J. **108**:33, 1973.)

The substitutions, however, also produce the side effects listed on p. 204. Whether this is related to the fluorine group is not yet known. It seems to be related to potency rather than specifically to fluorination.

***Vehicles.*** Topical glucocorticoids are now available in sprays, lotions, creams, ointments, gels (a modification of ointments), suspensions, powders, and possibly other forms as well. Stoughton has presented evidence that the newer gel formulations give greater steroid effect. However, the sophistication and complexity of modern vehicles require individualization of vehicles for individual glucocorticoids, and sometimes alterations for varying concentrations of steroids. No overall statements can be made. The advantage of the newer, more potent agents is chiefly in the rapidity of their action, enhanced effectiveness, and economy of use, particularly under plastic occlusion.

Only representative compounds and their relative effective concentrations are listed in Table 1.

Dilute forms are available for many of these compounds. *In general, our philosophy directs us to use 1% hydrocortisone when a weaker steroid or maintenance therapy is desired.* It is effective, less expensive, and free of side effects.

The very potent topical steroids are fast acting, expensive, able to clear otherwise unresponsive dermatoses, and likely to produce cutaneous side effects on long-term use. (See p. 204 for side effects of these drugs.)

The glucocorticoid creams show increased

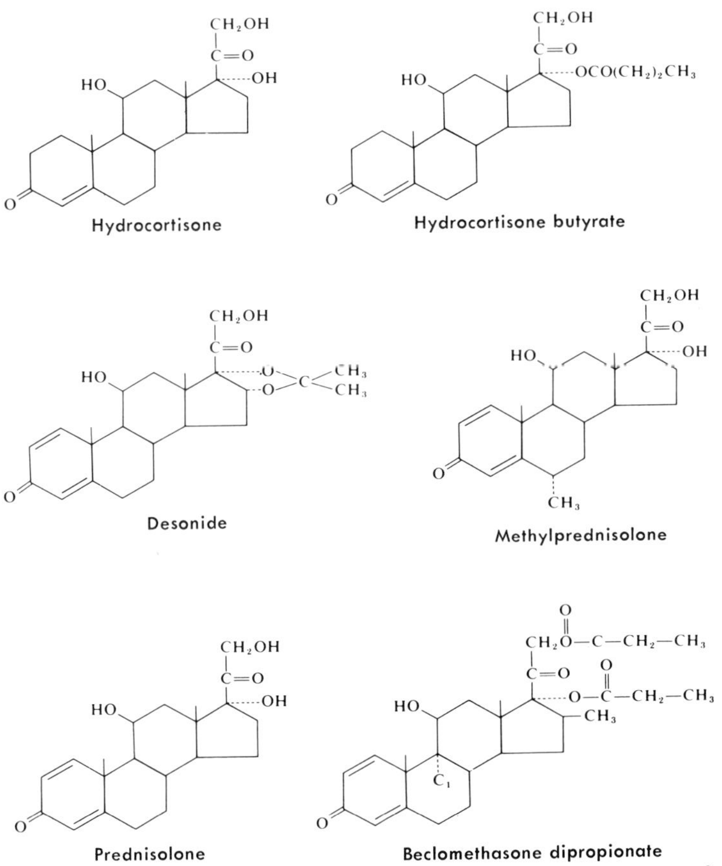


*Continued.*

**Fig. 2-2.** Substitutions to the basic hydrocortisone molecule for topical use. Compounds above are nonfluorinated, and compounds on facing page are fluorinated. Bulky side chains tend to enhance penetration.

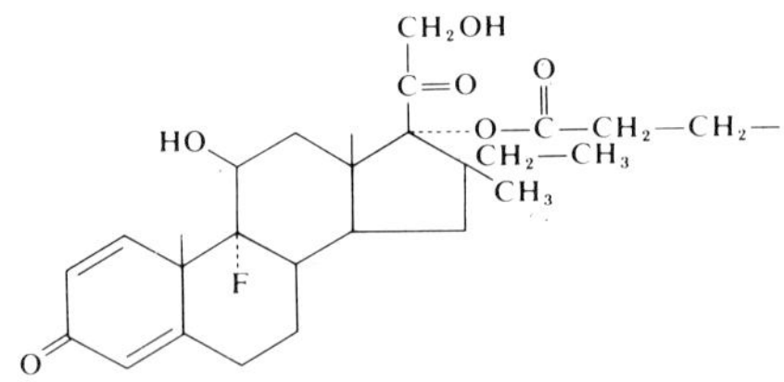

Betamethasone 17-valerate

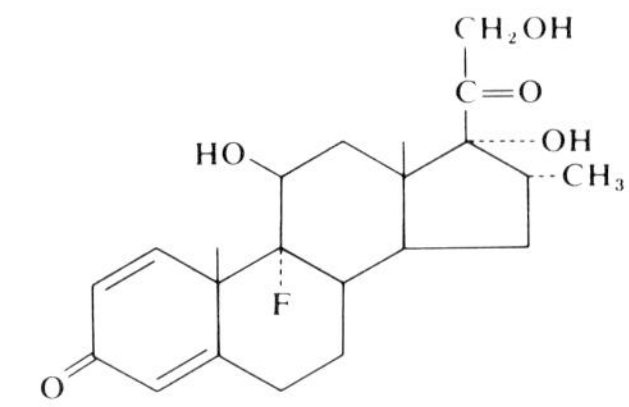

Dexamethasone

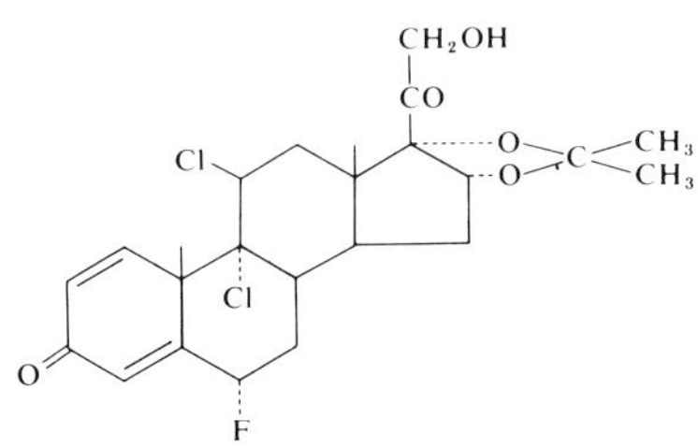

Fluclorolone acetonide

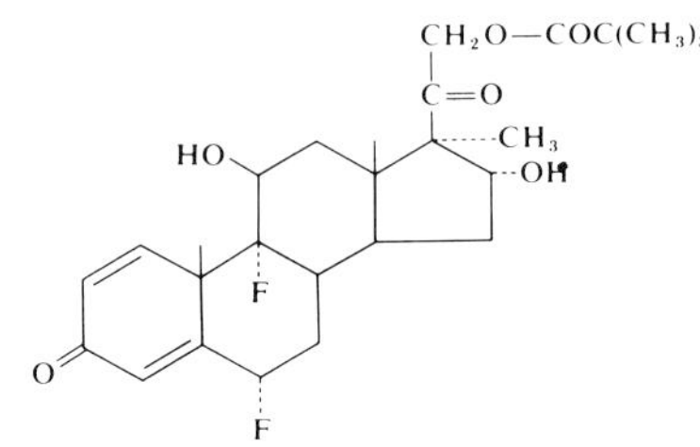

Flumethasone pivalate

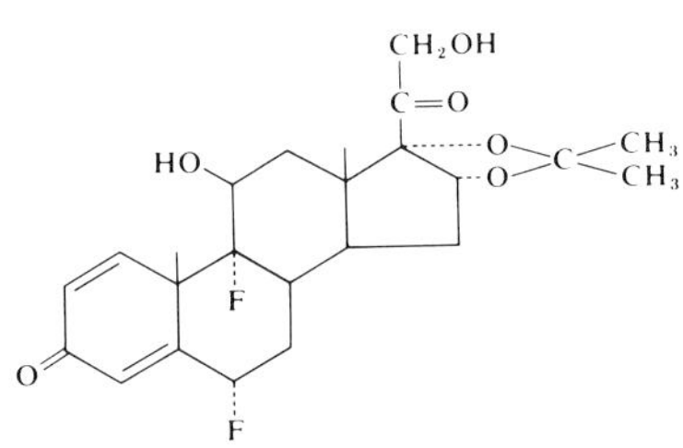

Fluocinolone acetonide

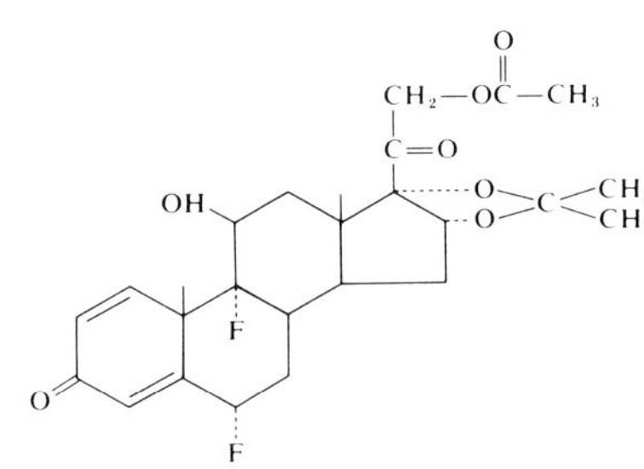

Fluocinonide

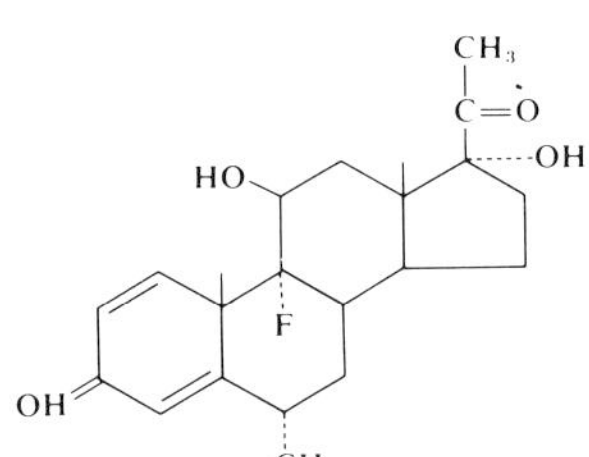

Fluorometholone

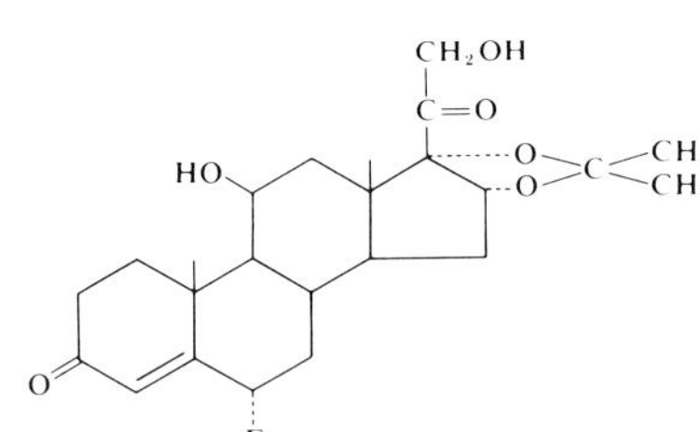

Flurandrenolone acetonide

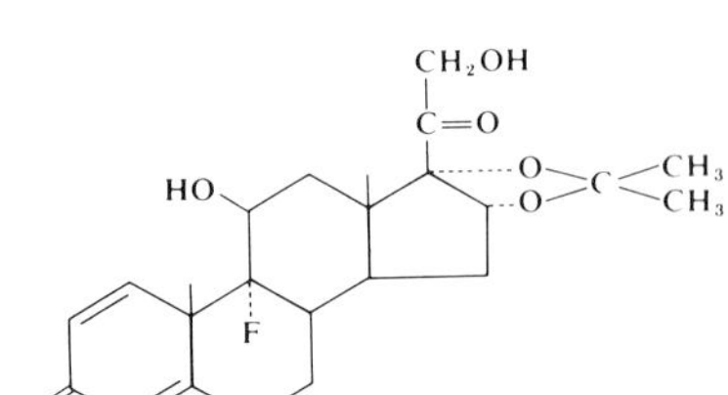

Triamcinolone acetonide

**Fig. 2-2. cont'd.** For legend see p. 65.

**Table 1.** Some available representative glucocorticoids

| Compound | Topical concentration |
|---|---|
| Effective | |
| Hydrocortisone (Cortisol, many others) | 1.0% |
| Prednisolone (many names) | 0.5% |
| Stronger | |
| Dexamethasone phosphate (Decaderm) | 0.1% |
| Desoxymetasone (Topicort) | 0.25% |
| Desonide (Tridesilon) | 0.05% |
| Fluorometholone (Oxylone) | 0.025% |
| Hydrocortisone butyrate (Locoid) | 0.1% |
| Hydrocortisone 17-valerate (Westcort) | 0.2% |
| Methylprednisolone acetate (Medrol) | 0.1% |
| Triamcinolone acetonide (Aristocort, Kenacort) | 0.1% |
| Potent | |
| Beclomethasone dipropionate (Propaderm) | 0.025% |
| Betamethasone dipropionate (Diprosone) | 0.05% |
| Betamethasone 17-valerate (Celestoderm V, Betnovate) | 0.1% |
| Clobetasol propionate (Dermovate) | 0.05% |
| Fluclorolone acetonide (Flucloronide) | 0.025% |
| Fluocinonide (Lidex, Topsyn) | 0.05% |
| Halcinonide (Halog) | 0.1% |
| Very potent | |
| Fluocinolone acetonide (Synalar) | 0.2% |
| Triamcinolone acetonide (Aristocort, Kenacort) | 0.5% |

penetration under occlusive, pliable plastic film dressings. With some, penetration is enhanced a hundredfold, producing a reservoir of active drug in the epidermis. This can, of course, also enhance the *systemic effects* of the topical steroids, particularly the newer, more potent varieties. Definite depression of adreno cortical function has been recorded. Hendrikse and Moolenaar have studied six patients on a long-term regimen of topical potent glucocorticoids under plastic occlusion. They showed incomplete pituitary-adrenal axis suppression. Stress (as tested with insulin) produced a rise in plasma cortisol levels, showing responsiveness of the system. For these reasons it seems wiser to use plastic occlusive therapy in localized areas, with minimal concentrations of medication. Weston has shown that topical application of fluorinated steroids on the skin of children without occlusion may unpredictably result in adrenal suppression. Children are more susceptible than adults to this unwanted effect. Also some of the newer compounds, that is, clobetasol propionate, are very likely to be quickly and effectively absorbed through the skin in very significant amounts.

## Intralesional therapy

The glucocorticoids are also used intralesionally. Sterile aqueous suspensions of agents such as triamcinolone can be injected into cutaneous lesions with a tuberculin or dental syringe and a fine-gauge needle. The medication is placed intracutaneously; the more superficial the injection, the more satisfactory is the result. Soluble steroid preparations are not used, since they are removed in tissue fluid and lymphatic channels too rapidly to have much therapeutic effect.

For intralesional injection we use 5 to 10 mg./2 ml. of triamcinolone diacetate diluted in lidocaine (Xylocaine) hydrochloride so that only the first injection into a plaque is painful.

Agents used include triamcinolone diacetate aqueous suspension, Kenalog or Aristocort, and betamethasone suspension 6 mg./ml. Only the relatively insoluble forms of the corticosteroids are suitable for intralesional use.

Intralesional therapy is indicated for *lichen simplex chronicus* (circumscribed neurodermatitis), *alopecia areata*, *granuloma annulare*, *chronic discoid lupus erythematosus*, *psoriasis vulgaris*, *indurated cystic lesions associated with acne vulgaris*, *myxoid cysts*, *keloid*, and *lichen planus*.

Side effects include pain, hemorrhage, atrophy, infection, some pigmentation, and adrenal suppression. The most significant is *atrophy*, although there is evidence of adrenal suppression from absorption of the deposit. There have, however, been reported cases of sudden obstruction of retinal and other small vessels after intralesional therapy of the face or scalp, caused by the injection of the insoluble material into a small blood vessel.

Atrophy can result from these medications, with visible depression of the injected area. This is usually reversible. The severity depends on the concentration of steroid deposited, with higher concentrations producing greater degrees of atrophy. (We have seldom produced atrophy when using a concentration of 10 mg./2 ml. intralesionally.)

## Systemic therapy

Glucocorticoid therapy, parenteral or oral, is very frequently used in dermatological maladies. Ordinarily, the doses used are considerably lower than those in endocrine disorders, arthritic disease, or cardiopulmonary disease. Exceptions are the doses necessary to control pemphigus, some acute bullous eruptions, and systemic lupus erythematosus. In these disorders maximum doses, given early and over a long period of time, are necessary to control the disease adequately and give the patient the best opportunity for survival.

For most steroid-responsive dermatoses, however, the dose ranges from 5 to 20 mg. of prednisone or its equivalent, to be tapered off as the disease subsides.

The chief indication for systemic use of glucocorticoids is in treating acute self-limited disorders such as acute contact dermatitis, exacerbations of atopic dermatitis, drug reactions, or exfoliative dermatitis when the cause is apparent. One must not fall into the trap of using glucocorticoids for a dermatitis and then finding that it is only partially responding and that the cause is not as yet determined.

Side effects to be observed in patients being treated with systemic steroids are as follows:

1. Euphoria, increased well-being
2. Peptic ulceration
3. Intercurrent infection, cutaneous or systemic (prophylactic antibiotics do not lessen this risk, indeed they may enhance it)
4. Exacerbation of hypertension
5. Exacerbation of diabetes mellitus
6. Thrombophlebitis.
7. Osteoporosis, associated with long-term therapy; less frequent in patients who have good protein intake and are active physically
8. Cushingoid features; acne, moon facies, hirsutism, and ecchymoses

Regular examinations of blood pressure and weight are indicated, and urinalysis and white blood cell counts should be carried out on all patients during more than minimal steroid therapy.

There is some evidence that intermittent therapy, that is, giving steroids on alternate days, produces fewer side effects and less adrenal suppression than daily therapy with equivalent dosage. For example, 20 mg. of prednisone given on alternate days is safer than 10 mg. given daily.

Tapering off a dose of systemic steroids is done slowly, particularly when the level approaches zero. Halving the dose at weekly intervals is a good rule of thumb. Many dermatoses will evince a flare-up as the dose is lowered or discontinued. The patient should then be maintained on the minimum effective dose, for several weeks, if necessary, until it is apparent that it can be lowered safely again.

Approximately equivalent oral doses of various steroids are as follows:

| | |
|---|---|
| Hydrocortisone | 20 mg. |
| Prednisone | 5 mg. |
| Prednisolone | 5 mg. |
| Methylprednisolone | 4 mg. |
| Triamcinolone | 4 mg. |
| Paramethasone | 2 mg. |
| Betamethasone | 0.5 mg. |
| Dexamethasone | 0.75 mg. |
| Fludrocortisone | 2 mg. |

## ACTH (CORTICOTROPIN)

Adrenocorticotropic hormone is ordinarily prepared for human use from the pituitary glands of pigs. It is used in dermatology in steroid-responsive dermatoses when oral corticosteroids cannot be given or retained, and it is also prescribed by some dermatologists who believe that it produces a more satisfactory response in some selected cases of chronic dermatosis, or exfoliative dermatitis. It is probably not of value when patients are already taking large doses of steroids by mouth, since the adrenal glands are then nonresponsive to pituitary stimulation, but here again there is room for argument, since ACTH may have some direct action on the skin.

ACTH is infrequently given intravenously, but more often is administered intramuscularly in a gel or repository form.

The usual dose is from 20 to 80 units daily. Available forms, with route and dose, are as follows:

| | |
|---|---|
| 1. Repository corticotropin (corticotrophin gel, Depo-ACTH, Synacthen depot)—intramuscular | 20-100 units/ml. |
| 2. Corticotropin in carboxymethylcellulose (Duracton)—subcutaneous | 40 I.U./ml. |
| 3. Corticotropin (Cortrophin-zinc), zinc hydroxide suspension—intramuscular or subcutaneous | 20-40 units/ml. |
| 4. Cosyntropin zinc hydroxide—intramuscular (1 mg. = 100 units, but lasts longer) | 1 mg./ml. |
| 5. Solution—intravenous (usually given as 25 units in 1,000 ml. of 5% glucose in water over an 8-hour period) | 10-80 units/ml. |
| 6. Lyophilized powder—intravenous | 25- and 40-I.U. vials |

#### REFERENCES


Hendrikse, J. C. M., and Moolenaar, A. J.: Adrenal and pituitary functions during long term topical steroid therapy, Dermatologica **144:**179, 1972.
**Partial suppression that appeared reversible over 2 to 5 years.**

Jarrett, M. T., Spark, R. F., and Arndt, K.: The effects of intradermal steroids on the pituitary adrenal axis and the skin, J. Invest. Dermatol. **62:**463, 1974.
**Unequivocal atrophy and adrenal suppression.**

Sim, A. W., Picton, W., Fox, P. K., et al.: The effect of topical corticosteroids on the metabolism of dermal collagen. In Wilson, L., and Marks, R., editors: Mechanisms of topical corticosteroid activity, New York, 1976, Churchill Livingstone.

Snyder, D. S., and Greenberg, R. A.: Evaluations of atrophy production and vasoconstrictor potency in humans following intradermally injected corticoids, J. Invest. Dermatol. **63:**461, 1974.
**First evidence occurred within a week.**

Stewart, W. D., Runikis, J. O., Verma, S. C., and Wallace, S. G.: Problems in selection of topical anti-inflammatory corticosteroids, Can. Med. Assoc. J. **108:**33, 1973.
**To fluorinate or not to fluorinate.**

Voorhees, J. J.: Personal communication, 1977.

Weissman, G., and Goldstein, I. M.: Effect of steroids on lysosomes. In Wilson, L., and Marks, R., editors: Mechanisms in topical corticosteroid activity, New York, 1976, Churchill Livingstone.
**Probably an important part of the counterinflammation effect of these compounds.**


# Dermatological techniques

## LOCAL ANESTHESIA

Topical anesthetic agents are unable to penetrate the intact stratum corneum to produce sufficient anesthesia for cutaneous surgery. They quickly penetrate mucous membranes, such as those of the lips, tongue, and glans penis, and produce enough anesthesia to allow introduction of a needle for deeper local anesthesia. Local anesthetics also penetrate fairly well in abraded, raw, or inflamed acute dermatoses. Here, however, they can be sensitizing and thus provoke greater irritation.

Lidocaine in ointment or viscous form is of low sensitizing potential and is rapid acting and satisfactory on mucous membranes. Anesthesia for dermatological surgical procedures can be achieved with 2% lidocaine or similar anesthetic of choice without epinephrine. It is injected intracutaneously with a dental syringe or a 26-gauge needle in a Luer-Lok or similar syringe, raising a wheal at the base of the lesion to be treated. Large lesions should be surrounded by wheals, and smaller lesions can be infiltrated thoroughly with the anesthetic. The Panjet apparatus is capable of introducing the local anesthetic into the epidermis by pressure without needle injection. It anesthetizes an area of approximately 1 $cm.^2$ with each jet.

## DIAGNOSTIC TECHNIQUES

### Wood's light*

Wood's light is a selected wavelength of light, 360 nm., that has had most visible light eliminated. It is so-called black light that produces fluorescence from many different objects, including some forms of dermatitis and some tumors. It is used chiefly in dermatology

*Named for R. W. Wood (1868-1955), former Professor of Experimental Physics, Johns Hopkins University.

to produce fluorescence in fungi; thus it is a quick diagnostic method in certain of these disorders. It is also used in photopatch testing to diagnose light sensitivities and light allergies from photosensitizing drugs. It can be used therapeutically in association with the oxypsoralens with which it produces an enhanced photodynamic effect. Long-term exposure to Wood's light can produce cutaneous atrophy.

## Skin scrapings

Skin scrapings are used for identification of fungal elements. When the diagnosis of fungal infection is considered, either because of suggestions in the history or in the appearance of the lesions, scrapings to aid in the identification of the fungus are indicated.

First the area is cleansed with alcohol and air dried so that a superficial, fine, dry scale is apparent. Then the scale is gently but firmly scraped with a sharp scalpel, and the scrapings are collected in a Wassermann blood collection tube or similar container. Nail clippings or infected hairs of the scalp should be similarly collected. Some of the skin scrapings are placed on a glass microscope slide, and a generous drop of 10% potassium hydroxide is applied and covered with a cover glass. This is left for 20 minutes and then examined under reduced light by microscope for fungal elements.

The remainder is cultured on Sabouraud's media for 3 weeks, and the colonies that appear on the surface are studied for identification of the fungus type involved. Containers for collection, slants of Sabouraud's media, and instructions for use are obtainable from private laboratories and are available for the convenience of the practicing physician.

## Punch biopsy

Biopsies of cutaneous lesions can be performed either by scalpel and subsequent suturing or by a dermal punch, which requires no suturing. If no sutures are used, healing takes place rapidly and there is essentially no danger of secondary infection except under very abnormal circumstances (Figs. 2-3 and 2-4).

The selection of a biopsy site is of the utmost importance. For *tumors* and *indurated lesions*, a mature or fully developed lesion reveals the most pathological information. For *bullous* or *vesicular lesions*, however, the first stages of the lesion formation are most significant, and new or newly forming lesions are the most desirable.

A 3- to 5-mm. punch is preferable, for it permits an adequate amount of tissue for examination. If areas of varying clinical appearance are present in one lesion, more than one biopsy may be desirable.

The specimen should be deep, including the full dermis, as well as some of the fatty tissue, if possible.

If the skin is slightly stretched at right angles to the lines of tension for that area while the punch is made, the resultant defect will be oval as the skin returns to its normal position, and the wound will heal with less defect.

After local anesthesia with lidocaine, the biopsy punch is twirled between the thumb and forefinger with a rotary motion, pressing lightly downward as it cuts through the skin. Practice will make the operator cognizant of the depth he attains and when to go deeper or stop. The pedicle of the biopsy core is then snipped off with scissors, and the bleeding is stopped with electrodesiccation or simple pressure. An antibiotic powder may be dusted on the area.

## Touch preparations

This technique is used when distinctive cells, diagnostic of the disease process, are present on the surface of the lesion.

A clean glass slide is touched firmly to the surface so that a layer of cells can adhere to it. A spray (Cytospray) similar to that used in the Papanicolaou technique is used to fix the cells so that they may be stained and examined later. Cells of mycosis fungoides and other erosive malignancies may be recognized by their morphology. Virus-produced cellular alterations (herpes simplex, varicella) may give a specific diagnosis when taken from the base of a blister, and acantholytic cells seen in pemphigus vulgaris may aid in the diagnosis.

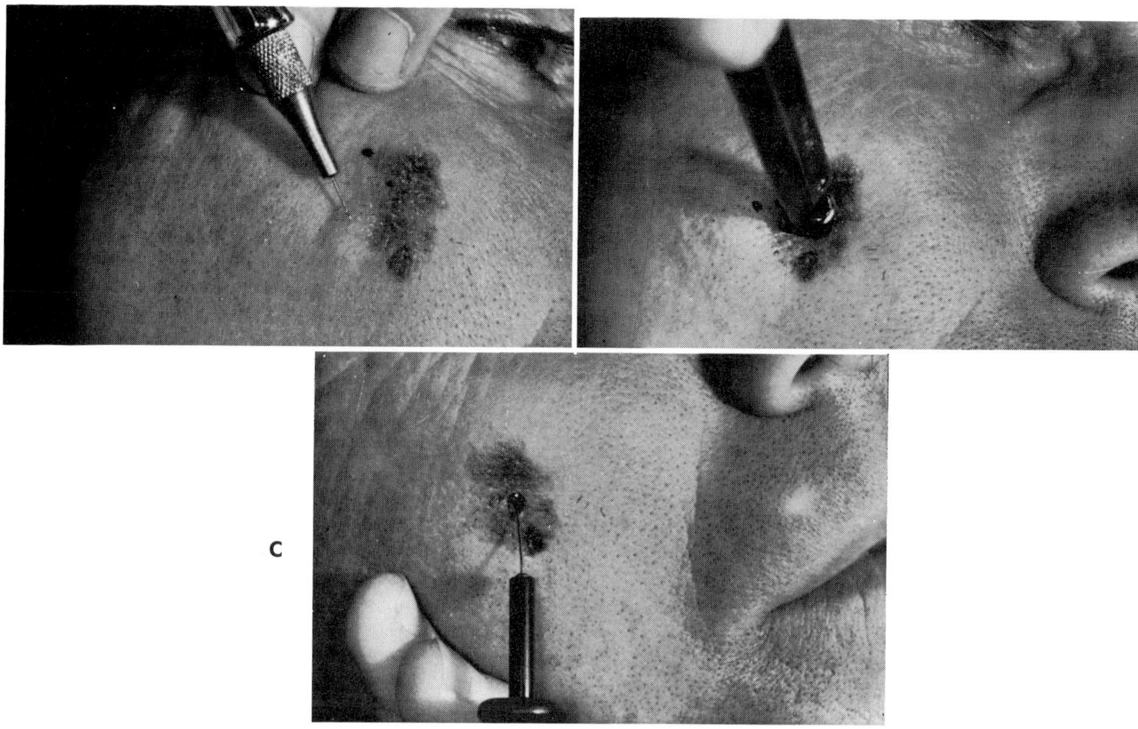

B

C

**Fig. 2-3. A,** Infiltration with local anesthetic. **B**, Punch biopsy from active nonnecrotic center of lesion. **C**, Electrodesiccation for hemostasis.

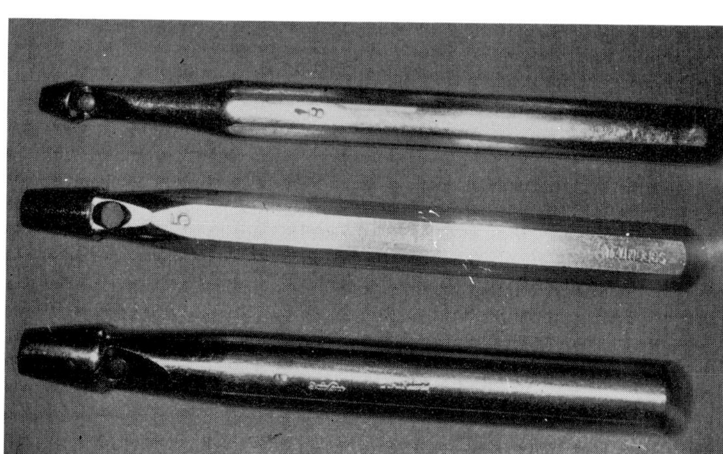

**Fig. 2-4.** Biopsy punches of varying sizes.

A

B

C

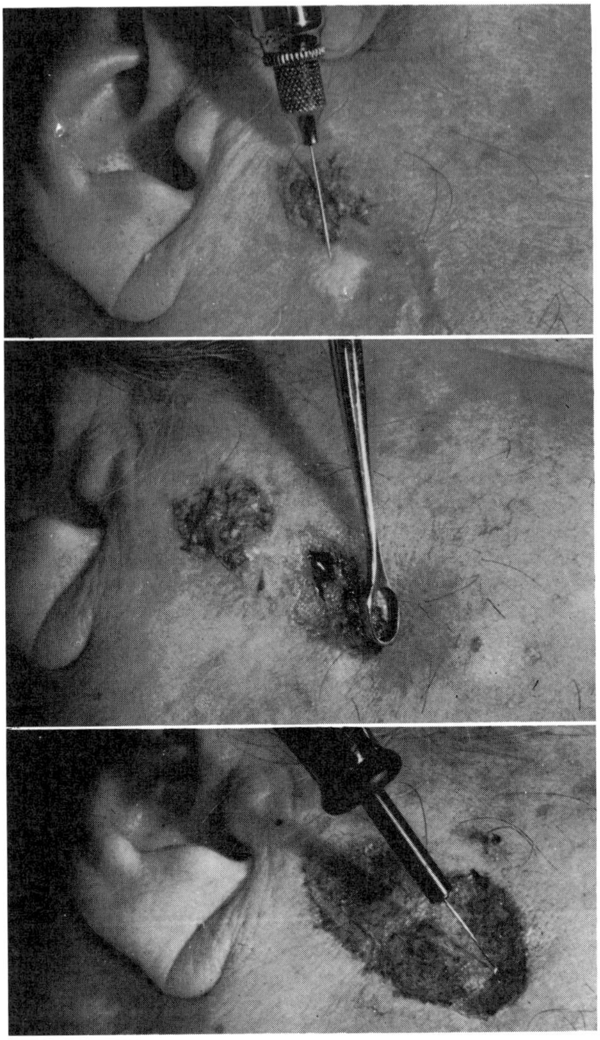

**Fig. 2-5. A,** Infiltration with local anesthetic. **B,** Curettage. **C,** Electrodesiccation for hemostasis.

## THERAPEUTIC TECHNIQUES

### Curettage

Curettage effects the removal of neoplastic or hyperkeratotic tissue and certain selected lesions by scraping with a dermal curet under local anesthesia. It is performed with firm pulling strokes toward the operator, who at the same time applies downward pressure. Its use in the treatment of basal cell epithelioma is enhanced by the operator's ability to feel the tissue he is curetting and to determine quite accurately the borders of neoplastic and normal tissue. The bleeding produced by curettage is halted by Monsel's solution (basic ferric sulfate solution) applied to the raw area to stop capillary bleeding, or by electrodesiccation (Fig. 2-5).

### Electrodesiccation

Electrodesiccation is carried out with a diathermy machine, which possesses a spark gap that controls the electric current so that a spark passes from the monopolar needle to the tissues. The spark can be selectively lessened or enlarged to produce the desired effect.

Individual bleeding points are sealed, and a

plane of cells is destroyed. This charred layer can then be curetted away, the next plane desiccated, and so forth, thus moving deeper into the tissue in a well-controlled manner.

Electrodesiccation is used in combination with curettage for treating the following lesions: *basal cell epithelioma, seborrheic keratosis, leukoplakia, skin tag, pyogenic granuloma, dermatofibroma, wart, nevus, actinic keratosis,* and *cutaneous horn.*

## Cryotherapy

Another destructive medium, cryotherapy, uses solid carbon dioxide (Dry Ice), the temperature of which is −79° C. Its degree of tissue damage may be judged by the fact that cryonecrosis begins around temperatures of −20° to −30° C. It is used with moderate pressure on the lesion for 3 to 20 seconds. A blister follows, and a lesion within 2 to 4 mm. of the surface will be destroyed. Keloids do not ordinarily form from this treatment.

Liquid nitrogen boils at −195° C., is quite easily obtained in most cities, and is widely used for the treatment of warts. It is often kept in a thermos bottle, preferably one designed for the purpose, and a container will usually last 2 or 3 days if kept covered between uses. Cotton swabs are dipped in the solution and applied to the wart for 10 to 20 seconds. It is painful, and blisters appear within 5 to 10 hours. One should first use it on himself to become familiar with its capabilities. Quite sophisticated tank, tube, and nozzle apparatuses are available for office use if one has a frequent need for it. Small tumors, hemangiomas, warts, pyogenic granulomas, seborrheic keratoses, and the like can be treated in this manner, which allows freezing effects to about 5 mm. in depth. Zacharian and others with considerable experience find a wide use and significant need for the procedure.

The following are common disorders amenable to cryosurgical procedures:

Cutaneous tags
Dermatofibromas
Molluscum contagiosum
Warts (excluding plantar warts)
Condyloma acuminatum
Granuloma pyogenicum
Seborrheic keratosis
Actinic keratosis
Discoid lupus erythematosus
Acne cysts
Malignancies (for which an experienced cryotherapist is required)

## Electrolysis

By means of a galvanic current generated by battery, a direct current is developed through a tiny needle, which can be used to coagulate the hair bulb, thus destroying terminal hair growth. Electrolysis is also used for eliminating telangiectatic blood vessels. It leaves no scar when properly performed.

## X-ray therapy

Conventional dermatological x-ray therapy is used for the treatment of malignancies that do not extend farther than a few millimeters beneath the epidermis. It is a mistake to use a beam that is too penetrating for the depth of the lesion to be destroyed. X-ray therapy is used with careful shielding to protect those areas that derive only harm from being exposed. Permanent atrophy, telangiectasia, malignancies, ulcers, depigmentation, and hyperpigmentation can arise from excessive therapy.

## Electron beam therapy

Beams of high-speed electrons can be used, just as x rays are used, for treatment of cutaneous malignancies. The beam ideally is uniform and is uncontaminated by x rays. X rays are derived from the interaction of the electrons and the atoms in the apparatus and the patient's tissues. The technique can provide homogeneity throughout the field, the total body receiving an equivalent dose of radiation, with the penetration depending on the energy of the electrons. The general range of energy used is 5.3 to 2.5 Mev, with penetration around 5 to 15 mm. Bone marrow and deeper organs are not affected. Total doses as used for mycosis fungoides range from 1,000 to 3,500 rads, with good patient tolerance. One course of 3,000 rads may take 6 weeks. Repeat courses can be given, but radioresistance of the tumor, subcutaneous fibrosis, and skin atrophy occur.

## Grenz-ray therapy

Grenz rays, so-called "soft" ionizing radiation, penetrate only a very short distance beneath the epidermis and thus can be used satisfactorily for those lesions involving the epidermis and not the deeper dermis. There are no side effects from these rays when they are used in the recommended dosages and durations. Excessive dosages can produce pigmentation, depigmentation, and atrophy. They should be used in intermittent dosage only and for carefully restricted periods.

## Ultraviolet light

An erythema-producing form of radiation, ultraviolet light (290 to 400 nm.) consists of waves or quanta, some segments of which react with DNA, purines, pyrimidines, enzymes, lysosomes, and proteins of the epidermis to produce proteoses that may stimulate a histamine-like reaction in the dermal papillae, as well as far-reaching changes in the vasculature and collagen of the deeper dermis. A very narrow range of ultraviolet light is absorbed by the biological compounds of the skin, and that narrow range is the part of the ultraviolet spectrum responsible for the damaging long-term effects of sunlight on the skin. The immediate reaction ranges from a mild erythema to a full epidermal thickness blister formation. Pigmentation follows. The following are sources of ultraviolet light used in clinical dermatology:

*Cold quartz*—254 nm.
EFFECT: Produces peeling and erythema

*Hot quartz*—sunburn range, not continuous
EFFECT: Produces benefit in acne, peeling, and erythema; pigmentation

*Sun lamp tube (fluorescent)*—280 to 350 nm. (sunburn range and over)
EFFECT: Pigmentation, therapeutic (antipsoriasis)

*Wood's lamp*—360 nm.
EFFECT: Diagnostic, therapeutic

*Black light tube*—365 nm.
EFFECT: Diagnostic, therapeutic

*Long-wave ultraviolet (UVA) tubes*—320 to 400 nm.
EFFECT: Therapeutic in combination with psoralens

Certain dermatoses, such as acne, psoriasis, pityriasis rosea, and parapsoriasis, may benefit from regular ultraviolet light treatments in carefully graded dosages. (See treatment sections for each.)

### REFERENCES

Caplan, R. M.: Medical uses of the Wood's lamp, J.A.M.A. **202**:123, 1967.

Epstein, E.: Skin surgery, ed. 4, Springfield, Ill., 1977, Charles C Thomas, Publisher.

Epstein, J., Fukuyama, K., and Fye, K.: Effects of ultraviolet radiation on the mitotic cycle, DNA, RNA and protein synthesis in mammalian epidermis in vivo, Photochem. Photobiol. **12**:57, 1970.

Zacharian, S. A.: Cryosurgery of tumors of the skin and oral cavity, ed. 2, Springfield, Ill., 1977, Charles C Thomas, Publisher.

Zacharian, S. A.: Cryosurgical advances in dermatology and tumors of the head and neck, Springfield, Ill., 1977, Charles C Thomas, Publisher.

PART THREE

# Specific dermatological disease entities

CHAPTER 3

# Acne vulgaris, hidradenitis, and rosacea

## Development, structure, and function of the sebaceous glands

### Embryology

In the twelfth-week embryo, an epidermal bulge of cells aligned at an angle to the developing hair tract appears on the posterior surface of each forming hair follicle to develop into a sebaceous gland (Fig. 3-1, *A*). The glandular cells acquire fat droplets by the seventeenth week, and the central cells degenerate to form a lumen leading to the surface, along the path of the future hair shaft (Fig. 3-1, *B*). The glands are well formed before the hair follicles, by the fourth intrauterine month, beginning on the face. Sebaceous gland development elsewhere on the skin continues through intrauterine life and after birth, and sebaceous differentiation can occur on mucosal surfaces and in salivary glands of adults. By birth the sebaceous glands are at a peak of activity but involute in the neonatal period to a much less active state lasting until puberty. The vernix caseosa, present at birth, is a sebaceous gland secretion.

### Anatomy

Sebaceous gland (Fig. 3-1) secretion is discharged onto the skin surface through the lumen of a hair follicle alongside the hair shaft. On the face and anogenital area, some sebaceous glands appear to open directly and individually onto the skin surface. These mostly have minute disproportionately small hair follicles and hairs, which fail to be shed to the outside. *This becomes terribly important in the pathogenesis of acne.* Ultrastructural studies of cellular sebaceous differentiation at the periphery of the gland indicate that a uniform lipid material is formed in the smooth endoplasmic reticulum and Golgi zones. Lipid-laden cells move slowly from the periphery of the gland to the centers of the lobules where degeneration of the cells occurs, and the resulting oil (sebum) is slowly and continuously disgorged without pressure through the short sebaceous duct and then alongside the hair shaft onto the skin surface. The lining of the hair follicle contributes keratin to the sebum, and farther along, clusters of bacteria, debris, and sloughed epidermal cell lipids and protein are added. These are *holocrine glands;* that is, the secretion contains the cells of the gland. No sebaceous glands are present on the palms and soles, but they are apparent everywhere else, with increased concentration on the forehead and face (500 ducts/cm.$^2$) fewer on the back (160 ducts/cm.$^2$), and fewer than 100/cm.$^2$ elsewhere. Modified sebaceous glands have developed in the ear canals, eyelids, and prepuce. As above noted, ectopic spontaneous sebaceous differentiation of epithelial cells takes place on mucous membranes and skin, a commonly known example of which are Fordyce's spots on the lip and buccal mucosa.

### Physiology and biochemistry

Sebum, the product of the sebaceous gland, exudes from the gland through the short sebaceous duct and then along the hair follicle, collecting by-products of epidermal keratinization along the way. It joins the fatty products of surface epidermal keratinization to form the lipid film at pH 4.2 to 5.6 on the skin surface. Although the film is resistant to bacterial action, its presence confers no confirmed advantage, and preadolescent skin appears satisfactorily functional without sebum.

Wax esters, squalene, glycerides, free fatty

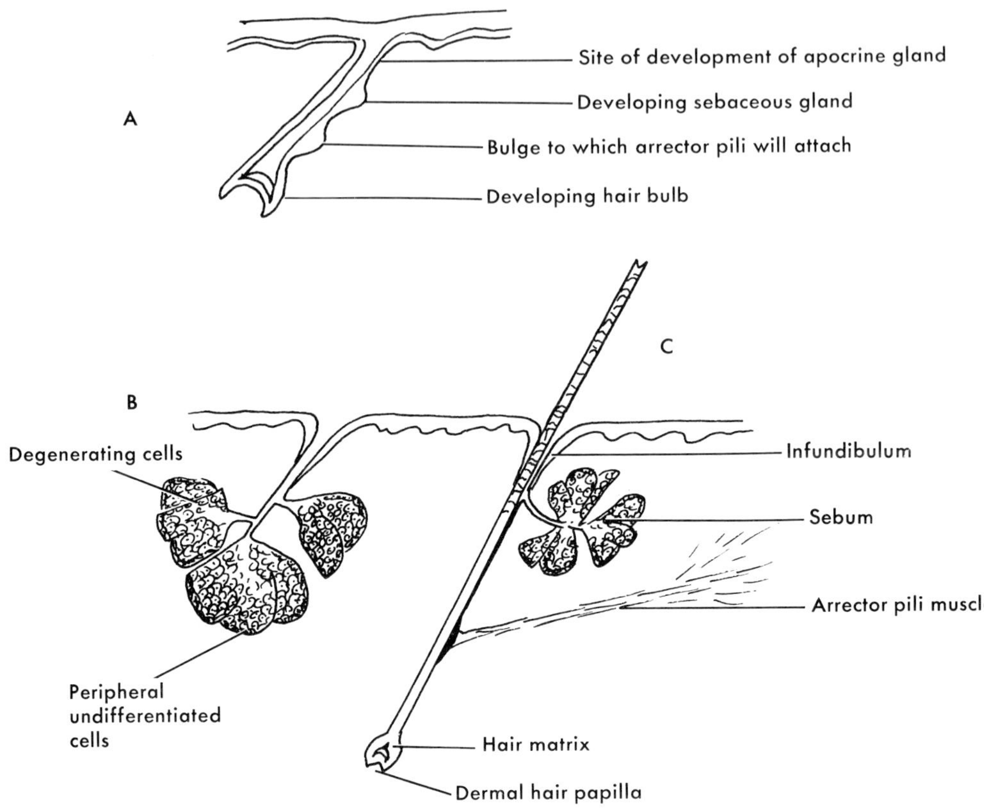


**Fig. 3-1.** Sebaceous glands. **A,** Developing pilosebaceous unit at 14 to 16 weeks of intrauterine life. **B,** Gland opening to skin surface. **C,** Gland opening to terminal hair follicle.

acids, sterols, sterol esters, and saturated hydrocarbons make up the components of sebum produced by sebaceous glands. A small proportion only arises from epidermal cell lipid. The components can be identified and measured by thin-layer or column-adsorption chromatography. Prepuberal children have more cholesterol and less wax ester and squalene than do adults, although neonates have lipid-surface film that more closely resembles adults. By 8 to 12 years, wax esters and squalene have risen close to adult levels. Although the rate of sebum synthesis is under hormonal control, the composition appears not to be affected by variations in hormonal stimulation. Starvation produces first an increased proportion of squalene and decreased triglycerides within a week. A 40% reduction in sebum production occurs after an average of 2 weeks on restricted diet.

Cutaneous lipogenesis is at variance with major pathways of lipid synthesis elsewhere in the body in the types of lipid produced and in the apparent absence of a homeostatic regulatory mechanism related to diet, as in other fat pools. The lipid in sebaceous glands and in epidermis obviously takes on a different form and purpose than does storage lipid such as subcutaneous fat. However, the purpose of sebum has not been clearly defined.

Males produce more sebum than do females, except between 10 and 15 years of age when both sexes produce equal amounts. The rate of excretion approximates 0.5 $\mu$g/cm.$^2$/min. (for females) to 1.2 $\mu$g./cm.$^2$/min. (for males). Male adult sebaceous glands appear to function at a near maximal level of activity normally.

Sebaceous gland size and sebum production is under hormonal control. There are no demonstrable neural controls. The pituitary gland exerts an important androgenic effect indirectly, with trophic hormones acting through gonads and adrenals, and may secrete an as-yet-unidentified sebotropic hormone. Thyroid-stimulating hormone and growth hormone add permissive effects to androgens, meaning that androgen in the presence of these hormones has a greater effect on sebaceous glands than in their absence.

Androgens, from gonads and adrenals in both sexes, stimulate sebaceous gland activity at physiologic dose levels. Topically applied androgens have not been shown to affect sebaceous glands. Sansone-Bazzano and Reisner (1974) indicated that the simple presence of androgen in serum may *not* be enough to "turn on" the gland. Other factors to be considered are its concentration, the amount and specificity of the cellular cytoplasmic and nuclear receptor proteins, their binding strengths, the presence of competing compounds or metabolites, and the like.

Estrogens inhibit sebaceous gland function and reduce glandular bulk, but only in high nonphysiologic doses. Male adult sebaceous glands appear to function at a near maximal level normally. Although topical estrogens in large concentrations do affect the glands, their response appears to arise from systemic rather than local influence; that is, distant glands respond as well. Progesterone imparts no effect on the glands. Glucocorticoids may be permissive, acting in concert with androgens to obtain a maximum response.

Specialized sebaceous glands in some animals perform sexual and cognitive functions. It is not known whether human sebum has, or had in the past, any similar role.

#### REFERENCES

Bell, M.: A comparative study of the ultrastructure of sebaceous glands of man and other primates. J. Invest. Dermatol. **62**:132, 1974.
**A superb correlation of function with ultrastructure.**

Downing, D. T., and Strauss, J. S.: Synthesis and composition of surface lipids of human skin, J. Invest. Dermatol. **62**:228, 1974.
**Human lipid composition is now known in detail, and thus deductions regarding their origin and synthesis can be made.**

Kligman, A. M.: The uses of sebum? In Montagna, W., Ellis, R. A., and Silver, A., editors: Advances in biology of skin. vol. IV. The sebaceous glands, Oxford, 1963, Pergamon Press, pp. 110–124.
**Undermined!**

Nicolaides, N., Fu, H. C., Ansari, M. N. A., and Rice, B. R.: The fatty acids of wax esters and sterol esters from vernix caseosa and from human skin surface lipids, Lipids **7**:506, 1972.
**A detailed discussion of the epidermal or sebaceous gland origin of branched chain acids, wax, and sterol esters.**

Sansone-Bazzano, G., and Reisner, R. M.: Steroid pathways in sebaceous glands, J. Invest. Dermatol. **62**:211, 1974.
**Steroid interconversions by sebaceous glands studied in vivo in rats and mice.**

Shuster, S., and Thody, A. J.: The control and measurement of sebum secretion, J. Invest. Dermatol. **62**:177, 1974.
**Intermediate lobe of pituitary assumes new importance in sebaceous gland control, along with other factors.**

Strauss, J. S., Pochi, P. E., and Downing, D. T.: The sebaceous glands: twenty-five years of progress, J. Invest. Dermatol. **67**:90, 1976.
**A very brief, but informed review of a massive subject and voluminous data.**

Also refer to the special edition of the Journal of Investigative Dermatology for March 1974 on sebaceous glands.

## ACNE VULGARIS

Almost all adolescents experience acne vulgaris in some manner. It is, however, a disease for the age group of 20's and 30's as well. Peak incidence appears to be near 14 years of age in girls and 16 in boys, but severe cases tend to occur in boys later than this. It is multifactorial and its course varies with cause and age.

### *Natural course*

Excluding infantile acne, a transient occurrence in the neonate, acne truly begins when sebaceous glands enlarge and start to function under androgen stimulation. Small, open comedones and a few papules begin to appear in the faces of many children from age 8 onward, but the presence of closed comedones, inflammation, and small pustules are the earliest signs of clinically significant acne. Open comedones are blackheads, with a black plug in the follicle, whereas closed comedones, or whiteheads, are nonmelanized plugged folli-

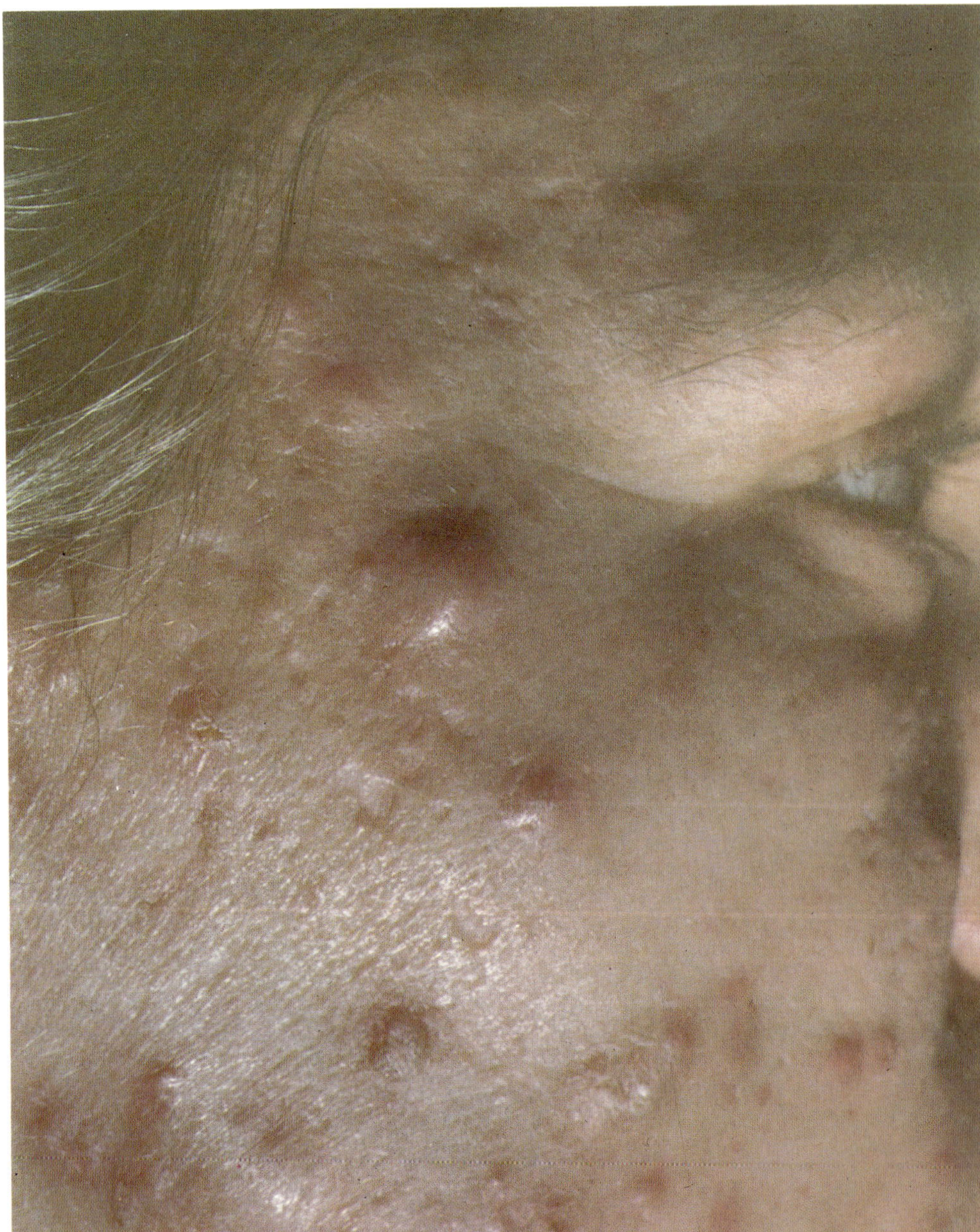

**Plate 8**

Acne vulgaris. Papules and cysts. Note central crateriform scarring from previous inflammatory lesions.

cles that are usually visibly distended. In some adolescents the acne process consists of nothing more than a few scattered pustules and comedones that have a relatively short duration and produce no permanent defect. Other adolescents develop more extensive acne that not only persists, but also produce permanent pits and scars. Emerson and Strauss's interesting survey of over 1,000 high school students with acne revealed that 2.2%

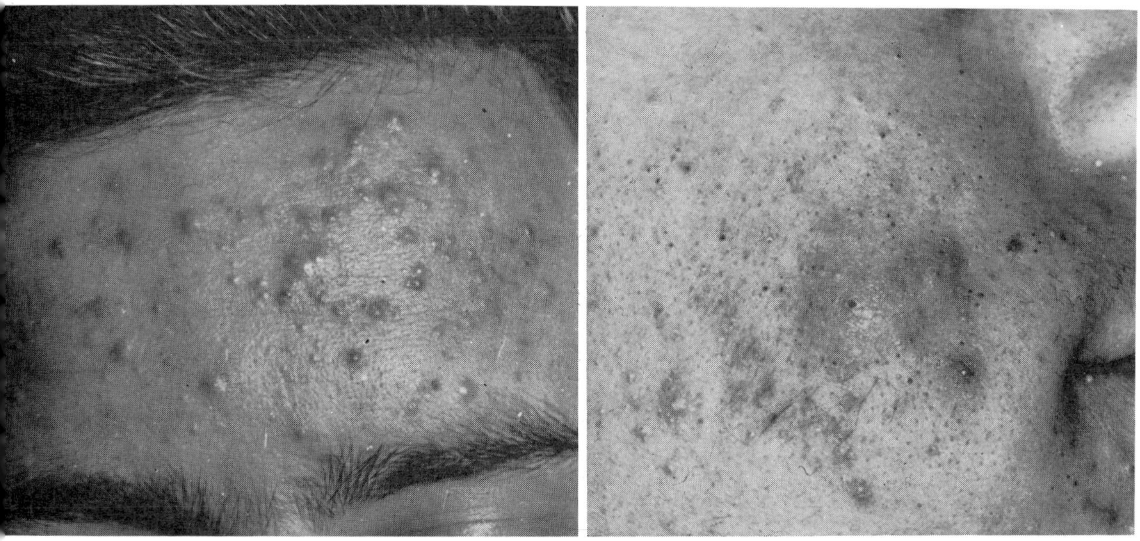

Fig. 3-2. Acne vulgaris. Papular pustules and comedones.

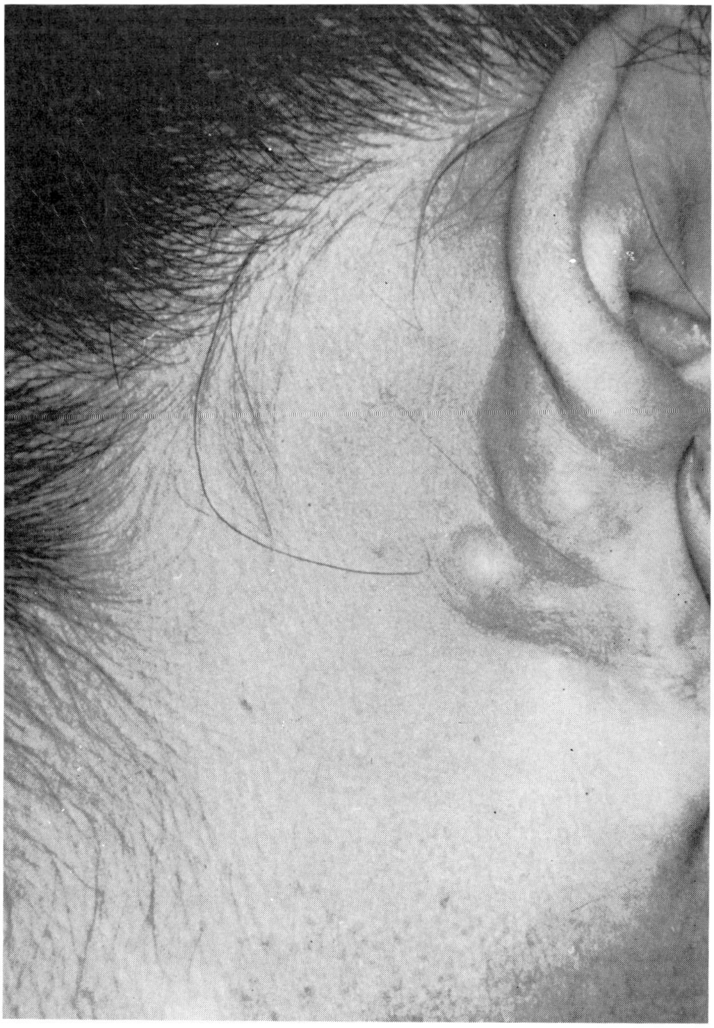

Fig. 3-3. Postauricular acne cyst.

have severe forms of the disease. The lesions that produce large scars are the tender, red pustules and cysts (Plate 8). It is this latter clinical group that needs proper dermatological care if scars of both the skin and the psyche are to be avoided. Small perifollicular scars are much more common, and less often identified. They usually affect most of the follicles overlying the malar prominences when they occur.

The clinical lesions that typify acne vulgaris are as follows: comedones, papules, pustules, cysts, and scars (Figs. 3-2 and 3-3). These lesions occur in the areas of greatest concentration of sebaceous glands: face, central chest, and upper back. Severely affected subjects may have arms, back of neck, lower back, buttocks, and thighs involved.

The clinical course of acne vulgaris fluctuates with the seasons. When teenagers living in temperate zones return to school in the fall, there may be an upswing or worsening of the acne as a result of the sharp reduction in sun exposure that occurs on the return to classes after a favorable summer. Sun plus tropical humidity, however, frequently produces severe, boggy acne lesions. A flare-up of acne usually occurs premenstrually. On occasion, some older patients, not infrequently women in the later 20's and early 30's, experience a recurrence of acne. There is also a group of patients who experience persistence of the disease from adolescence onward. Scarring can produce unsightly hypertrophic scars and keloids in predisposed individuals (Fig. 3-4).

Severe cystic acne seems to have a familial tendency. Kelly and Burns described three cases of very severe acne with associated febrile and joint symptoms.

There is less uniformity in regression than in onset. Most cases are insignificant by late teens, but some persist longer. Many are maintained by ill-advised use of cosmetics or self-manipulation, or both.

### *Pertinent information*

Sansone and Reisner showed that the sebaceous glands convert testosterone to a compound more active at the cellular level and that acne patients do this twentyfold more than do people without acne.

It is the effect of androgens on sebaceous glands that initiates acne. Without these hormones, adult sebaceous gland development and adult sebum productivity does not occur, and neither does acne. Four factors are responsible: (1) androgen stimulation of sebum

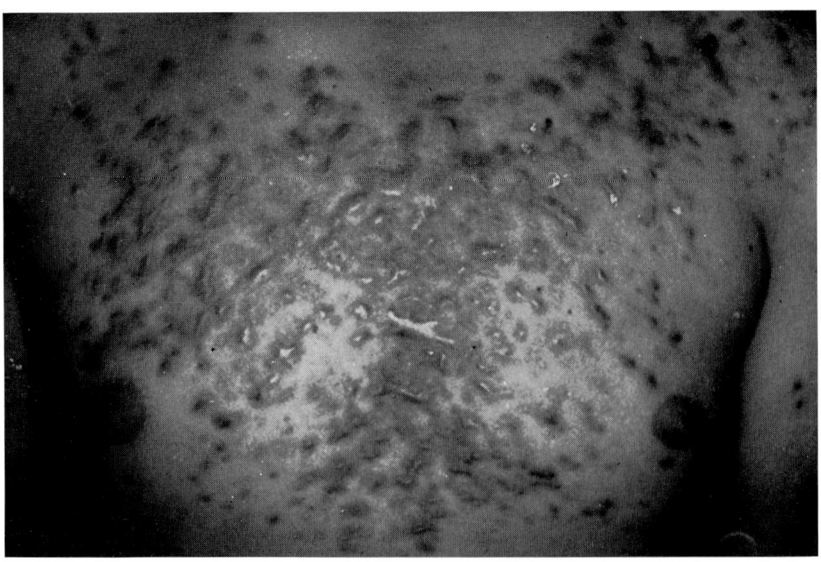

**Fig. 3-4.** Keloid scars resulting from acne.

production, (2) alteration of the border between the epidermal keratinization of the hair follicle and the sebaceous keratinization of the hair follicle and the sebaceous keratinization of the gland duct (Knutsen), (3) presence of masses of *Corynebacterium acnes* in the pilary canal, and (4) inadequacy of small vellus hairs to move the accumulating material out of the follicle. Despite the occurrence of acne in the pilosebaceous follicles in the bearded areas in males, one does not see hairs extruding through acne papules, pustules, cysts, or comedones.

The sequence of events appears to be as follows. The sebaceous gland increases in size and productivity under androgenic influence, accompanied by an alteration in the follicle lining as shown beautifully by Knutsen. This results in stagnation of sebum and comedo formation during which normally harmless *C. acnes* are attracted. Large masses of these organisms collect in the pilary canal. No inflammatory lesions are produced without these bacteria, and their presence is important in the production of the comedo. They produce hyaluronidase, which may facilitate weakening of the comedo wall. These bacteria hydrolyze sebum to short-chain fatty acids, the presence of which produces irritation. However, here some doubt arises. Physiologic amounts of these fatty acids do not produce inflammation. Also inflammatory acne lesions can be produced without free fatty acids and with only *C. acnes* present. The first and primary abnormality is the comedo, which, in functioning terminal hair follicles, is prevented from forming by the "pipe-cleaner" effect of the growing hair shaft. In small, fine hair follicles, the comedo is too fixed for the growing hair to budge (Fig. 3-5). Kligman has demonstrated multiple unshed hairs in comedones, indicating the age of the comedones and acting as evidence to their pathogenesis. In addition, the closed comedo develops internal pressure as its wall continues to proliferate, building up tension and pressure prior

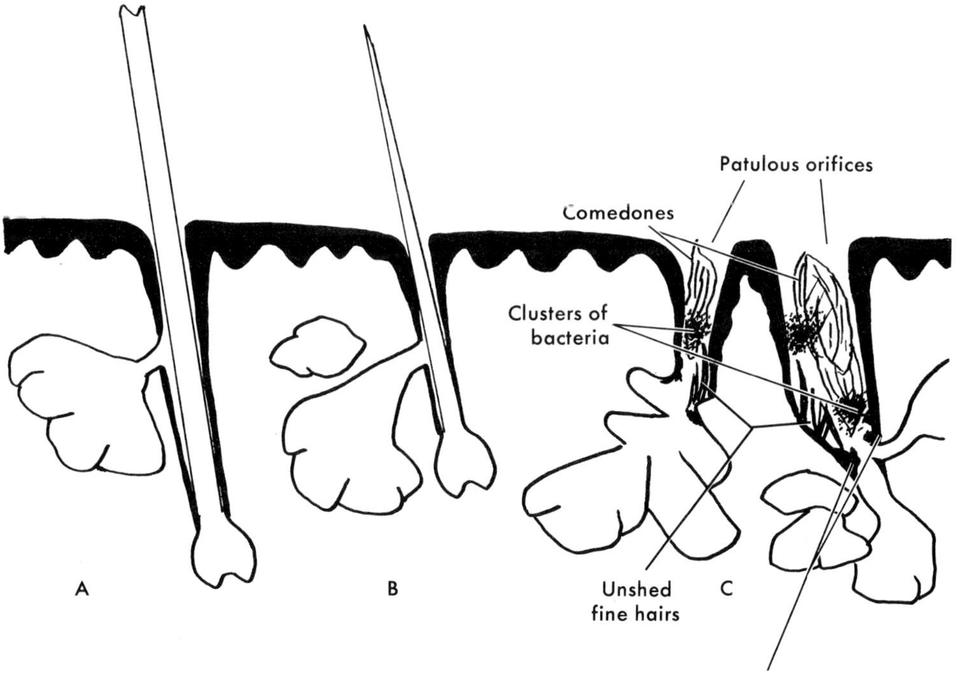


**Fig. 3-5.** Sebaceous glands in relation to acne pathogenesis. **A,** Terminal hair and sebaceous gland. **B,** Vellus hair and sebaceous gland. **C,** Patulous sebaceous follicle and fine unshed hair structures, with comedone formation.

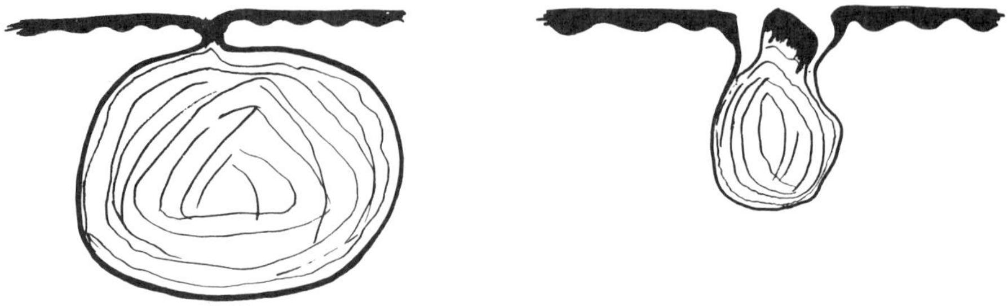


**Fig. 3-6.** Obstructed atrophic remnants of sebaceous glands. Keratinization is still taking place in walls. **A,** Whitehead or closed comedone. **B,** Blackhead or open comedone.

to rupture. Neutrophils begin to pass through the comedo wall, and when significant numbers collect, the wall softens and a microabscess forms. Later the area fibroses. Cysts are very large comedones. Inflammatory lesions derive from present or antecedent comedones (Knutson) (Fig 3-6).

Manipulating or squeezing the acne lesion plays a very important role in the perpetuation of acne. Oil or sebum production is a favorite villain on which to blame acne. However, the acne process subsides long before the increased oil production of the young adult begins to diminish.

Dietary factors are of less importance in the pathogenesis of acne than has previously been believed. Feeding acne patients excessive amounts of chocolate has shown little in the way of worsening of the disease. Grant first dissented from a set view on this subject, and Fulton and co-workers carried out convincing studies to refute the dietary effect of chocolate patients with acne.

The combination of heat and humidity that occurs in tropical areas produces severe acne in some individuals.

There is no disease that produces more psychic trauma, maladjustment, insecurity, and feelings of inferiority than does acne. There is no reason to believe that a patient's psychological makeup causes the lesions (Whitlock).

***Oil acne, chloracne.*** Certain occupational hazards give rise to acne. The oil- and grease-contaminated clothing of workers can produce acneiform papules and pustules, certainly over the thighs and forearms. Cutting oils, crude petroleum, and vegetable oils have been identified as comedogenic. Certain halogenated compounds used in the coating of electrical wires and in the lumber industry as wood preservatives produce numerous persistent acneiform lesions (chloracne) (Fig. 3-7) because of their comedogenic action. Polychlorobiphenyls, chlorobenzenes, polychlorinated dibenzofurans, and chloronaphthalenes are all chloracnegenic. Severe and extensive acne may be very difficult to treat. Also, new lesions may continue to appear after exposure has ceased. Taylor reported on 41 employees of an Ohio factory where 90% of the workers were affected, most within 1 to 2 months of their first exposure. Topical retinoic acid (vitamin A acid) may be beneficial in these cases, particularly the milder ones. Acne surgery is an aid as well.

***Cosmetic acne.*** Moisturizers, creams, and some cosmetics contain comedogenic compounds that add to the plugging of the follicles and frequently produce nonpigmented comedones and papules.

***Steroid acne.*** ACTH, androgenic steroids, gonadotrophins, anabolic steroids, and topical or systemic glucocorticoids may result in a form of acne with comedones, papules, and pustules. This form of acne does not seem to be associated with sebaceous hyperplasia. In certain predisposed individuals, this form of acne may be startlingly severe. It does not affect prepubertal or elderly individuals.

***Drugs.*** Bromides, iodides, diphenylhydantoin (Dilantin), phenobarbital, trimethadione, isoniazid, ethionamide, and rifampin can produce or aggravate existing acne vulgaris.

***Frictional or occlusive factors.*** Headbands,

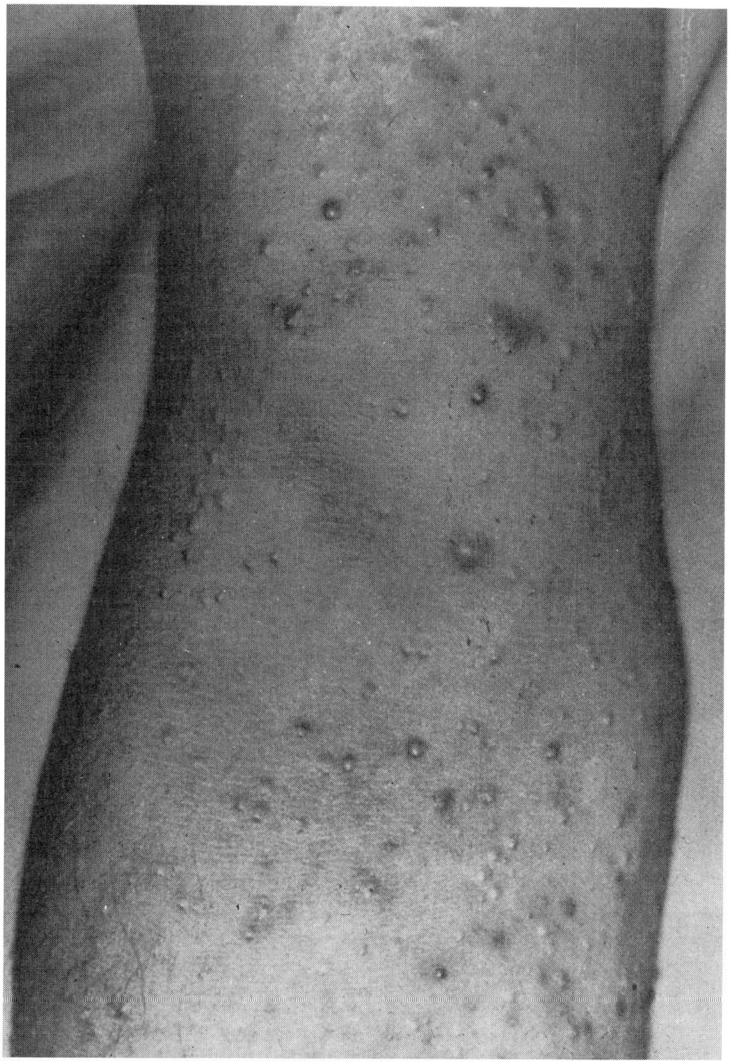

**Fig. 3-7.** Chloracne caused by chlorinated wood preservative.

shoulder straps, football shoulder pads, and other clothing that occludes acne areas may produce lesions, particularly with a hot environment.

***Hyperalimentation.*** Acne lesions resulting from deficiencies in hyperalimentation diets have resulted in explosive characteristic acne lesions. The reason for this is obscure.

### *Differential diagnosis*

***Furunculosis.*** Furunculosis (boils) consists of discrete, tender, pustular, indurated, erythematous lesions not limited to the acne distribution. Staphylococci can be cultured from the lesions.

***Rosacea.*** Rosacea occurs in patients in an older age group than that affected by acne. Pustules involve the central area of the face only, with a background of erythema.

***Folliculitis.*** Folliculitis occurs mostly in the bearded area in males, is associated with hair follicles, and consists of papules and pustules.

### *Treatment*

1. *Parents should be present at the first visit.*

2. The patient should be firmly told to avoid further squeezing or manipulation of the lesions.
3. An adequate and well-balanced diet should be encouraged.
4. It should be emphasized that sun exposure is beneficial.
5. Psychological factors play only a secondary role.
6. The patient should feel that he or she understands and can control the acne process. This requires careful explanation and repetition where needed.

**Treatment principle 1 (mild cases).** Regular shampooing of the scalp, at least twice weekly is desirable.

One of the abrasive soaps modified for use in acne should be used two times daily. Industrial hand cleansers such as Snap are inexpensive and satisfactory. Girls who are at first unused to soap will describe "tight" or "drawn" facial skin. This is only transient and will not be apparent in 2 or 3 weeks.

Absolutely no creams or moisturizers.

Exposure to natural sunlight should be recommended in moderation.

**Treatment principle 2 (moderate cases).** For comedones, papules, and pustules, a drying and peeling modality is recommended. If excessive or painful, frequency of application is decreased. Milder concentrations are used initially, and then stronger ones as needed, to maintain improvement.

***Expression of comedones.*** Careful expression of comedones is an acceptable procedure, as demonstrated by clinical studies, but only if properly carried out. It should be carried out by the physician. Inflamed comedones or pustules should not be touched. Reduction in the number of comedones reduces the number of subsequent papular and pustular lesions.

1. A powder-base *shake lotion containing resorcinol and sulfur* has a twofold purpose. It acts as a cosmetically acceptable covering agent, as well as mildly but actively treating the acne process.

| | |
|---|---|
| Neutracolor or skin-coloring agents | q.s. |
| Precipitated sulfur | 5% |
| Resorcinol | 3% |
| Glycerin | 15 Gm. |
| Zinc oxide | 10 Gm. |
| Talc | 15 Gm. |
| Alcohol | 40 ml. |
| Water | 40 ml. |

Apply with fingers three times daily.

There are dozens of more costly commercial products available with similar formulations. They should not be greasy or occlusive. Lotions are preferable.

2. An alternative preparation would be one available commercially that contains *benzoyl peroxide*, an old and established keratolytic and antibacterial agent. This peeling compound does produce redness as well, and especially for fair complexions it should be begun at 5%. Gels, creams, and lotions are available. Cost is a factor, as most are equally efficacious.

3. *Topical antibiotics.* In the past 2 or 3 years, topical erythromycin and topical clindamycin have been demonstrated to be effective in mild to moderate acne. Clindamycin phosphate in 1% solution has demonstrated a strong suppressive effect on *C. acnes* in open comedones. A 1% solution in ethyl alcohol and propylene glycol can be easily prepared from capsules of clindamycin hydrochloride that is stable for 6 months (Algra). We find this a very suitable substitute for oral tetracycline in less than severe cases of acne. We use it after washing, applied with fingertips twice daily.

Erythromycin base 2%, also in an alcohol–propylene glycol base, appears on clinical usage to be almost equally effective in our clinic.

We believe that, started early in the course of acne, the abrasive soaps and topical antibiotics can probably prevent perifollicular scarring. This is, however, a difficult question to answer because of the very frequent occurrence of this form of scarring.

4. *Retinoic acid (vitamin A acid).* Retinoic acid is now widely used in acne for its primarily irritant, drying, and peeling qualities. It is used topically in 0.05% to 0.1% in such preparations as propylene glycol and creams and may cause more lesions before improvement occurs. It is said to be effective in the cystic variety as well (Mills).

5. *Ultraviolet light.* In addition to natural

sunlight, our standard procedure for this and more severe forms of acne, is weekly exposure to minimal erythema doses (we do *not* find that strong erythema is necessary). More intense exposures ordinarily are necessary for back and chest than for the face.

If acne affects the back of the neck, the hair *must* be cropped in that area.

**Treatment principle 3 (severe cases).** For those pustular and cystic lesions that cause scarring, one of the following regimens of systemic therapy may be effective in addition to the above.

***Antibiotics.*** The only antibiotics that are effective in acne are those that reduce the numbers of *C. acnes*. These organisms rarely show resistance to tetracycline. Oral tetracycline is an effective safe treatment, and in severe cases may be the only effective method of preventing severe scarring. Erythromycin is a safe rational alternative. Other systemic antibiotics may have undesirable or unwarranted risks.

Tetracycline or erythromycin is given in a dosage of four 250 mg. tablets per day for 7 days and then two per day for 7 days. The dosage is then adjusted for the individual by maintenance of the minimal possible amount to control the acne, down to one capsule daily or even every other day. Capsules should be taken with water, and not just before bed, as regurgitation may irritate the esophagus.

Tetracycline should not be prescribed during pregnancy because of its effects of mottling the teeth of the fetus. Grossman and colleagues have calculated the amounts of tetracycline capable of producing darkening of permanent teeth in children before 6 to 8 years of age. We do not prescribe it before 16 years of age when bones and teeth are fully formed. Reisner suggests 12 years of age.

***Glucocorticoids.*** Apart from the Pochi and Strauss report, systemic glucocorticoids are rarely indicated even in severe inflammatory acne, because they are so closely related to androgens. In some individuals, they have some androgenic effect, for example, pigmented hair growth. ACTH is never advisable.

We use injection of triamcinolone diacetate (intralesional) 5 mg./ml. in lidocaine hydrochloride for unresponsive cystic acne lesions. An injection of 0.1 to 0.5 ml. into a cyst will often result in a rapid regression. This must be done with care, first, because the cyst ruptures easily under pressure, and second, because stretching the cyst capsule is exquisitely painful. Absorption and measurable blood levels occur after injection.

**Other treatment measures**

***Hormones.*** Although the response is unpredictable, a significant number of female patients will respond well to estrogen-progestogen medications prescribed in a cyclic monthly routine. The progestogen component of the anovulatory (or birth control) medication should be a nonandrogen, such as norethynodrel or ethynodiol diacetate. Contraceptives containing norethindrone and norgestrel are androgen dominant and should not be used in acne-prone individuals. Side effects of estrogens include thromboembolic disease, gallbladder disease, stroke, myocardial infarcts, hepatic tumors, hypertension, and endometrial cancer. These must be weighed against the benefits obtained.

***Antiandrogens.*** If it can be proved that this family of compounds is safe, the use of specially antiandrogen medications would be rational for treatment of severe acne. Ebling and his colleagues have confirmed earlier European reports that one of these compounds, cyproterone acetate, is effective in improving acne when given cyclically in women from days 5 to 14 of the menstrual cycle. Topical use is preferable, and lack of other hormone activity necessary, for the ideal antiandrogen.

***Ultraviolet light.*** Ultraviolet light produces peeling of the keratin layer and reduces sebaceous gland obstruction and comedone formation. It should be used in increasing dosages, at least once weekly, and forms a basic part of acne therapy. The duration of treatment should be kept at a level to produce a minimal erythema dose.

***Cryotherapy.*** Solid carbon dioxide or $CO_2$ slush for peeling acne-affected areas has been accepted therapy for decades. It became less necessary with the advent of antibiotics. More recently, the availability of liquid nitrogen and other refrigerants (Leyden) has revived an interest in this modality. Liquid nitrogen is used on a cotton swab dipped from a larger container for speeding the absorption of cysts. Increasing the pressure and the duration increases the effect. Avoidance of scars requires experience. Probes and sprays are available, with instructions for use. They enhance peeling. Cryosurgery can be used to benefit hypertrophic scars and keloids that result from acne (Zacarian).

***Minor surgery.*** The practice of draining cystic lesions by incision and evacuating pustular lesions has not proved beneficial and produces scarring. Fortunately, the use of improved topical medications, antibiotics, and steroids has resulted in a far superior therapeutic result without cosmetic impairment.

***Dermabrasion.*** A corrective plastic procedure, dermabrasion is useful in the treatment of selected patients with acne scars. This is not a treatment for active acne lesions. Much of the early enthusiasm has waned, and the result has been a more selective choice of patients.

***Chemosurgery.*** Caustic chemicals such as trichloracetic acid applied with skill to the areas scarred by acne may be gratefully accepted by the patient. Some good results have been obtained by evening out the sharper edged scars.

***X-ray therapy.*** Superficial x-ray therapy is no longer widely used in acne because of the efficacy of modern methods of treating this disease and the inescapable hazard of the biological effects of radiation.

## REFERENCES


Ad Hoc Committee on the Use of Antibiotics in Dermatology. Systemic antibiotics for treatment of acne vulgaris, Arch. Dermatol. **111**:1630, 1975.
**Safe effective long-term therapy in appropriate doses.**

Algra, R. J., Rosen, T., and Waisman, M.: Topical clindamycin in acne vulgaris, Arch. Dermatol. **113**:1390, 1977.
**How to prepare a stable potent 1% solution in alcohol and propylene glycol.**

Cunliffe, W. J., and Cotterill, J. A.: The acnes. Clinical features, pathogenesis and treatment, Philadelphia, 1975, B. Saunders Co.
**Current information on the clinical dermatology and experimental pathology of acne.**

Cunliffe, W. J., Williams, M., Edwards, J. C., et al.: Chloracne. An industrial hazard, Acta Derm. Venereol. **55**:211, 1975.
**Industrial acne and acne vulgaris compared.**

Ebling, F. J., Thomas, A. K., Cooke, I. D., et al.: Effect of cyproterone acetate on hair growth, sebaceous secretion and endocrine parameters in a hirsute subject, Br. J. Dermatol. **97**:371, 1977.
**Promising effects on decreased hair growth, diameter, pigment, sebum and acne. Why acne?**

Emerson, G. W., and Strauss, J. S.: Acne and acne care, Arch. Dermatol. **105**:407, 1972.

Fulton, J. E., Jr., and Pablo, G.: Topical antibacterial therapy for acne, Arch. Dermatol. **110**:83, 1974.
**2% topical erythromycin effective in reducing free fatty acids.**

Fulton, J. E., Jr., Plewig, G., and Kligman, A.M.: The effect of chocolate on acne vulgaris, J.A.M.A. **210**:2071, 1969.

Grant, J. D., and Anderson, P. C.: Chocolate as a cause of acne; a dissenting view, Mo. Med. **62**:459, 1965.
**The first such analysis.**

Grossman, E. R., Walchek, A. Freedman, H., and Flanagan, C.: Tetracyclines and permanent teeth: the relation between dose and tooth color, Pediatrics **47**:567, 1971.

Kaidbey, K. H., and Kligman, A. M.: The pathogenesis of topical steroid acne, J. Invest. Dermatol. **62**:31, 1974.
**Not in children or senior citizens. Negates any use of topical glucocorticoids in acne.**

Kelly, A. P.: Acute febrile ulcerative conglobate acne with polyarthralgia, Arch. Dermatol. **104**:182, 1971.

Kligman, A. M.: An overview of acne, J. Invest. Dermatol. **62**:268, 1974.
**Acnegenic importance of minute intrafollicular unshed hairs and *C. acnes*.**

Kligman, A. M., and Mills, O. H., Jr.: Acne cosmetica, Arch. Dermatol. **106**:843, 1972.
**Comedogenic cosmetics.**

Knutson, D. S.: Ultrastructural observations in acne vulgaris; the normal sebaceous follicle and acne lesions. J. Invest. Dermatol. **62**:288, 1974.
**A superb piece of work.**

Leyden, J. J., Mills, H. O., Jr., and Kligman, A. M.: Cryoprobe treatment of acne conglobata, Br. J. Dermatol. **90**:335, 1974.
**Painless cryoprobes hastened cyst resorption. Spray is less desirable.**

Mills, O. H., Jr., and Kligman, A. M.: Acne mechanica, Arch. Dermatol. **111**:481, 1975.
**Various physical traumas provoke lesions in acne patients.**

Mills, O. H., Jr., Marples, R. R., and Kligman, A. M.: Acne vulgaris; oral therapy with tetracycline and topical therapy with vitamin A, Arch. Dermatol. **106:**200, 1972.
**Good results.**

Pochi, P. E., and Strauss, J. S.: Sebaceous gland inhibition from combined glucocorticoid-estrogen treatment, Arch. Dermatol. **112:**1108, 1976.
**Impressive sebum reduction and acne improvement.**

Puhvel, S. M., and Reisner, R. M.: Effect of antibiotics on lipases of *C. acnes in vitro*, Arch. Dermatol. **106:**45, 1972.
**Bacterial numbers reduced and so lipase is reduced.**

Puhvel, S. M., and Sakamoto, M.: A re-evaluation of fatty acids as inflammatory agents in acne, J. Invest. Dermatol. **68:**93, 1977.
**Not the prime inflammatory agent in acne.**

Reisner, R. M.: Rational therapy of acne vulgaris, Cutis **7:**175, 1971.
**The best balance of factual information and thoughtful principles of treatment.**

Resh, W., and Stoughton, R. B.: Topically applied antibiotics in acne vulgaris, Arch. Dermatol. **112:**182, 1976.
**In small numbers of patients topical erythromycin base and clindamycin phosphate were very effective.**

Sansone, G., and Reisner, R. M.: Differential conversion rates of testosterone to dihydrotestosterone in acne and in normal human skin—a possible pathogenetic factor in acne, J. Invest. Dermatol. **56:**366, 1971.
**An important finding.**

Sauer, G. C.: Safety of long-term tetracycline therapy for acne, Arch. Dermatol. **112:**1603, 1976.
**325 patients took tetracycline for 3 years or more, hepatic and renal test findings reported and discussed. Conclusion in general: such therapy is safe.**

Schlappner, O. L. A.: Acute papulo-pustular acne associated with prolonged intravenous hyperalimentation, J.A.M.A. **219:**877, 1972.
**Intriguing.**

Serious adverse effects of oral contraceptives and estrogens, The Medical Letter **18:**5:21, Feb. 27, 1976.
**A sobering provocative review of the price paid for contraception.**

Taylor, J. S., Wuthrich, R. C., Lloyd, K. M., et al.: Chloracne from manufacture of a new herbicide, Arch. Dermatol. **113:**616, 1977.
**More than 90% of the workers affected, more than one fourth severely.**

Whitlock, F. A.: Psychophysiologic aspects of skin disease, Philadelphia, 1976, W. B. Saunders Co., p. 171.
**A careful weighing of the factual evidence.**

Zacarian, S. A.: Cryosurgery of tumors of the skin and oral cavity, Springfield, Ill. 1973, Charles C Thomas, Publisher, p. 118.
**The authority.**

## Development, structure, and function of the apocrine glands

Apocrine glands are far fewer, more localized, and larger than the eccrine sweat glands to which they are often compared. They develop as an attachment to the hair follicle, as do the sebaceous glands, but they are slightly later appearing, around 17 weeks, and they extend eventually the full length of the hair follicle. The face and scalp develop vestigial glands that later disappear normally. Glands develop and remain in the axillae, external auditory meatuses, areolae, nipples, mons pubis, and genital, perianal, eyelid, and scalp areas.

The apocrine glands are small at birth, but from midchildhood to adolescence, they enlarge to full-sized adult glands and, when they begin to function, emit a characteristic axillary odor. Each gland has a large secretory coil (Fig. 3-8), some up to 2 mm. in diameter, lying deep in the dermis or even into the subcutaneous fat. Secretory cells are interdigitated with myoepithelial cells, both of which may contact the thick limiting outer basal lamina. The secretory coil connects to a long straight duct that parallels the hair follicle and usually empties into it in the infundibulum above the sebaceous gland. Some open onto the skin surface.

Apocrine secretion is turbid, milky, and slightly yellow. The glands produce a tiny droplet at long intervals. Apocrine secretion occurs after both adrenergic and cholinergic stimuli. In the axilla, the more profuse eccrine sweat diffuses the distinctly odorous apocrine secretion over a wider area. Axillary odor arises from gram-positive bacterial degradation of the apocrine secretion.

***Chromhidrosis.*** The secretion of colored sweat occurs at times in otherwise normal apocrine glands and has been reported from axillae and periorbital facial areas. Colored axillary sweat is usually yellow, but green, blue, or blue-black are seen. The color is attributable to lipofuscins.

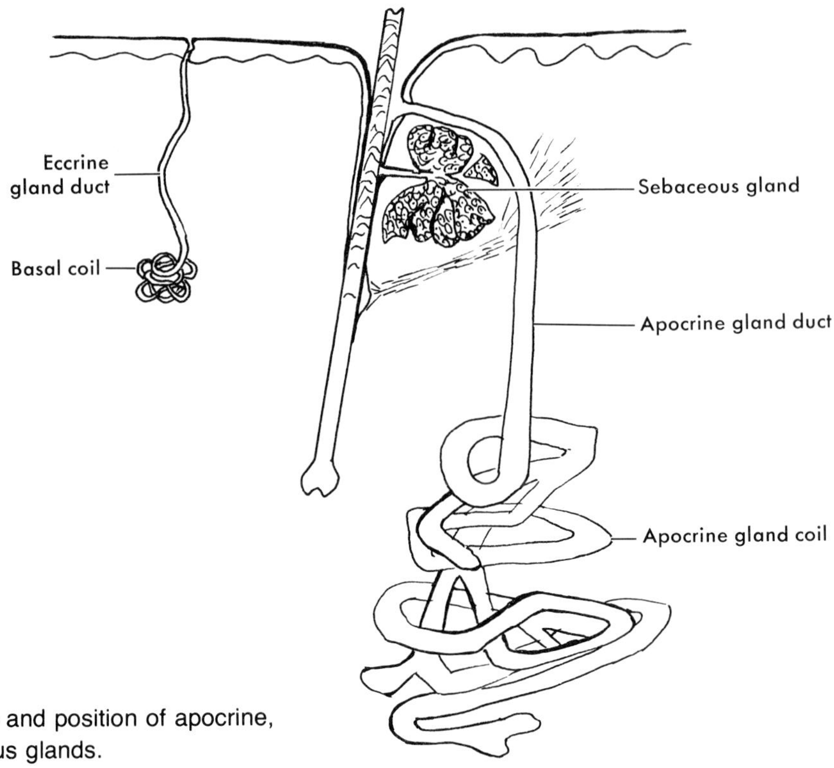


**Fig. 3-8.** Relative size and position of apocrine, eccrine, and sebaceous glands.

## HIDRADENITIS SUPPURATIVA

Hidradenitis suppurativa is an uncommon, painful, scarring, chronic, recurrent inflammatory disease of the apocrine glands.

The apocrine gland is first obstructed by a keratin plug. The lesion that begins as a tender red papule that rapidly evolves into a painful, deep-seated, reddish purple fluctuant tumor. This tumor may rupture, expelling a purulent discharge usually containing staphylococci. These invade the area obstructed by the keratin plug. Other organisms are present in large numbers, and no one consistent bacterial cause is apparent. The intense leukocytic reaction produces further inflammatory response. Adjacent lesions begin as isolated nodules, become confluent, and form a single, indurated, painful mass, limiting movement of the extremity (Fig. 3-9). The lesions may be multiple, chronic, and recurrent. In its early stages the disease may affect only a single site, but it may later go on to involve other apocrine gland–bearing areas. Because of the repeated attacks that are a major feature of this disease, the apocrine glands at the site are eventually destroyed and replaced with scar tissue, which may be extensive.

Most frequently this disease is seen in the axilla, less often in the perianal region. It occurs on the scrotum, vulva, or areola even more seldom. It can affect large areas of the body if allowed to progress. Dvorak was unable to demonstrate any host-defense defects, cellular or humoral.

### *Microscopic findings*

After the formation of the keratin plug, there is an infiltrate of neutrophils. The next stage is characterized by an infiltrate of chronic inflammatory cells associated with necrotic destruction of the apocrine gland and final replacement with scar tissue. The whole process occurs deep in the dermis in the vicinity of the deep convoluted secretory coil. Dense fibrosis and sinus tract formation are

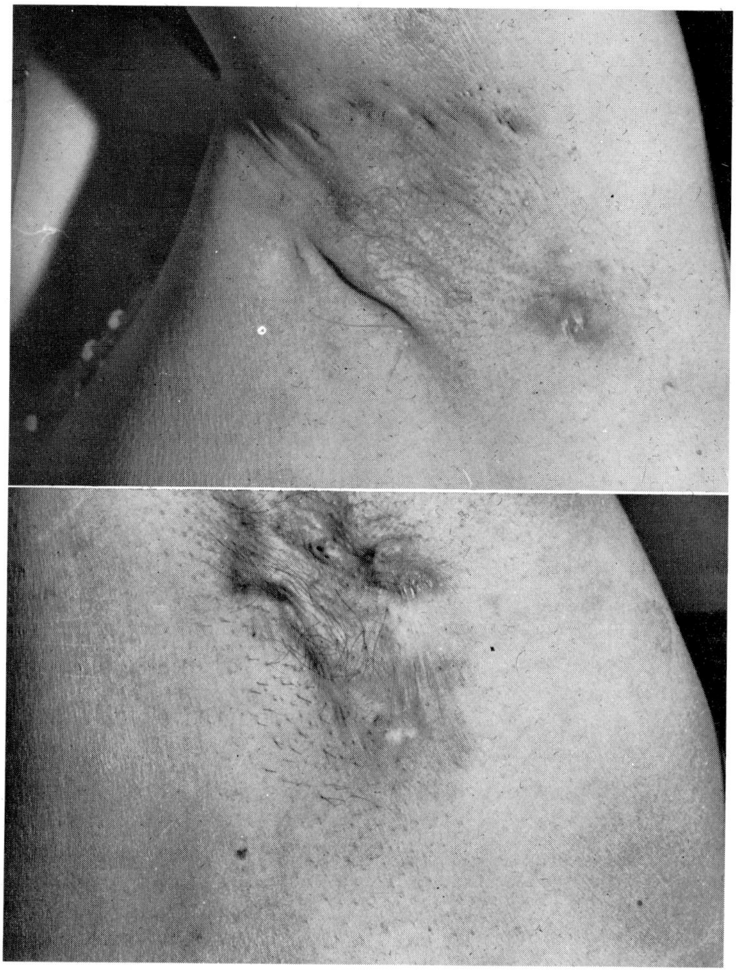

**Fig. 3-9.** Hidradenitis suppurativa.

common. Staphylococci are coagulase-positive; *Escherichia coli* and *Pseudomonas* are most commonly cultured.

### *Differential diagnosis*

***Furuncle.*** Furuncle clinically resembles hidradenitis suppurativa in the acute form only. It lacks the depth, chronicity, and destruction of hidradenitis.

***Cystic acne (acne conglobata).*** A severe form of acne to be differentiated from hidradenitis suppurativa consists of cystic lesions that become tender and indurated and are usually located on the face, neck, back, chest, outer aspect of the arms, and, occasionally, the buttocks.

***Sebaceous cyst.*** Sebaceous cyst is a skin-colored, nontender nodule that may be found on the scalp, back, chest, or scrotum.

### *Treatment*

Treatment can be difficult because of the inveterate tendency to recurrence and the appearance of new areas of involvement. Prompt and aggressive management is essential to avoid extensive scar formation.

Regular use of antiperspirants and deodorants should be discouraged in the involved axilla. Manipulation of lesions and shaving the area are to be avoided. Antiseptics containing hexachloraphene, chlorhexidene, or Betadine cleanser can be substituted.

Systematically administered wide-spectrum antibiotics should be prescribed according to culture and sensitivity studies of the exudate. It is usually necessary to prescribe high dosages, for example, 2 Gm. daily of tetracycline, erythromycin, and cephalosporin (1 to 1.5 Gm.) for 1- to 2-week periods.

Refractory cases may respond to supplementation of antibiotics by oral steroid therapy. As soon as it is apparent that recurrences and extension are not controlled by initial topical and systemic measures, a surgical approach should be entertained. Early rather than late, complete excision or exteriorization with removal of all diseased tissue will produce successful results. Incision and drainage is of no value.

#### REFERENCES

Dvorak, V. C., Root, R. K., and MacGregor, R. R.: Host defence mechanisms in hidradenitis suppurativa, Arch. Dermatol. **113**:450, 1977.
**No host-defence defects identified.**

Hurley, H. J., and Shelley, W. B.: The human apocrine sweat gland in health and disease, Springfield, Ill., 1960, Charles C Thomas, Publisher.
**The classic source of information.**

Masson, J. K.: Surgical treatment for hidradenitis suppurativa, Surg. Clin. North Am. **49**:1043, 1969.
**Early in the disease.**

Montagna, W., and Parakkal, P. F.: The apocrine glands. In The structure and function of the skin. New York, 1974, Academic Press, Inc., p. 332.

Newell, G. B., Voelter, W. W., and Mullins, J. F.: Treatment of hidradenitis suppurativa, J.A.M.A. **223**:556, 1973.
**Chronic cases do well with exteriorization and removal of all infected tissue.**

Reller, H. H., and Luedders, W. L.: Pharmacologic and toxicologic effects of topically applied agents on the eccrine sweat glands. In Marzulli, E. N., and Maibach, H. I., editors: Advances in modern toxicology: vol. IV, Dermatotoxicology and pharmacology, Washington, D.C., 1977, Hemisphere Publishing Corp.
**How deodorants work.**

Shelley, W. B., and Cahn, M. M.: The pathogenesis of hidradenitis suppurativa in man, Arch. Dermatol. **72**:562, 1955.
**Experimental blockage reproduced the disease.**

## ROSACEA

One of the most striking causes of a red face, rosacea combines pustules and erythema, sometimes causes enlargement of the nose, and often affects the conjunctivae.

### *Natural course*

The disease begins insidiously with intermittent redness of the face, usually affecting a person of one of the two predisposed types described below. The episodes of redness become more frequent and prolonged and are particularly evident around the blush areas of the central face, nose, forehead, and chin. Gradually a permanent redness and secondary telangiectasia develop.

At this stage or sometimes earlier the pustules, the second component of rosacea, make their appearance. These occur also around the central forehead, nose, malar areas, and central chin (Fig. 3-10). They are tender and ordinarily erythematous. Each lasts for several days. These may also affect the eyelids a condition that is never seen in acne.

If the person has a tendency toward seborrhea and oily skin, he will slowly develop a bulbous enlargement of the nose (rhinophyma) because of underlying sebaceous gland hyperplasia, although no increased sebum excretion rates seem to occur.

There may be an associated severe keratitis, with corneal vascularization and opacity. Blepharitis and conjunctivitis are frequently present; iritis occurs less commonly.

### *Pertinent information*

The illness tends to occur in two general types of persons: (1) the easy blusher, a person who has reddened easily from an early age, often for very little reason, and (2) the person who becomes red very easily from brief sun exposure.

Most commonly affected are women in their 40's and 50's. Rhinophyma is a late occurrence and is seen more often in men.

The etiology is undetermined, and although the obvious suggestion of a psychosomatic etiology has been made, detailed psychiatric studies have failed to convincingly reveal a personality type or disorder responsible for the clinical findings. A labile vasomotor system is operative, producing vasodilatation after exposure to heat and after ingestion of spices, vinegar, alcohol, and hot beverages. The exact mechanism of blushing remains poorly explained.

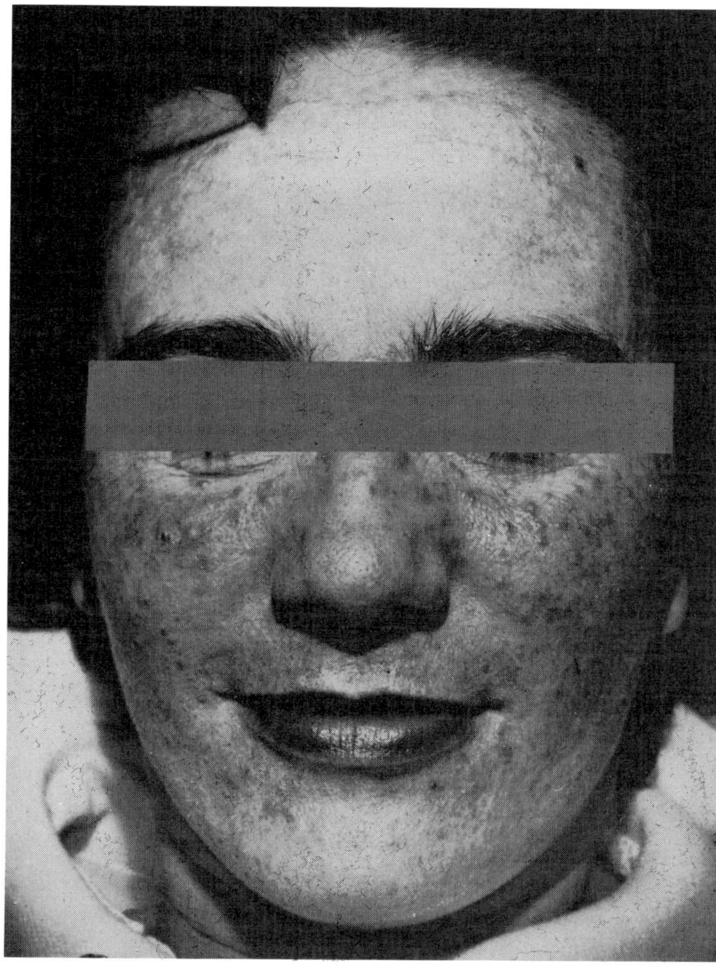

**Fig. 3-10.** Rosacea. There is no associated rhinophyma here.

There is no doubt that topical potent fluorinated *glucocorticoids* applied to the face will lead to rosacea. The difficult problem is to have the patient discontinue the steroid and suffer through at least 3 weeks of very much more severe rosacea, until subsidence begins to be apparent.

Sneddon and subsequently many others have described a suppression and then worsening of rosacea from the use of topical potent glucocorticoids. Sneddon and several British authors in fact attribute the *cause* of some forms of rosacea *entirely* to these agents. We now recognize the worsening of clinical rosacea with increased erythema, telangiectasia, and pustule formation as one of the adverse effects of potent topical glucocorticoids. Hydrocortisone, does not appear to worsen or produce this problem.

Marks reviewed 90 cases of rosacea and from studying them has concluded that the pathogenesis does not include bacterial, psychological, gastrointestinal, seborrheic, or extreme climatic causes. He found no important blood vessel abnormalities. Whitlock states: "A psychological component is more likely to be a consequence than a precursor of the eruption."

A mite that lives comfortably in the sebaceous follicles of the face, *Demodex folliculorum*, is found very frequently in rosacea patients. No one seems to have been able to make much of this, although several have tried. Grosshaus believes that it may be the cause of a sarcoid reaction seen microscopically in rosacea.

### *Microscopic findings*

In long-standing cases capillary and venular dilatation, a nonspecific inflammatory cell infiltration in the dermis, and scarring and fibrosis in the older lesions are seen. There is sometimes an epithelioid cell component with a tuberculoid pattern. The nose shows sebaceous gland hypertrophy and hyperplasia, sometimes to a remarkable degree.

### *Differential diagnosis*

***Acne vulgaris.*** The average age of the patient with acne vulgaris is far lower than that of the rosacea group. Acne does not include a noticeable erythema. Acne, however, may precede rosacea in later life.

***Seborrheic dermatitis.*** The oiliness and erythema but not the pustules may be seen in seborrheic dermatitis. Seborrhea may accompany rosacea.

***Folliculitis or staphylococcal pyoderma.*** Neither folliculitis nor staphylococcal pyoderma is associated with diffuse erythema or telangiectasia.

### *Treatment*

All topical fluorinated glucocorticoid applications are forbidden.

1. All factors leading to facial hyperemia should be avoided by the patient. These include ingestion of hot liquids and foods, spicy foods, alcohol, exposure to external irritants, and excessive environmental heat or cold.
2. Tetracycline, 250 mg., two or three times daily for 1-to 2-week periods, is prescribed at intervals frequent enough to prevent pustule formation. The tetracycline dosage may have to be doubled initially to control the more severe cases.
3. Sulfur applied topically has for years been accepted as having a beneficial effect. The following topical medications are recommended:

| | |
|---|---|
| Precipitated sulfur | 20% |
| Hydrocortisone | 1% |

Apply sparingly to affected areas twice daily.

4. The hair should be shampooed frequently to reduce oiliness.
5. The hyperplastic sebaceous glands deforming the nose may be successfully shaved off or removed by cryotherapy or dermabrasion by an operator skilled in any of these procedures. This produces a very satisfactory cosmetic result.
6. If the eye and its surrounding structures show a significant degree of involvement, ophthalmological consultation should be obtained.
7. Excessive sun exposure should be avoided, particularly in those individuals in whom minimal exposure produces redness.

#### REFERENCES


Burton, J. C., Meyrick, G., and Shuster, S.: The sebum excretion rates in rosacea, Br. J. Dermatol. **92**:541, 1975.

**No difference between 55 patients and 126 controls.**

Grosshaus, E. M., Kremer, M., and Maleville, J.: *Demodex folliculorum* and histogenesis of granulomatous rosacea, Hautarzt **25**:166, 1974.

Marks, R.: Concepts in the pathogenesis of rosacea, Br. J. Dermatol. **80**:170, 1968.

Marks, R., and Ellis, J.: Comparative effectiveness of tetracycline and ampicillin in rosacea; controlled trial, Lancet **2**:1049, 1971.

Sneddon, I.: Adverse effects of topical fluorinated corticosteroids in rosacea, Br. Med. J. **1**:671, 1969.

Weber, G.: Rosacea-like dermatitis; contraindications or intolerance reaction to strong steroids, Arch. Dermatol. **105**:541, 1972.

Whitlock, F. A.: Psychophysiological aspects of skin disease. Philadelphia, 1976, W. B. Saunders Co.

**A marvelous book.**

CHAPTER 4

# Cutaneous immunological diseases

## BASIC IMMUNOLOGY

The immune system consists of small uncommitted lymphocytes, committed or programmed lymphocytes, plasma cells, monocytes, macrophages, Langerhans cells, and complement. Other tissue and circulatory cells, neutrophils, basophils, mast cells, and eosinophils are called in to help as the occasion arises.

The cellular components of the immune system are able to recognize and destroy invading microorganisms, recognize and respond to offending simple foreign chemicals, identify elements of the body tissues that are altered by age or disease, and attack them as well. The cells produce antibodies that attach to the specific antigen that initiated their manufacture, enhance phagocytosis, and initiate inflammation. The attack on invading cells is largely mediated by complement initiated by these antibodies. The substances attacked are immunogens, or antigens. To be strongly antigenic, a compound needs to be a chemically complex foreign protein with a molecular weight over 10,000. However, a great variety of compounds quite different from these criteria may be antigenic.

The functions of the immune system include (1) surveillance of normally working tissue components of body functions, (2) warning of threats to normal function by foreign or internal antigens, (3) mobilization of body defense forces against a new antigen or against a new invasion by a recognized foreign antigen, (4) attack and destruction of the foreign or internal antigen.

Cutaneous disease of this system then falls into four categories:

1. A normal immune system misdirected against a foreign nonthreatening agent (allergy)—allergic contact dermatitis.
2. A normal immune system misdirected against the body's own antigens (autoimmunity, autosensitivity)—lupus erythematosus.
3. A deficient immune system—thymic aplasia, phagocytic dysfunction.
4. An immune system activated by unclear mechanisms and remaining functional—rheumatoid disease, Reiter's syndrome.

### Humoral immunity

After introduction to the body, antigen is taken up by macrophages and catabolized if possible. There is some evidence that the Langerhans cells in the epidermis may give warning of introduction through the skin of allergenic substances. If it cannot be degraded completely and rendered harmless, the fragments and conjugates of the antigen are capable of stimulating an immune response. This may be either humoral (antibody formation) or cellular (committed specifically programmed lymphocytes). If humoral, for example, in response to bacterial invasion, large lymphoblasts and plasma cells are produced upon antigen exposure. These are known as B-lymphocytes or B-cells, so named because of their phylogenetic counterparts in birds where their origin is from the bursa of Fabricius.

Upon stimulation by the antigenic conjugates, changes in lymphoid tissues of the body occur, with the formation of large numbers of antibody-secreting plasma cells and B-lymphocytes, largely contained in the paracortical and medullary areas of lymph nodes. From the time of first contact with an antigen, any significant antibody formation takes a minimum of 5 days. After development of the immune state, circulating antibodies are always

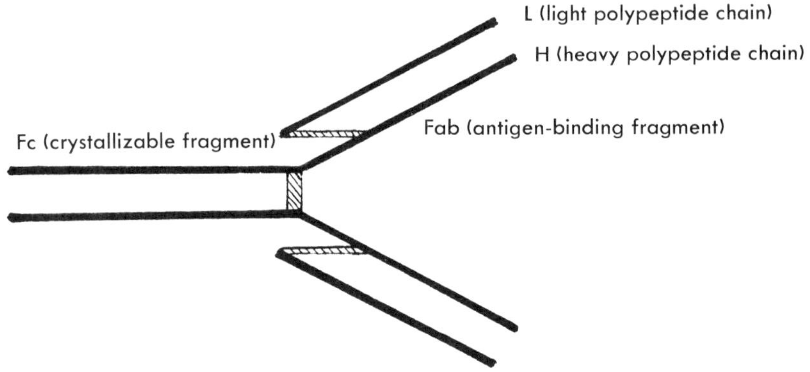


**Fig. 4-1.** Antibody structure. Basic unit or monomer of immunoglobulin $IgG_1$. *Hatched areas,* Disulfide bonds.

present and are capable of rapid supplementation on recontacting the antigen. *These are immune reactions of the immediate type.*

Antibodies are formed from B-lymphocytes and their progeny plasma cells and are referred to as *immunoglobulins.* They are subdivided into at least five classes, identified as IgG, IgA, IgM, IgD, and IgE. Antibodies have a variety of chemical characteristics and are dissimilar even within classes. They are composed of a family of closely related proteins, with overlapping physical and chemical properties. Each immunoglobulin molecule can be thought of as a Y-shaped structure or basic unit of *Fab,* or antigen-binding fragments with four polypeptide chains of amino acid sequences, and an *Fc,* a fragment that seems to retain complement fixation and other effects of the molecule (Fig. 4-1).

***Antibody classes.*** IgG is 75% of adult immunoglobulins. It has four genetically controlled subclasses—$IgG_1$, $IgG_2$, $IgG_3$, $IgG_4$. It can pass the placental barrier, is present in milk, uses complement, and is found in tissue fluid and plasma in nearly equal amounts. The higher the IgG level, the more rapidly it is destroyed. It is important in antibacterial activity, cytolysis, agglutination, precipitation, immune complex formation, and innumerable other areas.

IgA does not activate complement. It has antiviral and antibacterial activity. It is synthesized locally in secretions that are in contact with the external environment, saliva, gastrointestinal secretions, colostrum and prostatic fluid. It patrols respiratory and gastrointestinal membranes for known offending agents. It comprises 15% of total serum immunoglobulin.

IgM has an antibacterial effect and is mobilized early in the immune response. It has a molecule several times larger than the other immunoglobulins, and as a result is largely contained within blood vessels. IgM has a protective activity, combines best with larger antigens, and combines with complement to lyse antigens. It is a naturally occurring blood group antibody. It is 10% of adult serum immunoglobulin.

IgD is small in size and amount and is largely intravascular. Its activity is not well known. Predominant immunoglobulin on B-lymphocyte surfaces comprises 0.2% of total immunoglobulins.

IgE is a heat-labile, skin-sensitizing antibody and also has been identified as reagin. It is responsible for allergic disease, that is, most anaphylaxis and reactions in asthma, hay fever, and atopy. It also forms antibodies to parasites. It does not fix complement or cross the placenta. It is chiefly in tissues, being only transiently in the serum and has a particular ability to bind to mast cells and basophils. When antigen is present, the resultant IgE-antigen reaction causes discharge of histamine, bradykinin, and other vasoactive substances from the mast cell granules. cAMP and GMP are involved to modulate the speed and completeness of the histamine release (Fudenberg et al.). IgE is found, like IgA in secretory areas such as the nose, tonsils, adenoids, bronchioles, gastrointestinal mucosa, and urinary bladder. In the serum it constitutes 0.004% of total immunoglobulins.

## Cellular immunity

The second and distinct type of immunity is characterized by a delayed reaction time of 24 to 48 hours to maximal effect, between antigenic contact and allergic response, even after initial sensitization has taken place. This involves *cell-mediated* or *delayed immunity*. Circulating antibodies are not involved, although the two forms of immunity are closely related. Each is necessary for the normal functioning of the other. The ability to react with the antigen rests primarily with T-lymphocytes, or thymus-dependent cells that originally derived their integrity from that source. They are long-lived "memory" cells, and they carry cell-mediated immunity as opposed to their counterparts, the B-lymphocytes, which are non–thymus derived, short-lived antibody producers. The ratio of T-cells to B-cells is roughly 4:1. The T-cells are immunologically competent cells that after the initial antigen sensitization, which takes a minimum of 5 days, become "committed" lymphocytes, capable of reacting with antigen, which is usually tissue fixed. They participate in cyto toxic "killer cell" functions, homograph rejections, tuberculin sensitivity, contact type of dermatitis, fungal sensitivity, reactions to parasites, and some drug reactions.

When sensitized lymphocytes meet their specific antigen, they produce lymphokines, or effector substances. These attract and hold macrophages (MIF), and polymorphonuclear leukocytes (LIF), cause proliferation and antibody production of "noncommitted" lymphocytes (LMF), and transfer delayed hypersensitivity to them (transfer factor). There are also cytotoxic factors, interferons, erythema-producing agents, and other factors that participate in the immune response to the presence of the antigen. cAMP, histamine, and other compounds affect the production of these mediators.

The immunological memory of the antigen is passed on from the initially sensitized cells to other, distant nodes until the whole skin is alerted and sensitized, with the nearer areas achieving the earliest sensitization.

Cross-sensitization occurs when a substance closely related chemically to the original antigen sets off the immune reaction and an inflammatory response to the related chemical is established.

The basic immune mechanisms have been described. Recent work has demonstrated refinements of these functions. In T- and B-lymphocyte function, it has become apparent that T-cells have subpopulations of

1. helper T-cells, which
   a. amplify antibody synthesis by B-cells
   b. amplify cytolytic activity of T-cells
2. suppressor T-cells, which moderate both B and T, all functions.

Some B-cells accentuate and encourage T-cell killer function, whereas others may directly or indirectly block the reaction. This emphasizes the interdependence of these two facets of the immune effector system (Fig. 4–2).

## Complement system

This is a series of more than 15 protein components that together act as the primary effector of antigen-antibody reactions. Each component is present in the serum as a precursor of the active form and must be activated sequentially for the reaction to progress. Activation of complement leads to cell membrane damage; cell lysis; release of kinin, histamine, and lysosome enzyme; chemotaxis; B-cell activation; and preparation of cells for phagocytosis (Fig. 4-3).

Components are numbered $C_1$, $C_2$, $C_3$, etc., in the classic activation process, and those in the alternate, or more recently described properdin pathway, are lettered IF, P, B, D. Fragments of the components are sub-lettered $C_4$, $C_{4a}$, $C_{4b}$.

This is an integrated system that has a major physiologic role in maintenance of health and in localizing and destroying offending agents in disease. It is controlled and inactivated by serum proteins and by self-limiting character of its components. It is activated by a variety of substances including IgG and IgM. These

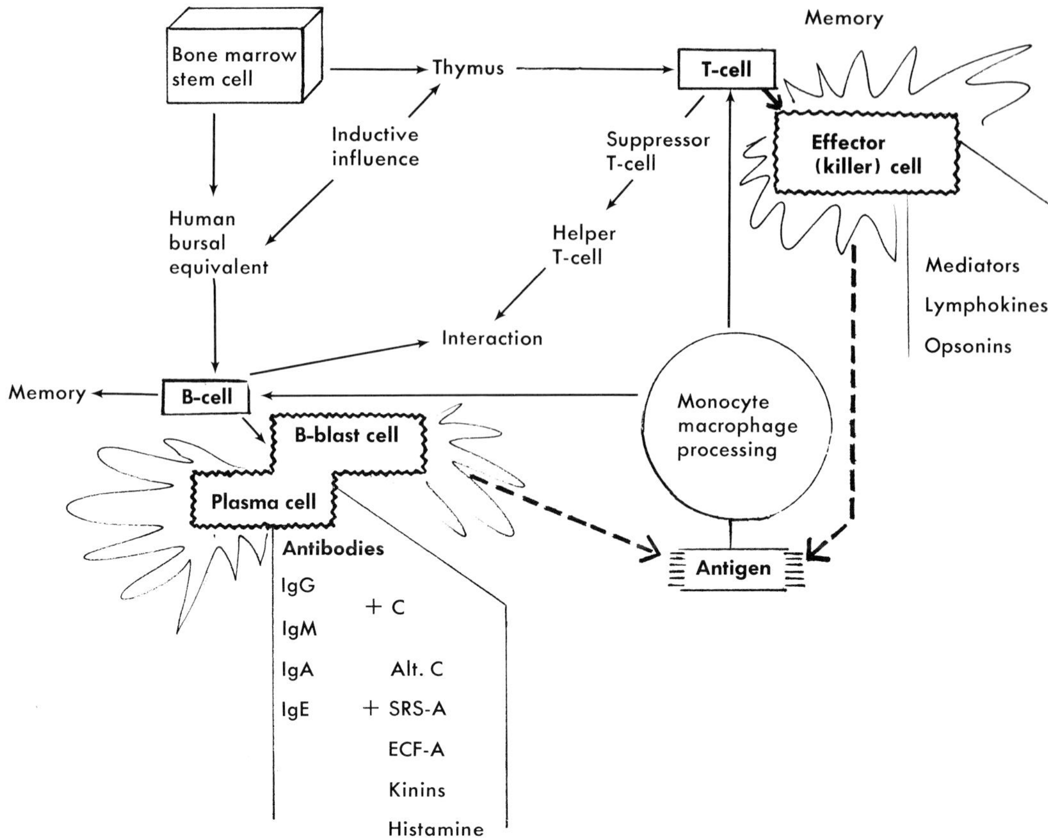


**Fig. 4-2.** Some interdependent aspects of the immune response.

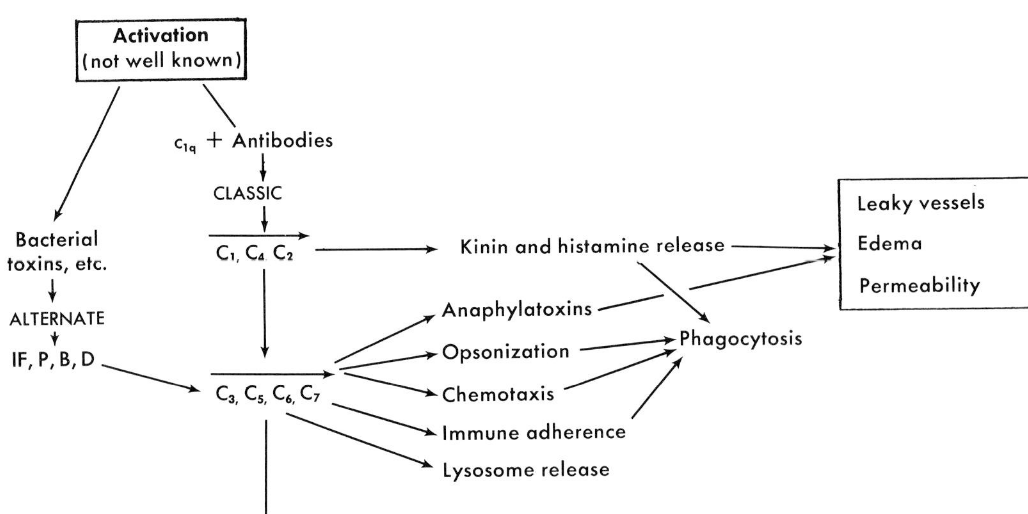


**Fig. 4-3.** Effects of complement system upon activation. *IF,* Initiating factor.

antibodies identify the offender by linking with it. The resulting antigen-antibody complex specifically activates the intricate complement system that then effects its destruction.

## HL-A system

The system by which a person receiving a graft recognizes the foreign nature of that graft, is the HL-A antigen system. These antigenic determinants are products of a closely linked cluster of genes on chromosome 6. This region is the major histocompatability region from which self-identifying protein markers arise, which are embedded on surfaces of most cells. These antigens give the tissues of each individual their own chemical identity. They are present through evolution back to the first vertebrates. There are many HL-A antigens in humans, some of which are strong and some are weak. The strong antigens, after graft recognition, cause the graft to be destroyed within 14 days. Weaker antigens take longer.

The structure of the HL-A antigens closely resembles some portions of the antibody molecule. If they are normally formed, the cell upon whose outer membrane they are embedded, is safe. If, however, one of these antigens is transformed, either by virus action, or by other disease processes, the lymphocytes will recognize them as foreign and identify them to the killer T-cells, who will attack and destroy them, as they would a foreign graft.

These antigens can be used to identify individuals, families, and races. They are important in identifying inherited diseases that show a high association with an HL-A pattern, such as ankylosing spondylitis and HL-A B27. Their future usefulness will be profound. However, at present, they are primarily used for identification of donor-recipient pairs for organ transplantation.

## Autoimmunity (immunologic self-injury)

Autoimmunity is a major immunologic phenomenon that identifies the immune response to aging, viral infections, and other situations where normal structures are altered so that they are not recognizable as "self" by the patrolling surveillance lymphocytes. It may result in cell or host death, or in transient mild illness. It may be transient or permanent.

To produce self-injury, immunologic tolerance to tissue and cellular self-antigens must be lost or overcome. This involves the self-identifying HL-A system by which all cells are marked as self. Certain virus infections may produce host-virus tissue antigens that are intolerable, or an imbalance in the delicate T-cell regulation of immune surveillance may be the initiating factor. Possible autoimmune disorders include Hashimoto's thyroiditis, thyrotoxicosis, some encephalopathies, atrophic gastritis, vitiligo, halo nevus, alopecia areata, polyarteritis nodosa, lupus erythematosus, pemphigus, pemphigoid, herpes gestationis, and the like.

## Types of immune reaction

***Type I: immediate reactions.*** Anaphylaxis is an antigen-antibody reaction that is immediate; that is, it may take place in minutes from the time of reexposure to the antigen.

The antigens include environmental proteins such as antiserum pollens, food, and drugs. The antibody is IgE. These are allergic reactions in which antibody is surface bound to the mast cell or basophil, and with antigen contact, histamine or kinins are released together with other vasoactive substances such as slow-reacting substance of anaphylaxis (SRS-A), eosinophil chemotactic factor of anaphylaxis (ECF-A), and prostaglandins. The effect ordinarily passes in 6 weeks as IgE persists at the site for that duration.

The reaction includes discharge of histamine and kinins from mast cells and basophils as well as substances from leukocytes and other sources. The reaction may involve not only the skin, but also other organs or tissues. Swelling, wheezing, abdominal pain, and other symptoms may be produced. The reaction may be fatal, but is ordinarily transient and short lived. Examples are *urticaria, anaphylactic drug reaction, asthma,* and *hay fever.*

***Type II: cytotoxic reactions.*** Humoral reactions can be cytotoxic, mediated by IgG or

IgM affecting the tissue site or cell membrane. Complement is fixed and cell lysis, inactivation, or phagocytosis occurs. Some type II reactions, however, result in cell stimulation (for example, long-acting thyroid stimulator, LATS) or blocking antibody effects. Reactions in which the antibody is specifically shaped to attach to cellular antigens so that the cell is rendered vulnerable to destruction by the antibody-antigen union, are cytotoxic reactions. *Purpura* caused by apronalide (Sedormid) sensitivity, some hemolytic anemias, hemolytic disease of the newborn, and some autosensitization effects are examples of this type of reaction. The homograft rejection response is in this category.

***Delayed-sensitivity reactions.*** In some reactions the clinical response to the antigen-antibody union is not immediate, but becomes apparent only after 48 to 72 hours. The cutaneous reaction is erythematous or indurated and is associated with a mononuclear cell infiltration that begins in a perivascular localization and takes time to accumulate. It is a cell-mediated response. Examples of delayed sensitivity reactions are *bacterial infections* (for example, tuberculosis), *fungal infections* (for example, coccidioidomycosis), *allergic contact dermatitis* and *homograft rejection response*. Organ transplants are subject to this type of reaction and to a cytotoxic effect as well. The reaction is accelerated and more intense if performed a second time, when the sensitized cells are again confronted with tissue or cells from the same donor.

***Type III: Arthus reactions.*** These are local reactions in the sensitized tissues between circulating antibodies and antigen in excessive concentration at the local site. Complement is activated. Chemotactic and vasoactive substances are liberated, with leaky vessels produced. Lysosomes of the leukocytes are damaged, and their contents produce the local damage. Fibrin is deposited in vessel walls. Repeated injections of *foreign protein*, such as serum, are one cause. Other examples are *serum sickness type of reactions*, *poststreptococcal glomerulonephritis*, and some form of *vasculitis*.

*Serum sickness.* Three to 21 days after injection of foreign serum, it produces urticaria, fever, malaise, and arthralgia often with erythematous patches. Lymphadenopathy may be noted. It is attributable to intravascular soluble immune complexes.

*Immune complex diseases.* These immune complex diseases (Fig. 4-4) are the most important disorders of the human immune sys-

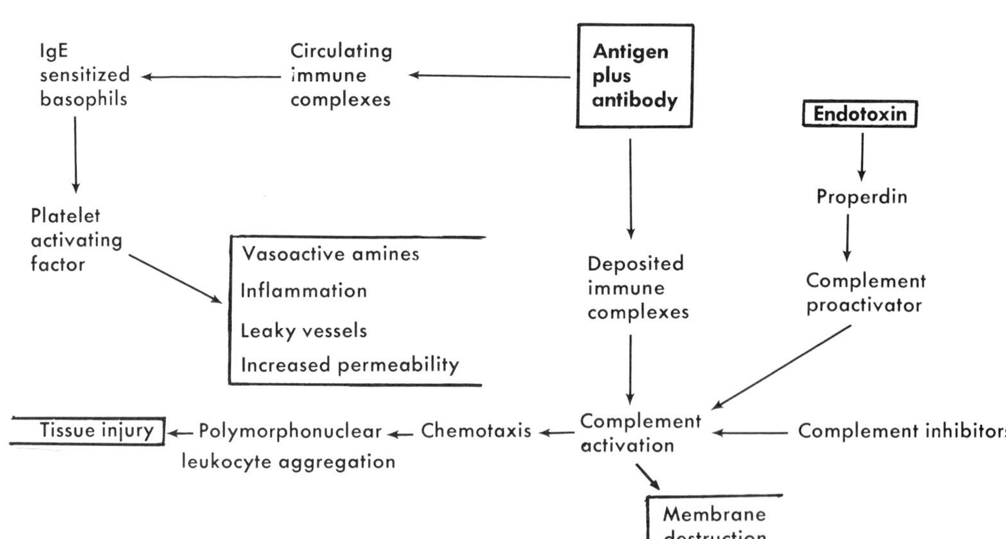


**Fig. 4-4.** Immune complex disease.

tem. Their mechanism is similar to that in Arthus and serum-sickness reactions, but the presentation of the antigen may be continual, as from endogenous nucleic acid antigens from damaged cells, or infection from a persistent source. IgG and IgM participate and form dynamic, constantly changing antigen-antibody complexes, which may activate complement.

The renal glomeruli are the chief site of deposition of immune complexes. Diseases related are bacterial and viral infections, parasitic infestations, autoimmune disorders, cancer, drug reactions, dermatitis herpetiformis, and ulcerative colitis.

***Type IV: cell-mediated reactions.*** These reactions develop 24 to 48 hours after antigen contact with sensitized lymphocytes. The reaction is produced by lymphokines, other cellular elements and cell products, recruitment of further lymphocytes so that the inflammation and tissue damage may extend beyond the destruction of the original focus. Cytotoxic killer cells are activated. Complement is not involved.

These mechanisms of immune reactions are amplified and enhanced by vascular changes, blood coagulation system, kinin system, and the fibrin-fibrinolysin system, each of which affect, and is affected by, inflammation.

## Transfer factor

As our understanding of the mechanism and functioning of the immune system has increased, it has become more feasible to intervene therapeutically in diseases of overfunction and underfunction. Transfer factor is a dialyzable extract of immune leukocytes that transfers positive cellular immunity between individuals. Taken from a specific antigen-reactive donor and given to a recipient with no delayed reaction to the same antigen, the recipient will from then demonstrate a positive cellular immune response to that specific antigen.

Transfer factor enhances reactivity of lymphocytes now specifically and may assist in recruiting noncommitted cells. Its mechanism of action, however, is not well defined.

Problems have prevented accurate assessment of its effects and rational selection of donors. Reproducible in vitro tests for assessment of immune function have not been available.

It is prepared from isolated blood leukocytes, one unit being defined as the dialysate from $5 \times 10^8$ leukocytes and is given subcutaneously in normal saline.

Its side effects are local pain, slight fever, and mild fatigue. Its use has been confined to immunodeficiency diseases, infections, and tumors, and cases as yet are too few or incomplete to be accurate regarding its benefit.

## Immune system deficiency

Recurrent cutaneous infections in children may be the clinical sign of defective leukocyte function because of immune system disease. Persistent vesicular dermatitis in flexures, apart from atopy, are present in some immune system diseases, and a child with recurrently infected recalcitrant nonhereditary eczema should be investigated for failure of immune defenses.

Oral candidosis and subsequent persistent unresponsive cutaneous candidosis in infants past 6 months should arouse suspicion of T-cell deficiency. Resistant infantile inability to resist deep-seated staphylococcal infection, with large cervical lymph nodes, cutaneous abscesses, sinus tracts, and facial granulomas in the modern hospital must make one think of a disorder of granulocyte or phagocyte function such as chronic granulomatous disease of childhood. This introduces the close interrelationships between leukocyte and phagocyte function and the integrity of the immune system, well described by Weston.

### REFERENCES


Adler, L. M., Reich, N. E., and Clough, J. D.: Transfer factor and the immune system, Cleveland Clin. **41** (3): 127, 1974.

**Amplifier of immune response, measured by immunofluorescence production.**

Buckley, R. H.: The functions and measurement of human B and T lymphocytes, J. Invest. Dermatol. **67**:381, 1976.

**Depressed cell-mediated immunity in eczema unexplained.**

Co-operative study: Uses for immunofluorescence tests of skin and sera, Arch. Dermatol. **111**:371, 1975.
**Are you making enough use of the immunofluorescence facilities available to you?**

Fudenberg, H. H., Stiles, D. P., Caldwell, J. L., and Wells, J. V.: Basic and clinical immunology, Los Altos, Calif. 1976, Lange Medical Publications.
**Clearly explained and well diagrammed.**

Gigli, I.: Immunochemistry and immunobiology of the complement system, J. Invest. Dermatol. **67**:346, 1976.
**108 references.**

Good, R. A., and Fisher, D. W.: Immunobiology: current knowledge of basic concepts in immunology and their clinical applications, Stamford, Conn., 1971, Sinauer Associates.
**A classic.**

Henney, C. S.: Killer T-cells, New Engl. J. Med. **291**:1357, 1974.
**Once they are committed, how do we subvert these determined killers?**

Hong, R., and Amman, A. J.: Cutaneous signals of host defense failure, Int. J. Dermatol. **16**:627, 1976.
**Warning diagnostic signs of immune decompensation.**

Rocklin, R. E.: Mediators of cellular immunity, their nature and assay, J. Invest. Dermatol. **67**:372, 1976.
**Seventeen of them.**

Roitt, I. M., Greaves, M. F., Torrigiani, C., et al.: The cellular basis of immunological responses, Lancet **2**:367, 1969.
**Expressed with a clarity that cannot be improved.**

Weston, W. L.: Disorders of phagocyte function, Arch. Dermatol. **112**:1589, 1976.
**Leukocyte-phagocyte B and T cell interrelations.**

## ALLERGIC ECZEMATOUS CONTACT DERMATITIS

An acute inflammatory reaction of the skin, allergic eczematous contact dermatitis is attributable to simple, direct contact with a substance to which the skin has become allergic (Plate 9). It is a cell-mediated type 4 form of immunity. It is an allergy because the antigen is environmental.

### *Natural course*

***Initial lesion.*** Erythema, sharply limited to the area of contact with the causative agent, is the first apparent change in the skin. Depending on the duration of contact and the intensity of the reaction, this inflammation may develop quite rapidly into an intense inflammatory response, with a moist surface and localized edema. With the erythema, small pruritic papules may form. Vesicles then begin to appear and enlarge, rupture, and crust over. If the process is severe enough, the vesicular reaction proceeds to the formation of large bullae.

Without further contact with the agent and without complications, healing occurs over a period of a few days to a few weeks. Further contacts with the causative agent, however, produce an intensification of the reaction, making it both more rapid and more severe. The process is intensely pruritic and is accompanied by a burning, stinging sensation that dispels sleep and rest and demands attention. This frequently results in the patient's applying various home remedies, many of which are irritating and some of which are allergenic. These very often aggravate and complicate the clinical picture. Because of the moist surface, the lesion is often colonized by staphylococci and a mild or significant secondary infection is superimposed.

***Spread.*** If the original area of dermatitis is repeatedly irritated, new sites of similar-appearing dermatitis will appear. These may be adjacent to the original site at first but will soon develop in areas distant from it. In this way, a generalized, acute, cutaneous inflammation can be seen to develop from a small, initial, localized patch of contact dermatitis.

***Severity.*** Generally speaking, the severity of the reaction depends on the duration of contact. For instance, an article of clothing with a dye or finish to which the patient is allergic will produce a more severe reaction if worn for 8 hours than one worn for a few minutes only.

Most individuals are repeatedly exposed without becoming sensitized, and some will become sensitive only after years of exposure; but after the development of sensitivity, the causative substance will produce an allergic dermatitis in from minutes to hours after contact. The history of the onset of the dermatitis is thus very important for determining the causative substance. The more frequent the contact, the more rapidly the subsequent reaction will follow, and the more violent the reaction will be.

An allergic contact dermatitis is enhanced

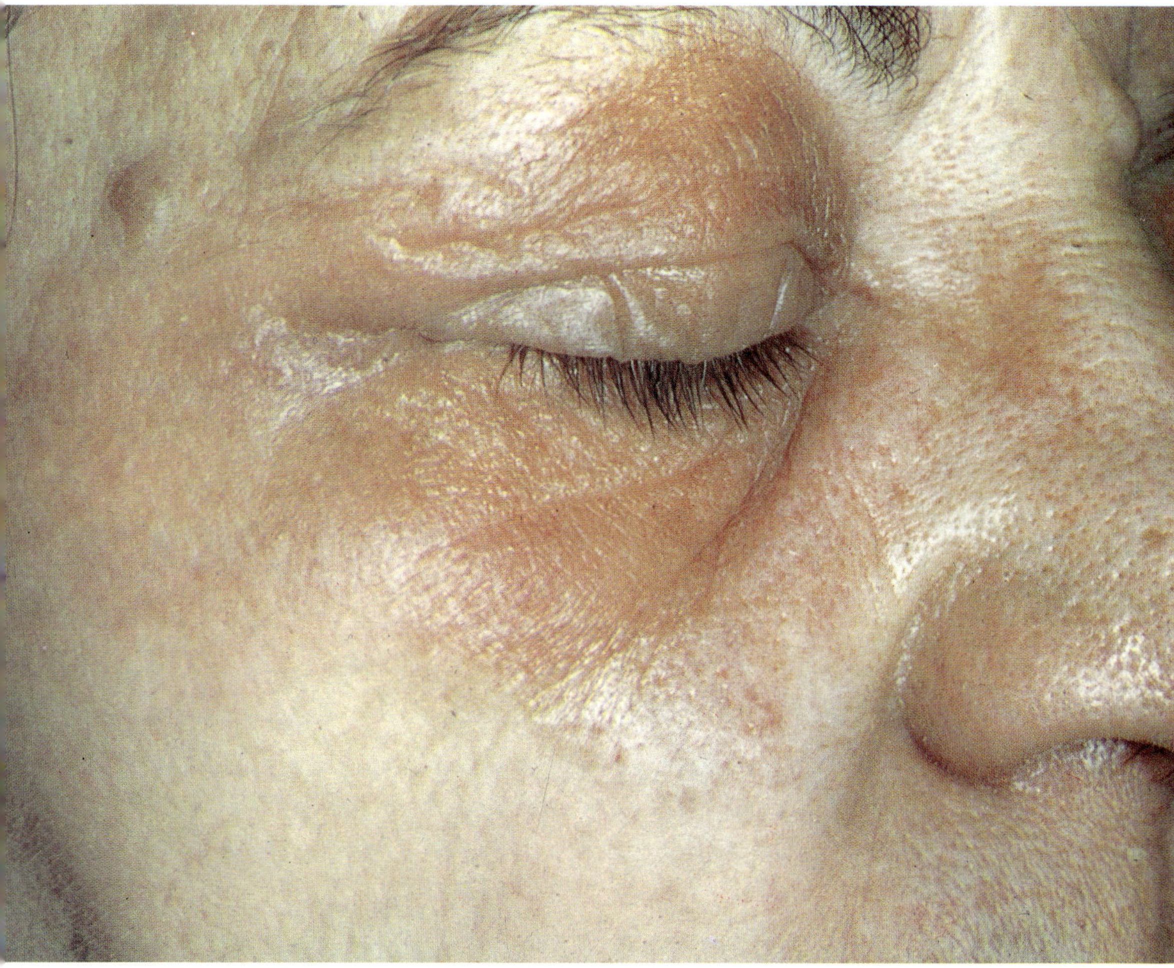

**Platc 9**

Allergic contact dermatitis caused by ointment. Note erythema, edema, and vesiculation.

by friction and pressure, so that when these factors are added to simple contact, the reaction is more severe.

***Chronicity.*** An allergic response may persist for 7 to 10 days after a single exposure. In *prolonged* or *recurrent* cases the sites of contact with the causative substance may become thickened, dull, erythematous, scaling, and chronically pruritic. These lesions become more difficult to clear satisfactorily because a general, nonspecific, increased susceptibility to irritation of all kinds develops. This "polyvalent sensitivity" to any and all irritants develops into a chronic irreversible dermatitis, and *the individual becomes badly handicapped.*

Sensitivity persists and may be heightened with reexposure but lessens and may even disappear with complete lack of contact with the allergen. Potent allergens, though, do produce a degree of sensitivity that is most likely to persist. It seems that a strong immune reaction is most likely to remain in immunological "memory."

However, there are instances in which workmen with an allergic contact dermatitis may become tolerant to the allergenic substance on repeated and continued exposure to it. This is referred to as *hardening* and is well known to those who work with sensitizing chemicals. This does not occur in all individuals, and it may disappear if the exposure is discontinued for any length of time. Mitchell has reviewed this area, as well as the genetic aspects of immunological tolerance.

***Sweat retention*** (p. 505). During recovery from a contact dermatitis the complication of sweat retention may occur. This is produced by obstruction of the sweat duct openings, with rupture of the duct and extrusion of sweat into the surrounding tissue, where it produces a pruritic response. This is often

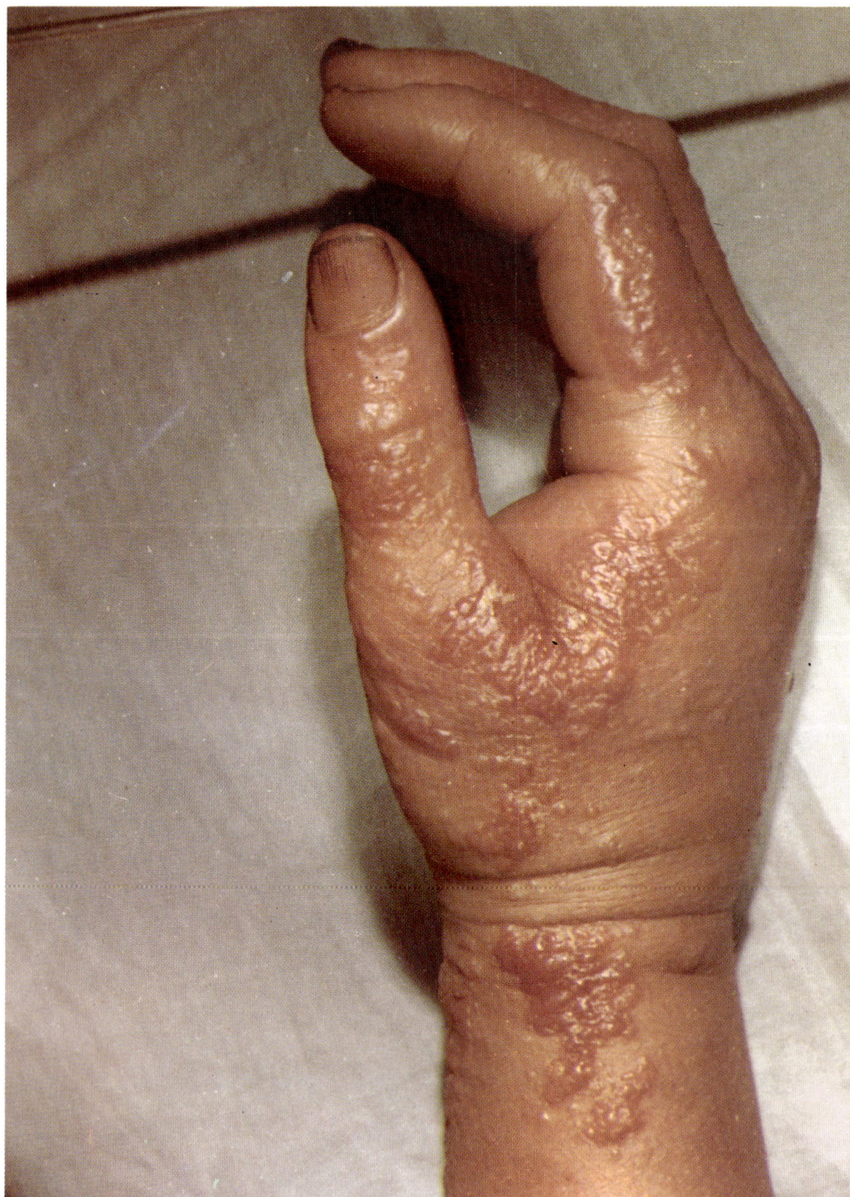

**Plate 10**

Acute allergic contact dermatitis caused by onion.

mistaken clinically for a recurrence of the allergic dermatitis, because there is an increase in inflammation and pruritis. Rubbing and further external irritation intensify the process of sweat retention. To prevent this complication, one must avoid exposure to excessive heat, increased perspiration, friction, and occlusive bandages and must use well-ventilated covering or clothing, cool baths, and soothing lotions.

***Mechanism of production of signs.*** Allergic contact dermatitis is a misdirected massive reaction of an apparently normal immune system to a trivial foreign invader. The chemical offender may be a simple compound and needs to combine with an epidermal protein in order to act as an antigen. Such a compound is called a *hapten*. After the hapten penetrates the stratum corneum, it is probably first processed and conjugated to protein by Langerhans cells (Shelley, 1977) and then a delayed cellular immunity reaction is set in motion. Langerhans cells or macrophages transport the hapten-protein complex to the regional nodes. Committed lymphocytes develop and are attracted to the presence of further antigen, where they will release lymphokines. Shortly after, macrophages appear to become the predominant cell. After the appearance of the mononuclear cells, 8 hours or so after antigen application, one sees intercellular edema, spongiosis, and then intracellular edema and gross vesicle formation. There is also increased vascular permeability and edema, endothelial, pericyte and mast cell changes, and fibrin deposition (Dvorak). The inflammation may be severe (Plate 10). Basophils and mast cells participate in the reaction as well.

### *Etiology*

***Chemicals commonly causing allergic contact dermatitis*** (Fig. 4-5). Common causes of allergic contact dermatitis vary somewhat as life styles change and new chemicals are brought into our clothing, leather goods, cosmetics, medications, and daily environment. The North American Contact Dermatitis Group in 1975 reported on the allergens that produced positive patch test reactions in some 3,200 patients tested (Table 2).

All allergens do not sensitize with equal incidence. Some, such as paraphenylenediamine, found in hair and textile dyes, will produce allergy in a greater number of individuals than will many other compounds (Plate 11). Formaldehyde is similarly a potent sensitizer, and unexpected sources of strong antigens in shoe dermatitis are chromate solution, rubber (in glues), and formaldehyde, and Dahl has shown that these are the most common shoe sensitizers. Some compounds, such as dinitrochlorobenzene, are used experimentally with the expectation that they will produce sensitivity. Certain individuals are more prone than others to develop allergic contact dermatitis. Walter and colleagues present evidence to show that there is a genetic individual predisposition to the development of allergic sensitivity. If only certain members of the resting lymphocyte population can react to specific antigens, and the numbers of these lymphocytes are genetically determined, then the basis for genetic predisposition to specific allergens is apparent.

Patients having one episode of allergic contact dermatitis have a greater than average potential for developing further episodes to other allergens. Also, some individuals are resistant to sensitization. This may be attributable to genetic factors related to the immune mechanism. Some skins are less amenable to penetration by the contacting allergen because of pigmentation (blacks are less susceptible), degree of perspiration, and so forth. Children appear to be less susceptible than adults (for example, shoe dermatitis in children is rarely caused by allergy).

***Hand dermatitis.*** Although hand dermatitis is most often attributable to primary irritation in industry and in housewives, Sinha and colleagues have shown the importance of allergic reactions to common vegetables. They found garlic, onion, tomato, and carrot reactions most often in a series of 53 patients, all cooks. Selected cases of hand dermatitis may be attributable to nickel or chromate sensitivity and has been shown to be at least partly dependent on oral ingestion of these metals. Other causes of exacerbations of contact hand eczema by ingestion include cinnamon, hydroxyquinolones, thirams, quinine, antihistamines, sulfonamides, antibiotics, nickel,

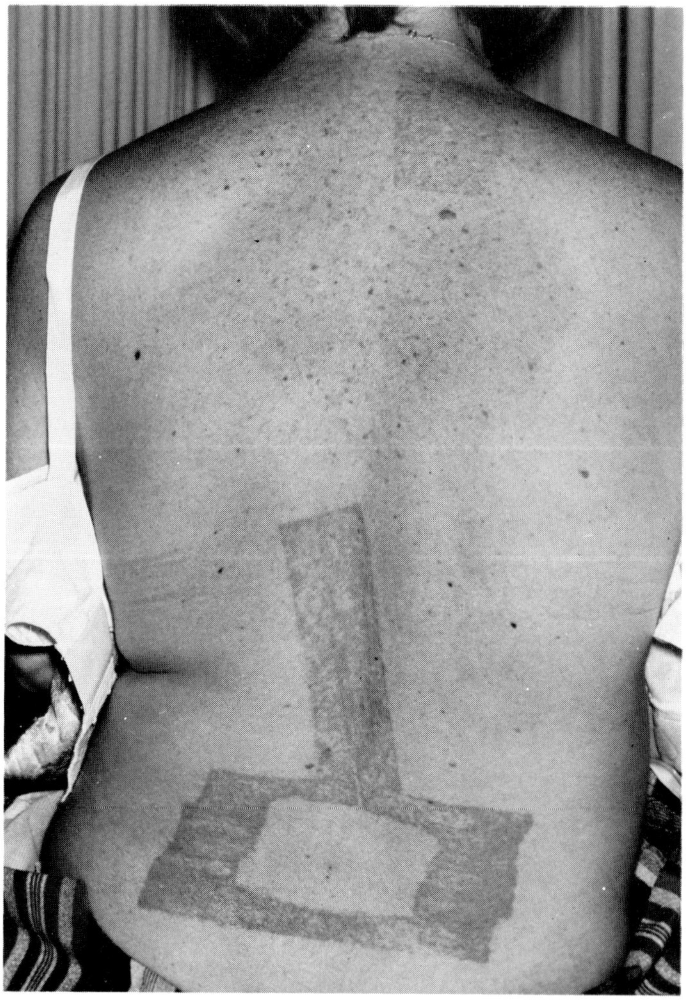

**Fig. 4-5.** Allergic contact dermatitis from tape adhesive. Patch test reaction to components was positive.

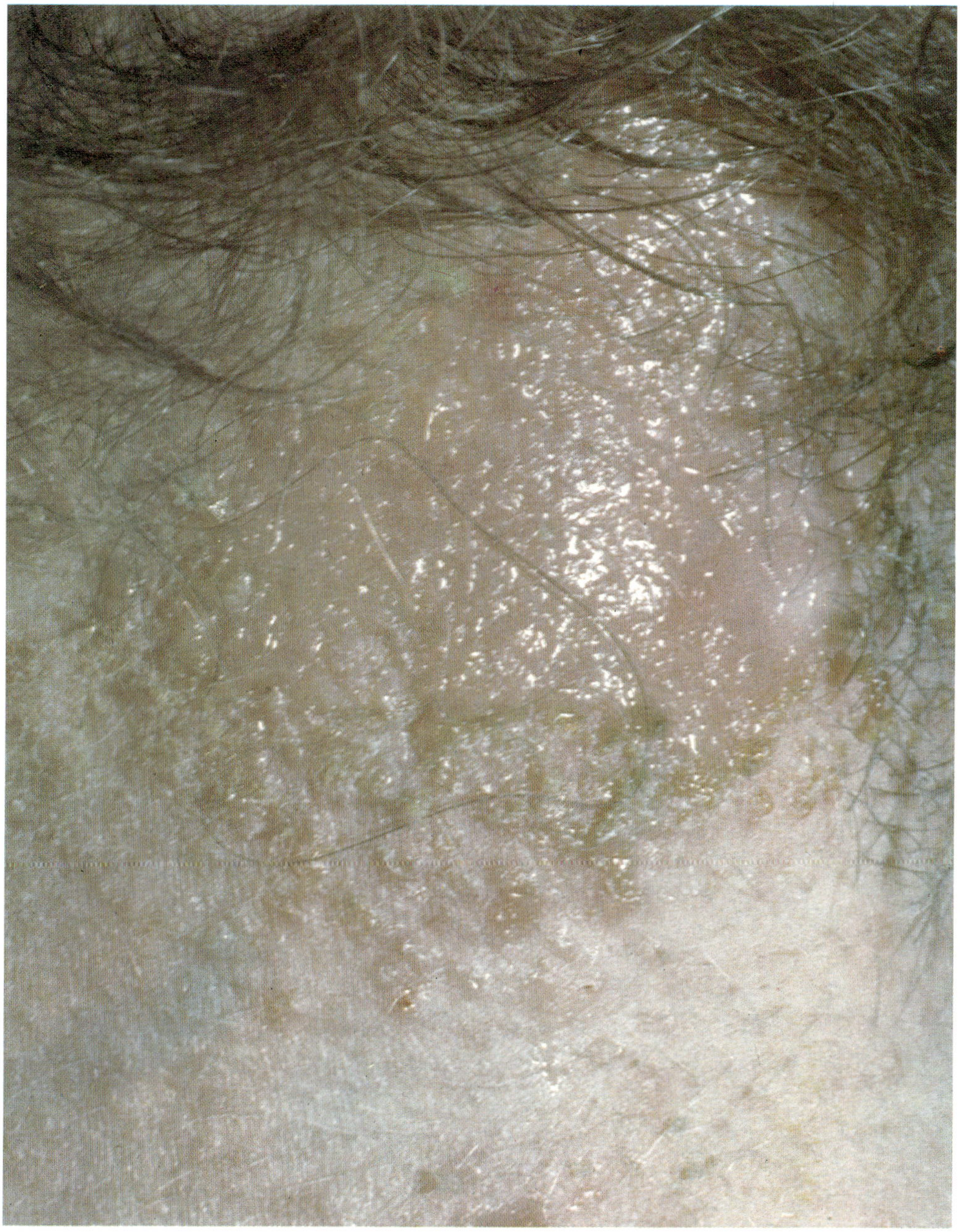

**Plate 11**

Allergic contact dermatitis of neck caused by hair dye.

**Table 2.** Chemicals commonly causing allergic contact dermatitis*

| Chemical | Most common source | 1972-1974* % positive reaction |
|---|---|---|
| Nickel sulfate† 2.5% | Metal jewelry, fasteners | 13.0 |
| Potassium dichromate 0.5% | Leather products, shoes | 7.8 |
| Neomycin sulfate 20% | Topical medication, deodorants, cosmetics | 4.7 |
| Ethylenediamine hydrochloride 1% | Topical agents, antihistamine cream, aminophylline | 6.0 |
| Thimerosal 0.1% | Preservatives | 6.5 |
| Ammoniated mercury 1% | Topical agents, antiseptics, industries, cosmetics | 4.6 |
| Paraben mixture 15% | Preservatives, cosmetics | 3.5 |
| Formaldehyde 2% | Clothing, shoes, soaps | 3.4 |
| Paraphenylenediamine 1% | Hair dyes, leather | 6.1 |
| Turpentine peroxides 1% | Paints, thinners, polishes, waxes | 2.2 |
| Wool wax alcohols 30% | Lanolin | 2.7 |
| Thiram 1% | Rubber | 5.0 |
| Mercaptobenzothiazole mixture 1% | Rubber | 3.0 |
| Caine mixture 8% | Local anesthetics, creams, lozenges, suppositories | 8.4 |
| Naphthyl mixture 1% | Rubber | 1.4 |
| Carba mixture 3% | Rubber | 2.9 |
| Epoxy resin 1% | Plastic and household glues | 2.8 |
| Paraphenylenediamine mixture 0.6% | Leather and hair dyes | 2.2 |
| Balsam of Peru‡ 25% | Creams, ointments | 7.2 |

*Data from Rudner, E. J., Clendenning, W. E., Epstein, E., et al.: Contact Dermatitis **1**:277-280, 1975.
†Stainless steel earrings and surgical implants do not cause sensitization to nickel.
‡Cross-reaction between perfumes and balsam of Peru are significant.

and chromium, the last two of which are released in cooking by stainless steel and salt or acid (Fregert).

Dermatitis from plastics and auxiliary substances are reviewed by Malton, those from acrylics by Rycroft, and dermatitis from topical vehicle ingredients by Fisher. Fregert's manual is very useful for brief specific accurate general information on contact dermatitis.

***Allergic contact dermatitis caused by plants.*** Plants and plant products are among the commonest causes of allergic contact dermatitis. Plant dermatitis is caused by several of the most potent contact allergens now known. By far the most prevalent cause of plant dermatitis is the *Rhus* plants, which are poison ivy, poison oak, and poison sumac, belonging to the Anacardiaceae family, of which there are more than 400 members and which are virtually ubiquitous in North America. Kligman states that 25% to 60% of North Americans are sensitive to these plants. One of the very few areas in which poison ivy does not grow is the coastal area of the Pacific Northwest, where poison ivy dermatitis is seen only in individuals contacting it elsewhere. Other forms of allergic dermatitis from plants arise from contact with chrysanthemums, primulas, tulip and daffodil bulbs, hops, tobacco plants, and many other plants. Some plants produce a *photocontact dermatitis requiring sun exposure* in addition to contact; others cause a primary irritant dermatitis from oils on their surface (buttercups, clematises). *Ragweed* may cause an exposed surface dermatitis from airborne pollens. Hjorth and Fregert discuss these pollens thoroughly, with complete references and related known chemistry of offending substances. Mitchell has shown that causative chemical allergens are common to many varieties of plants responsible for dermatitis. Mitchell and Rook describe the six distinct clinical patterns of dermatitis resulting from plant allergies.

Although exceedingly variable, most plant

dermatitis is, first of all, *erythematous* and *vesicular* or *bullous* (Plate 10). It is limited to the site of contact and therefore is found in patches or streaks, primarily on extremities. It can be transferred to face, ears, neck, or elsewhere from hands or fingers. Chronic long-standing cases are thickened, dusky, red, and pruritic, involving exposed surfaces.

One can carry out patch testing for dermatitis from plants by crushing the flowers, leaves, or stems of the supposedly offending plant and applying portions in the routine manner. However, there is no point in testing with known irritants. Controls should be tested as well to establish an irritancy standard (Mitchell and Rook). A 10% extract appears safe. *Patch testing to Rhus (or poison ivy) and Frullania plants should not be done,* since it is such a potent sensitizer that patch testing alone causes production of allergic sensitivity in approximately 10% of previously nonsensitive individuals. Herbicides, as well as plants, are potent sources of allergens in an agricultural setting.

*Treatment of poison ivy dermatitis.* If exposure has occurred, the oil can be washed off with soap and water, provided that it is done immediately. This unfortunately is not often possible.

Application of a drying alcoholic shake lotion is best in mild cases.

| | |
|---|---|
| Menthol | 0.5% |
| Phenol | 0.5% |
| Zinc oxide | 15 Gm. |
| Talc | 15 Gm. |
| Glycerin | 10 ml. |
| Alcohol | 40 ml. |
| Water | 40 ml. |
| Apply with fingers | q.2h. |

For intense reactions, potent fluorinated topical glucocorticoids such as betamethasone, fluocinolone acetonide, or flurandrenolone creams may be *used every 2 hours.* Systemic glucocorticoids can be used with great benefit if no contraindication exists. The dosage would be in the range of 20 to 30 mg. daily in divided doses, tapering off to zero in 3 to 4 weeks.

*Hyposensitization to poison ivy.* For highly sensitive individuals who must be exposed to poison ivy, a prophylactic partial desensitization can be carried out. This consists of daily ingestion of small measured amounts of *Rhus* oleoresin.* The procedure takes at least 6 months, and, if successful, the dermatitis resulting from poison ivy contact is milder and shorter than before. The sensitivity often returns after treatment is stopped. Mitchell noted that this was the technique used by the American Indian in his attempts to solve the same problems our foresters and other woodsmen face today.

***Contact urticaria*** (p. 113). Immediate reactions to potatoes, fish, shellfish, cheese, nuts, and flour have been reported occurring from handling these food products. Urticarial wheals are the manifestation and can be demonstrated by patch tests carefully done, since the reaction is sometimes quite violent.

### *Distribution of allergic contact dermatitis*

Items used for months or even years without causing cutaneous irritation may eventually result in allergic contact dermatitis. Some of the commonly encountered agents and the associated affected sites are listed below. Maibach has dramatically demonstrated the difference in reacting potential, of two different anatomic areas in a sensitized individual.

| Site | Causative agents |
|---|---|
| Exposed areas | Airborne sprays, fumes, pollens, weeds (ragweed) |
| Scalp | Hair dyes, tints, rinses (paraphenylenediamine present in blond as well as dark hair rinses) |
| | Ointments and medications |
| Face | Cosmetics, ointments, soaps |
| | Photocontact from plants |
| Eyelids | Nail polish, hand lotions, hair dyes |

*Obtainable from Hollister-Stier Laboratories, Box 3145 T.A., Spokane, Wash. 99220, or 1345 Fewster Drive, Mississauga, Ontario.

| | |
|---|---|
| Lips | Lipsticks, creams, medications |
| Neck | Collars, necklaces, fur, hair dyes (Plate 11), nail polish |
| Female breasts | Clothing dyes and finishes, foam rubber, brassiere linings |
| Axillae | Deodorants |
| Abdomen, hips, thighs | Corset and girdle materials, textile finishes, rubber, metal fasteners |
| Genitalia, perianal area | Contraceptive creams, rubber, paper dyes and resins, personal hygiene items, ointments for hemorrhoids |
| Hands | |
| Dorsa | Lotions, ointments, industrial contacts, plants, leather, rubber gloves |
| Palms | Nickel, chrome, and solid objects |
| Feet | Shoe dyes and glues, stocking dyes and finishes |
| Forearms, legs | Plants |
| Mucous membranes | Toothpastes, anesthetics, surgical dressings |

### *Differential diagnosis*

Keep in mind that allergic eczematous contact dermatitis can be superimposed on any other dermatosis.

***Primary irritant contact dermatitis.*** Primary irritant contact dermatitis may appear identical to allergic contact dermatitis, but is produced by primary irritation of the skin rather than allergy. Usually it is caused by soaps, cleansers, bleaches, and so forth, used by the housewife in the home. Patch tests are negative.

***Atopic dermatitis.*** The patient with atopic dermatitis usually has a personal or family history of hay fever, asthma, or eczema. The characteristic distribution of the dermatitis involves the face, neck, hands, and antecubital and popliteal fossae.

***Seborrheic dermatitis.*** Usually a long-standing condition, seborrheic dermatitis involves the forehead, central face, scalp, ears, sternum, and umbilicus.

***Light-sensitivity dermatitis.*** Light-sensitivity dermatitis is ordinarily present over the exposed areas of face, neck, and hands, and there is a history of sun exposure just prior to the onset of the dermatitis.

***Fungal infection.*** Superficial fungal infections, particularly when they involve the toes, feet, and hands, may mimic a contact dermatitis. Scrapings from the area show fungal elements on microscopic examination or culture.

***Hypostatic dermatitis.*** Localized to the lower one half of the legs, as a rule, hypostatic dermatitis is a chronic, slowly developing, inflammatory disorder associated with disturbed venous return from the legs. Intermittent edema of the ankles and pigmentation are associated findings. Allergic contact dermatitis is often superimposed on this disorder because of allergies developing to topical ointments.

### *Patch testing*

A standardized technique is used for the confirmation of the role of suspected causative agents in producing an allergic contact dermatitis. The technique produces a small controlled reaction, the degree of which can be measured. Cronin has concluded from reviewing 1,000 patch tests that this procedure is essential, over and above clinical expertise, in diagnosing contact allergens.

*It must be emphasized that patch test results, like other investigative procedures, are only valid if the technique is standardized and evaluation is accurate and controlled.*

Primary irritant reactions are lessened by dilution of those substances capable of producing irritation to nonirritating dilutions.

**Technique.** The suspected material is applied to 1 $cm.^2$ squares of filter paper. Liquids are applied directly; solids are first dampened with water. Most potentially irritating or concentrated substances can be diluted to 0.1% to 1% in water, alcohol, or acetone, otherwise petrolatum can be used.

The patch is applied to a normal skin surface uninvolved by the dermatitis for at least 1 month. It is secured by tape to keep it from slipping. Keep in mind that many patients have reactions to plain adhesive tape (Fig. 4-5). For these patients, *Scotch* or *Blenderm tape* may be tried as an attempt to overcome this difficulty. Aluminum test patches (Al test) covered with plastic are currently used as a standard and are available from Astra Chemical Limited (Pharmaceutical Division, Middlegate Road, Mississauga, Ontario, Canada) or Imeco Astra Agency Falk. (Stockholm 42, Sweden). A control patch with no test material must always be used for comparison.

The patch is left on for 48 hours, then removed, left open to the air for 15 minutes, and read. The results are indicated as follows (criteria of the North American Contact Dermatitis Group):

| | |
|---|---|
| Plus 1 | Erythema |
| Plus 2 | Erythema, edema, vesicles |
| Plus 3 | Erythema, edema, pseudopods, bullae, ulceration |
| IR | Irritant reaction |

The areas are reexamined in 5 days to note persistence of reaction, seen in strong-positive and delayed-reacting cases, and to rule out irritant reactions.

*Patients with active acute contact dermatitis should not be tested.* If the causative agent is used, the primary areas of the dermatitis caused by this agent will be made much worse immediately. Patch tests must be deferred until the acute phase subsides.

The following are nonirritating concentrations of substances used in patch testing:

| Substance | Concentration to be used |
|---|---|
| Adhesive tape | As is |
| Aluminum chloride | 25% in water |
| Auto lubricating oils | 60% in olive oil |
| Balsam of Peru | 25% in petrolatum |
| Benzalkonium chloride | 0.1% to 0.01% aqueous |
| Benzocaine | 5% in petrolatum |
| Boric acid | Pure powder |
| Carbon paper | As is, wetted with acetone |
| Chromic acid | 0.5% to 1% in water |
| Clothing | As is |
| Cosmetics | As is |
| Crude coal tar | 5% to 10% in petrolatum |
| Deodorants | As is |
| Furs | As is |
| Lanolin | As is |
| Leather | Test with extracts |
| Lipstick | As is |
| Lysol | 1% in water |
| Metals | As is |
| Nail polish | As is |
| Neomycin | 20% in petrolatum |
| Oil paints for walls | 50% in petrolatum |
| Paraphenylenediamine (constituent of hair dyes) | 2% in petrolatum |
| Plants (except poison ivy) | 10% aqueous |
| Plastics | As is |
| Polishes (furniture) | 10% and 50% in petrolatum |
| Proprietary medications | As is |
| Rubber | Test with components |
| Turpentine | 50% in olive oil |

Patch tests may be used despite concomitant use of oral glucocorticoids up to 20 mg. daily by the patient being tested. Chemicals for use in patch testing may be obtained from Hollister-Stier Laboratories (P.O. Box 3030, Calgary, Alberta, Canada, and in the United States, 3525 Regal, Spokane, Washington 99207).

**Patch phototesting.** This technique, available to the confirmation of diagnosis of photoallergic contact dermatitis, introduces light exposure to one of two identical patch test areas. It should be performed and interpreted by an expert in the field.

### *Management*

**Diagnosis.** *When an allergic contact dermatitis is suspected, all potential etiological agents must be removed from the patient's environment to prevent reexposure and worsening of the dermatitis.* Nowhere is a detailed and carefully taken history of more use in establishing the causative agent than in this disorder. All possible sources for a causative contact allergen should be queried.

The area of skin involved must be taken into consideration and a list made of agents contacting that area within a day or so of the onset of the dermatitis. This list must be kept for use as a reference in possible future patch testing.

**Prevention.** When the diagnosis of an allergic contact dermatitis has been confirmed, all efforts must be made to avoid further contact with the causative agent, lest a chronic recalcitrant dermatitis is produced by repetitive exposures.

Hygiene is important. Soaps and waterless cleansers can be used to remove allergens before they act. In some situations allergen substitutions may be made. Some cleansers can be dispensed with in favor of less damaging agents. Knowledge of the source of the dermatitis allows avoidance.

### *Treatment*

For topical therapy, cold *compresses* are essential if there is oozing or crusting. The most satisfactory medication is Burow's solution in a dilution of 1:20. It can be prepared from tablets or powders, by use of a tablet or packet of powder to 1 pint of cool water for compressing, four times daily for 15-minute periods. The area is allowed to dry and a glucocorticoid cream applied sparingly, without excessive rubbing. Either 0.1% betamethasone or 0.025% fluocinolone, or their equivalent, should be applied until the acute inflammation has subsided. Then, because of the complications of the potent topical steroids, a tapering off with 1% hydrocortisone is recommended.

If the inflammation is severe, oozing, and spreading, and if the health of the patient offers no contraindication, *glucocorticoids* can be administered orally. These will promptly relieve the symptoms and ameliorate the disease. Dosage used should be adequate to suppress the inflammation and should be tapered off within 2 to 3 weeks with topical steroid therapy used only for the subsiding dermatitis. Any of the standard glucocorticoid creams, the equivalent of 1% hydrocortisone or stronger, is satisfactory.

Studies are in progress that attempt removal of the allergenicity of specific chemicals to the individual by use of methods to induce tolerance in patients, by removal of specific patient reactivity to chemicals by adsorption, by alteration of biological processes to prevent debilitating allergic reactions, and the like. However, for the present, avoidance of the causative allergen, by all means at our disposal, seems to be the only practical method. To this end it is most important that the specific causative chemicals in any individual case be identified and thus can be substituted or avoided by the patient. Fisher discusses allergen replacement and delineates some very practical substitutes for common contact dermatitis problems including topical medications.

#### REFERENCES

Christensen, O. B., and Möller, H.: External and internal exposure to the antigen in the hand eczema of nickel allergy, Contact Dermatitis **1**:136, 1975.
**5.6 mg. of oral nickel aggravated hand eczema in minutes in selected cases.**

Christensen, O. B., and Möller, H.: Nickel allergy and hand eczema, Contact Dermatitis **1**:129, 1975.
**Pompholyx with periodic activity in 52% of nickel allergies.**

Cronin, E.: Clinical prediction of patch test results. Trans. St. John's Hosp. Dermatol. Soc. **58**:153, 1972.
**Over 1,000 patch tests.**

Dahl, M. V.: Allergic contact dermatitis from footwear. Shoe dermatitis in 42 patients, Minn. Med. **58**:871, 1975.
**Rubber adhesives, chromate solution and formaldehyde most common.**

Dvorak, A. M., Mihm, M. C., Jr., and Dvorak, H. C.: Degranulation of basophilic leucocytes in allergic contact reactions in man, J. Immunol. **116**:687, 1976.
**60% of viable basophils degranulated by 72 hours.**

Dvorak, H. F.: Delayed hypersensitivity. In Zweifach, B., editor: The inflammatory process. ed. 2, New York, 1974, Academic Press, Inc., p. 291.
**Several new pathologic mechanisms described.**

Fisher, A. A.: Allergen replacements in allergic dermatitis, Int. J. Dermatol. **16**:319, 1977.
**Substitutes for allergens in shoes, clothing, rubber, cosmetics, hair dyes, topical medications, and drugs are presented.**

Fisher, A. A.: Contact dermatitis, ed. 2, Philadelphia, 1973, Lea & Febiger.
**The source.**

Fisher, A. A.: New advances in contact dermatitis, Int. J. Dermatol. **16**:552, 1977.
**Diagnosis, prevention, new allergens, new mechanisms, new treatments.**

Fregert, S.: Manual of contact dermatitis, Copenhagen, 1974, Munksgaard, Year Book Publications.
**An excellent quick reference manual for those treating, but not specializing in contact dermatitis.**

Hjorth, N., and Fregert, S.: Contact dermatitis. In Rook, A. J., Wilkinson, D. S., and Ebling, R. J. E., editors: Textbook of dermatology, Oxford, 1972, Blackwell Scientific Publications Ltd., p. 356.

**Clinical features, identification, testing, and differential diagnosis.**

Iden, D. L., and Schroeter, A. L.: Allergic contact dermatitis to herbicides, Arch. Dermatol. **113**:981, 1977.
**Grass and weed killers alachlor and propachlor caused positive reactions in 7 of 22 patients.**

Kaaber, K., and Veien, N. K.: The significance of chromate ingestion in patients allergic to chromate, Acta Derm. Venereol. **57**:321, 1977.
**Ingestion of 2.5 mg. of chromium caused worsening of 11 of 31 patients with chromate dermatitis.**

Maibach, I. H., and Prystosky, S. D.: Glutaraldehyde allergic contact dermatitis, Arch. Dermatol. **113**:170, 1977.
**A striking variation in tolerance between soles and arms.**

Malten, K. E.: Occupational dermatoses in the processing of plastics, Trans. St. John's Hosp. Dermatol. Soc. **59**:78, 1973.
**Good technical information.**

Mitchell, J. C.: The angry back syndrome. Eczema creates eczema, Contact Dermatitis **1**:193, 1975.
**Positive tests from negatives because of concomitant strong reactions.**

Mitchell, J. C.: Hardening in allergic contact dermatitis and immunological tolerance, Trans. St. John's Hosp. Dermatol. Soc. **55**:141, 1969.
**Puts it all into perspective.**

Mitchell, J. C., and Rook, A. J.: Diagnosis of contact dermatitis from plants, Int. J. Dermatol. **16**:257, 1977.
**A plan for investigation of suspected plant dermatitis.**

Rudner, E. J., Clendenning, W. E., Epstein, E., et al.: The frequency of contact sensitivity in North America 1972-74, Contact Dermatitis **1**:277-280, 1975.
**Revealing findings from the North American Contact Dermatitis Group.**

Rycroft, R. J. G.: Contact dermatitis from acrylic compounds, Br. J. Dermatol. **96**:685, 1977.
**These are used in artificial nails, bone and adhesive tape cements, splints, and photoprinting processes that produce acrylic polymerization under ultraviolet light.**

Shelley, W. B., and Juhlin, L.: Selective uptake of contact allergens by the Langerhans cell, Arch. Dermatol. **113**:187, 1977.
**These active cells process, transform, and conjugate foreign haptens that successfully pass the stratum corneum barrier.**

Sinha, S. M., Pasricha, J. S., Sharma, R. C., and Kandhari, K. C.: Vegetables responsible for contact dermatitis of the hands, Arch. Dermatol. **113**:776, 1977.
**Hyperkeratosis and fissuring of fingertips caused by garlic, onion, tomato, and carrot allergies.**

## URTICARIA (EXCLUDING FAMILIAL ANGIOEDEMA)

Urticaria is a common dermatosis in which pruritic transient wheals or welts, variable in size and sometimes of allergic origin, are produced by local histamine release. IgE antibodies attached to mast cells effect the release of histamine in allergic cases.

### *Natural course*

Urticaria begins with sensations of pruritus or numbness of a localized area. The wheal follows within minutes, lasts for minutes to hours, and subsides; subsequent wheals then appear elsewhere. A skin area is refractory to further wheal formation for some 24 hours after an urticarial lesion has subsided. The wheal is a sharply bordered pale or pink area of localized edema with a palpable elevated edge and a diffuse erythematous background. The lesions tend to occur on points of pressure from clothing, belts, shoulder straps, or girdles. If the urticarial lesions involve the lips, mucous membranes, periorbital area, or eyelids, there may be simply a diffuse swelling of the involved area. Urticarial lesions of the lips, tongue, or buccal mucosa may rarely be associated with laryngeal edema and airway obstruction.

The gastrointestinal mucosa may be involved with urticarial lesions, with the production of cramps, nausea, or vomiting.

There are three clinically distinct forms of urticaria: the acute immediate allergic type, the acute delayed type, and the chronic form.

***Acute contact urticaria.*** The allergen, coming in contact with skin or mucous membranes, produces a severe swelling at the site of contact within seconds or, at most, minutes. It may be allergic or nonallergic and can be produced by a wide variety of compounds that include foods, cosmetics, medications, commercial chemicals, and plants. The offending substance penetrates the skin or membrane to release the mediator of the reaction at the site. Some housewives' dermatitis is of this type. Open patch tests are positive to the offending item.

***Acute delayed urticaria.*** In acute delayed

urticaria the urticarial reaction occurs hours after exposure to the causative factor. The lesions are generalized rather than localized, and the causative factor may be a food, inhalant, or other substance. It is not a consistent reaction occurring with each exposure to the causative agent; thus, identifying the initiating substance may be very difficult. It is probably not always an allergic reaction, and skin tests are usually negative.

***Chronic urticaria.*** This type of "hives" is probably rarely allergic in nature. The lesions are usually less severe, less extensive, and always more persistent than in the previous forms. A few lesions may be present at any one time, but they may involve only a small area such as one hand, or even one finger. Causative agents are rarely found in chronic urticaria. It may continue for months, or even years.

Occasionally after an acute allergic reaction to penicillin, chronic urticaria may persist in gradually lessening intensity for months, despite lack of exposure to penicillin. Other drugs and chemicals may result in chronic urticaria, even if taken intermittently and in

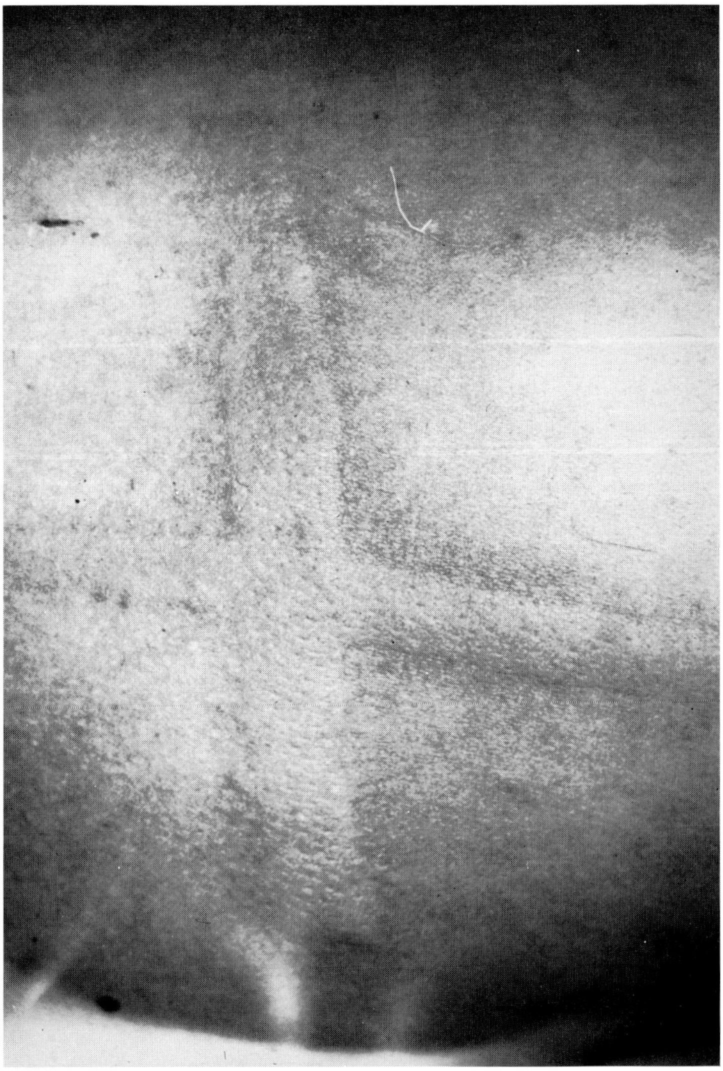

**Fig. 4-6.** Dermographism.

small amounts over prolonged periods, probably because of concomitant ingestion of other urticariogenic compounds such as salicylates. Neither may produce hives alone, but in combination they may do so.

***Urticaria caused by physical agents***

*Dermographism.* Dermographism is a cutaneous urticarial response to stroking the skin (Fig. 4-6). It may arise in minutes or take an hour or so to develop. The whealing is pruritic and often uncomfortable. The patient with dermographism finds it produced by clothing, bra straps, belts, and cutaneous pressures not significant to a normal individual. More severe trauma, such as a whiplash, will however produce wheals in a normal person. Aoyama has demonstrated the role of IgE and histamine in the production of dermographism. It is present without apparent cause in 1% of normal individuals.

*Cold contact urticaria.* Cold urticaria occurs locally, within seconds or minutes of an area's exposure to cold. The source may be cold air, cold glass, metal, ice, or any similar

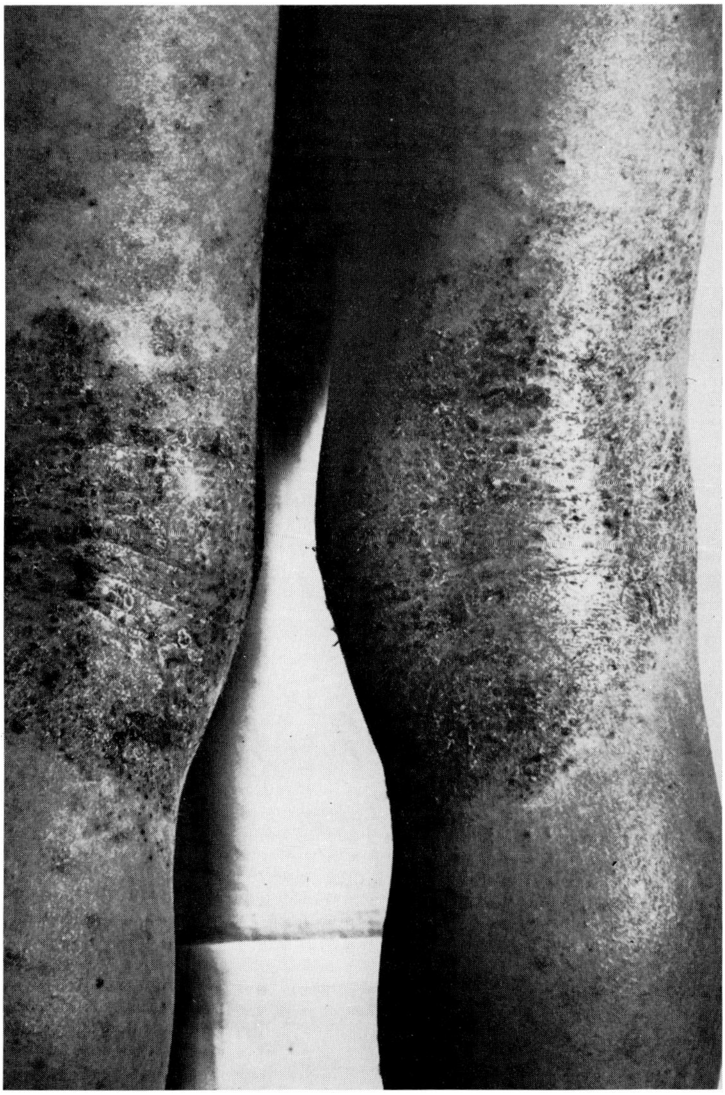

**Fig. 4-7.** Atopic dermatitis with characteristic flexural involvement and crusting.

substance. The lesion is often exceedingly pruritic.

*Heat contact urticaria.* This is completely analogous to cold urticaria. The skin responds within seconds to minutes to a contact temperature usually above 39° C.

*Solar urticaria.* Solar urticaria is an unusual form in which a specific wavelength of light produces urticarial lesions on the skin surface exposed to it.

*Cholinergic urticaria.* The lesion pattern in cholinergic urticaria is different from that of other physical forms and is recognizable (Fig. 4-7). It consists of small (less than 1 cm.) lesions studded over the skin surface. Diffuse external heat or heat from cutaneous flushing and exercise is the causative factor.

*Aquagenic urticaria.* Most dermatologists have observed this clinical entity in which a water (of varying temperature) exposure produces hives that may be follicular.

*Urticaria in systemic disease.* Urticaria is rarely caused by internal disease, but these few cases should not be overlooked. It may be a clinical finding in acute rheumatic fever, juvenile rheumatoid arthritis (Still's disease), lupus erythematosus, serum hepatitis, internal malignancy, Hodgkin's disease, amebiasis, and rarely, in association with foci of infection. It may also be caused by intestinal parasites.

### Pertinent information

Histamine is produced and stored in the granules of the mast cells, which, when once depleted, require 24 hours or more to replenish their stores. An antigen-antibody union involving IgE can release histamine and result in urticaria, but so can many other agents. Kinins, prostaglandins, and slow-reacting substance of anaphylaxis (SRS-A) can produce urticarial wheals, and complement may institute the histamine release rather than IgE. Venoms, toxins, jellyfish stings, proteolytic enzymes, serums, surface-active agents (Tween 20), histamine liberators (compound amine 48/80), and certain drugs (morphine, codeine, aspirin, polymyxin, quinine, curare) can all produce histamine release apparently without the help of IgE.

A variety of physical agents as well may result in urticaria as noted by the variety of "triggers" described above in the physical urticarias. Histamine in blood has been found elevated on challenge in cold urticaria. Greaves and Yamamoto investigated the immunopharmacology of histamine release and suggested cAMP as a regulator of this system dependent on intracellular temperature, energy, and calcium. The studies of Greaves and his colleagues indicate the possibility of a qualitative abnormality of basophil-bound IgE in chronic urticaria.

Michaëlsson and Juhlin, and subsequently Doeglas, demonstrated the success of a salicylate-free diet in most patients with chronic urticaria, cholinergic urticaria, and pressure urticaria, who responded positively to salicylate challenge. Noid, Schulze, and Winkelmann have supplied a salicylate-free diet that we find very helpful. It seems most urticariogenic agents are additive, and if provocative compounds such as aspirin, other salicylates, penicillin, morphine, codeine, and tartrazine can be eliminated, hives may disappear.

Penicillin was the most common cause of urticarial drug reactions in Kauppinen's records of a 10-year period. The small amounts of penicillin in dairy products cannot be overlooked.

Aoyama transferred serum from patients with acute urticaria to normal controls by intradermal injection and produced localized dermographism. Anti-IgE serum eliminated this response, showing that IgE was at least in part, causative.

Whitlock confirms that urticaria patients in general are stable normal individuals. Although there is an overready tendency to invoke psychological factors, emotion can act as a precipitant of chronic urticarial lesions.

The author (WDS) remembers the case of a fellow medical student developing urticaria on the morning she was to give a clinic lecture on hives!

### Microscopic findings

Microscopic examinations reveal edema of the dermis, and it is often difficult to demonstrate.

### *Differential diagnosis*

***Erythema multiforme.*** The appearance of lesions of erythema multiforme is often very similar to urticaria. Urticarial lesions are evanescent, lasting from minutes to a very few hours, whereas lesions of erythema multiforme last for several days. "Iris" lesions are present in erythema multiforme.

***Insect bites.*** Insect bites are persistent, small papular lesions, often with central puncta and a tendency toward grouping. They frequently have a superimposed urticarial element.

***Renal disease.*** Renal disease, as well as other forms of edema producing puffy eyelids and periorbital areas, can be confused with urticaria. Urinalysis and hematological studies should be performed in doubtful cases.

### *Investigation*

***Initial procedures.*** A detailed history, including a careful survey of foods, inhalants, and environmental contact factors (best done with a *detailed, methodical diary recording foods, activities, and contacts*) correlated with the condition of the skin, is important as a first step in treatment. This diary can be reviewed by the physician at weekly intervals, with suggestions for avoiding causative items. Repeated and persistent questioning is essential to elicit all potential causative factors, for example, drugs (particularly aspirin), home remedies, and sprays. In persistent cases, a physical examination and history specifically for evidence of systemic disease, arthralgias, liver disease, infection, parasites, or presence of *Candida*, *Trichomonas*, or *Entamoeba* should be carried out. As Shelley points out, a search for purulent foci is important in unusual cases.

Laboratory tests, including white blood cell count, sedimentation rate, urinalysis, stools for parasites and ova, and chest x-ray films should be performed. Biopsy (see Soter) should be done if the erythrocyte sedimentation rate is elevated or the lesions are at all unusual so that a venulitis is not overlooked.

*In many cases a careful history gives the most help in managing a case of urticaria.*

***Secondary procedures.*** Chiefly arising from positive initial investigations, secondary procedures should include the following:

- Challenge testing is used in our institution when urticaria is unresponsive to salicylate deprivation, careful history taking for causes, and a nonresponse to treatment over 3 months. The patient is placed in the hospital and challenged with acetylsalicylic acid, tartrazine, sodium benzoate, penicillin, and yeast in increasing doses. When performed with caution, we find this helpful.
- Antistreptolysin titer, rheumatoid factor, liver function tests, LE cell test, x-ray studies of teeth and sinuses, or, where indicated, serum proteins.
- Cold urticaria necessitates testing for cryoglobulins, cold agglutinins, and syphilis

### *Treatment*

Administration of *antihistamines* remains the most satisfactory treatment in all forms of urticaria except acute laryngeal edema.

***Acute immediate allergic urticaria with laryngopharyngeal involvement.*** Drug therapy consists of *epinephrine* in a concentration of 1:1,000 given subcutaneously in a dose of 10 to 20 minims and repeated in 15 minutes if necessary. This is a histamine antagonist and its effect is immediate. It also may be given by inhalation. Alternately, *ephedrine* may be used orally in a 25 mg. dose, two to three times daily. Intravenous or intramuscular *antihistamines* should be added to prevent more histaminic effects from occurring. Soluble parenteral *glucocorticoids* administered intramuscularly or subcutaneously will have a much slower effect and will not produce a consistent response. Greaves states that the glucocorticoid effect in urticaria is complex and not well understood.

***Acute and chronic urticaria.*** Adequate dosage of an antihistaminic drug, either in prolonged-release form or standard tablets, should prove effective. The side effect of drowsiness must be discussed with the patient so that hazards from driving or working with machinery are foreseen. This drug should be maintained for more than 2 to 3 weeks after symptoms have subsided. If one antihistamine has less than the desired effect, a representative from another group may be tried. There are five groups and miscellaneous examples. Yellow tartrazine-coated tablets should be avoided. A representative from each group is as follows:

Diphenhydramine hydrochloride (Benadryl)
Tripelennamine (Pyribenzamine)
Chlorpheniramine maleate (Chlor-Trimeton)
Cyclizine (Marezine)
Promethazine hydrochloride (Phenergan)
Hydroxyzine (Atarax) (shown by more than one study to be superior)

Avoidance of aspirin and a salicylate-free diet is important and should be maintained for 6 weeks, in association with a daily hive count, before it is given up.

***Physical urticarias.*** For treatment one should use a combination of an antihistamine in adequate dosage, protection or avoidance of the physical factors, and a reduction in environmental exposure to known urticariogenic agents. *Solar urticaria* will be helped by sunscreens (p. 62).

All types of urticaria will benefit by elimination of all strong urticariogenic agents from their environment, as the effect of these compounds is known to be additive.

### REFERENCES

Aoyama, H.: IgE as a dermographism-inducing principle of urticaria factitia. Jpn. J. Dermatol, Series B **81**:266, 1971.
**An exaggerated normal mechansim.**

Doeglas, H. M. G.: Reactions to aspirin in food additives in patients with chronic urticaria, including the physical urticarias, Br. J. Dermatol. **93**:135, 1975.
**27 on salicylate-free diet; 17 good to excellent results.**

Greaves, M. W., Plummer, V. M., McLaughlin, P., and Stanworth, D. R.: Serum and cell bound IgE in chronic urticaria, Clin. Allergy **4**:265, 1974.
**Perhaps chronic urticarial patients have a basophil cell surface alteration that affects histamine release.**

Greaves, M. W., and Yamamoto, S.: Immunopharmacology of the immediate allergic response in skin, Clin. Exp. Dermatol. **1**:83-90, 1976.
**Glucocorticoids may decrease mast cell secretion of histamine.**

Johnson, A. R., Moran, N. C., and Mayer, S. E.: Cyclic AMP and histamine release in rat mast cells, J. Immunol. **112**:511, 1974.
**A controlling factor that suppresses histamine liberation.**

Kauppinen, K.: Cutaneous reactions to drugs, Acta Derm. Venereol. **52**(suppl. 68):16, 1972.
**A remarkably helpful series of observations by a courageous woman on a large selected patient series.**

Michaëlsson, G., and Juhlin, L.: Urticaria induced by preservatives and dye additives in food and drugs, Br. J. Dermatol. **88**:525, 1973.
**Yellow turns out to be a poor color for antihistamines.**

Monroe, E. W., and Jones, H. E.: Urticaria. An updated review, Arch. Dermatol. **113**:80, 1977.
**Good brief update.**

Noid, H. E., Schulze, T. W., and Winkelmann, R. K.: Diet plan for patients with salicylate induced urticaria, Arch. Dermatol. **109**:866, 1974.
**Potatoes, tomatoes, peppers, almonds, yellow dyes, and mint have the most.**

Odom, R. B., and Maibach, H. I.: Contact urticaria: a different contact dermatitis. In Marzulli, F. N., and Maibach, H. I., editors: Advances in modern toxicology. Vol. 4. Dermatotoxicology and pharmacology, New York, 1977, John Wiley & Son, Chap. 15.
**Etiologic mechanisms of contact urticaria; over 50 recorded causative items.**

Shelley, W. B.: Urticaria of nine years' duration cleared following dental extraction, Arch. Dermatol. **100**:325, 1969.
**A reminder.**

Soter, N. A.: Chronic urticaria as manifestation of necrotizing venulitis, N. Engl. J. Med. **296**:1440, 1977.
**Biopsy urticaria with abdominal pain, arthralgia, and elevated erythrocyte sedimentation rate.**

Warin, R. P., and Champion, R. H.: Urticaria, Philadelphia, 1974, W. B. Saunders Co.
**Excellent. Emphasis is on basic mechanisms but new practical applications are drawn. A first rate publication.**

Whitlock, F. A.: Urticaria in psychophysiological aspects of skin disease, Philadelphia, 1976, W. B. Saunders Co, p. 154.
**An unemotional assessment of an emotional subject on emotion as a cause.**

## ATOPIC DERMATITIS

With our changing concepts, the diagnosis of atopic dermatitis in an individual now identifies a person with a skin that is abnormally susceptible to environmental irritants, that has certain specific vasomotor alterations, that is susceptible to a few specific viral, bacterial, and fungal infections, and that tends to demonstrate ichthyosis. There is usually a personal and family history of eczema, asthma, or hay fever. IgE production appears to be increased. The disease affects between 0.1% and 0.5% of the general population (Rajka).

### *Natural course*

Atopic dermatitis follows a clinical course that has several distinct patterns.

The age of onset of atopic dermatitis varies, but about 4 months appears to be the median. The typical clinical pattern of atopic dermatitis consists of the following stages:

1. Vesicular, oozing and crusted infantile atopic dermatitis occurring at approximately 4 months of age, followed by a tendency toward spontaneous clearing between the second and fourth years
2. The appearance of the typical flexural type of eczema during the prepubertal and adolescent period
3. The more localized or persistent regional patches of atopic dermatitis in older children and adults

A common thread throughout is the gradual clinical improvement that occurs with the passage of time. The majority of these patients are essentially free of dermatitis by 30 years of

A

B

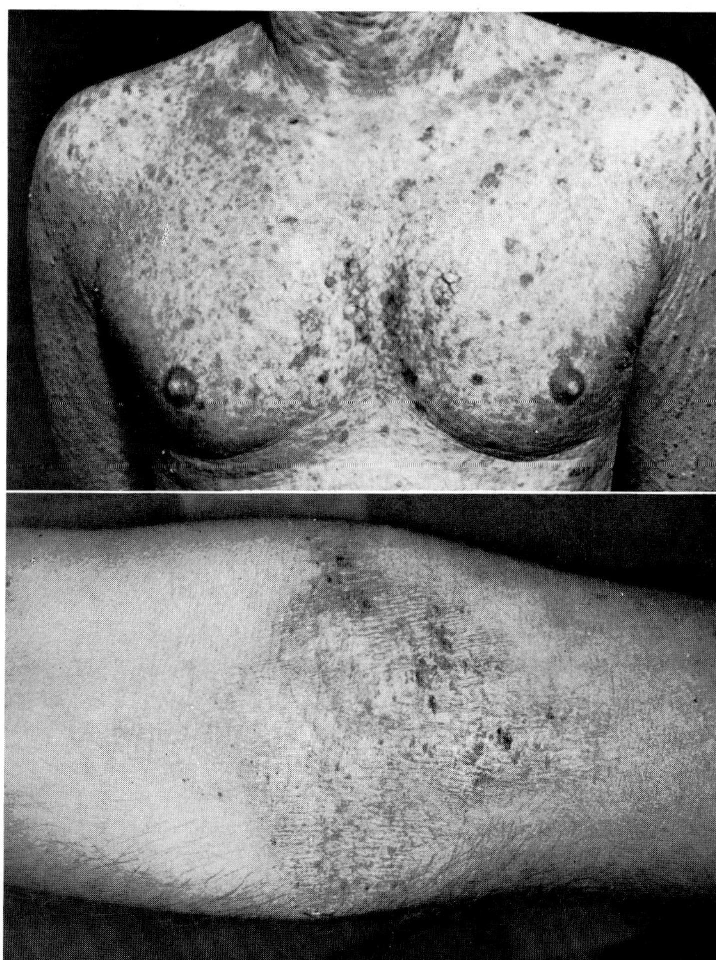

**Fig. 4-8. A,** Atopic dermatitis—severe adult form. **B,** Lichenification and antecubital involvement.

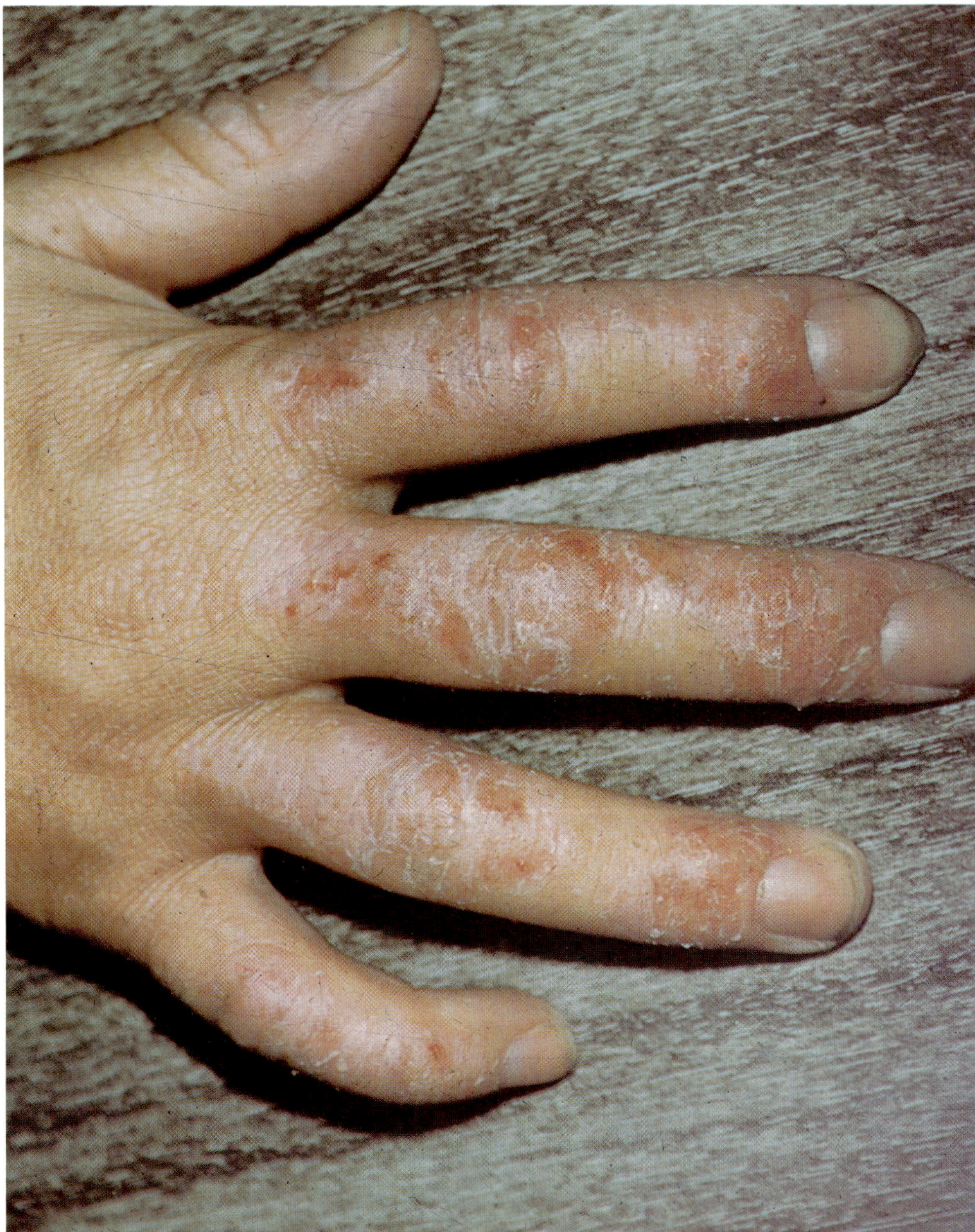

**Plate 12**

Atopic dermatitis—localized form.

age. However, some patients retain symptoms. Thus, in Roth and Kierland's 20-year study, it was found that one third of the patients still had eczema, one fourth had bronchial asthma, one half had allergic rhinitis, and one fourth had no allergic manifestations.

***Infantile form (infantile eczema).*** This dermatological problem may first appear soon after birth, often by the fourth month of life. The face, scalp, neck, and diaper area are the areas of predilection. Frequently, the manifestations of infantile atopic dermatitis are limited to a localized eczematous involvement of the flexural areas (Fig. 4-7) and the cheeks. However, with an exacerbation, which is characteristic of this disease, the localized process spreads to involve a large part of the skin surface. The process may be red, dry, slightly scaly, cracked, and excoriated, or it may be moist and oozing. Pruritis is the major complaint. Bacterial infection from staphylococci or streptococci is frequently apparent as impetigenization of the affected site. In less than half of these patients the disease spontaneously clears completely by 4 years of age, and even then the disease may occur at a later age. The dermatitis in older children tends to blend into the adult form.

***Adult form.*** The more classical features of the disease become clinically apparent as the patient grows older. The antecubital and popliteal areas are the sites of predilection. In some cases the hands, feet, and face may be involved. Here again, pruritus is the main complaint. The involved sites are usually dry, erythematous, and excoriated and demonstrate accentuation of the normal skin markings (lichenification) with bacterial crusting and redness. An accompanying secondary lymphadenopathy is not unusual. (See Fig. 4-8.) There is a seasonal fluctuation in the severity of the disease, which tends to improve with summer and worsen in winter and shows exacerbations in both extremes of climate.

***Localized form.*** Not infrequently, the patient may demonstrate recurring or persistent localized areas of involvement. The localized areas are most often found over the wrists, ankles, hands, (Plate 12), feet, perianal region, scrotal sac, or vulva. Möller's "winter feet" are a classic example of this localized form in older children. The persistence of the eczema and a previous family or personal history of infantile or flexural involvement or other atopic disease may be the only clues. Patients with atopic disease may be the only clues. Patients with atopic dermatitis usually demonstrate an associated xerosis (dry skin), which is particularly prone to external irritation from heat, perspiration, soap, and external irritants.

### *Pertinent information*

The incidence of personal or family histories with a positive atopic aspect ranges around 20% of the general population.

Thirty percent of patients with atopic dermatitis have asthma or hay fever, or both. Allergic rhinitis or urticaria, or both, occur in about 15%, whereas more than 70% give a family history of atopy (hay fever, asthma, and atopic dermatitis).

What is the definition of an atopic individual? A clinical appreciation of this concept can be stated in this way: "A person who by heredity is more predisposed than others (1) to acquire immediate type of sensitizations to common allergens, (2) to develop, together with other members of his family, asthma, hay fever, or atopic dermatitis, and (3) to have skin that is easily inflamed by such common external factors as heat, wool, or soap."

***IgE.*** In atopy there is a hereditary abnormal immune mechanism that produces increased IgE antibody, although there is some question whether serum IgE is elevated in atopic dermatitis. Clendenning, Stone, Jones, and Rogge have demonstrated a significant correlation of serum IgE with the extent and severity of skin involvement. Also IgE can be produced locally in tissues without appearing in serum. From these findings, correlated with clinical experience, one can conclude that an elevated serum IgE may be significant in the diagnosis and management of atopic dermatitis, but negative findings are of no help.

***Delayed cell-mediated immunity.*** Lobitz first demonstrated depressed cell-mediated immunity in patients with atopic dermatitis. This suppression of cell-mediated immunity worsened during an exacerbation of the disease. The depressed immunity may be correlated with increased viral and fungal infections in patients with atopy.

Rogge and Hanifin documented decreased leukocyte function, depressed cell-mediated immunity, increased IgE, and infection with bacteria and fungi in 14 cases of severe atopy. Thus in severe atopic dermatitis, at least, and during exacerbations, there is a defect in cellular immunity that results in a susceptibility to viral infection of vaccinia and herpes simplex, perhaps to warts, to ringworm, and to staphylococcal skin infections. Chemotaxis of the polymorphonuclear neutrophil leukocyte and monocyte group is depressed as is lymphocyte transformations, but all these parameters improve as the dermatitis improves.

Atopic patients are less likely to develop *allergic* contact dermatitis (for example, poison ivy) than are nonatopic patients.

***Vasomotor changes.*** There is altered peripheral cutaneous vasoconstriction of the affected skin in atopic patients, with decreased response to cooling and warmth and increased sweat production in flexural areas. There are paradoxical vasomotor changes in response to acetylcholine, nicotinic acid esters, and histamine. A curious blanch phenomenon occurs on stroking, replacing the red flare in normal individuals *(white dermographism)*. These changes may be seen in eczematous skin caused by contact dermatitis.

***Emotional factors.*** Whitlock assesses the current status of knowledge of this etiology of atopic dermatitis. He concludes that the influence of psychological factors is unquestionable at least as a modifying factor in the day-by-day symptoms. There seems to be no good confirming evidence for a major etiological role.

***Diet.*** In the past, diet was presumed to play a more significant role in the production of atopic dermatitis than is now believed. Although in infants there may be some association of exacerbations with certain foods, this appears to be a short-lived effect.

***Skin tests.*** After long clinical trial, it is now apparent that once frequently used skin tests with various extracts have not proved of benefit in determining individual causative factors in this disease. The atopic patient may demonstrate a positive, immediate type of wheal response to a large number of proteins that often have *no clinical significance*. Kaufman has demonstrated clearly that atopic infants have multiple positive skin reactions to common antigens that are clinically irrelevant. These positive reactions seem to be the result of high concentrations of tissue IgE attached to mast cells. The RAST test measures serum IgE antibodies and is not clearly related to activity in the individual patient.

### *Making the diagnosis*

***History of patient.*** A careful family or personal history will reveal a background of asthma, hay fever, or allergic rhinitis in a high percentage of the cases. Questioning of the adult patient will usually bring out a past history of infantile eczema and of lifelong dry skin. History will reveal the seasonal fluctuation of the clinical signs and symptoms, with the tendency to improve with the warmth and dryness of summer and to worsen during the winter season.

***Clinical observation.*** Clinical observation will reveal the typical areas of involvement: (1) the face and neck in infants, (2) the flexural sites in children and young adults, and (3) the localized areas (perianal, perivulvar, and scrotal regions, and hands, feet, wrists, and ears) in many patients. The atopic skin generally, even in uninvolved areas, is dry and finely scaling (Plate 13).

### *Complications associated with atopic dermatitis*

***Sweat retention.*** Sweat retention is one of the most common complications. The skin of an atopic patient is excessively susceptible to occlusion of sweat pores from such factors as excessive soap and hot water, friction of rubbing and scratching, and sunlight.

***Exfoliative dermatitis.*** Overtreatment, external irritants, excessive heat and perspiration, infection, and other exacerbating factors can turn a generalized atopic dermatitis into

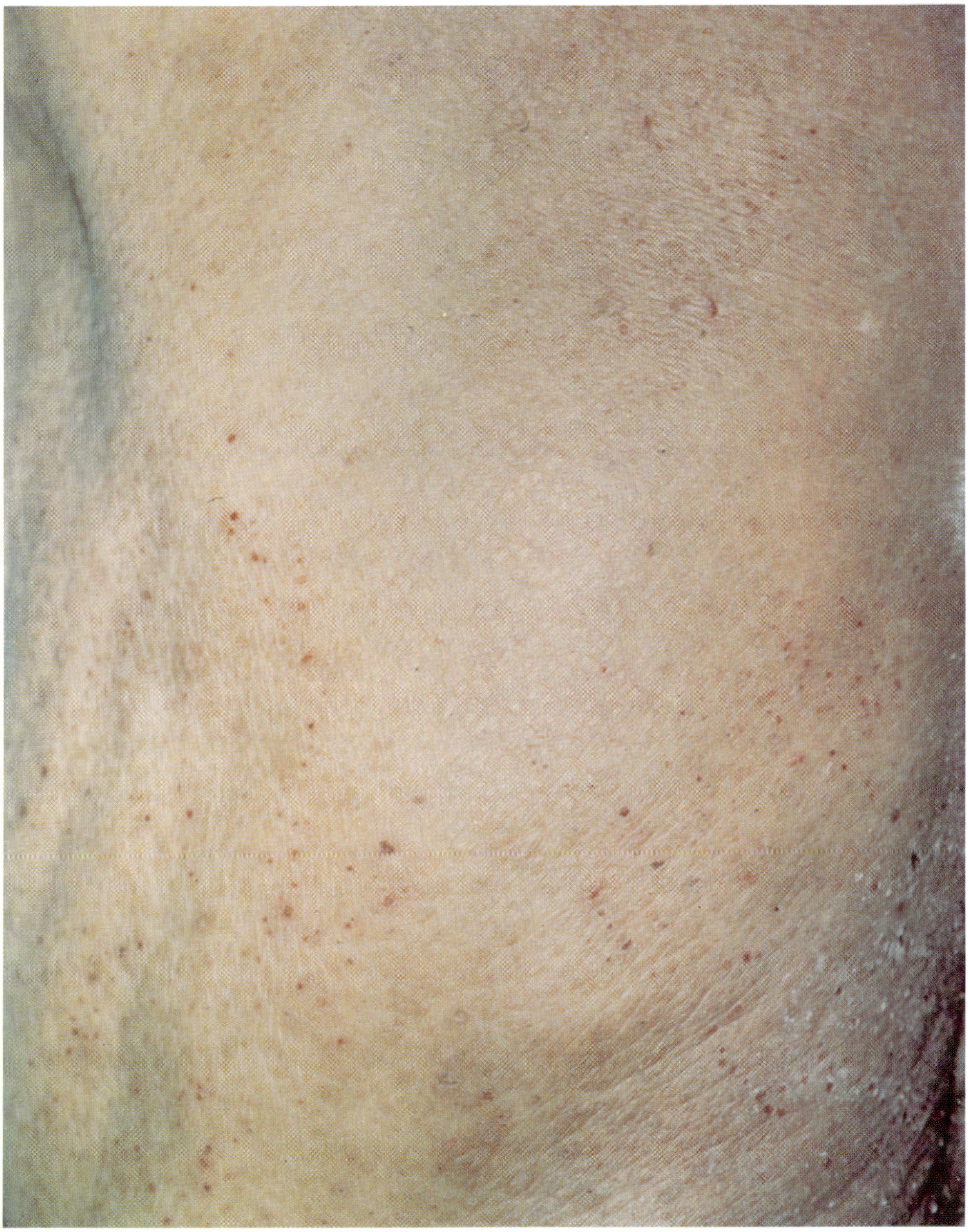

**Plate 13**

Atopic dermatitis of lateral thorax—adult form.

an exfoliative dermatitis, either in children or adults.

***Cataract formation.*** The incidence of cataracts may exceed 12% in patients with severe atopic dermatitis. The cataracts associated with atopic dermatitis mature rapidly and occur at a younger age than do senile cataracts.

***Viral infection.*** A most feared development in atopic individuals is *Kaposi's varicelliform eruption*, a clinical syndrome resulting from the hematogenous spread of herpes simplex virus or vaccinia virus to the areas involved by the dermatitis and then to the entire skin surface. The spread of these vesicular and pustular lesions may be associated with high fever and generalized systemic symptoms. The syndrome occurs chiefly in infants and children and may end fatally. *Patients with active atopic dermatitis should not be vaccinated.* It is considerably safer to vaccinate these individuals at a time when no active lesions are present and pruritis is well controlled.

### *Microscopic findings*

The appearance will vary with the stage of the disease. If the stage is acute, intercellular edema and spongiosis are present. The capillaries are dilated and often have an associated perivascular infiltrate. In the chronic stage, hyperkeratosis, parakeratosis, and acanthosis are the paramount features. The findings are not diagnostic.

### *Differential diagnosis*

***Allergic eczematous contact dermatitis.*** Allergic eczematous contact dermatitis is an eczematous process that is localized at the site of contact with the allergy-producing agent.

***Primary irritant dermatitis.*** Primary irritant dermatitis is an eczema caused by excessive exposure to primary irritants such as soaps and detergents.

***Seborrheic dermatitis.*** Seborrheic dermatitis consists of scaly, erythematous patches over the scalp, midsternal region, and hair-bearing parts of the body.

***Lichen simplex chronicus.*** In lichen simplex chronicus, a localized, pruritic, lichenified plaque occurs, usually on the occipital area of the scalp or on the shins, sacral area, or forearm.

***Nummular eczema.*** Frequently nummular patches (discrete, circular) develop in children or adults with atopic dermatitis and imitate nummular eczema.

### *Treatment*

There are few more gratifying experiences in dermatology than of controlling adequately the continued pruritis that has become the lifelong companion of the atopic patient. Children particularly are changed individuals, with a "new lease on life" after relief of their inexorable itching.

The parent or patient, or both, should be made aware of the nature of atopic dermatitis; a simple explanation of the various trigger mechanisms should be given. *The cardinal treatment principle in the management of atopic dermatitis is control of pruritis.*

***Practical instructions for the patient.*** The patient should be made aware of the long course of this disease and the vital importance of faithfully following instructions regarding precautionary measures.

Clothing should be as soft and light as allowed by the environmental temperatures. Cotton or corduroy materials are preferable. Wools and coarse heavy synthetics are to be avoided. Wool fibers should not touch the skin because their pointed ends mechanically irritate the sensitive surface. Atopics are rarely, if ever, allergic to wool.

Heat from any source can be provocative. The work, play, and sleeping areas should be cool and well ventilated.

Washing and bathing procedures must be modified for the atopic dermatitis patient. Indiscriminate use of soap and hot water in a tub bath or shower must be omitted. The use of a colloid or tar type of bath may be soothing and beneficial, but of greatest importance is the regular use of lukewarm, brief baths or showers not to exceed 5 minutes with soap kept to a minimum.

Primary irritants should be avoided at all times; paints, cleansers, solvents, and chemical sprays and dusts can adversely affect the skin of atopic patients.

These patients are believed to have an increased incidence of immediate type 1 reactions to penicillin, oral or parenteral.

Infection and fever can cause a flare-up of this disease.

Changes in climate influence the severity of atopic dermatitis. During the summer, the patient frequently improves. Conversely, the patient with atopic dermatitis is worse during the winter season. The physician may, in selected cases, suggest a change of residence that permits the severely afflicted patient the benefit of a different climate. Warm, dry, temperate, unvarying climates without extremes of temperature are most desirable.

***Topical measures.*** If the process is acute, wet, or crusted, bacterial cultures should be taken. Then wet compresses of Burow's solution offer a convenient approach in prepackaged tablets or powders, with one tablet or package added to 1 pint of cool water, used for compressing three times daily for 10-minute periods.

If the process is acute and generalized, a colloidal or tar bath is beneficial when used as a cool, brief bath.

***Antiseptics.*** Antibacterial cleansers, such as Betadine and Hibitaine, can be very beneficial if frequent impetigenization is seen.

The *regular application* of a glucocorticoid cream in effective concentration (see p. 67) three times daily is the single most effective modality for long-continued control of atopic dermatitis. For localized areas, such as hands, flexures, or lichenified areas, potent steroid creams should be used either every 3 to 4 hours, or daily, under plastic, occlusive, pliable dressings. For larger areas, 1% hydrocortisone in Unibase or similar vehicle, four times daily, should be used. Topical adverse effects of glucocorticoids and systemic effects from absorption must be monitored.

Topical medications must be prescribed in adequate amounts to ensure their continued use. An average is 4 oz. every 2 weeks. Topical glucocorticoids are effective if there is no continuing external irritation, if infection is not present, or if the disease is not too generalized and severe.

***Systemic measures***

*Antipruritic agents.* Antipruritic agents are very important in controlling the sleep-disturbing pruritus. Trimeprazine tartrate 2.5 to 5 mg. tablets, and cyproheptadine, 4 mg. tablets, may be helpful when given three times daily. They may produce drowsiness. In children particularly, elixir of trimeprazine, 2.5 mg. per teaspoon, is very helpful an hour before sleep and if necessary in the morning as well.

Tranquilizers and barbiturates may be used as adjuvant therapy, but they are not very effective antipruritic agents. If tranquilizers or sedatives are necessary, the choice of a drug must be decided on an individual basis. Adequate rest at night is essential to the well-being of these patients. This can be aided by the use of chloral hydrate and acetylsalicylic acid for combined sedative and antipruritic effect. Although attempts at daytime sedation may be justifiably resented by busy active individuals.

*Antibiotics.* These individuals have increased bacterial colonization of their skin and may be nasal, scalp, or perineal carriers of staphylococci. Skin trauma is often followed by infection and increased pruritis. Culture and sensitivity studies with suitable oral antibiotic therapy will produce a remission.

*Glucocorticoids.* The systemic use of the glucocorticoids is justified only if they are deemed necessary because of severity or nonresponse to topical medication and if the following necessary precautions are taken:

1. Superficial infection is eliminated.
2. The dosage must be absolutely minimal and ordinarily for limited periods. (Complete clearing of the skin lesions is *not* necessary so long as a normal pattern of living is attainable, sleep is undisturbed, and clothing causes no untoward pruritus.)
3. The drug should not be administered in the presence of any contraindications (for example, diabetes, peptic ulcer, and hypertension).
4. Medical surveys of blood pressure, urine, and general health are mandatory at regular intervals.

***Dry skin.*** Many atopic patients have an associated ichthyosis with generalized dryness of all parts of the skin, which adds to the pruritus. We have found the following to be worthwhile:

| | |
|---|---|
| Hydrocortisone | 0.5% to 1% |
| Urea | 10% to 20% |
| Unibase | 4 to 8 oz. |

To be applied in a thin layer to the moist skin immediately after bathing, or once daily.

## REFERENCES


Clendenning, W. E., Clack, W. E., Ogawa, M., and Ishizaka, K.: Serum IgE studies in atopic dermatitis, J. Invest. Dermatol. **61**:233, 1973.
**Significant as to extent of disease.**

Dahl, M. V.: Dermatologic manifestations of immunodeficiency, Progr. Dermatol. **10**:9, 1976.
**Many are similar to atopic dermatitis.**

Hanifin, J. M., and Lobitz, W. C.: Newer concepts of atopic dermatitis, Arch. Dermatol. **113**:663, 1977.
**An attempt to put it all into perspective.**

Hanifin, J. M., and Rogge, J. L.: Staphylococcal infections in patients with atopic dermatitis, Arch. Dermatol. **113**:1383, 1977.
**Pustules, chiefly on extremities and face, in severe cases.**

Huggins, K. E., and Brostoff, J.: Local production of specific IgE antibodies in allergic rhinitis patients with negative skin tests, Lancet **2**:148, 1975.
**And not measurable in serum.**

Jones, H. E.: Allergic contact sensitivity in atopic dermatitis, Arch. Dermatol. **107**:217, 1975.
**Reduced.**

Jones, H. E., Inouye, J. C., McGerity, J. L., et al.: Atopic disease and serum IgE, Br. J. Dermatol. **92**:17, 1975.
**Elevated.**

Kaufman, H. S.: Diet and heredity in infantile atopic dermatitis, Arch. Dermatol. **105**:400, 1972.
**Unrelated to diet.**

Leyden, J. J., Marples, R. R., and Kligman, A. M.: *Staphylococcus aureus* in lesions of atopic dermatitis, Br. J. Dermatol. **90**:525, 1974.
**Exudative lesions yielded *Staphylococcus* in 100% of attempts; from plaques, 90%.**

Lobitz, W. C., Honeyman, J. F., and Winkler, N. W.: Suppressed cell-mediated immunity in two adults with atopic dermatitis, Br. J. Dermatol. **86**:317, 1972.
**The first dermatologic confirmation.**

Möller, H.: Atopic winter feet in children, Acta Derm. Venereol. **52**:401, 1972.
**A common clinical presentation.**

Rogge, J. L., and Hanifin, J. M.: Immunodeficiencies in severe atopic dermatitis: depressed chemotaxis and lymphocyte transformation, Arch. Dermatol. **112**:1391, 1976.
**Alter with successful treatment of the skin.**

Roth, H. L., and Kierland, R. R.: The natural history of atopic dermatitis, Arch. Dermatol. **89**:209, 1965.
**500 patients over 20 years.**

Stone, S. P., Muller, S. A. and Gleich, G. J.: IgE levels in atopic dermatitis, Arch. Dermatol. **108**:806, 1973.
**Elevated.**

Sulzberger, M. B., and Witten, V. H.: Atopic dermatitis. In Loewenthal, L. J. A., editor: The eczemas. London, 1964, E & S Livingstone, Ltd.
**The entire clinical picture.**

Uehara, M., and Ofugi, S.: Abnormal vascular reactions in atopic dermatitis, Arch. Dermatol. **113**:627, 1977.
**Requires a clarification of unaffected skin.**

Whitlock, F. A.: Psychophysiologic aspects of skin disease, Philadelphia, 1976, W. B. Saunders Co., p. 130.
**Vasomotor, sweat, and allergic responses augment itching in atopy, but their emotional content needs assessment.**

# CHAPTER 5
# Bullous diseases

## DEVELOPMENT AND STRUCTURE OF THE EPIDERMIS
### Embryology

The stratified squamous epithelium of the human epidermis is derived from the ectoderm, which envelops the embryo. Ectodermal cell surfaces in contact with the amniotic fluid exhibit some cilia and microvilli. The cells possess tangled cytoplasmic, filamentous skeins, which may be for structural support. When two layers develop at the fourth to fifth week, the outer periderm and the inner germinative layer remain functionally distinct. Desmosomes appear intracellularly at condensations of the plasma membranes in apposing sites of adjacent cells. Tonofilaments appear for the first time opposite the sites of desmosome formation, and hemidesmosomes appear subsequently.

The outer periderm is not just passively protective, but an important active metabolic layer, involved with compound exchanges with amniotic fluid up to 16 weeks. It then flattens to a chiefly filamentous cellular layer but does not form keratohyalin granules nor does it keratinize. Melanocytes and Langerhans cells begin to be found among the proliferating epidermal cells around the third to the fourth month of intrauterine life. By the third month, the cutaneous appendages and ridges of the dermoepidermal border have begun to form. From the fourth month on, the future epidermis becomes several cell layers thick.

In higher vertebrates, two distinct types of keratin are formed as an end product of epidermal cells, the hair or alpha type, and the feather or beta type. Higher vertebrates also demonstrate an ability to form complex epidermal appendages from localized epidermal downgrowths into condensations of the adjacent mesenchyme. These, under the mesenchymal influence, differentiate into distinct patterns of cutaneous organs, such as hair follicles, sebaceous glands, apocrine glands, and eccrine sweat glands. In addition, regional epidermal characteristics such as the number of layers, the overall thickness, or the extent of keratinization are strongly dependent on adjacent connective tissue influences (Flaxman and Maderson). Throughout cutaneous organogenesis, interactions between epidermis and dermis are important, complex, and interdependent. The specific stage of the overall organism's development has an important bearing on the outcome of these interactions (Slavkin). The epidermal changes occur as a result of mesenchymal influence that extends over a distance of 50 to 100 μm and as a result the importance of the actual cell contact as a part of this influence has been considered unnecessary. However, it has more recently been reconsidered as an important regulatory influence in cutaneous organ development. Small electrically charged molecules may pass directly between cells, thereby establishing intercellular communication (Slavkin). Also, cell surface phenomena, such as recognition and adhesion between cells, may be important in organogenesis.

### Anatomy

The epidermis varies between 0.5 to 1.5 mm. in thickness, normally becomes thicker on the soles and palms, and shows local areas of thickening in response to friction and pressure. The undersurface of the epidermis consists of varying patterns of ridges and pockets, fitting intimately with corresponding craters and protuberances of the dermis. The size and number of these irregularities vary

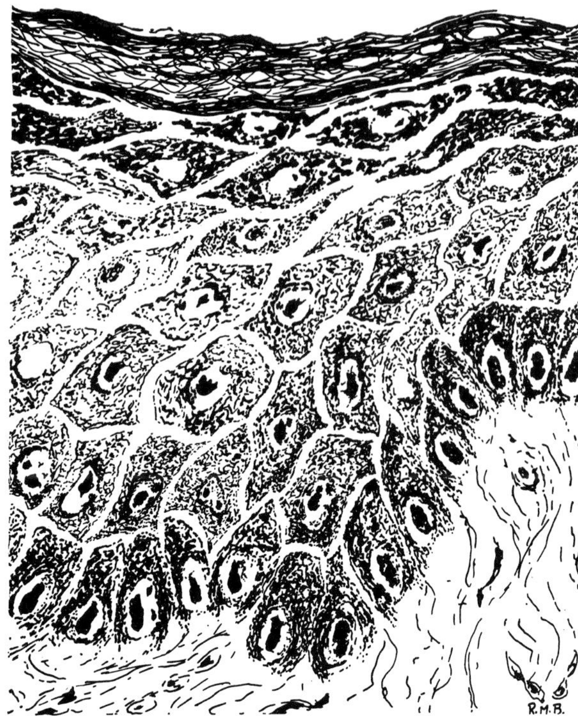


**Fig. 5-1.** Layers of the skin. After mitosis, basal cells migrate upward as components of each layer, finally reaching the surface.

with the epidermal thickness and anatomical location, and they are more prominent in areas of greater environmental stress.

The epidermis contains no blood vessels or lymph channels of its own and is dependent on the vascular and tissue fluid supply of the dermis for its sustenance.

Although microscopic examination reveals that the dead, fixed, and stained epidermis is apparently separable into four areas—basal cell layer, prickle cell layer, granular cell layer, and cornified layer—representing transitional stages in the keratinization of the epidermal cell as it moves toward the surface (Figs. 1 [p.4] and 5-1), the concept of the living epidermis as "layered" is neither desirable nor correct, since it is functionally a unit, composed of large numbers of actively dividing and maturing cells oriented vertically in columns rather than horizontally. These cells are called *keratinocytes* for their main role, which is the manufacture of keratin, the chief component of the surface layer of the skin.

The actively proliferating cells of this tissue are the basophilic erect columnar epidermal cells with large oval dark nuclei along the dermoepidermal junction in the bottom layer. These basal cells rest on the basement membrane, which consists of a condensation of PAS-positive polysaccharides 1 nm. thick overlying a thinner submicroscopic band of reticulin fibers. Both bands are demonstrable only by special stains. The attachment of the epidermis to the dermis is considered in detail in respect to blistering diseases on p. 130. The basal keratinocytes form a single layer and are interconnected with each other and with the overlying keratinocytes by intercellular bridges or *desmosomes*. Half-desmosomes are present along the base of the keratinocyte at its contact with the basement membrane. A desmosome consists of a discrete electron-dense attachment plaque within the cell adjacent to the cell membrane, from which termination fibrillar protein strands *(tonofibrils)* spread out into the cell cytoplasm. This forms the basis of the future surface keratin, which can be shown to be alpha type by x-ray diffraction in vertebrates and beta type in reptiles and birds.

Desmosomes or intercellular bridges appear as rigid structures in stained tissue fixed by routine methods where cell bodies are shrunken, just as the epidermis artificially appears as a layered structure. One must, however, contemplate the activity of these cells in the living state where they exhibit continued movement outwards, individually, as do persons elbowing their own way through a crowd going in the same direction. As with most groups, some move more and faster than others, and desmosomes are released and realigned to conform to individual cell movements (Epstein and Maibach).

Although normal mitotic activity is confined to the basal cell layer, trauma to the epidermis produces a burst of mitotic activity in all the lower layers of the epidermis within 24 to 36 hours. Immediately above the erect columnar basal row, the cells begin to round out and show a streaming tendency in their migration to the surface. This is the *prickle cell* or spinous zone, so named for the intercellular attachments. In fixed stained section, the shrunken cells take on diamond shapes with a "pavement stone" appearance. They possess in vivo a tetrakaidecahedron shape, the most efficient for surface contact in the context of their cellular environment. There are five to ten layers in this zone, the outer layers consisting of flatter cells as they near the surface.

The cells migrate from the spinous into the *granular zone,* which varies in thickness from one to ten layers, in proportion to the overall epidermal thickness. It is easily identified by the large number of dense granules that fill the cytoplasm of each cell. These keratohyaline granules probably become the final amorphous glue within the membranes of the flat, dead cell of the outer tough protective surface. The granular layer is most prominent where the process of keratinization or maturation of the epidermal cell is most active. There is no granular layer in the oral mucous membranes.

The final step in the maturation of the surface-bound migrating epidermal cell is its transition abruptly to an anuclear fibrous keratin pancake with no organelles and thickened tough outer cellular envelope. These flat cells are closely adherent, interdigitating plates that are longer, independent structures, but form a tight, compact, but flexible layer that is able to resist many malevolent influences that would otherwise be life destroying (Fig. 1, p. 4). Through most of this "cradle-to-grave" course of migration from basal layer to corneal surface, the keratinocyte is actively synthesizing protein and lipid. Although flat, it does have elevations on its surface that make it roughened, more so in areas of greater movement and friction. The compact layer formed by these flat cells retains water within it and guards the body from entry by threatening substances, although it is only 0.05 to 2 mm. thick in various parts of the body. It becomes much more fragile and easily penetrated when water soaked, and Montagna and Parakkal describe a greater susceptibility to damage from alkalis, water, and trauma when wet.

***Dendritic epidermal cells.*** There are other normal cellular epidermal inhabitants. These are *dendritic cells,* or cells possessing dendrites—hollow extensile processes that reach out between the surrounding keratinocytes. There are three types of dendritic cells:

*Melanocytes.* These cells with dark shrunken nuclei surrounded by a "clear" zone (largely fixing artifact) rest on the basement membrane between basal keratinocytes. They are concerned with manufacturing melanin and distributing it to the surrounding keratinocytes. (See p. 413 and Fig. 24-1.)

*Langerhans cells.* These dendritic cells remain mysterious. They rest in the upper epidermis and can be identified assuredly only by electron microscopy. They are independent and metabolically active. There has been recent evidence that they may be active in phagocytosis or processing of antigens absorbed through the epidermis. They may form part of an "early-warning" network with a surveillance function.

*Indeterminate dendritic cells* are identifiable in the epidermis, but their function is unknown.

*Merkel cells.* These unusual cells are neural

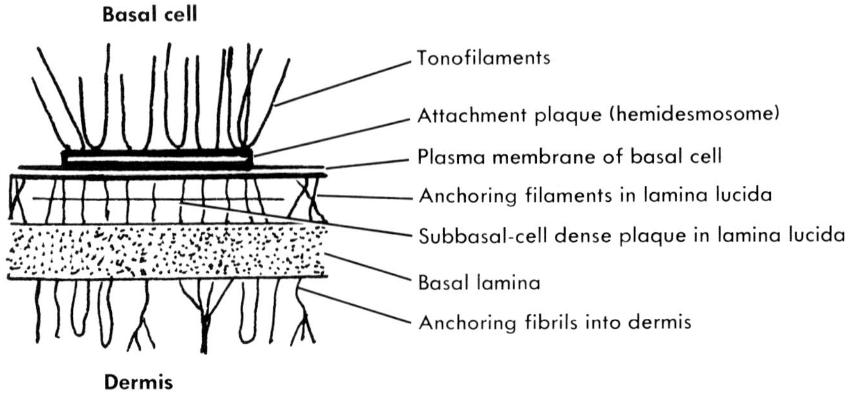


**LOCALIZATION OF PATHOLOGIC CHANGES BY IMMUNOFLUORESCENCE IN SPECIFIC BULLOUS DISEASES**

| | | |
|---|---|---|
| Lupus erythematosus | Anchoring filaments | IgG |
| Pemphigoid | Lamina lucida | IgG |
| Dermatitis herpetiformis | | |
| Papillary dermis | Subbasal lamina | IgA |
| Linear | Anchoring fibrils | IgA |
| Herpes gestationis | Lamina lucida | IgG |
| Epidermolysis bullosa | | |
| Lethal | Lamina lucida | — |
| Recessive | Anchoring fibrils | — |

**Fig. 5-2.** Fine structure of dermoepidermal junction.

and ectodermal and have chromaffin cell–like granules (Winkelmann). They underlie the keratinocytes. Although their purpose is not clear, they have intrigued numerous investigators who are convinced their function is a significant one.

Epidermal cells are joined to one another by desmosomes. Half-desmosomes or hemidesmosomes attach the basal cells to the underlying basal lamina. The upright basal cells are lined up in a row upon the basal lamina, which forms a component of the basement membrane. This structure, a thin zone of neutral polysaccharide can be seen under the light microscope, with special stains. It is not ordinarily visualized by routine staining. Under the electron microscope, the following individual components of the basement membrane are seen (Fig. 5-2): (1) the basal lamina, a 40 nm. thick electron-dense layer that is separated from (2) the basal plasma membrane of the epidermal basal cell by a clear space, (3) the lamina lucida. It is believed that the basal lamina is formed by the epidermal cells. Hemidesmosomes, which appear to serve as areas of attachment for the basal cell to the basal lamina, are seen to be the centers for a concentration of tonofibrils, which radiate from the hemidesmosome out into the cytoplasm of the cell. In the lamina lucida, there is a series of anchoring filaments. There are larger anchoring fibrils, formed by fibroblasts, which extend from the basal lamina into the collagen fibers of the dermis. At this level, there are collections of fiber groups, some of which stain with silver and are called reticulum fibers and some of which are fine elastic fibers. The specific function of each of these types of fibers is not clear, but each forms a part of the fine structure making up the complex attachments of the epidermis to the underlying dermis.

The significance of these fine structures in clinical dermatology becomes apparent in the study of bullous diseases when it is found that the initial malfunction for each type of blister formation affects a specific structure in or adjacent to the dermo-epidermal junction.

### REFERENCES

Breathnach, A. S.: Embryology of human skin. A review of ultrastructural studies, J. Invest. Dermatol. **57**:133, 1971.

**A brief but cogent synthesis of what is known and what is conjectured on early skin structure and function.**

Epstein, W. L., and Maibach, H. I.: Cell renewal in human epidermis, Arch. Dermatol. **92**:462, 1965.

**Labeled epidermis cells migrate at varied speeds, defying apparent hindrance from intercellular bridges.**

Flaxman, B. A., and Maderson, P. F. A.: Growth and differentiation of skin, J. Invest. Dermatol. **67**:8, 1976.

**An intensely interesting review of available knowledge on mechanisms controlling development of skin and its appendages.**

Lever, W. F., and Schaumberg-Lever, G: Histopathology of the skin, ed. 5, Philadelphia, 1975, J. B. Lippincott.

**Histogenesis is given as much emphasis as histopathologic description, written with a clinician's understanding.**

Menton, D. N.: A liquid film model of tetrakaidecahedron packing to account for the establishment of epidermal cell columns, J. Invest. Dermatol. **66**:283, 1976.

**Like interdigitating soap bubbles floating to the surface.**

Slavkin, H. C., and Breulich, R. C.: Extracellular matrix influences on gene expression, New York, 1975, Academic Press, Inc.

**Mesenchymoepithelial interactions as demonstrable controlling factors in skin development.**

Winkelmann, R. K.: The Merkel cell system and a comparison between it and the neurosecretory or APUD system, J. Invest. Dermatol. **69**:41, 1977.

**An imaginative role for these cells that appear to be touch receptors with endocrine potential.**

## CLINICAL DISORDERS

Bullous diseases present a clinical appearance that is so unmistakable that they have traditionally been classified in a group, despite widely differing etiologies (Fig. 5-3). This disparity grows with the years as new knowledge of causes accumulates. We have continued, however, to group bullous disorders together for the simple reason that it still seems less confusing to do so. Much of the material herein has been brought up to date based on Roger W. Pearson's superlative review of blistering diseases in the Year Book of Dermatology for 1977 (edited by Frederick D. Malkinson and Roger Pearson, Year Book Publishers Inc., Chicago).

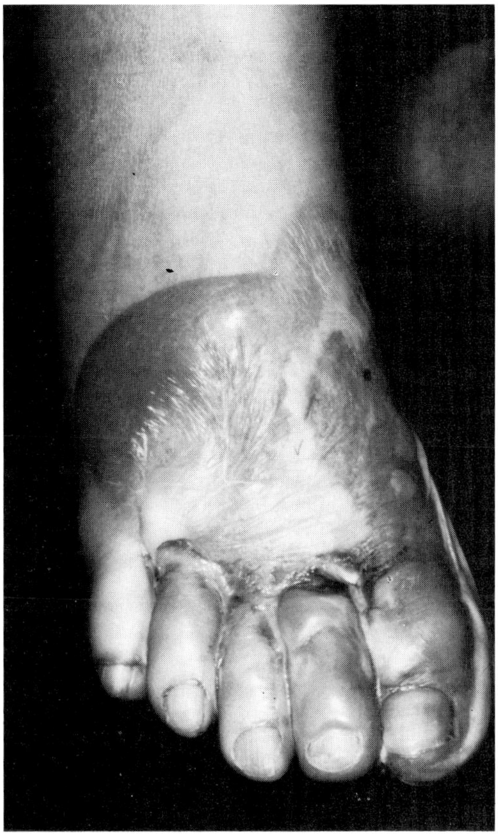

**Fig. 5-3.** Pressure bullae in barbiturate-induced coma.

The following are the causes of bullae:

**impetigo** Can produce bullae in children, chiefly on extremities (p. 242).

**insect bites** May produce bullae in susceptible patients (p. 332).

**plant dermatitis** Contact allergy from poison ivy and other plants (p. 108).

**drug eruptions** Any degree of severity from a small group of small bullae to extensive involvement and mucous membrane ulceration (p. 199).

**barbiturate-induced coma** Bullae appear on areas of pressure (see Fig. 5-3).

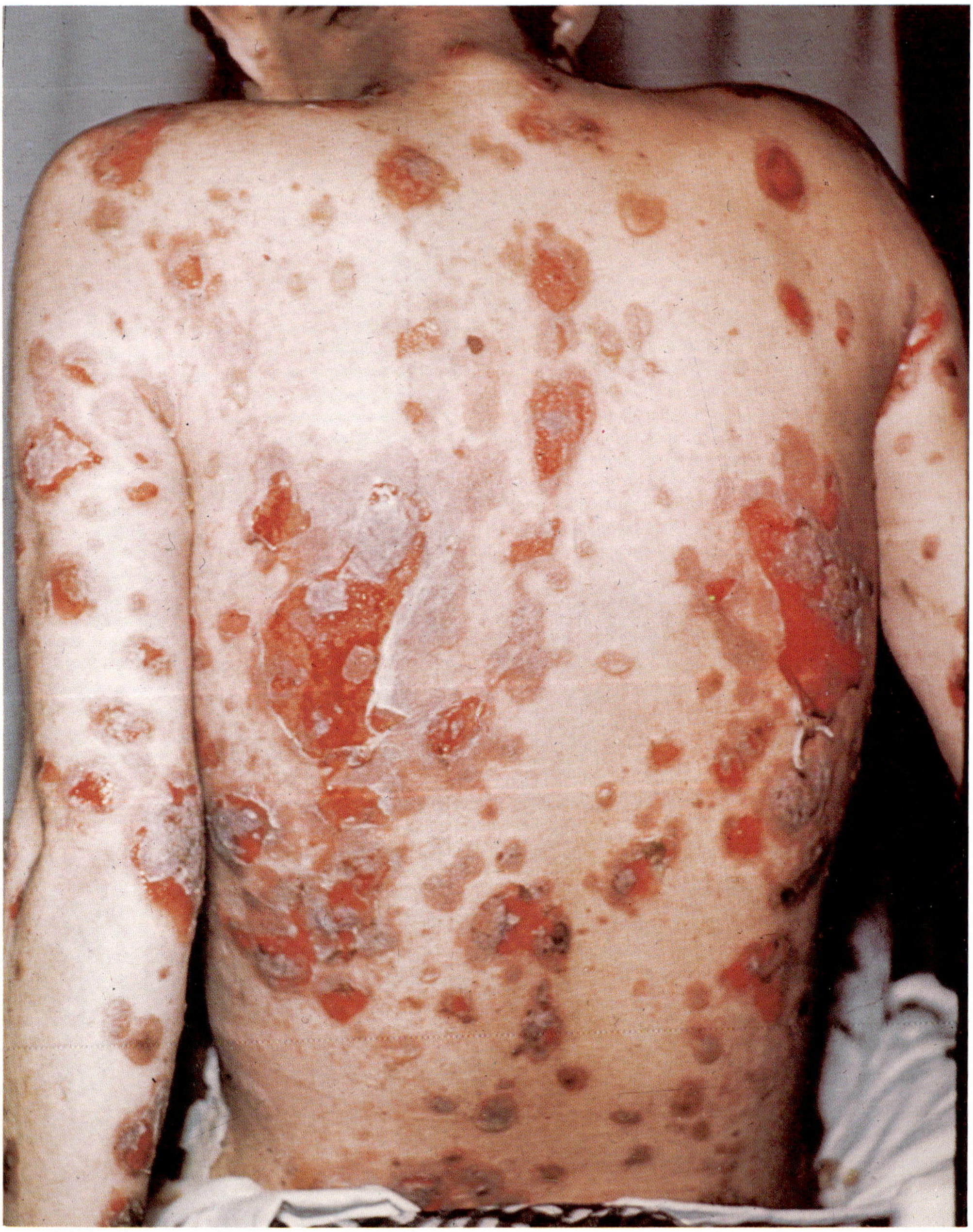

**Plate 14**

Pemphigus. (Courtesy Professor Shigeo Ofugi, Faculty of Medicine, Kyoto University.)

**physical trauma** Extremes of heat, cold, and friction produce bullae.
**erythema multiforme** Severe forms are bullous (p. 212).
**pemphigus** (below).
**pemphigoid** (p. 137).
**cicatricial pemphigoid** (p. 139).
**dermatitis herpetiformis** (p. 140).
**epidermolysis bullosa** (p. 142).
**congenital ichthyosis** (p. 344), **infantile urticaria pigmentosa** (p. 562), **toxic epidermal necrolysis** (p. 144).

## PEMPHIGUS

Bullae in pemphigus are first small and then enlarge, but are unilocular or single chambered throughout. The bullae appear in crops on the skin and mucous membranes (Plate 14).

The basic abnormality lies in the destruction of the mucopolysaccharide protein complex of intercellular cement that Hashimoto and Lever have explored. The normal intercellular contact between epidermal cells is lost, and the unattached rounded cells are a notable feature of the splitting process (acantholysis).

Pemphigus is divided into groups by the level and type of splitting in the epidermis and by differences in the course of the disease. There are some transitions in the epidermis.

***Pemphigus vulgaris.*** In pemphigus vulgaris, bullae appear in crops on nonerythematous, normal-appearing skin and mucous membranes. Erosions of the buccal mucosa and lips are often the first indication of the

A

B

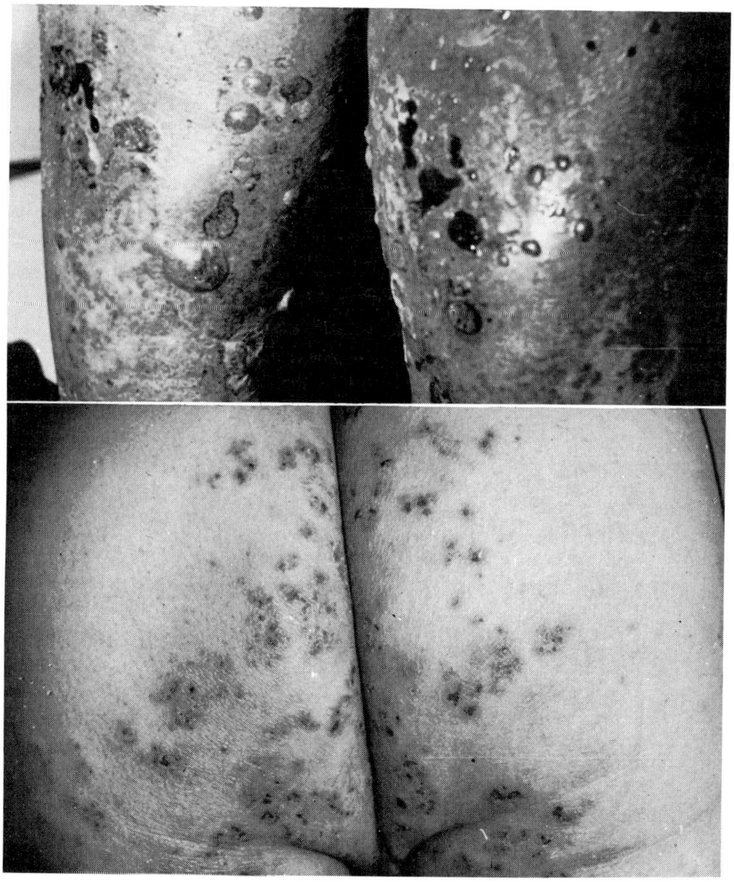

**Fig. 5-4. A,** Pemphigus vulgaris. **B,** Dermatitis herpetiformis affecting buttocks.

disease and are rarely absent sometime in its course. Cutaneous lesions appear on any part of the body as tense, fluid-filled bullae that become flaccid, rupture easily, ooze, and bleed, leaving a raw surface as new lesions form (Fig. 5-4, *A*). Intact skin surfaces are easily damaged by friction or rubbing, which separate the outer layers. All lesions heal very slowly.

Other organs or systems are not involved, except secondarily from pneumonia, septicemia, or other complications.

The untreated course is progressively toward a fatal outcome, with greater and greater involvement. With the introduction of glucocorticoid therapy the mortality from bullous diseases has fallen to one third of the presteroid levels.

Middle-aged persons of Jewish descent and those of Mediterranean extraction are chiefly affected. The incidence in Beutner and Chorzelski's review of 234 North American cases was 5.5 times higher in young females (under 20) than males, but sex incidence was equal after the second decade. Eighty percent of cases were between 31 and 70. A variety of factors seem to be operative in initiating the misdirected immune response against epidermal structures. Minor burns, x-ray burns, sunburn, injury, and drugs are recorded. Patients with Brazilian pemphigus live in a very limited geographic area. Familial factors occasionally seem important.

It is not determined whether the disease represents an abnormal immune response or an abnormal antigenic stimulus.

***Pemphigus vegetans.*** Initial bullous lesions in pemphigus vegetans develop in the characteristic sites of oral or nasal mucous membranes, axillae, inguinal folds, genitalia, or perineum. Overgrowths of soft fungating, crusting lesions are then superimposed. The course often has long remissions, but in general parallels pemphigus vulgaris.

***Pemphigus foliaceus.*** Very superficial bullae are characteristic of pemphigus foliaceus. They enlarge to produce extensive areas of skin with a moist, red, edematous, exfoliating appearance. The oral mucosa is rarely involved. The course is relatively benign.

***Pemphigus erythematosus (Senear-Usher syndrome).*** The lesions in pemphigus erythematosus are unique in that they are erythematous, moist, and crusted over the nose and malar areas. Bullae also occur on the rest of the cutaneous surface, but are few in number. This is a relatively more benign type of pemphigus. Recent immunological evidence indicates that this disease is a combination of lupus erythematosus and pemphigus, which the two clinicians who described the disease in 1926 originally suggested from clinical grounds alone.

### *Microscopic findings*

The tonofibrils within cells become disorganized and detached from desmosomes. This is followed by a dissolution of intercellular bridges in the epidermis just above the basal cell layer. This leads to separation of epidermal cells so that the bulla is formed within the epidermis, with a minimal amount of inflammation. Rounded, free, unattached epidermal cells are found on the floor of the bulla (acantholysis).

### *Pertinent information*

Immunofluorescent studies in patients with pemphigus vulgaris demonstrate circulating IgG antibodies to epidermal intercellular protein that are related to active lesions and severity of the disease.

Complement $C_1$, $C_3$, $C_4$ components and properdin have been identified in the epidermal intercellular spaces, and serum from patients with active pemphigus have a circulating IgG antibody to a component of the intercellular cement material. Injection into rabbits of high-titer pemphigus serum has resulted in bulla formation.

IgG coats the outer layer of the affected epidermal membrane at the pathologic site. IgG antibodies have been shown to produce and sustain intercellular damage in human epidermal cultures. The cause of the clinical lesions seems to be the circulating antibodies, but the cause of their production is unclear. Minor trauma is not uncommon prior to the onset of the disease.

Associations with rheumatic arthritis,

myasthenia gravis, and pernicious anemia have been reported. Penicillamine, rifampin, phenylbutazone, and irgapyrin have been ingested at the onset of the disease. Pemphigus-like antibodies may be found in the serum of patients on some drugs who have experienced drug reactions and in some skin diseases other than pemphigus. They have been seen in burn patients.

***Pemphigus and cancer.*** There have been reports of a number of patients with pemphigus and tumors. Krain and Bierman described a 12% incidence of internal malignancy and thymomas in 42 pemphigus patients. Their review turned up 19 other cases in the literature, half of which had neoplasms of the lymphoid-reticular system.

Katz and co-workers have shown that HL-A 13 occurs more frequently in pemphigus patients than would be expected.

## *Differential diagnosis*

### *Cutaneous surface lesions*

ERYTHEMA MULTIFORME BULLOSUM. Characteristic iris lesions, febrile onset, and initial distal distribution of lesions are helpful in differentiating erythema multiforme bullosum.

PEMPHIGOID. Pemphigoid is usually distinguished from pemphigus by the minimal mucous membrane lesions, histological examination, the patient's age, and the slow progress and benign nature of the lesions.

DERMATITIS HERPETIFORMIS. An intense, burning pruritis, polymorphic lesions, grouped vesicles, and bullae are present in dermatitis herpetiformis. The oral mucosa is not involved.

PLANT DERMATITIS. Vesicular and bullous lesions, usually localized, pruritic, and sudden in onset are found in poison ivy and other forms of plant dermatitis.

INSECT BITES. On occasion, insect bites may form as discrete bullae, usually on the ankles or legs of susceptible individuals.

DRUG ERUPTIONS. Drugs producing a bullous type of eruption include sulfonamides, phenylbutazone, penicillins, aspirin, iodides, bromides, and barbiturates.

BULLAE CAUSED BY PHYSICAL FACTORS. Extremes of heat and cold can produce local bullae. Unconscious, epileptic, or syncopal episodes can result in pressure necrosis and bullae. Barbiturate overdose, producing a comatose patient, may also produce pressure bullae.

### *Mucous membrane lesions*

APHTHOUS STOMATITIS. Lesions are small, painful, recurrent canker sores rather than large erosions.

STEVENS-JOHNSON SYNDROME. The Stevens-Johnson form of erythema multiforme has an acute febrile onset, leukocytosis, and, often, characteristic distal iris lesions on the extremities.

CICATRICIAL PEMPHIGOID. The oral lesions in cicatricial pemphigoid are difficult to distinguish from those of pemphigus, but are often nonpainful; they occur in elderly individuals. Conjunctivae and periorificial skin are affected. The disease goes on to chronic scarring, and adhesions develop.

## *Immunofluorescence tests related to cutaneous disease*

### Specimen taking

***Indirect test.*** *Serum* samples are tested for circulating antibodies to cellular or tissue antigens, most often cutaneous structures. At least 8 ml. of blood without anticoagulants is collected and centrifuged to leave cell-free serum. Clotted blood can be used if no hemolysis is present. Freezing will hemolyze the red cells.

***Direct test.*** *Biopsies* are tested for antibody either in normal tissue or diseased tissue depending on the disease. The specimen, which need not be more than 2 mm., should extend to middermis and is placed immediately in Michel's *N*-ethylmaleimide buffer transport medium, or quick frozen by wrapping it in foil and putting it in liquid nitrogen.

### Method of testing

***Indirect immunofluorescence test.*** Patient's serum is allowed to react with selected tissue sections such as monkey esophagus, or the like. One can then identify the antibody-antigen combinations after washing off unattached proteins, by allowing fluorescein-labeled antihuman IgG antibodies to react with the tissue-serum specimen. The serum antibodies that have fixed to the tissue structure antigens can be clearly identified under a fluorescence microscope.

***Direct immunofluorescence.*** The direct immunofluorescence examination is performed by addition of the fluoroscein-labeled antihuman globulin antibody directly to the tissue, and then by washing off the unattached protein. Immediate examination under the fluorescence microscope identifies the site of the antibody-antigen combinations, usually epithelial cell, basement membrane, or papillary dermis. The type of immunoglobulin present is important (IgA, IgG, IgM, etc.), and whether complement is present and which fraction ($C_3$, properdin, etc.).

**Investigation**

***Direct immunofluorescence (biopsy)***

Intercellular fluorescence present.

Pemphigus erythematosus may show basement membrane fluorescence as well.

***Indirect immunofluorescence (serum)***

Circulating antibodies against intercellular cement present in concentrations proportional to the disease activity.

Pemphigus erythematosus may show circulating antinuclear antibodies as well.

Serum studies for circulating antibodies against intercellular substances are indicated in all forms of pemphigus for diagnosis and for follow-up to assess the activity of the disease as modified by treatment. A rise or fall in titer is significant over two doubling dilutions.

Biopsies for immunofluorescence are particularly indicated if indirect antibodies are not found or are equivocal. A new small bulla with some normal peripheral skin should be selected, and part of the specimen sent for hematoxylin and eosin staining, and the normal skin is placed either in liquid nitrogen or Michel's transport medium for immunofluorescence study.

Routine biopsy studies will also differentiate the intraepidermal bullae, provided that a fresh, small blister is taken.

Smears from the base of these bullae stained with Wright's stain will demonstrate the characteristic acantholytic epidermal cells.

***Treatment***

Pemphigus should preferably be managed from the first by a dermatologist, in a hospital environment.

Large doses of corticotropin or glucocorticoids are given to eliminate the signs of the disease. Treatment should be early and of high dosage, in the range of 150 to 300 mg. daily for 6 to 8 weeks and then 40 mg. per day for a week (Lever). Precautionary measures must be taken to minimize the undesirable side effects of high dosage and prolonged administration of glucocorticoids. These are now probably a more likely cause of serious complications and death then the primary disease process.

After initial suppressive prednisone therapy, immunosuppressives, methotrexate, azathioprine, cyclophosphamide, selected for the individual patient, are used.

With the addition of the immunosuppressive drug, prednisone dosage is lowered and cautiously kept at a minimum. In Rosenberg's 107 patients over 20 years, half the deaths occurred in the first year, and all but one was within the first 3 years. Eventual dosage of corticosteroids was 0 to 15 mg. per day for most.

Penneys initiated and then reviewed gold therapy in 18 patients after 3 years with considerable success. It was commenced after the initial corticosteroid-suppressive treatment in all but three patients.

Topical corticosteroids must not be neglected since they can greatly reduce the dosage of oral corticosteroid needed for control.

Symptomatic treatment is used for eroded mucous membranes and cutaneous surface. A suggested formula is as follows:

| | |
|---|---|
| Soluble betamethasone tablets (0.5 mg.) | 28 |
| Zephiran hydrochloride (21.3%) | 1 drop |
| Peppermint oil | 1 drop |
| Lidocaine hydrochloride | 3% |
| Tragacanth | 4.8 Gm. |
| Distilled water | to make 4 oz. |

1/4 tsp. of mixture to be swirled around mouth q.3h. (gives 0.1 mg. of betamethasone per dose)

Fluid balance and nutrition must be maintained and secondary infection avoided. Large quantities of starch in beds of those uncomfortable patients may help.

Topical application of potent glucocorticoid creams is most beneficial in pemphigus foliaceus and erythematosus.

#### REFERENCES


Beutner, E. H., and Chorzelski, T. P.: Studies on etiologic factors in pemphigus, J. Cutan. Pathol. 3:67, 1976.
**Familial, aging, traumatic, and drug factors may help to initiate antibody formation.**

Hashimoto, K., and Lever, W. F.: An ultrastructural study of cell junctions in pemphigus vulgaris, Arch. Dermatol. **101**:287, 1970.
**Loss of intercellular cement.**

International Co-operative Study: Uses for immunofluorescence. Tests of skin and sera, Arch. Dermatol. **111**:371, 1973.
**A most useful source of information for all.**

Jordan, R. E., Schroeter, A. L., Rogers, R. S., and Perry, H. O.: Classic and alternate pathway activation of complement in pemphigus vulgaris lesions, J. Invest. Dermatol. **63**:256, 1974.
**Complement consumed at lesion site.**

Jordan, R. E., Triftshauser, C. T., and Schroeter, A. L.: Direct immunofluorescent studies of pemphigus and bullous pemphigoid, Arch. Dermatol. **103**:486, 1971.
**IgG, IgM, or IgA in nearly all cases.**

Katz, S. I., Dahl, M. V., Penneys, N. S., et al.: HL-A antigens in pemphigus, Arch. Dermatol. **108**:53, 1973.
**HL-A 13 increase.**

Krain, L. S., and Bierman, S. M.: Pemphigus vulgaris and internal malignancy, Cancer **33**:1091, 1974.
**Five to eight of 42 UCLA pemphigus patients had neoplasms. Previous world cases reviewed.**

Lever, W. F.: Methotrexate and prednisone in pemphigus vulgaris: therapeutic results in 36 patients between 1961 and 1970, Arch. Dermatol. **106**:491, 1972.
**The first combined therapy.**

Lever, W. F.: Pemphigus, Medicine **32**:1, 1953.
**The classic.**

Michel, B., Milner, Y., and David, K.: Preservation of tissue fixed immunoglobulins in skin biopsies of patients with lupus erythematosus and bullous diseases. Preliminary report, J. Invest. Dermatol. **69**:449, 1973.
**A transport medium that makes immunofluorescence far more easily available to all.**

Pearson, R. W.: Advances in the diagnosis and treatment of blistering diseases: a selective review. In Malkinson, F. D., and Pearson, R. W., editors: Yearbook of dermatology, Chicago, 1977, Year Book Medical Publishers, Inc.
**Selective and authoritative.**

Penneys, N. S., Eaglestein, W. H., and Frost, P.: Management of pemphigus with gold compounds, Arch. Dermatol. **112**:185, 1976.
**14 of 15 successfully managed. Long remissions in 8 of 15.**

Rosenberg, F. R., Sanders, S., and Nelson, C. T.: Pemphigus: A 20 year review of 107 patients treated with corticosteroids, Arch. Dermatol. **112**:962, 1976.
**If the first year and especially the third year are successfully gained, mortality falls to insignificance. One third required no therapy when last seen.**

Savin, J. A.: International mortality from bullous diseases since 1950, Br. J. Dermatol. **9**:179, 1976.
**A decrease in mortality concomitant with steroid use.**

Schiltz, J. R., and Michel, B.: Production of epidermal acantholysis in normal human skin in vitro by the IgG fraction from pemphigus serum, J. Invest. Dermatol. **67**:254, 1976.
**Pemphigus IgG antibodies initiate and sustain acantholysis in human skin explants.**

Senear, F. E., and Usher, B.: An unusual type of pemphigus combining features of lupus erythematosus, Arch. Dermatol. Syph. **13**:761, 1926.
**Great clinical acumen.**


## PEMPHIGOID (BULLOUS PEMPHIGOID)
(Fig. 5-5)

Pemphigoid occurs chiefly in elderly persons, although cases have been reported in children. It is twice as common as pemphigus. There is no racial prevalence. The bullae appear in inguinal areas and flexural sites but do not enlarge. They are transient and heal usually without scarring. The disease follows a more benign, if somewhat prolonged, course compared with that of pemphigus. Recently a greater variety of types of pemphigoid have been described, including scarring, drug-related, and mixed forms. There is a definite mortality connected with the disease, and this mortality is the indication for intensive therapy. Some cases are localized and transient. Some demonstrate only a few continuing lesions although more extensive cases are completely covered. The oral mucosa may only occasionally be involved.

There is a suggested association with rheumatoid arthritis, polymyositis, systemic lupus

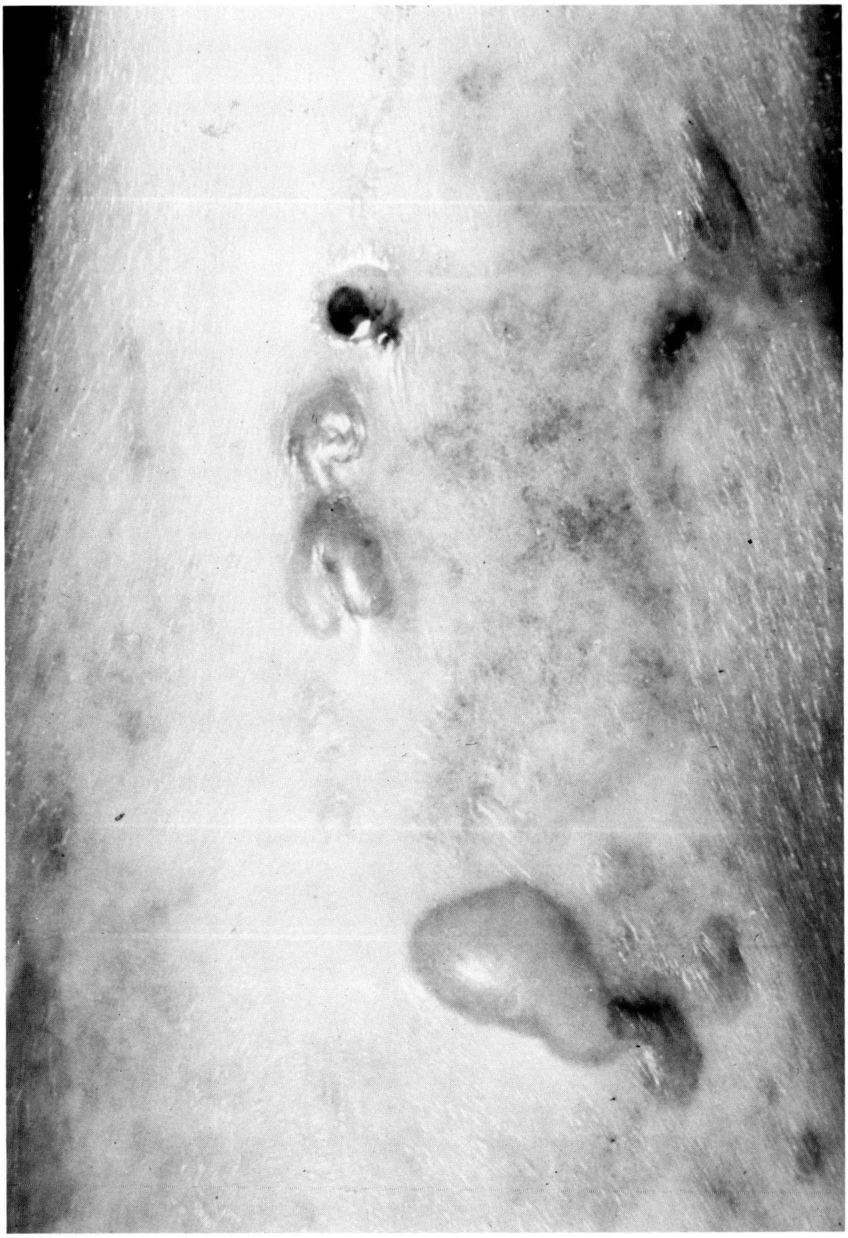

**Fig. 5-5.** Pemphigoid. Bulla arising on noninflamed elderly skin.

erythematosus, and chronic pancreatitis. Lesions have been produced locally by external trauma and by ultraviolet light, on previously unaffected patients. Localized forms occur spontaneously as well. Disruption of the dermoepidermal junction may be a complex injury, capable of producing a variety of antibody-antigen mechanisms as a result. The Honeymans and Lobitz described a fascinating alternation between dermatitis herpetiformis and bullous pemphigoid. Other similar types of change seem to occur with bullous pemphigoid. Similarities exist between bullous pemphigoid and herpes gestationis as well.

Immunofluorescent studies demonstrate

circulating IgG autoantibodies that show a specificity for dermoepidermal basement membrane, the exact site of the microscopic lesion in this disorder. However, the titer of the antibodies does not correlate with activity of the disease or with therapeutic response.

### *Diagnosis*

Biopsies should be taken of small fresh blisters. Microscopically, there is subepidermal bulla formation with no acantholysis. The dermoepidermal basement membrane remains intact on the dermal surface of the blister.

***Indirect immunofluorescence tests.*** Circulating antibodies to basement membrane are found in over 80% of cases and are highly specific.

***Direct immunofluorescence tests.*** Biopsies for these studies should be taken from normal skin adjacent to a blister. Deposits of complement and IgG are present.

### *Treatment*

Treatment with glucocorticoids forms the basis of therapy, but the doses required are lower than those given in pemphigus. Immunosuppressive drugs, methotrexate, azathioprine, and cyclophosphamide are also used associated with glucocorticoids and as a steroid-sparing measure. Ahmed and his colleagues have most convincingly demonstrated the benefit of such combined therapy. Dapsone has also been used successfully.

#### REFERENCES

Ahmed, A. R., Maize, J. C., and Provost, T. T.: Bullous pemphigoid, Arch. Dermatol. **113**:1043, 1977.
**Combined azathioprine and prednisone produced fewer side effects in more severe disease than prednisone alone.**

Honeyman, J. F., Honeyman, A., Lobitz, W. C., Jr., et al.: The enigma of bullous pemphigoid and dermatitis herpetiformis, Arch. Dermatol. **106**:22, 1972.
**First it's one and then the other!**

Lever, W. F., and Hashimoto, K.: The etiology and treatment of pemphigus and pemphigoid, J. Invest. Dermatol. **53**:373, 1969.
**Evidence favors autoimmune cause, and so immunosuppressives are rational.**

Pearson, R. W.: Advances in the diagnosis and treatment of blistering diseases: a selective review. In Malkinson, F. D., and Pearson, R. W., editors: Yearbook of dermatology, Chicago, 1977, Year Book Medical Publishers, Inc., p. 15.
**Illustrates the heterogeneity of this disorder.**

Person, J. R., and Rogers, R. S.: Bullous pemphigoid and psoriasis. Does subclinical bullous pemphigoid exist? Br. J. Dermatol. **95**:535, 1976.
**Apparently lesions are produced by trauma.**

Person, J. R., and Rogers, R. S.: Bullous pemphigoid responding to sulfapyridine and the sulfones, Arch. Dermatol. **113**:610, 1977.
**Another unusual feature of this disease called an enigma by the Honeymans and Lobitz.**

Person, J. R., Rogers, R. S., and Perry, H. O.: Localized pemphigoid, Br. J. Dermatol. **95**:531, 1976.
**A multitude of factors are being considered as provocative in this disease.**

## CICATRICIAL PEMPHIGOID (BENIGN MUCOUS MEMBRANE PEMPHIGOID)

Scarring occurs as a result of this bullous disease of mucous membranes usually in elderly individuals (we have seen it in the second decade). The conjunctiva, buccal mucosa, pharynx, genitals, and anus may be involved, with occasional skin lesions. The process is inflammatory, erosive, and scarring with adhesions (Fig. 24-2). It has been described frequently recently in association with drugs, notably practolol, a beta-receptor blocker and cardiac drug.

The course is benign, but prolonged, and it produces a great deal of discomfort during eating in individuals who may have few other pleasures remaining to them. Lesions are said to be painless, but we have not found this to be true.

Bullae are superficial to the basement membrane, but it may be destroyed or damaged in the process. This probably activates a different group of antigens than do other bullous disorders, one of which results in scarring.

*Indirect immunofluorescence* had demonstrated circulating antibodies to basement membrane.

*Direct immunofluorescence* reveals IgG and complement on basement membrane in affected areas.

### *Treatment*

Systemic glucocorticoids have been used most. Doses required are half or less those required in pemphigus. Azathioprine (Imuran) and cyclophosphamide have been used as well. Topical glucocorticoids must be given a thorough trial in adequate concentration. We have found them of help.

REFERENCES

Bean, S. F.: Cicatricial pemphigoid: immunofluorescent studies, Arch. Dermatol. **110**:552, 1974.
**Positive direct and indirect immunofluorescence with IgG.**

Harder, K. M., Perry, H. O., Pingree, G. C., and Kirby, T. J.: Benign mucous membrane pemphigoid, Arch. Dermatol. **104**:467, 1971.
**One fourth resulted in blindness. Doses of 40 to 60 mg. prednisone daily were successful.**

Susi, F. R., and Shklar, G.: Histochemistry and fine structure of the oral lesions of mucous membrane pemphigoid, Arch. Dermatol. **104**:244, 1971.
**The bulla is clearly shown at or above the basement membrane.**

## DERMATITIS HERPETIFORMIS

Dermatitis herpetiformis is a hereditary chronic, intensely pruritic, vesiculobullous skin disorder associated with patch, coeliac disease, and IgA immunopathy.

### *Natural course*

The disease usually has an insidious onset, although an intense burning pruritis is apparent from the earliest appearance. It infrequently affects children; most patients are males, middle aged or older.

The lesions characteristically are of more than one type. The usual form is vesicular, with the small, tough-walled vesicles occurring in groups. There are papules and macular lesions as well. Each of these is pruritic, with a characteristic penetrating, burning, stinging quality. The lesions heal with pigmentation, so that the affected area at any one time demonstrates active lesions, excoriations, and pigmentation (Fig. 5-4, *B*). The distribution of lesions is very characteristic. They are bilaterally symmetrical, grouped, and concentrated in the interscapular and sacral areas of the back and on the buttocks, the extensor aspect of the forearms, and the scalp (Fig. 5-6). In severe cases the vesicles progress to form bullae.

In most cases exacerbations and remissions occur, but lesions rarely clear completely. The disease becomes less severe and tends to "burn itself out" after an average of 10 years.

### *Pertinent information*

Immunofluorescence shows IgA present either along the basement membrane or on the dermal side of the papillae. The earliest change visible microscopically is vesicle formation in the papillae adjacent to the basement membrane followed by anchoring fibril destruction. Complement is activated.

A gluten-sensitive enteropathy is also present as a patchy involvement of the duodenojejunum. If carefully looked for, it is present in 97%. However, only 60% of those with demonstrable changes present gastrointestinal symptoms (diarrhea, large bulky stools, etc.). The enteropathy differs in no way from adult coeliac disease, including the tendency to have HL-A B8 (90%) and cell-surface antigens $B_1$ and $W_1$. One might think about this as coeliac disease with a marker of skin disease that, because of its pruritic nature, calls attention to the coeliac disease before it becomes advanced.

### *Differential diagnosis*

***Scabies.*** The distribution of the lesions in scabies shows a concentration in interfinger webs and on wrists and genitalia.

***Insect bites.*** Grouped pruritic lesions that fade in a few days characterize insect bites. Usually these consist of well-formed, small bullae.

***Erythema multiforme bullosum.*** In erythema multiforme bullosum, the bullous lesions are preceded by the characteristic target lesions, and mucous membranes are involved early.

***Pemphigoid.*** Pemphigoid may be difficult to differentiate from dermatitis herpetiformis. The lesions are homogeneous rather than varied in appearance like those in dermatitis herpetiformis. The patients are elderly.

***Pemphigus.*** In pemphigus, bullae arise on normal skin. The disease usually begins on the buccal mucosa and causes no pruritus. The patient is severely ill.

A

B

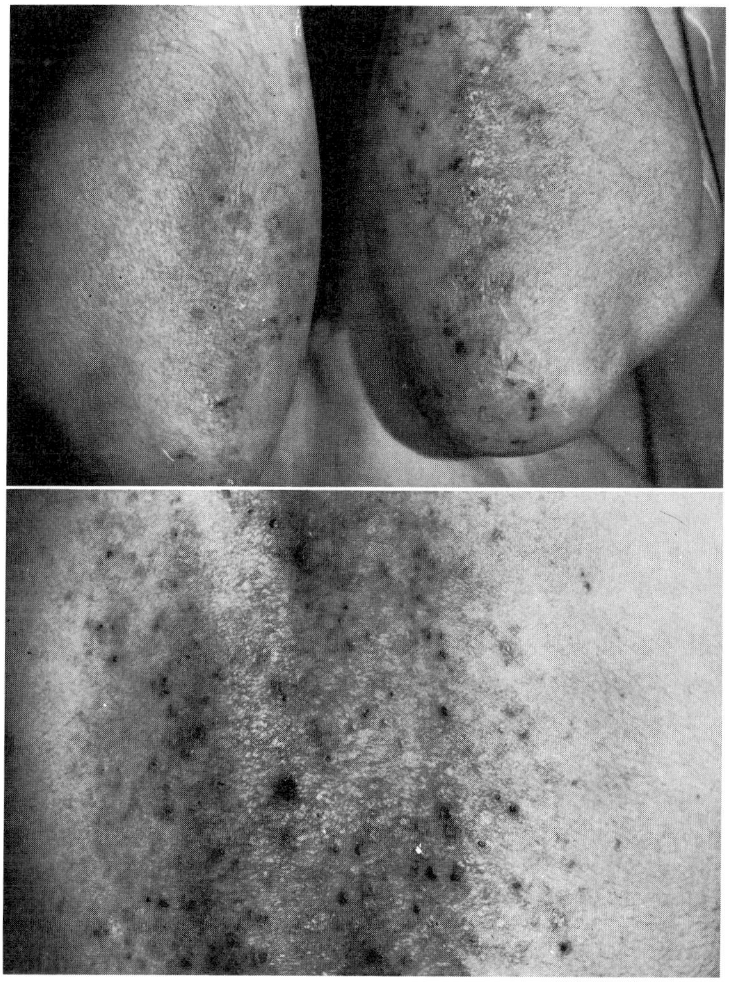

**Fig. 5-6. A,** Dermatitis herpetiformis on elbows. **B,** Dermatitis herpetiformis in midback region.

### *Investigation*

***Initial.*** Biopsy of small, newly forming bulla gives the best specimen for hematoxylin and eosin staining and microscopic differentiation from other bullous diseases. Another biopsy, this time from the uninvolved, normal-appearing skin of a buttock, must be examined by immunofluorescence for granular IgA deposition in the papillary dermis (86%) or in a linear pattern along the dermoepidermal junction (12%). Complement, IgG, or IgM may be present.

***Secondary.*** Duodenojejunal biopsy may show villous atrophy or lymphocytic accumulation, particularly if a high gluten diet is given.

### *Treatment*

***Diet.*** Evidence is accumulating that the requirements of dapsone or sulfapyridine for control of pruritus lessen with a gluten-free diet. Fifty percent of patients respond within a year and all within 5 years. Whether a gluten-free diet alone will suffice to eliminate all pathologic physiology remains to be seen. It certainly is the most rational approach so far, and decreases the dangers of dapsone and sulfa by enabling a reduction and discontinuance of these drugs. Over 6 months to 1 year, the skin lesions will respond to this diet in our experience.

A gluten-free diet requires abstinence from all wheat and grain products; corn or potato flour may be substituted for bread making. Most diet manuals now describe a satisfactory gluten-free diet. The patient must be provided with the motivation to stay on the diet at first.

***Drug therapy.*** To control the intolerable pruritus and clear the lesions, some medication is necessary until the diet can exert its effect. Relief from the two major drugs occurs within a week.

Sulfapyridine, 0.5 gm., is given four times daily at the beginning, and twice daily as a maintenance dose. White blood cell counts and urinalyses should be performed at weekly intervals for a month and then less frequently, to determine hematological or renal effects.

Dapsone (Avlosulfon) may be used as an alternative to sulfapyridine with equal success. It may cause a hemolytic anemia, and hemoglobin levels should be watched for a month or two after therapy is started.

Patients with hereditary glucose-6-phosphate deficiency are at risk to developing a hemolytic anemia on dapsone.

#### REFERENCES

Fry, L., Seah, P. P., Riches, D. J., et al.: Clearance of skin lesions in dermatitis herpetiformis after gluten withdrawal, Lancet **1**:288, 1973.
**Months to years on the diet is essential.**

Harrington, C. I., and Read, N. W.: Dermatitis herpetiformis: effect of gluten-free diet on skin IgA and jejunal structure and function, Br. Med. J. **1**:872, 1977.
**Six of 10 patients able to stop drug therapy within 1 year of diet.**

Mann, D. L., Katz, S. I., Nelson, D. C., et al.: Specific B-cell antigens associated with gluten-sensitive enteropathy and dermatitis herpetiformis, Lancet **1**:110, 1976.
**$B_1$- and $W_1$-antigen incidence identical in the Z group of patients.**

Marks, J.M.: Dogma and dermatitis herpetiformis, Clin. Exp. Dermatol. **2**:189, 1977.
**120 patients with dermatitis herpetiformis from 1966 to 1976 reviewed in all aspects.**

Riches, D. J., Martin, B. G., Seah, P. P., et al.: The utrastructural changes in the skin in dermatitis herpetiformis after withdrawal of dapsone, Br. J. Dermatol. **94**:31, 1976.
**The primary changes are vacuole formation in the dermis.**

Seah, P. P., and Fry, L.: Immunoglobulins in the skin and their relevance in diagnosis in dermatitis herpetiformis, Br. J. Dermatol. **92**:157, 1975.
**Two distinct patterns of IgA deposition. Positive in all cases.**

## HERPES GESTATIONIS

A rare bullous disease of pregnant women, usually affecting the last two trimesters and disappearing after delivery. It may persist, however. It does not affect the fetus. Subsequent pregnancies are often affected more severely.

The bullae are very pruritic, widespread, subepidermal, and nonscarring and do not usually affect mucous membranes. With direct immunofluorescence, complement can be found along the dermoepidermal basement membrane. The initial site of damage is the interior or lamina lucida of the multilayered basement membrane, the same location as in bullous pemphigoid. A circulating IgG HG (herpes gestationis) factor has been identified.

Treatment is with glucocorticoids, in as low a dose as possible to avoid adrenal suppression.

#### REFERENCES

Carruthers, J. A., and Black, M. M.: Further studies in herpes gestationis, Br. J. Dermatol. **95**(suppl. 14):19, 1976.
**Herpes gestationis factor is characterized.**

Jordon, R. E., and Provost, T. T.: The complement system and the skin. In Malkinson, F. D., and Pearson, R. W., editors: Year book of dermatology, Chicago, 1976, Year Book Medical Publishers, Inc. p. 7.
**Our knowledge to date of complement activation in selected skin disorders.**

Katz, S. I., Hertz, K. C., and Yaoita, H.: Herpes gestationis. Immunopathology and characterization of the HG factor, J. Clin. Invest. **57**:1434, 1976.
**The complement-binding factor, clearly a thermostable IgG, the antigen responsible, has not been identified.**

## EPIDERMOLYSIS BULLOSA

Epidermolysis bullosa is a group of six hereditary bullous disorders in which there are abnormalities in the basal cell layer, the basement membrane zone, and the dermis. These

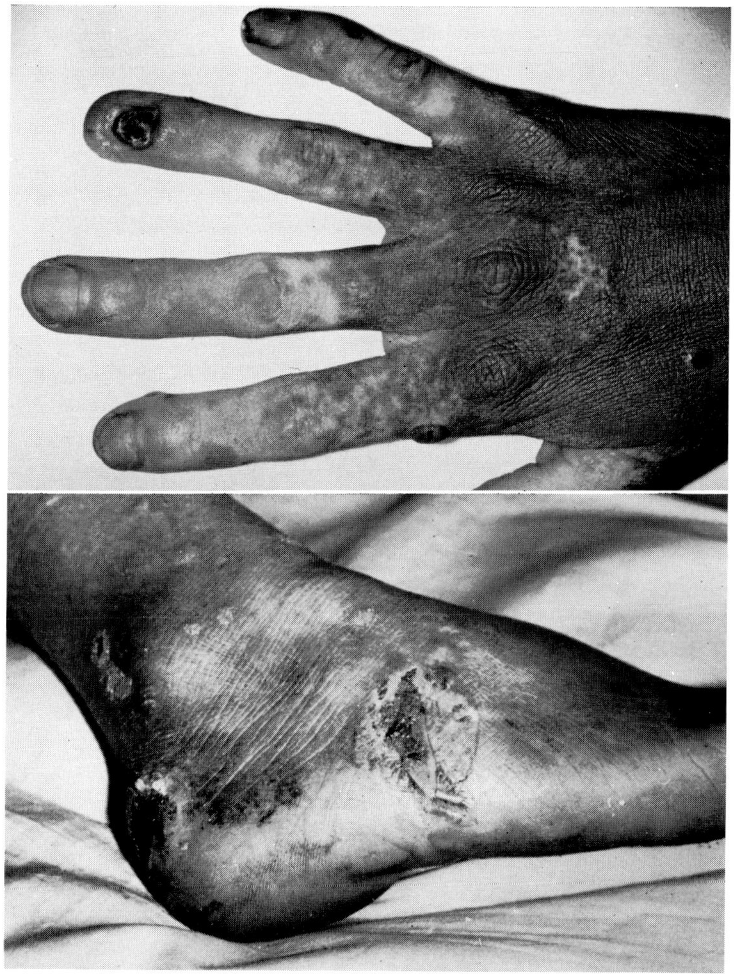

**Fig. 5-7.** Epidermolysis bullosa in characteristic areas of involvement, with bullae, scarring, and nail changes.

are named (1) simple, (2) recurrent, (3) lethal, (4) dystrophic dominant, (5) dystrophic recessive, (6) dystrophic acquired.

The superficial forms of the disease are the milder nonscarring varieties. These are the simple and the recurrent categories. A deeper form is the lethal group in which the blistering occurs at the basement membrane. It is recessive and nonscarring, but extensive with mucous membranes affected. Death occurs often shortly after birth. The deepest forms are the dystrophic group in which blisters affect the dermis and produce scars and chronic mucocutaneous orificial erosions. Bullae affect chiefly distal extremities (Fig. 5-7).

The hereditary disease usually first manifests itself in the newborn period, producing blebs at sites of the child's first trauma from bed sheets and crawling, with bullae on the feet, on extensor surfaces of the extremities, and over joints. Lesions tend to be more numerous during the summer months. In these forms in which the mucous membranes are frequently involved, subsequent scars, adhesions, leukoplakia, and malignancies are seen.

The recurrent, superficial form may not become apparent until adult life. It is limited to the feet and hands, on which bullae form in association with unusual trauma, such as military marches in hot weather.

Depending on the pattern of inheritance

and the level of involvement, the lesions will either heal satisfactorily, or will form scars, produce strictures, and lead to severe mutilations.

### *Treatment*

Used with skill and experience, glucocorticoids administered both orally and topically have somewhat changed the outlook in certain cases of this dreadful disorder. The diagnosis necessitates a consultation and direction of care by those skilled in the demanding, continuous special nursing practices required to maintain life and minimize scarring and deformities. Bacterial and candidal secondary infection must be curbed.

Since Ivan Price presented his complicated patient with epidermolysis to the Canadian Dermatological Association in 1962 to show the beneficial effect of oral vitamin E, there have been further reports such as Michaelson's on its successful use in this disorder. Most have been of the dermal dystrophic variety, and the dose varies from 200 to 3,200 I.U. daily.

#### REFERENCES

Gedde-Dahl, T., Jr.: Epidermolysis bullosa. A clinical, genetic, and epidermological study, Baltimore, 1971, Johns Hopkins Press.

Michaelson, J. D., Schmidt, J. D., Dresden, M. H., et al.: Vitamin E treatment of epidermolysis bullosa, Arch. Dermatol. **109:**67, 1974.
**Success with three patients.**

## STAPHYLOCOCCAL SCALDED-SKIN SYNDROME AND TOXIC EPIDERMAL NECROLYSIS

*Toxic epidermal necrolysis* (Fig. 5-8) is a severe life-threatening disease in which extensive reddened indurated patches of skin may peel off to reveal a *"scalded-skin" syndrome*. The disease is chiefly caused by staphylococcal infection in children in whom it begins with crusting and erythema in the perioral area, spreading to the torso. Recovery follows in 3 or 4 days. Cloxacillin is the treatment of choice where necessary because recovery may be spontaneous. Drugs such as sulfamethoxypyridazine, phenylbutazone, and antibiotics produce toxic epidermal necrolysis

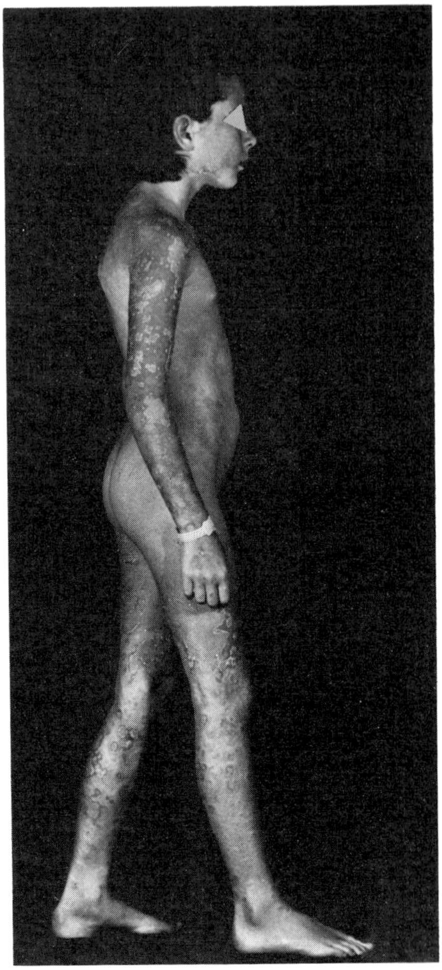

**Fig. 5-8.** Toxic epidermal necrolysis in a 10-year old girl. Extremities completely affected, with healing bullae.

in adults in whom the process is deeper and more toxic. Erythema gives way to bulla formation and epidermal necrosis with which there is much loss of fluid. Nursing care and constant attention are essential; dialysis may be necessary. Mortality is high. Many drugs have been indicted in this disorder, including penicillin, barbiturates, aspirin, diphenylhydantoin (Dilantin), phenolphthalein, dapsone, and thiabendazole, and the alcoholic drink gin and tonic. (See p. 197.)

Rapid initial hospitalization, knowledge, skilled nursing care, and good treatment are essential.

**REFERENCES**

Elias, P. M., Fritsch, P., and Epstein, E. H.: Staphylococcal scalded skin syndrome, Arch. Dermatol. **113**:207, 1977.
**SSSS in children versus TEN in adults**

Pearson, R. W.: Advances in the diagnosis and treatment of blistering diseases. A selective review. In Malkinson, F. D., and Pearson, R. W., editors: Yearbook of dermatology, Chicago, 1977, Year Book Medical Publishers, Inc., p. 7.

## BULLOUS ERUPTIONS OF LEGS AND FEET

Bullous eruptions of the legs and feet are mentioned here separate from the foregoing simply because they frequently present such diagnostic difficulties. Björnberg and Moliacken described 15 patients, most of whom were elderly, and five had diabetes, in whom immunofluorescent findings were not helpful, and the subepidermal bullae were present on abnormal skin with circulatory insufficiency, venous or arterial. Some forms of epidermolysis bullosa (familial) affect the pretibial areas. Impetigo and insect bites, as well as some phototoxic eruptions may result in the appearance of bullae on exposed portions of legs. Contact dermatitis of allergic origin can produce bullae, and much less commonly, metabolic disorders such as amyloid and lichen sclerosus cause bullae on legs. Bullosis diabeticorum is seen in long-term diabetes, affecting toes, fingers, and feet in areas of neuropathy. Friction blisters and pressure blisters may be the initial sign of neurologic disease or the result of aging skin and heat. They may arise from immobility and pressure in unconscious patients, in whom anoxid is the chief factor.

**REFERENCES**

Arndt, K. A., Mihm, M. C., and Parrish, J. A.: Bullae: a cutaneous sign of a variety of neurologic diseases, J. Invest. Dermatol. **60**:312, 1973.
**Frequently unrecognized.**

Björnberg, A., and Moliacken, H.: Recurrent bullous eruptions on the lower legs, Acta Derm. Venereol. (Stockh.) **56**:405, 1976.
**15 patients with puzzling bullous leg lesions.**

## CHAPTER 6

# Connective tissue diseases

### DERMIS

The dermis is derived from mesenchyme. At first it consists of spindle-shaped cells that become *fibroblasts*. It begins to demonstrate procollagen fiber formation by the second to fourth intrauterine month and elastic fiber formation from the sixth month on, continuing after the time of birth. Coarse fibers become apparent in the deeper dermis close to the subcutaneous tissue, whereas fine, horizontally oriented fibers develop in the papillary layer, adjacent to the epidermis. The mature dermis retains this division into easily identifiable superficial *papillary* and deep *reticular* areas.

The dermis then becomes the connective tissue layer intimately associated with the overlying epidermis. It serves as a source of nutrition for the epidermis and at the same time exerts a controlling influence on its growth and maintenance and on the form and location of epidermal structures. The embryonal bud of each developing structure grows by the help of a condensation of activated mesenchyme.

The dermis possesses several components: collagen fibers, reticulin fibers, elastic fibers, ground substance, and cellular elements.

***Collagen.*** Collagen bundles distinguishable by eye are *fibers* ($100^{+}$ μm.), by light microscopy are *fibrils* (10 to 15 μm.), and by electron microscopy are *microfibrils* (30 to 60 nm.) made up of filaments (3 to 5 nm.), whereas a single molecule will be about 1 to 1.4 nm. Coiled coils predominate through all structures.

Collagen has a molecular weight of 345,000 daltons ($1.65 \times 10^{-24}$ gm.) and is 290 nm. by 1.4 nm. The well-known spaced cross striations in the collagen fiber are produced by the positioning of individual collagen molecules, each 290 nm. long, with "charged" regions 68 nm. apart that have an affinity for selected stains.

*Formation of collagen.* Within the fibroblast, procollagen is formed by assembly of 3-polypeptide chains, synthesis of hydroxyprolene and hydroxylysine, addition of galactose and glucose, sulfhydryl bond formation, and the final twist, or formation of the characteristic helical coil. The structure is then excreted from the cell. Two nonhelical pieces are removed from either end, and the bare triple-helix molecule of tropocollagen remains. Fibers are formed in the extracellular gel and then cross-links between adjacent molecules, to produce the three-dimensional network of insoluble collagen. Ascorbic acid is required for the intracellular synthesis of hydroxyprolene and hydroxylysine.

*Types.* Four types of collagen are normally present. Type 1, the most abundant, is in dermis, tendon, bone, and dentine. Type 2 is in cartilage. Type 3 is in dermis, mixed with Type 1, and is in heart valves, arteries, and synovial membrane. Type 4 is in basement membranes. Mature collagen becomes increasingly resistant to degradation with age. Trauma, however, causes increased destruction of collagen and then new collagen formation. Collagen destruction is achieved by collagenases, which are continuously present, as are their natural inhibitors. These components allow for a continual modification, modeling, and turnover of available collagen.

***Reticulin fibers.*** Reticulin fibers are finer than the fibrils of collagen, demonstrate branching, have similar components to collagen, but in different proportions, and appear surrounded by an amorphous matrix. These fibers are numerous in wound healing and some pathological states, but are sparse in normal adult dermis. They have the same 64 nm. axial periodicity as collagen.

***Elastic fibers.*** Fine elastic fibers extend from contact with basal cells into the dermis. They anchor and wrap arrector pili muscles and support sweat glands and blood vessels in position. Elastic fibers consist of an inner homogeneous medulla of elastin, a fibrillar cortex. The empty hollow cortex has been perceived lying in grooves along fibroblasts. These hollow tubes are filled with a homogeneous elastin that is synthesized and secreted by the fibroblast. Lysine is an important precursor. Cross-linkages of desmosine and isodesmosine are added as elastic tissue ages. Aging elastic tissue can also calcify.

***Glycosaminoglycans.*** Formerly called "ground substance," the glycosaminoglycans are hydrophilic and bind water. These extracellular components of the dermis are in the form of a gel, more fluid near the dermoepidermal boundary. The gel is in intimate relationship to the forming and degrading collagen, the reticulin fibers, the elastic fibers, cells, and their metabolites. It is an intensely active physicochemical milieu, difficult to conceptualize from stained sections. Major components of the glycosaminoglycans are hyaluronate chondroitin sulfate, dermatan sulfate, and keratin sulfate. These are polysaccharides, straight-chain molecules composed of repeating disaccharide units, bound to a protein core. The fibroblast synthesizes both components.

***Cellular elements***

*Fibroblasts.* Fibroblasts are the master cells of the connective tissues of the body traveling under many guises and specialized forms. They are responsible for synthesis of the fibrous and the amorphous components of connective tissues. Their appearance in dermis varies considerably with their degree of activity. When active, they are large, with a generous amount of cytoplasm, extensive rough endoplasmic reticulum, multiple Golgi complex vesicles, filaments, vesicles, and vacuoles. When inactive, they are long and thin, consisting mostly of nucleus.

*Histiocytes.* Some histiocytes arise from blood monocytes. The epithelioid cell is an end-stage histiocyte. They possess destructive lysosomal enzymes for phagocytosis, and they ingest hemosiderin, melanin, foreign material, dead cells, and debris. They synthesize and degrade lipids. They participate in immune responses such as allergic contact dermatitis by transporting antigenic substances to regional lymph nodes for processing.

*Mast cells.* Coarse granular cells that are usually found around blood vessels. The granules contain heparin and histamine and release these compounds under a variety of conditions. Heparin affects blood clotting, fat transport, and glycosaminoglycans, and histamine increases capillary permeability, contracts smooth muscle, attracts phagocytes, and initiates a variety of cellular activities.

The dermis undergoes aging, which can be assessed by an increased coarseness of collagen fibers, an increased proportion of insoluble collagen, an increase in cross-linkages, and an increase in numbers and sizes of elastic fibers and elastin. The overall amount of collagen decreases, and the metabolic activity of the glycosaminoglycans decreases.

#### REFERENCES

Bentley, J. P.: Excelsior: a retrospective view of collagen, J. Invest. Dermatol. **67**:119, 1976.

**The current state of knowledge of collagen biosynthesis in four pages.**

Grant, M. E., and Prockop, D. J.: The biosynthesis of collagen, N. Engl. J. Med. **286**:194, 242, 291, 1972.

**A lucid historical and current deposition.**

Montagna, W., and Parakkal, P. E., editors: The structure and function of skin, ed. 3, New York, 1974, Academic Press, Inc.

**All known aspects described and a few personal deductions added.**

Pearce, R. H., and Grimmer, B. J.: Age and the chemical constitution of the human dermis, J. Invest. Dermatol. **58**:347, 1972.

**Collagen content and cell population decreases, but water and elastin increase with aging.**

## LUPUS ERYTHEMATOSUS

### Discoid lupus erythematosus

Discoid lupus erythematosus is a chronic, recurrent, scarring dermatitis in exposed areas of autoimmune origin.

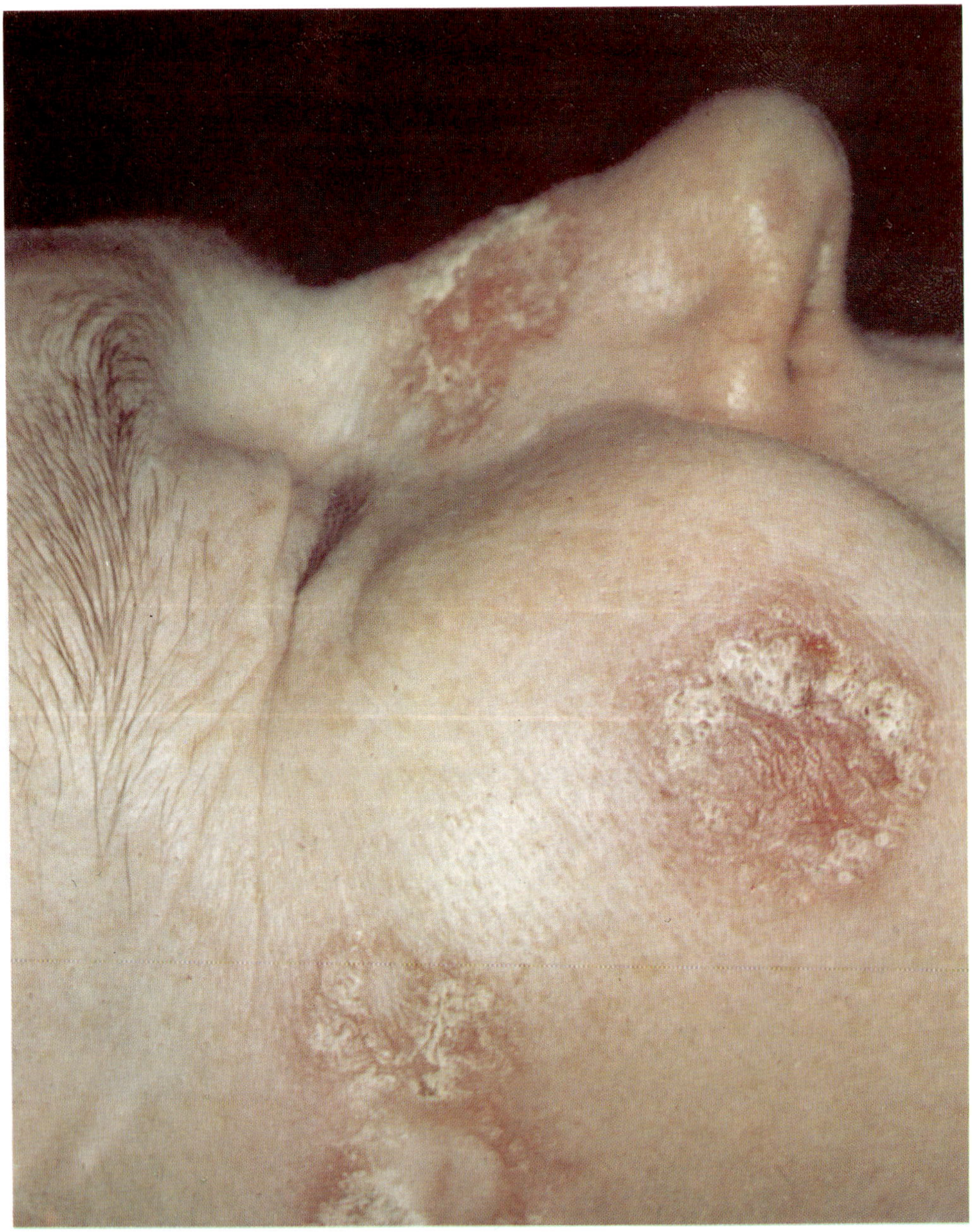

**Plate 15**

Discoid lupus erythematosus. This patient had an 18-year history of untreated disease. She had no systemic involvement.

*Natural course*

Cutaneous manifestations of discoid lupus erythematosus begin with scaling erythematous macules distributed over the bridge of the nose, malar area, forehead, and temples (Plate 15). Ordinarily it starts insidiously with a single small lesion; later, more and larger discrete lesions slowly appear and involve the neck, ear, scalp, and more rarely, upper mid-back, arms, forearms, and backs of hands. Atrophic erythematous, sharply bordered lesions of the periorificial skin of the ears are typical.

The lesions progress through a heavily scaling phase, with horny "tacks" extending from the scale into follicular openings. There is atrophy, characterized by pallor, depression, and scarring at the center of the lesions. Scalp lesions are erythematous, moist, and crusted, leading to early scarring and permanent alopecia of the area involved (Fig. 6-1).

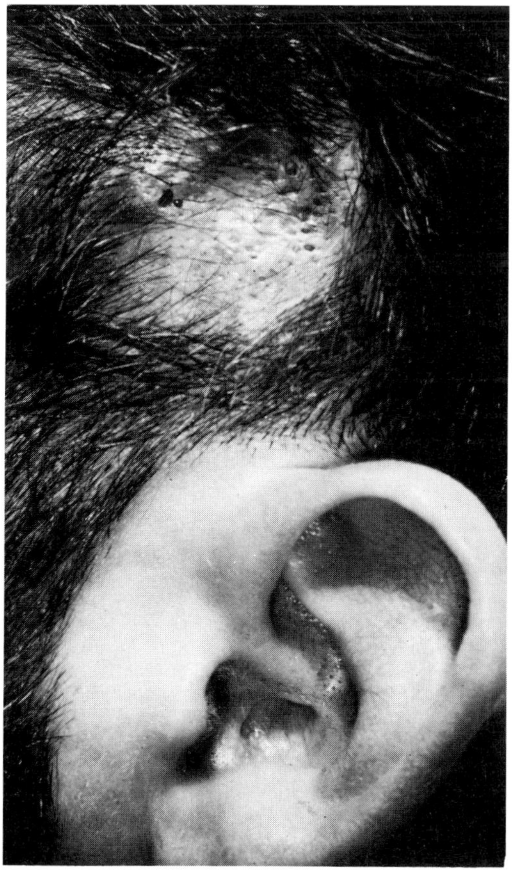

**Fig. 6-1.** Discoid lupus erythematosus. Scarring alopecia and classic periorificial external ear lesions.

Lesions of the mucous membranes are seen most commonly on the lips, where there is crusting, scaling, and erythema, usually of the lower lip. There may be dilated capillaries at the border. Occasionally lesions of the buccal mucosa are present. Conjunctival lesions also occur.

Some systemic symptoms of joint pains, malaise, weight loss, and Raynaud's phenomenon may be seen in some cases of discoid lupus erythematosus.

Fluorescent antibody studies have shown that there are antinuclear antibodies present in many discoid lupus cases, emphasizing the relationship between the two forms of the disease. Exposure to sunlight may precipitate the appearance of new lesions and worsen those already present, but this is true in less than half of the cases.

Spread of existing lesions, widening distribution of new lesions, and palm and sole involvement may indicate that a cutaneous case is becoming systemic.

*Pertinent information*

Discoid and systemic lupus erythematosus may be separate genetic disorders. It has been suggested that proliferation of "forbidden" clones of lymphocytes may be responsible for the development of the autoimmunity believed to cause both diseases, each occurring separately in predisposed individuals. Most evidence, however, indicates that discoid lupus erythematosus is at the benign end of the spectrum of the disease and that there are interrelationships between various forms of the disease. Environmental factors play an important part in the disease. Sun, trauma, stress, infection, cold, and so forth are significant as initiating causes.

This is a disease of autoimmunity. Immunoglobulins IgG, IgA, IgM, properdin, and $C_3$ and $C_4$ fractions of complement have been shown to be present at the involved dermoepidermal junction in active stages of the disease. The basal cell appears to be at the site of primary injury. The immunofluorescent appearance of inactive systemic lupus erythematosus is similar to discoid lupus erythematosus. Some evidence indicates that complement deposition at the basement membrane is by an alternate pathway in discoid lupus erythematosus and the classical pathway in systemic lupus erythematosus.

Also, an abnormal relationship between suppressor T-cells and B-cells may be part of the disturbance in lupus erythematosus with the discoid form demonstrating a B-cell proliferation (Gilliam) and the systemic form, a suppressor T-cell impairment (Abdou).

### *Microscopic findings*

There are several characteristic microscopic changes: hyperkeratosis, a degeneration of the basal cell layer, distinct but irregular lymphocytic cellular infiltrate beneath the basal layer and around the appendages, and a degeneration of the dermal collagen.

### *Differential diagnosis*

***Seborrheic dermatitis.*** In seborrheic dermatitis there are scaling diffuse patches of erythema of the paranasal areas, eyebrows, and eyelids, associated with scaling and erythema of the scalp. There is no atrophy.

***Psoriasis.*** In psoriasis, a heavy scale and sharp borders to the lesions are confusing, but there is no atrophy, and the lesions are benefited by sun exposure.

***Tuberculosis cutis (lupus vulgaris).*** A rare disorder, tuberculosis cutis characterized by pale, red-brown papular lesions that occur on the face and then crust, scar, and spread peripherally. Biopsy will differentiate this disease from discoid lupus erythematosus.

***Tinea corporis.*** Fungal infection may simulate lupus erythematosus with a circular scaling lesion and an actively spreading border. Culture with microscopic examination of scrapings will identify the fungus.

### *Investigation*

Active lesions should undergo biopsy for routine microscopy. Nonscarred, inflamed areas are best.

Systemic involvement must be ruled out by examination and history (Raynaud's phenomenon, joint disease, pneumonitis, fever, convulsions, and poorly defined illnesses) and by laboratory procedures (complete blood count, sedimentation rate, biopsy with light microscope and immunofluorescent studies, VDRL test, and serum electrophoresis). The differentiation is not clear-cut in some cases, and dogmatic classification into one or the other type may not always be possible.

***Direct immunofluorescence.*** Of discoid and systemic lupus erythematosus cases 90% demonstrate a granular or lumpy pattern of fluorescence at the dermoepidermal junction of active lesions, which indicates IgG, complement, and DNA. This is also found in the normal sun-exposed skin of 60% of patients with systemic lupus erythematosus. Antinuclear fluorescence may be found in cases of cutaneous lupus erythematosus.

***Laboratory.*** Anemia, leukopenia, elevated sedimentation rate, and increased gamma globulin levels may be found. Occasionally the LE cell test may be positive.

### *Treatment*

Scarring and facial disfigurement result from untreated lesions. Surgical removal of lesions can be complicated by recurrence of the immune process at the surgical site.

Local use of a fluorinated glucocorticoid ointment such as 0.1% betamethasone, 0.025% fluocinolone acetonide, or flurandrenolone under plastic dressing is good therapy. If no response is obtained, 0.2% fluocinolone administered topically under occlusion may be used. Triamcinolone acetonide, 5 mg./ml. in lidocaine (Xylocaine) hydrochloride can be injected intralesionally. Rarely, systemic glucocorticoids may be necessary to control the disease.

The most satisfactory treatment has been with one of the antimalarial drugs, chloroquinine phosphate; a 250-mg. tablet is given twice daily, reducing dosage to one tablet daily if possible. Other medications are hydroxychloroquine (Plaquenil) sulfate, amodiaquin (Camoquin) hydrochloride, and quinacrine (Triquin). However, the side effects of these drugs on the retina in certain patients and specifically in patients receiving total doses exceeding 8 gm./kg., producing toxic and irreversible changes leading to blindness, are so severe that they should be used only after full consideration of the risks and consequences. There should be regular 3 monthly examinations by and consultations with an ophthalmologist for each patient taking these medications. Other side effects include corneal opacities, nausea, vomiting, and headache.

For those patients with sun sensitivity, avoidance of sun exposure and an effective sunscreening cream for outdoor use are important. The rays affecting patients with lupus erythematosus are in the erythema producing range. A good sunscreening agent is the following:

| | |
|---|---|
| Para-aminobenzoic acid | 5% |
| Ethyl alcohol (Pabanol) | q.s. |

Liquid is applied prior to sun exposure and reapplied after heavy perspiration, bathing, or washing.

## Systemic lupus erythematosus

A widespread disease of connective tissue, systemic lupus erythematosus varies in severity from a mild, chronic condition to a fulminating, rapidly fatal disease affecting any organ and usually progressing by a pattern of remission and exacerbation. Major manifestations of the disease are joint involvement, inflammation of one or more serous membranes, cutaneous lupus erythematosus–like eruption, renal involvement, pneumonitis, and central nervous system disturbances.

### *Natural course*

Most patients are women between 10 and 40 years of age.

Joint disturbances are the most frequent initial finding, and if anything about this variable disease is characteristic, it is arthritis and arthralgia, which occur in over 90% of cases at some time during the course of the disease. There is typically a symmetrical migratory polyarthritis. Skin lesions develop first in only one fifth of the patients, but are present at some time in more than four fifths. The lesions center around the facial and upper chest areas, are similar to the discoid variety in some 15%, but are transient, erythematous, and nonspecific in most. The "butterfly rash" of the nose and malar area is present in at least half of those with the disease, though often for only a short time. Purpura, Raynaud's phenomenon, and photosensitivity are common. A history of worsening by sun exposure occurs in one third or more of cases.

Telangiectatic lesions appear at the nail folds and over knuckles. Palmar and fingertip dusky red lesions may be present. Purpura, atrophy, ulceration, and scarring are evidences of vasculitis.

Fever, weight loss, cardiopulmonary symptoms, and lymphadenopathy and, less often, central nervous system (CNS) symptoms and renal disease make up the next most common combinations of signs and symptoms. *Renal disease is the most significant involvement, since it is very resistant to therapy, and progressive renal failure is one of the most common causes of death.*

*Laboratory studies* reveal a pattern of mild to severe anemia, leukopenia, elevated sedimentation rate, abnormal serum proteins, abnormal liver function, and positive antinuclear factor. A biological false-positive serological test for syphilis may be present for years before systemic lupus erythematosus manifests itself (present in 10% to 20%). Latex fixation test for rheumatoid factor is present in 25% to 30%.

Urinalysis is performed to determine whether red blood cell casts or protein is present, all of which may indicate renal involvement. If protein is present, identification of light chains is important as a strong indicator of renal disease.

Lowered serum complement has been associated with active renal disease but may reflect widespread cutaneous deposition.

The fulminating variety of the disease may be rapidly fatal and results in a high mortality. The more chronic cases, however, reveal a prolonged course with many exacerbations and remissions and a greatly reduced mortality.

*The precipitation of lupus erythematosus by drugs is well known.* Hydralazine hydrochloride (Apresoline), phenylbutazone, diphenylhydantoin (Dilantin) sodium, mephenytoin (Mesantoin), griseofulvin, isoniazid, methylthiouracil, para-aminosalicylic acid, procaine amide, propylthiouracil, penicillin, streptomycin, sulfamethoxypyridazine, sulfonamides, reserpine, progestogens, trimethadione (Tridione), and an increasing list of others may cause a lupus erythematosus–like syndrome.

Some cases are a dissemination of a previous discoid lupus erythematosus, but these are not usual.

### *Pertinent information*

Reduced serum complement and anti–double stranded DNA antibodies are the distinguishing findings and represent the basic autoimmune process. Circulating immune complexes of DNA and anti-DNA antibodies are considered responsible for complement activation, and complement fraction deposition in normal skin of patients with systemic lupus erythematosus (SLE) was shown to correlate with disease activity.

There are, however, many forms of circulating antibodies to tissue and plasma components in this disorder. Lymphocyte stem cell or plasma cell mutations that are responsbile for the production of autoantibodies are at war with the surveillance protection mechanisms. Lymphocytoxic antibodies with specific attraction for T-cells may kill or impair these cells, which ordinarily are responsible for immunologic tolerance. T-cell impairment has been recorded in SLE. Trauma, sun exposure, infection, drug effects, stress, pregnancy, and so forth adversely affect the process. Soluble circulating immune complexes can produce serum sickness–like disease with vasculitis and glomerulitis. Anti-DNA, DNA, and complement have been shown in glomeruli in lupus nephritis. This is significant because 70% of SLE patients with lupus nephritis have cutaneous basement membrane deposits of immune complexes in non–sun exposed normal skin. Serum complement levels are related to activity of lupus nephritis. A fall denotes an increased activity, but whether it is attributable to increased complement consumption or decreased synthesis is not clear. A fall in complement also denotes an increase in anti-DNA antibody. Antinuclear, anti-gamma globulin, anticoagulants, anti–red blood cells, antileukocyte, antiplatelet, antithyroglobulin, and circulating antibodies have all been demonstrated. Antiplatelet antibodies occur in most patients who have SLE and may induce thrombocytopenia. Antibodies to double-stranded RNA may indicate viral involvement. Suspicion is growing that there may be a viral etiology to lupus erythematosus.

A recent study by Estes and Christian showed a 5-year survival rate of 77% and a 10-year survival rate of 60%. One third of their series of 150 patients died in the 8-year study period.

Evidence now suggests that lupus erythematosus, dermatomyositis, and progressive systemic scleroderma represent disorders involving a sensitization to DNA in all three diseases. Relatives of patients with systemic lupus erythematosus have a higher incidence of related abnormalities than would be expected, and identical twin and familial cases are on record.

### *Microscopic findings*

Cutaneous lesions in the acute fulminating form of lupus erythematosus are characterized by fibrinoid degeneration in the connective tissue of visceral organs and less in the dermis and in the small blood vessels. Sclerosis of collagen is seen, as well as endothelial proliferation of various-sized arterioles. There are changes similar to those in discoid lupus erythematosus, but with a difference in degree. These include epidermal atrophy, liquefactive degeneration of the basal cell layer, and inflammation around cutaneous appendages.

Earliest ultrastructural changes, as in discoid lupus erythematosus are basal cell damage and dermoepidermal junction. The basal lamina is multilayered, and anchoring fibrils are damaged very early.

### *Investigation*

Direct immunofluorescent (IF) studies of biopsies from active lesions and non–light-exposed normal skin are usually diagnostic.

Tuffanelli biopsies the exposed nonaffected forearm skin for diagnosis and the nonaffected unexposed skin for prognosis. Positive direct immunofluorescence of normal nonexposed skin is correlated with a high incidence of renal disease.

Examination for indirect antinuclear fluorescence is essential as well. The pattern of nuclear fluorescence, if diffuse or peripheral, is significant. It is the diffuse pattern of the antinuclear antibody (IgG) that is responsible for the LE cell test, positive in 75% to 80% of patients with SLE. Antinuclear antibodies are virtually always present in SLE, but they should be titered, as low titers may be present in other diseases.

Anti-DNA antibodies may be *anti–single stranded DNA* (not specific), *anti–double stranded DNA* (mean active lupus nephritis or extensive skin involvement), or *anti–single and double stranded DNA*. For practical purposes, anti–double stranded DNA is virtually specific for SLE. Anti-RNA antibodies are present and perhaps related to a viral etiology.

Leukopenia, anemia, thrombocytopenia, elevated sedimentation rate, and alpha and gamma globulin are present. A false-positive VDRL test and positive sheep cell agglutination are shown in some cases. Pulmonary, cardiac, central nervous system, renal, or hepatic function may be impaired.

SLE may be confused with other collagen diseases. Differentiation is often difficult early in the disease with an insidious onset. Some aspects of rheumatoid arthritis, systemic sclerosis, or dermatomyositis may be present in SLE.

### *Treatment*

Hospitalization, thorough assessment, and skilled management are required. A thoroughgoing history for all possible trigger mechanisms is essential.

Renal disease occurs in perhaps 50% of SLE cases. It may be focal membranes or diffuse, of which the latter is the most serious (Tuffanelli).

The modern forms of therapy have allowed a more hopeful outlook for patients with systemic lupus erythematosus by improving the prognosis and prolonging the course of the disease. However, a Toronto study indicates that prolongation of life in SLE by glucocorticoids may lead to increased atherosclerosis and myocardial infarcts. Earlier deaths tend to be attributable to infection (Urowitz). Oral glucocorticoids have serious disadvantages and the degree to which they alleviate the pathologic alterations of SLE requires review.

Caution and judgment are essential; Estes reported that 12 out of 53 deaths caused by systemic lupus erythematosus are caused by therapy or are contributed to by therapy. Central nervous system complications of SLE are *not* helped by glucocorticoids (Sergent). Rest and salicylate therapy, antimalarial drugs, nitrogen mustards for renal involvement, azathioprine (Imuran), and other immunosuppressive agents all have a part in the management of these difficult cases. Each is individualized, and therapy must be carefully planned for each patient. Sharon et al., in a study of the effects of azathioprine withdrawal in stable SLE, produced exacerbations on an average of 3 months later. One died.

Following serum complement levels may be essential for assessment of therapeutic achievement in lupus erythematosus nephritis cases although it may be related only to widespread skin involvement. Pregnancy should be avoided in all SLE patients with clinical or serologic evidence of disease activity.

Causes of death in Dubois' large series have changed somewhat since 1950, but not dramatically. Infections are different, now consisting of nocardiosis, cryptococcosis, coccidioidomycosis, pneumocystosis, and cytomegalic inclusion disease. Atherosclerosis, neoplasms, and suicides are probably steroid related. Median age at death has increased from 30 to 45 years.

#### REFERENCES

Abdou, N. I., Sagawa, A., Pascual, E., et al.: Suppressor T-cell abnormality in idiopathic systemic lupus erythematosus, Clin. Immunol. Immunopathol. **6**:192, 1976.

**Correlation between SLE disease activity and B-cell suppression by T-cells.**

Alarcon-Segovia, D.: Drug induced antinuclear antibodies and lupus syndromes, Drugs **12**:69, 1976.
**Two categories of drugs, the direct lupus activators and the immunity activators.**

Dubois, E. L., Wierzchowiecki, M., Cox, M. B., and Weiner, J. M.: Duration and death in systemic lupus erythematosus, J.A.M.A. **227**:1399, 1974.
**249 deaths in 491 patients with SLE since 1950.**

Estes, D., and Christian, C. L.: The natural history of systemic lupus erythematosus by prospective analysis, Medicine **50**:85, 1971.
**Valuable review of all aspects in 150 patients with SLE.**

Gilliam, J. N., and Hurd, E. F.: Comparison of circulating T- and B-lymphocytes in discoid versus systemic lupus erythematosus, Clin. Immunol. Immunopathol. **6**:149, 1976.
**SLE has reduced number of T-cells. DLE has B-cell proliferation, perhaps because of attempts to bind autoantigens.**

Marshall, D. A., Nesbitt, L. T., and Biundo, J. J.: Serum complement related to skin lesions of systemic lupus erythematosus, South. Med. J. **67**:1275, 1973.
**Serum B and C levels depressed in six SLE patients with skin but not renal activity.**

Paty, J. G., Jr., Sienknecht, C. W., Townes, A. S., et al.: Impaired cell mediated immunity in systemic lupus erythematosus, Am. J. Med. **59**:769, 1975.
**Decreased peripheral T-cells related to antilymphocytic antibodies in 23 patients with SLE.**

Schrager, M. A., and Rothfield, N. F.: Clinical significance of serum properdin levels and properdin deposition in the dermal-epidermal junction in systemic lupus erythematosus, J. Clin. Invest. **57**:212, 1976.
**Increased deposition of dermoepidermal proteins correlates with increased disease activity.**

Schrager, M. A., and Rothfield, N. F.: Pathways of complement activation in chronic discoid lupus, Arth. Rheum. **20**:637, 1977.
**Properdin (alternate pathway of complement activation) demonstrated on basement membranes of discoid LE and inactive SLE lesions.**

Sergent, J. S., Lockshin, M. D., Klemper, M. S., et al.: Central nervous system disease in systemic lupus erythematosus. Therapy and prognosis, Am. J. Med. **58**:644, 1975.
**Not helped by large doses of corticosteroids.**

Sharon, E., Kaplan, D., and Diamond, H. S.: Exacerbation of systemic lupus erythematosus after withdrawal of azathioprine therapy, N. Engl. J. Med. **288**:121, 1973.
**Seven of nine demonstrated exacerbation in an average of 3 months.**

Tuffanelli, D. L.: Management of the patient with lupus erythematosus, Prog. Dermatol. **8**:5, 1974.
**Cutaneous, systemic, renal, and obstetrical management.**

Tuffanelli, D. L.: Cutaneous immunopathology, recent observations, J. Invest. Dermatol. **64**:143, 1975.
**Direct immunofluorescence is more sensitive and more specific in differentiating lupus from clinically similar cutaneous diseases than is routine microscopy.**

Urowitz, M. B., Bookman, A. A. M., Koehler, B. E., et al.: Mortality pattern of systemic lupus erythematosus, Am. J. Med. **60**:221, 1976.
**Infection early and atherosclerosis late cause death in successfully treated SLE.**

## MIXED CONNECTIVE TISSUE DISEASE

Sharp and colleagues have described 25 patients with signs and symptoms of SLE with overtones of scleroderma or polymyositis. The course, by common agreement, seems to be benign. They possess antibody to extractable nuclear antigen (ENA), which is ribonuclease sensitive, and this is present in high titer. They have hypergammaglobulinemia. They demonstrate severe arthralgias, sclerodermatous changes, Raynaud's syndrome, lymphadenopathy, nonscarring focal alopecias, sclerodactyly, and discoid lupus erythematosus lesions. Speckled nuclear staining was present in all, including 15 patients reported by Gilliam. This disease may have a more serious implication in children.

They showed a good response to corticosteroids.

### REFERENCES

Gilliam, J. N., and Prystowsky, S. D.: Mixed connective tissue disease syndrome, Arch. Dermatol. **113**:583, 1977.
**Further definition of a less aggressive "collagen" disease.**

Sharp, G. C., Irwin, W. S., Tan, E. M., et al,: Mixed connective tissue disease: apparently distinct rheumatic disease syndrome associated with a specific antibody to an extractable nuclear antigen (ENA), Am. J. Med. **52**:148, 1972.
**A distinct syndrome that appears to have a good prognosis.**

Singren, B. H., Bernstein, B. H., Kornreich, K. H., et al.: Mixed connective tissue disease in childhood, J. Pediatr. **90**:893, 1977.
**Significant cardiac and renal involvement in children as opposed to adults.**

## DERMATOMYOSITIS

Dermatomyositis, an uncommon disease closely related to systemic lupus erythematosus on the one hand, and to progressive scleroderma on the other, involves chiefly the striated muscle and skin.

### *Natural course*

Reports of various series of patients with dermatomyositis tend to lack clarity in their definition of the disease. Because of the poorly controlled series in the literature and a lack of prospective studies, we have few firm facts about the natural course of this disease (Bohan).

Dermatomyositis affects persons of all ages, but most patients are women between 20 and 50 years of age. The disease is not uncommon among young children.

The onset is insidious, with the appearance of an unusual erythema of the eyelids and periorbital areas. It is of a "heliotrope" hue and may be associated with edema (Plate 16). Other symptoms and signs may be present or develop later and consist of muscle weakness and cutaneous changes. The muscle weakness is first noticed in the larger muscle groups, such as in the thighs and low back. Any striated muscle can be involved, including cardiac and sphincter muscles.

Dysphagia results from involvement of the hypopharynx, with difficulty in initiating the swallowing process.

An acute course of the disease is characterized by rapidly spreading progressive weakness, febrile course, and death. The more usual, chronic course follows an intermittent but progressive pattern to fibrosis and contracture of muscles after the initial inflammation. The end result is extreme atrophy, ankylosis, and ulceration at pressure points.

Cutaneous lesions, aside from eyelid involvement, include a petechial-erythematous combination of lesions over the knuckles and joints on extensor surfaces. The fingernail fold shows telangiectasia. There may be patchy, purpuric, and erythematous lesions on the thorax and in other areas. These are often followed by pigmentation and sometimes depigmentation. Subcutaneous deposits of calcium are not unusual in later stages.

### *Pertinent information*

If one includes dermatomyositis in the larger groups of polymyositis cases, then it fits as one of the following five categories (Bohan):

1. Idiopathic polymyositis
2. Idiopathic dermatomyositis
3. Polymyositis-dermatomyositis with malignancy
4. Childhood dermatomyositis-polymyositis
5. Polymyositis-dermatomyositis with other collagen diseases

Dermatomyositis-polymyositis is surely a disease of autoimmunity. There is polyclonal hypergammaglobulinemia and affected patients produce a muscle-toxic lymphokine.

*The disease in adults seems to be associated with internal malignancy of some variety in about one fifth or more of the cases.* In male patients, over 40 years of age, the association may approach 50%. The types of malignancy involve lung, breast, urogenital area, gastrointestinal tract, lymphoreticuloses, and others. Wong's startling incidence of 75% of associated malignancies attributable to epidermoid carcinoma of the nasopharynx in Hong Kong patients, where this disease seems relatively common, has not, to our knowledge, been reported in North America.

Degos and colleagues reviewed the cause of the disease in 31 adults over a 20-year period. About half of the patients died. Cancer caused half of the deaths; therapy caused one death and produced serious complications in others. One fourth of the patients were cured.

The disease in children is not associated with malignancy and has a better prognosis for spontaneous cure, but it also involves some of the most protracted and difficult instances of wasting disease.

Laboratory findings include elevated serum glutamic oxaloacetic transaminase (SGOT) and serum creatine phosphokinase (CPK) levels during the acute phase. These are the most useful current tests in following the course of the disease. Biopsy of muscle tissue may be of help in determining the diagnosis and should be taken from a muscle clinically involved, preferably early in its involvement.

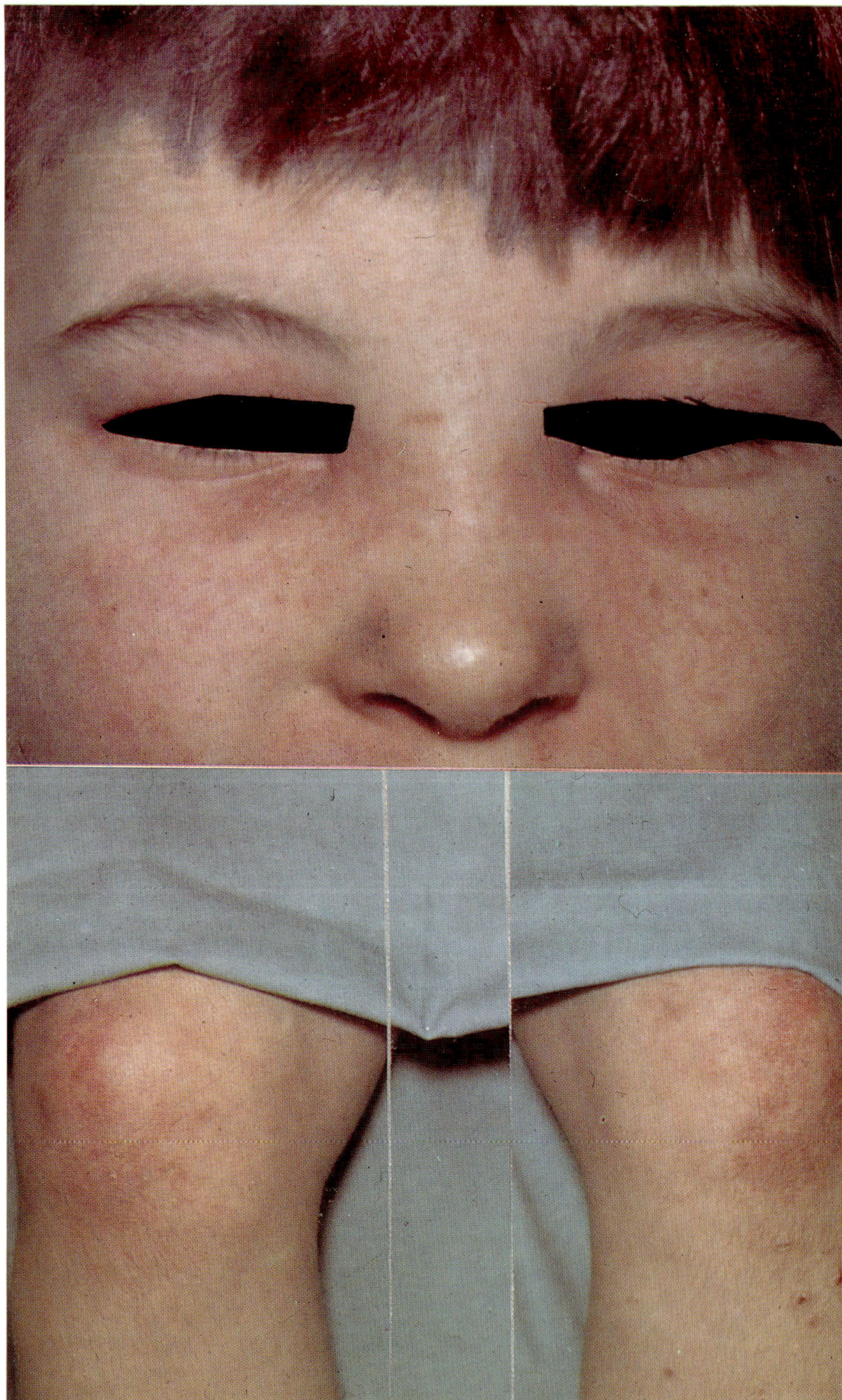

**Plate 16**

Dermatomyositis.

Intravascular, intramuscular, IgG, IgM, and complement have been observed by immunofluorescent studies. A new and perhaps very significant finding, reported by Leddy, is a total absence of $C_2$ complement in dermatomyositis, which would preclude activation of the classic pathway.

### *Microscopic findings*

There is a patchy degeneration of muscle fibers, together with extreme variation and regeneration of muscle cells. An infiltrate of inflammatory cells is seen in the area. In the skin, changes are often of a nonspecific nature, but may resemble those seen in lupus erythematosus, and a vasculitis involving small cutaneous vessels is common, especially in children.

### *Investigation*

Studies for the disease include the following: thorough evaluation for muscle weakness and serial retesting of this function; sedimentation rate, often moderately elevated, SGOT, CPK, serum aldolase, 24-hour urinary creatine levels; skin and muscle biopsy of involved areas; electromyography; x-ray study of distal phalanges for bony absorption and of soft tissues for calcinosis; and thorough investigation of all patients over 40 with confirmed dermatomyositis, for internal malignancy.

### *Differential diagnosis*

Diseases to be included in the differential diagnosis and which may show muscle weakness are systemic lupus erythematosus, scleroderma, polyarteritis nodosa, acute rheumatic fever, rheumatoid arthritis, sarcoidosis, mixed connective tissue disease, hyperthyroidism, muscular dystrophy, and drug-induced myopathy.

### *Treatment*

Hospitalization and thorough evaluation of the patient are mandatory. A search for malignancy in adults is essential.

Glucocorticoids in adequate and well-maintained dosages (prednisone, 60 to 80 mg./day), appear at the present time to offer the best hope for palliation and remission in those cases not associated with internal malignancy. In children, an aggressive, prompt, and sustained oral glucocorticoid regimen produced good results with no deaths over 5 years in 18 children. Physical therapy after the initial acute phase is an essential part of the treatment.

A good response with the use of methotrexate, azathioprine, and combined therapy in selected cases has been reported, although it is curious to recommend use of immunosuppressive agents in a disease so subject to association with cancer. The acute symptoms tend to subside on removal or treatment of an associated malignancy in adults.

#### REFERENCES

Barnes, B.: Dermatomyositis and malignancy. A review, Ann. Intern. Med. **84**:68, 1976.

**Females preponderate; cancer occurs younger than general population and is five to seven times more common.**

Bohan, A., and Peter, J. B.: Polymyositis-dermatomyositis, N. Engl. J. Med. **292**:344, 403, 1975.

**A very realistic assessment of the available facts on this disorder, which reveals a discouraging lack of good information.**

Degos, R., Civatte, J., Belaich, S., and Delarve, A.: Prognosis of adult dermatomyositis, Trans. St. John's Hosp. Dermatol. Soc. **47**:98, 1971.

**One half died in first 3 years, one half from cancer.**

Leddy, J. P., Griggs, R. C., and Klemperer, M. R.: Hereditary complement deficiency with dermatomyositis, Am. J. Med. **58**:82, 1975.

**Very carefully investigated study indicating dermatomyositis lesions can occur in association with classic complement-activation pathway deficit.**

Metzger, A. L., Bohan, A., Goldberg, L. S., et al.: Polymyositis and dermatomyositis. Combined methotrexate and corticosteroid therapy, Ann. Intern. Med **81**:182, 1974.

**17 of 22 patients improved, 10 of 22 excellent or clear.**

Sullivan, D. B., Cassidy, J. T., Petty, R. E., and Burt, A.: Prognosis in childhood dermatomyositis, J. Pediatr. **80**:555, 1972.

**1 to 2 mg./kg. of prednisone daily for 4 weeks, then half that for 4 weeks, then maintenance. Excellent results.**

Wong, K. O.: Dermatomyositis: A clinical investigation of 23 cases in Hong Kong, Br. J. Dermatol. **81**:544, 1969.

**75% of associated malignancies were nasopharyngeal.**

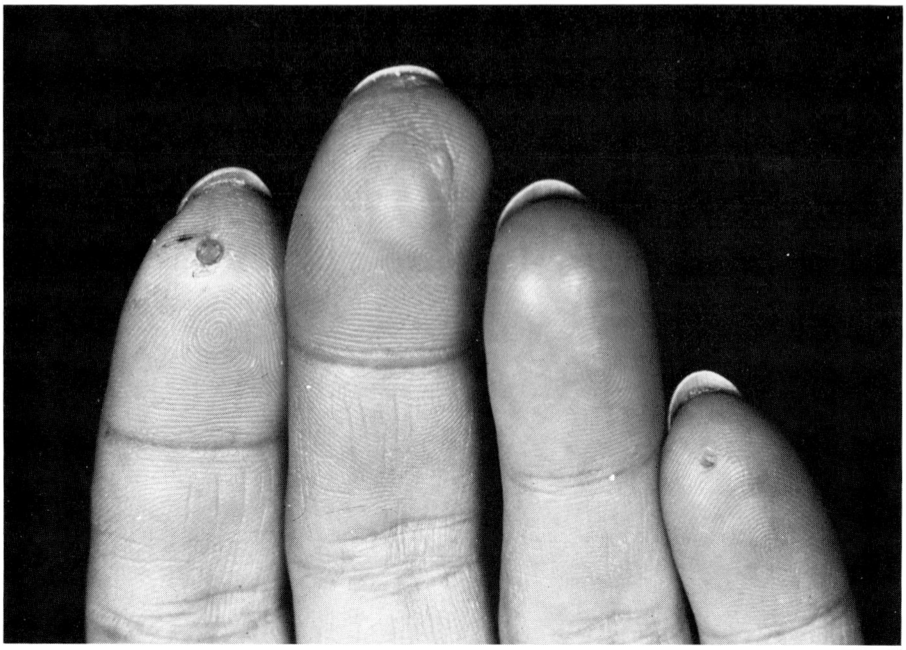

**Fig. 6-2.** Scleroderma. Early fingertip ulcerations.

## PROGRESSIVE SYSTEMIC SCLEROSIS (SCLERODERMA)

Progressive systemic sclerosis is a disease of connective tissue that follows a prolonged and disabling course, with increasing limitation of motion caused by a binding down of the skin to the underlying inelastic dense connective tissue.

### *Natural course*

Systemic scleroderma is more common in women and is seen most frequently in those between 20 and 50 years of age. The course and prognosis, however, is worse for males.

The commonest onset is a gradually immobilizing process beginning in the distal aspects of the upper extremities, with a pallid, temporary edema and then vasospastic changes, cyanosis, and Raynaud's phenomenon. This process is slowly followed by cutaneous changes leading to smoothing out of the skin markings and folds of the fingers, inelasticity of the skin, and flexion deformities. Dilated capillaries may be seen on the nail folds. Ulcerations (Fig. 6-2) develop on the exposed joint surfaces, calcium deposits are frequent, and eventually cutaneous atrophy is apparent. Telangiectasia is important and diagnostic. Angular 1 to 5 mm. mats are seen on the face, hands, and oral mucosa (Fig. 6-3). Telangiectases are also seen on nail folds. Pigmentation and depigmentation appear in about 50% of patients with systemic scleroderma.

The process may remain localized or may spread to affect the face, where the jaw, perioral areas, and nose become inelastic and "bound down." Mucous membranes of the mouth and pharynx are also affected.

The esophagus is involved in almost 75% of cases, manifested by symptoms of dysphagia. Dilatation and disturbed peristalsis are seen radiologically. The small intestine demonstrates x-ray changes of disordered mobility in almost half the cases. The colon may show "square" diverticula.

Malabsorption symptoms including iron, fat, and vitamin $B_{12}$ deficiences occur with and without skin changes. Pulmonary function is affected by testing in over 90% of cases, but 25% only show clinical pulmonary impairment. In Rowell's series, respiratory failure was the chief cause of death. There may be

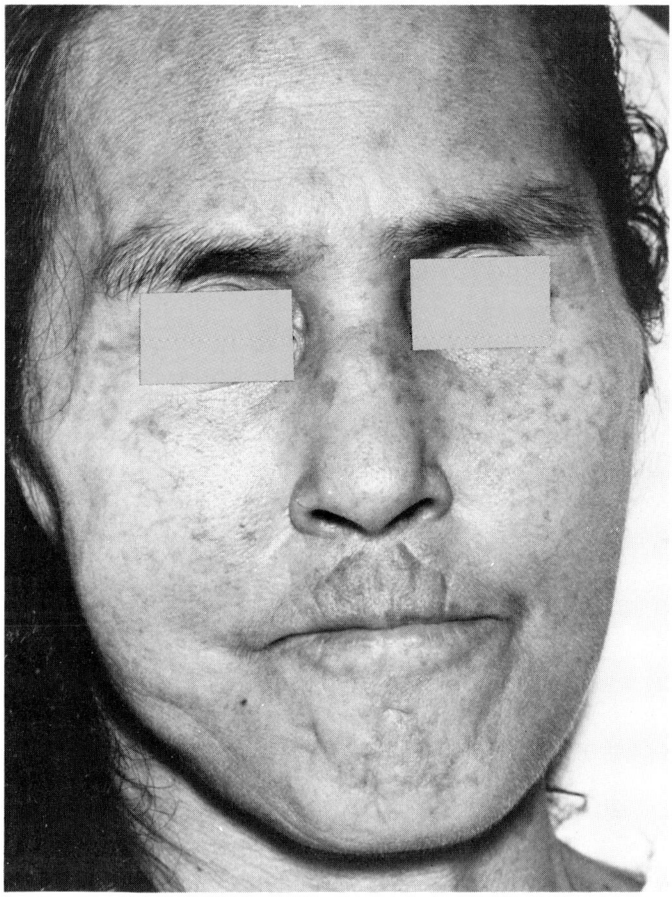

**Fig. 6-3.** Scleroderma. Note flat telangiectatic mats with angular configuration over malar areas and nose.

myocardial fibrosis, and renal involvement is not infrequent. Progressive renal failure causes death in more than 10% of affected patients.

There are records of spontaneous improvement and even disappearance of the disease. Studies indicate a 70% 5-year survival from time of diagnosis and a 50% survival in 10 years.

There is a true, but as yet unclear, association between discoid lupus erythematosus, lupus erythematosus, rheumatoid arthritis, dermatomyositis, and, of course, morphea, as reported by Dubois and co-workers.

***Diffuse progressive scleroderma.*** In the diffuse progressive form of the disease the course is variable, but may be much more rapid, and the prognosis is poor. Cutaneous sclerosis may appear only on the thorax, but internal organs are involved early, and widespread cutaneous involvement with binding down of the skin generally follows rapidly. Progressive gastrointestinal, cardiac, and renal lesions occur. Laboratory findings do not correlate well with the clinical findings of the disease.

Classic skin hardening and inflexibility of joints may be minimal. Cases also are seen with no cutaneous changes, but with severe gastrointestinal involvement. Bone changes characteristic of scleroderma, with terminal phalangeal absorption may be seen in these cases, as in those with cutaneous changes, and serve as an early diagnostic sign of the disease. Yune describes these changes in 52 patients.

### Pertinent information

***Immunofluorescence.*** *Indirect:* Serum studies for antinuclear antibodies are positive in a high percentage of cases. They are usually speckled or nucleolar. *Direct:* Uniformly negative.

There is no good direct evidence for an immunologic etiology for this disorder despite intensive efforts to show one, although Fleischmajer believes that the cellular infiltrate indicates that both cellular and humoral immunity probably play an important role. The unique aspect of progressive sclerosis that it marks it as different from systemic lupus erythematosus, dermatomyositis, rheumatoid arthritis, and related disorders, is the preponderant sclerosing effect that Winkelmann associates with vascular dysfunction. Raynaud's phenomenon, which can be recognized early in 90% of cases of clinical scleroderma, and usually precedes it, must participate in the production of thickened sclerotic bound-down fingers, which are the result of the process. Winkelmann has emphasized that the sensitive, hyperactive vessels in scleroderma always result in diminished circulation. They overrespond to cold and to serotonin.

Stachow has demonstrated good evidence for an abnormal metabolism of the precurser of serotonin, tryptophan, in both systemic and localized scleroderma. Many studies and clinical observations confirm the sclerosing effect of serotonin (MacDonald, Fries), and if enzymes for degradation of serotonin are impaired, this effect may be prolonged.

### Microscopic findings

Highly active fibroblasts are seen, together with increase in new, thin collagen fibrils. Collagen synthesis is more apparent in the deeper dermis than the upper layers. An increase in glycosaminoglycans is also apparent.

### Investigation

Hypertension, azotemia, and proteinuria are significant predictors of renal sclerodermatous involvement. Studies should be undertaken to determine presence of involvement of the heart, lungs, small or large intestine, or kidneys. Bennett and others have shown visceral involvement at the time of initial diagnosis to be a factor in adverse prognosis. Malabsorption as a result of visceral disease should be considered. Radiological studies of distal phalanges of the fingers may show changes.

### Differential diagnosis

***Raynaud's disease.*** The vasospastic phenomenon of Raynaud's disease are similar to those in progressive systemic scleroderma, and the skin of the fingers may show color changes, atrophy, and ulceration. The slow flexion deformities and "bound-down" appearance do not occur.

***Acrocyanosis.*** There are phalangeal color changes, but no flexion deformities or atrophy.

***Scleredema adultorum.*** This is a self-limited, rare disease characterized by woody induration and cutaneous swelling involving the neck, thorax, and face. It produces no permanent changes.

***Morphea, localized scleroderma.*** This is ordinarily a benign disorder, can be extensive, and may be confused with progressive sclerosis. There is no tendency toward an acral distribution (Fig. 6-2).

***Mixed connective tissue disease.*** These patients show sclerodermoid changes in fingers, arthritis, muscle weakness, and Raynaud's syndrome. They have positive antinuclear antibody (ANA) and extractable nuclear antigen (ENA) tests.

### Treatment

There is no satisfactory treatment for progressive systemic scleroderma. Many forms of therapy have been tried, without significant success.

Cold in all forms should be avoided. Rest and avoidance of overexertion is also important. Salicylate therapy for arthralgias is indicated. Glucocorticoids, although they do not worsen the disease, do not seem to alter the course. Correction of malabsorption may be achieved by tetracycline, oxytetracycline, or ampicillin therapy, according to Kalm and colleagues.

Paraffin baths and physiotherapy may maintain mobility.

Low molecular weight dextran has been used for symptoms of acrosclerosis and is given intravenously in short courses, a 10% solution in 2,000 ml. over a 2- or 3-day period. The patient has a feeling of warmth and improvement of the involved fingers, and ulcers may be healed with this therapy. Renal complications have occurred with this therapy.

#### REFERENCES

Bennett, R., Bluestone, R., Hold, P. J., et al.: Survival in scleroderma, Ann. Rheum. Dis. **30**:581, 1971.
**Measured from time of initial diagnosis. Steroids do not affect survival.**

Dubois, E. L., Chandor, S., Frion, G. J., et al.: Progressive systemic sclerosis (PSS) and localized scleroderma (morphea) with positive LE cell test and unusual systemic manifestations compatible with systemic lupus erythematosus (SLE): presentation of 14 cases including 1 set of identical twins, 1 with scleroderma and the other with SLE: Review of the literature, Medicine **50**:199, 1971.

Fleischmajer, R., Perlish, J. S., and West, W. P.: Ultrastructure of cutaneous cellular infiltration in scleroderma, Arch. Dermatol. **113**:1661, 1977.
**Electron micrographs of systemic and localized cases indicate immune mechanisms operative.**

Fries, J. F., Lindgren, J. A., and Bull, J. M.: Scleroderma-like lesions and the carcinoid syndrome, Arch. Intern. Med. **131**:550, 1973.
**Serotonin may cause localized edema and fibrosis.**

Kinder, R. R., and Fleischmajer, R.: Systemic scleroderma. A review of organ systems, Int. J. Dermatol. **13**:382, 1974.
**Clinical, pathological and radiological aspects of the organs involved.**

MacDonald, R. A., Robbins, S. L., and Mallory, G. K.: Dermal fibrosis following subcutaneous injections of serotonin creatinine sulfate, Proc. Soc. Exp. Biol. Med. **97**:334, 1958.
**Experimentally induced in rats.**

Rowell, N. R.: The prognosis of systemic sclerosis, Br. J. Dermatol. **95**:57, 1976.
**84 patients studied to find the prognosis worse in males. Respiratory failure chief cause of death.**

Stachow, A., Jablonska, S., and Skiendzielewska, A.: 5-Hydroxytryptamine and tryptamine pathways in scleroderma, Br. J. Dermatol. **97**:147, 1977.
**High tryptophan dose in patients with systemic and localized scleroderma was not excreted as well as in normals.**

Winkelmann, R. K.: Pathogenesis and staging of scleroderma, Acta Derm. Venereol. **56**:84, 1976.
**Primary lesion is noninflammatory fibromucinous endothelial proliferation in small vessels of skin and viscera.**

Winkelmann, R. K., Goldyne, M. E., and Linscheid, R. L.: Hypersensitivity of scleroderma cutaneous vascular smooth muscle to 5-hydroxytryptamine, Br. J. Dermatol. **95**:51, 1976.
**Hyperresponsiveness to serotonin may contribute to the vascular and fibrous changes in scleroderma.**

## LOCALIZED SCLERODERMA

Localized scleroderma (Plate 17) is a disorder of connective tissue characterized by localized inflammation, proceeding to atrophy, hardening, and depigmentation of the skin and often atrophy of underlying tissues.

***Morphea.*** Morphea occurs chiefly in young adults, beginning as indurated, erythematous plaques from a few to many centimeters in size (Fig. 6-4). The plaques may be single or multiple. They occur usually on the thorax and over a period of weeks fade from red to depigmented, atrophic, residual lesions. A few disappear without trace. There are no systemic symptoms.

***"En coup de sabre."*** Although it affects the same age group of young adults as morphea, this form of scleroderma involves the scalp rather than the thorax. Almost all these lesions progress to permanent atrophic changes. The involvement begins with erythema or pigmentation in a diagonal, linear distribution over anterior scalp and forehead, extending to the eye (Fig. 6-5). It may seriously affect the eye and even the face. The process progresses to cutaneous, subcutaneous, and even bony atrophy, resulting in a "coup de sabre" lesion with a depressed, hairless, linear scar. Electroencephalographic changes may be associated.

***Linear scleroderma.*** This form of localized scleroderma usually affects a single extremity, most often the leg. Occasionally hemiatrophy of the body is seen. A preceding erythematous or hyperpigmented, indurated phase advances on the limb, followed by a greater or lesser degree of atrophy of subcutaneous tissue, muscle, or bone. Severe deformity may result. Although spontaneous clearing occurs, it is unwise to conclude that the process is stopped because of lack of activity—it may

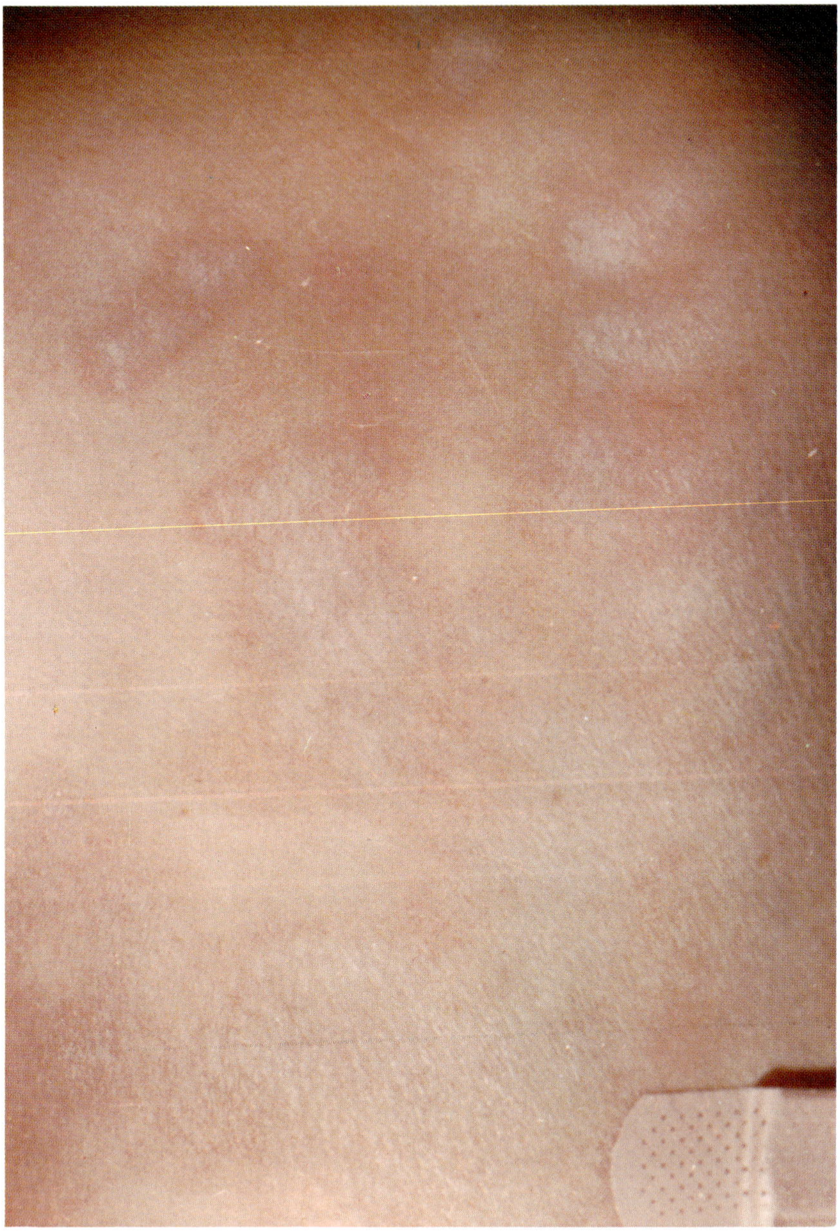

**Plate 17**

Localized scleroderma (morphea). Note white atrophic centers and violaceous peripheries.

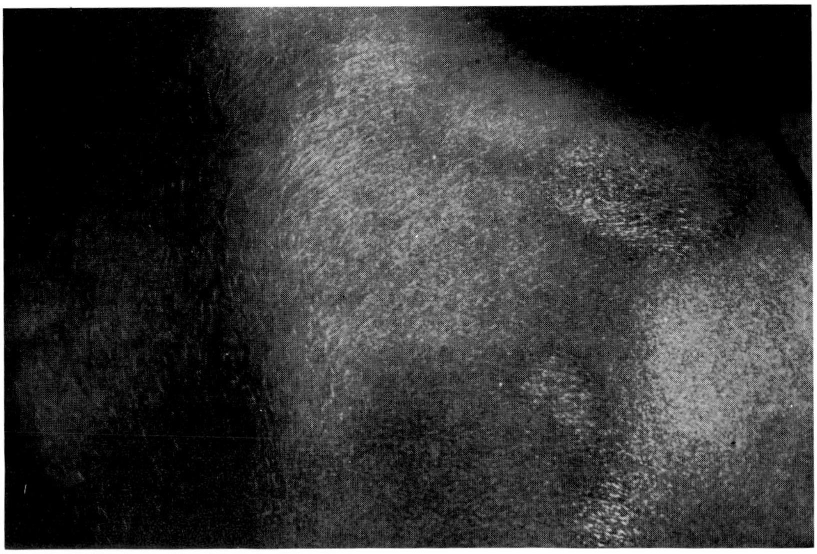

**Fig. 6-4.** Localized scleroderma (morphea).

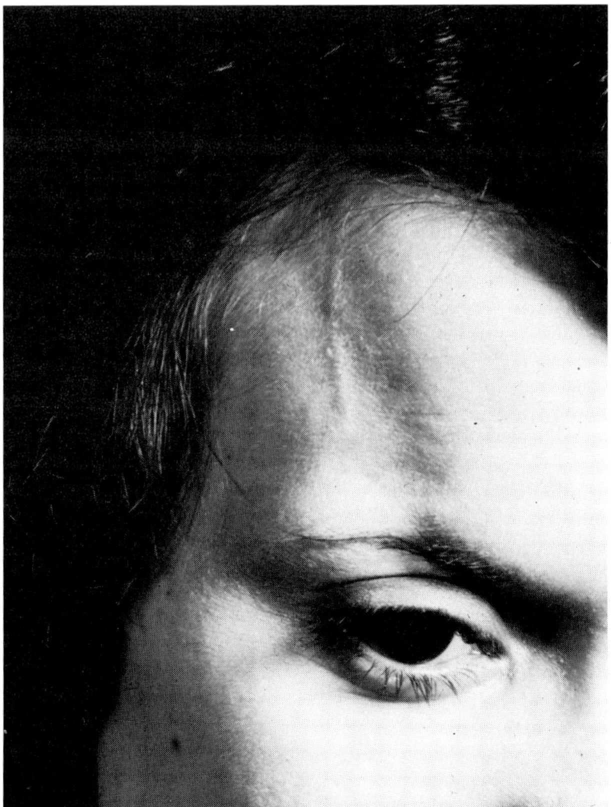

**Fig. 6-5.** Scleroderma "en coup de sabre." Atrophy may extend into bony structures.

recommence and continue intermittently for years.

### *Differential diagnosis*

***Lichen sclerosus et atrophicus.*** Lichen sclerosus et atrophicus produces atrophic, nonindurated areas of depigmentation of the upper back. There are usually shiny-topped white papules at the periphery of the lesion. Some cases have features of both diseases and may be difficult to differentiate.

### *Treatment*

Morphea may clear if treated in the early inflammatory phase with an effective, fluorinated glucocorticoid used under an occlusive plastic dressing. Most cases will, however, clear completely if left untreated.

Treatment of "en coup de sabre" and linear scleroderma does not ordinarily alter the course of the disease, which is locally progressive.

#### REFERENCE

Christianson, H. B., Dorsey, C. S., O'Leary, P. A., and Kierland, R. R.: Localized scleroderma, Arch. Dermatol. **74**:629, 1956.

**Morphea, linear scleroderma, and "en coup de sabre" without systemic manifestations.**

## LICHEN SCLEROSUS ET ATROPHICUS

Lichen sclerosus et atrophicus is an unusual disorder of dermal connective tissue of unknown etiology.

### *Natural course*

Lesions begin as small, irregularly shaped, ivory-white macules or grouped papules on the upper back and chest, shoulders, neck, thighs, or perivulvar areas (Fig. 6-6). These may or may not be preceded by an erythema-

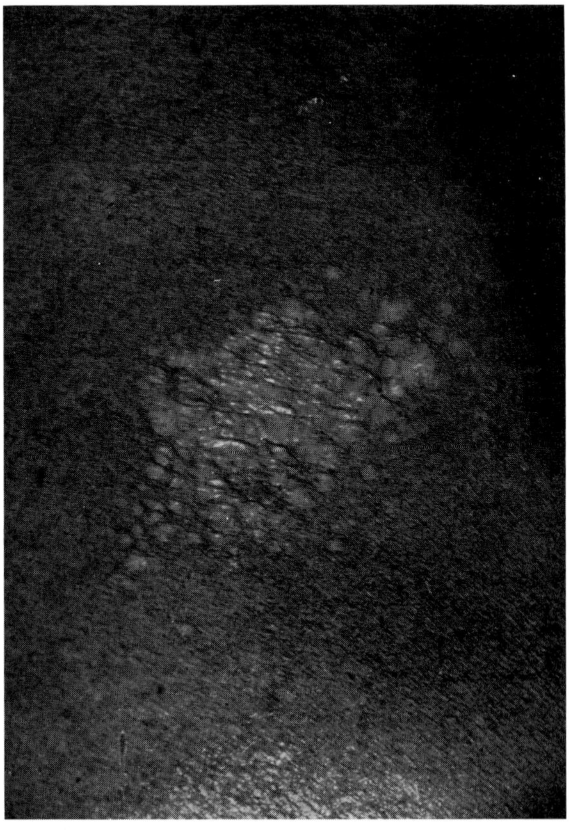

**Fig. 6-6.** Lichen sclerosus et atrophicus, posterior aspect of shoulder.

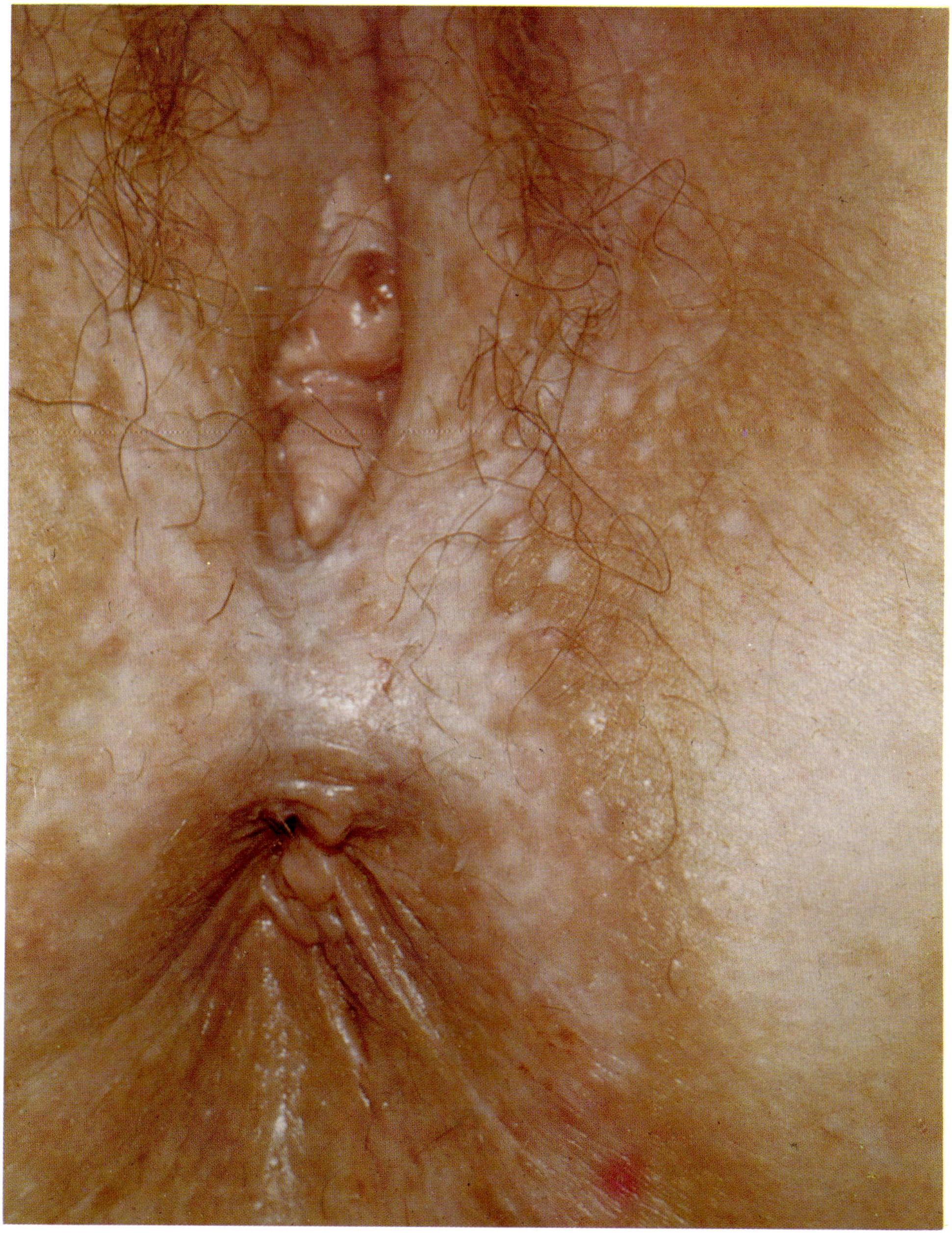

**Plate 18**

Lichen sclerosus et atrophicus of perineum. Itching and dyspareunia were present.

tous, inflammatory phase. They slowly enlarge and are associated with symptoms of pruritus. The small lesions become confluent and progress to an atrophic stage in which the overlying skin becomes wrinkled and thin. A pale depressed scar results. Around the vulva, atrophy of the labia minora ensues, and the vaginal orifice becomes stenotic. The process frequently extends to the perianal region also. Soreness, itching, dysuria, and dyspareunia are common and dispiriting symptoms. A few small lesions regress spontaneously, leaving no trace (Plate 18).

The disease occurs at any age, is six times more common in women, and most frequently appears in the preadolescent and postmenopausal periods. It most often affects the vulvar area and may or may not be associated with cutaneous lesions elsewhere. The vulvar lesions are not infrequently mistaken for leukoplakia. *This emphasizes the necessity for biopsy of these lesions prior to operative procedures.* This disorder either progresses to leukoplakia and then to the development of carcinoma or can be associated with these processes.

When lichen sclerosus et atrophicus occurs in men, it may attack the glans penis, possibly with resulting meatal stenosis. In this location it is referred to as *balanitis xerotica obliterans.*

### Microscopic findings

Hyperkeratosis occurs first, followed by a curious homogeneous edema in a very well-defined band in the upper dermis, immediately beneath which there is a band of inflammatory cells. The basal cell layer undergoes an irregular degeneration, and bullae may form beneath the epidermis. All cutaneous layers become thin and vascular. Abnormal collagen metabolism is present, and melanocytes show degenerative changes. Genital lesions must be watched for cellular atypia.

### Pertinent information

Some confusion arises in the definition of "white patch" vulvar disease as understood by those in various specialties. Gynecologists, pathologists, and dermatologists each view these processes differently and are familiar with their own names and meaning, but not always with others. Gynecologists and pathologists frequently include lichen sclerosus et atrophicus in a poorly defined group of vulvar disorders entitled "kraurosis vulvae."

H. J. Wallace, one of the world authorities, has recently reviewed this disorder in 380 patients of whom 290 were adult women with an average age of 54 years. Girls with the disease were from 2 to 6 years of age, and two thirds of the patients showed involution of the disease before onset of menses.

Leukoplakia occurred in one half of all cases biopsied, and squamous cell carcinoma was present in 4.4% of all patients. Hart's series showed "leukoplakia-like" changes in nearly half, and five of 92 had coexistent squamous cell carcinoma.

Three of 44 men had urethral strictures requiring surgery.

### Differential diagnosis

***Localized scleroderma.*** Localized scleroderma occurs chiefly on the thorax and abdomen and produces induration with some pigmentation. In its later atrophic stages, it is distinguished from lichen sclerosus only with difficulty. Some cases showed manifestations of both disorders concomitantly.

***Lichen planus.*** Atrophic forms of lichen planus may be similar to lichen sclerosus initially, but the characteristic violaceous color remains in lichen planus lesions. Biopsy differentiates these entities.

***Postmenopausal vulvar atrophy.*** The shrinkage of the vulva generally and the mucous membrane changes are not so pronounced nor so sharply defined as in lichen sclerosus et atrophicus. Stenosis does not occur.

***Leukoplakia.*** Leukoplakia is primarily an epidermal thickening in localized patches occurring on the labia of adult women beyond middle age. Biopsy is essential to establish the diagnosis.

***Pruritus vulvae.*** For differentiation of pruritic vulvar lesions, see the section on pruritis vulvae (p. 447).

### *Treatment*

Local application of fluorinated glucocorticoid ointments every 3 hours or under an occlusive thin plastic film for longer periods is the most satisfactory treatment for vulvar lesions, although atrophy occurs with prolonged use.

*Intralesional* glucocorticoid injections (for example, with triamcinolone, 5 mg./ml. by needle or jet injectors) may be helpful, and in some cases estrogen therapy may be beneficial.

Zelle and other gynecologists have treated these patients with 2% testosterone cream, once or twice daily. It is freely absorbed and should not be applied frequently. It has caused regression of some lesions in our experience.

Testosterone propionate 2.5% ointment has been used with startlingly good results on the glans penis by Pasieczny. He also states that where exclusively urethral involvement in males occurs, he favors the diagnostic term *obliterative urethritis* to identify those cases where there is a higher risk of malignancy.

## GRANULOMA ANNULARE

Granuloma annulare is an asymptomatic papulonodular eruption of unknown etiology that exhibits a characteristic appearance.

### *Natural course*

The primary lesion is a skin-colored to pale reddish purple papule that enlarges peripherally, leaving a depressed center. The resulting lesion is circular, crescentic, or linear, since some parts become more persistent than others. The process is obviously beneath the epidermis, the surface of which is not altered over the lesion (Plate 19). It tends to follow a chronic course, with steady, slow enlargement, but eventually heals without scarring or residual defect. Individual lesions may disappear shortly after onset or may last for months. Most will clear spontaneously within 2 years. The sites of predilection are the dorsa of the feet and hands, the fingers, and the ankles (Fig. 6-7).

Frequently the lesions are multiple, but usually they are not numerous. Rarely, one sees lesions of sufficient number and size to

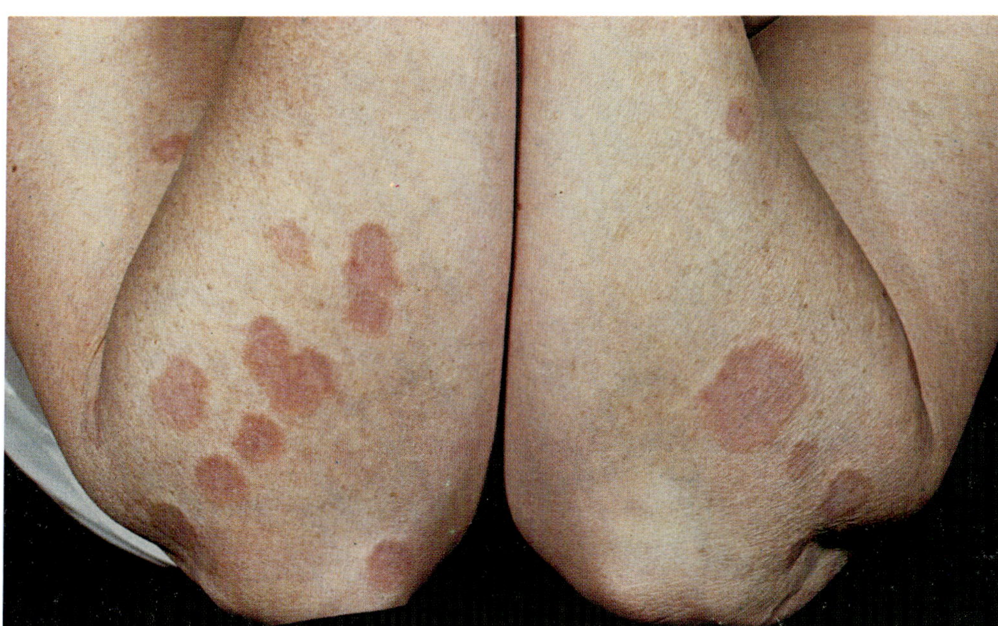

**Plate 19**

Granuloma annulare. Annular lesions with elevated border and intact epidermis.

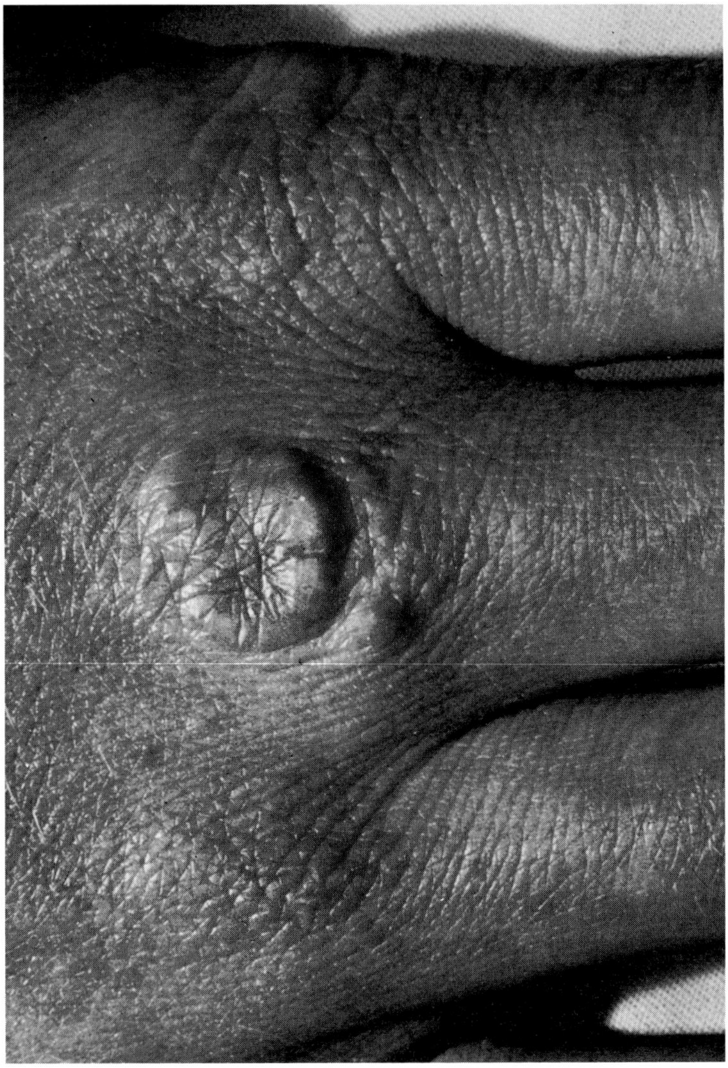

**Fig. 6-7.** Granuloma annulare.

cover the entire skin surface, a condition referred to as *disseminated granuloma annulare*.

Granuloma annulare is observed twice as often in women as in men, and the patients are usually under 30 years of age, often preadolescents. There are no subjective complaints. There appears to be a greater than expected incidence of diabetes in these patients.

### *Microscopic findings*

The principal cells are histiocytes, ranging from monocytes to epithelioid cells, and fibroblasts, both of which are metabolically very active. Some cellular patterns simulate sarcoidosis with epithelioid cell nodules. Areas of fragmentary focal collagen degeneration occur. At times giant cells may be present. Umbert and Winkelmann describe a very small vessel vasculopathy and obliteration, and Dahl found evidence of an immunoglobulin-related vasculitis.

It is interesting that the microscopic appearance of granuloma annulare is strikingly similar to that of rheumatoid nodules, necrobiosis lesions, and sarcoidosis, although they possess no known common etiological factors.

### *Differential diagnosis*

***Urticaria.*** The individual lesion of urticaria is transient and migratory, whereas granuloma annulare lesions are persistent.

***Erythema multiforme.*** In erythema multiforme, the iris and target lesions are more erythematous than those of granuloma annulare, are usually multiple, and are also more transient.

### *Treatment*

Most lesions do not require treatment.

Cryotherapy in the form of light pressure with solid carbon dioxide for 15 to 20 seconds will result in disappearance of some of these lesions.

Intralesional injection of a glucocorticoid compound (for example, triamcinolone suspension, 5 mg./ml.) by needle or jet injector, or topical application of a similar ointment under an occlusive plastic film, will ordinarily produce a disappearance of the lesion quite rapidly.

In the disseminated form systemic glucocorticoids may be successful in eliminating the disorder.

## NECROBIOSIS LIPOIDICA

An unusual disorder, necrobiosis lipoidica consists of persistent atrophic plaques on the lower extremities, sometimes associated with diabetes mellitus.

### *Natural course*

The lesions begin as rather dark red, scaling, circular plaques, sometimes with a slightly elevated border but often flat. They are asymptomatic. There is a slow but steady enlargement, first with an overlying scale; then, as the lesion progresses, it develops an atrophic depressed center with a yellow cast. The epidermis and dermis become atrophic and transparent, so that the finest details of the underlying blood vessels are readily visible. (See Plate 6, p. 52.)

Lesions are multiple but not symmetrical; they are most frequently observed on the anterior of the legs but may be seen occasionally on the forearms or on the thighs, hands, face, and scalp. The disease is seen chiefly in women under 50 years of age (Fig. 6-8).

### *Pertinent information*

The disease is linked to diabetes in that approximately 35% of patients with necrobiosis have diabetes mellitus. It occurs in about 3% of diabetic patients. The vascular changes in the lesions of necrobiosis have been compared with those found in diabetes, but no firm agreement has been reached regarding their essential similarity. Of the nondiabetic patients with this disorder, almost 50% show evidence of prediabetes or have relatives with diabetes.

### *Microscopic findings*

Two types of reaction are seen—a necrobiotic process with degenerating collagen replaced by a mucinous material, seen chiefly in the leg lesions, and a granulomatous response in other areas, often without necrobiosis, that has been likened to sarcoidosis. These variations seem more a function of geographical difference in response than anything else. Granuloma annulare, rheumatoid nodules, and sarcoidosis have similar microscopic changes in the granulomatous lesions. Foreign body giant cells are present. The blood vessels in the area may demonstrate thickening with internal proliferation and small vessel thrombosis. Fat is present in some of the areas of degenerating collagen.

### *Treatment*

Treatment of the local lesions is unsatisfactory, but produces partial clearing of the process. Fluorinated glucocorticoid ointment under occlusive plastic film is helpful, and the dressing should be changed every 24 hours. Intralesional injection of 1 ml. of 5 mg./ml. of triamcinolone acetate, by needle or by jet injection, is an alternative treatment. If further atrophy is produced by these steroids, they should be discontinued.

## PSEUDOXANTHOMA ELASTICUM

An uncommon hereditary disorder beginning in childhood, pseudoxanthoma elasticum involves the elastic tissue of the dermis and

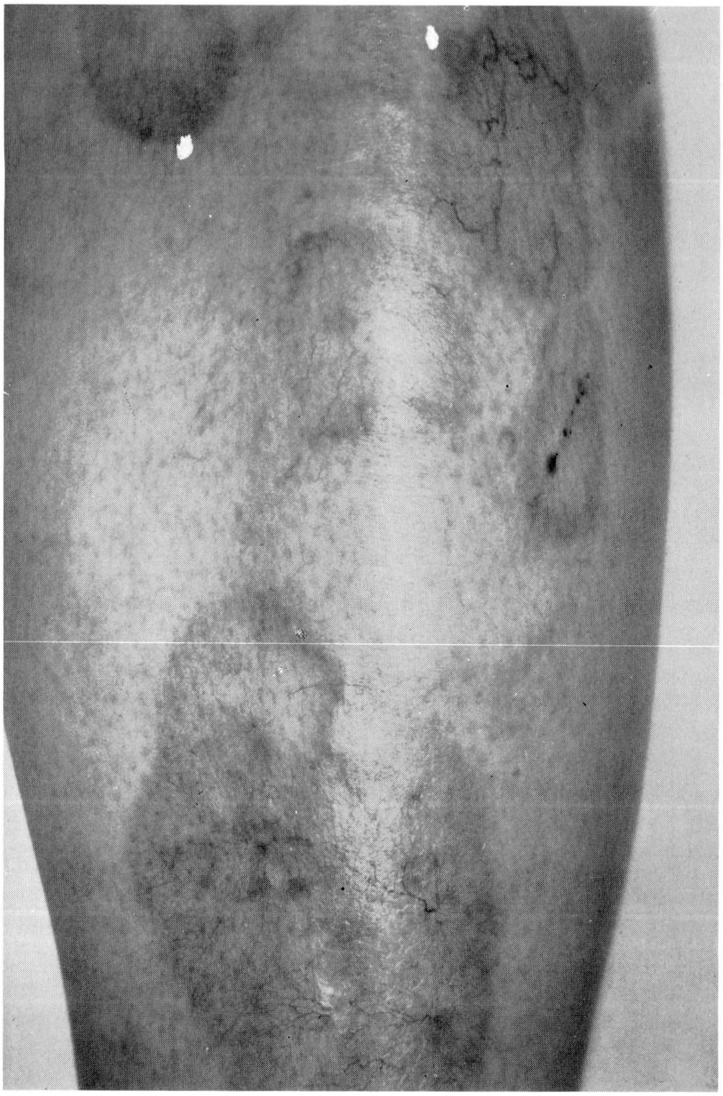

**Fig. 6-8.** Necrobiosis lipoidica; multiple lesions on the anterior aspect of leg.

may also involve the eyes and the larger arteries. The disease may be dominant or recessive, and the clinical findings rest on this (Pope).

The cutaneous lesions consist of small, closely set, yellowish papules in a darker-surfaced skin (Fig. 6-9). They give a weathered appearance. These areas are in plaques and streaks, usually localized to the sides of the neck, axillary areas, perineum, and sometimes other flexural areas. Skin folds may become redundant. The diagnosis is made by biopsy of the lesions. Mucosal surfaces also may be affected.

***Pertinent information***

Pope has carefully described two families with a total of 182 affected individuals and delineated two separate clinical patterns of dominant disease, as well as two separate types of recessive disease. The dominant forms are (1) with vascular disease and ret-

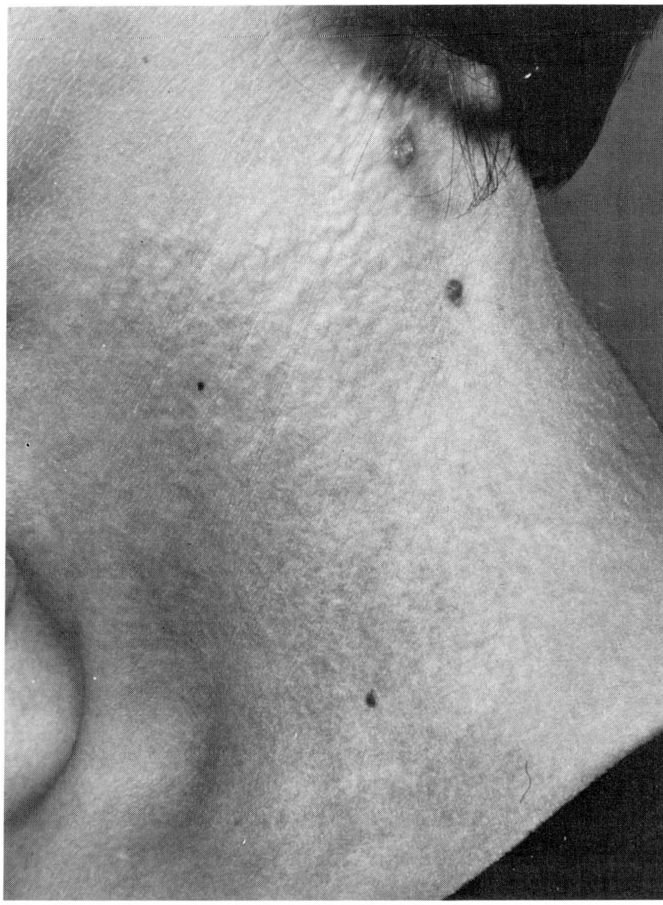

**Fig. 6-9.** Pseudoxanthoma elasticum. Closely set yellowish papules on the side of neck.

inopathy and (2) without these. The recessive forms are (1) with mild vascular disease and mild retinopathy and (2) total cutaneous elastic degeneration, but no systemic complications.

Martinez-Hernandez has beautifully demonstrated mineral deposits and polyanionic material in elastic fibers in the dermis of patients with pseudoxanthoma elasticum, prior to calcium deposition in the fibers. Collagen fibers were normal. Gordon developed a test of calcium uptake by biopsy, using excised dermis as an aid in diagnosis.

The significance of the eruption is its association in many cases with degenerative changes in the elastic tissue of the eye and visceral vessels. Retinal angioid streaks, which consist of radiating gray to brown lines that extend indistinctly out from the optic disc, are present in both dominant and one recessive form. There may be other degenerative ophthalmological changes and resulting loss of vision.

The involved elastic and muscular arteries of the body show decreased pulsation, localized narrowing, and medial calcification. Symptoms of insufficiency such as intermittent claudication, angina, and decreased peripheral pulses are found. Aortic aneurisms and hypertension may develop.

Gastrointestinal bleeding appears in 10% or more of these individuals. Visualization of the

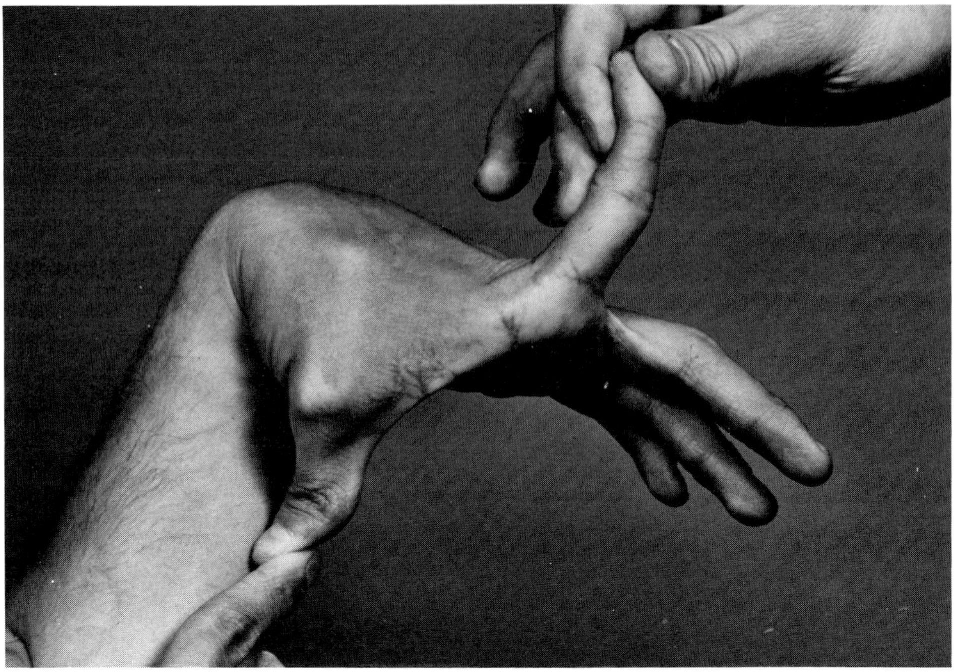

**Fig. 6-10.** Ehlers-Danlos syndrome. Note hyperextensibility of joints.

intestinal mucosa reveals yellow plaques and papules in the submucosa.

*Paget's disease of bone* is associated with some of these cases, as are blue sclerae and loose jointedness.

### Treatment

The diagnosis of pseudoxanthoma elasticum, which must be confirmed by biopsy and microscopic examination, warrants a thorough vascular work-up, including studies of peripheral vessels for calcification and insufficiency. There is no satisfactory treatment. Genetic counseling is now feasible.

## CUTIS HYPERELASTICA (EHLERS-DANLOS SYNDROME)

An uncommon hereditary syndrome, cutis hyperelastica includes fragility of the skin and cutaneous blood vessels, hyperelasticity of the skin, hyperextensibility of the joints, and development of nodular tumors (Figs. 6-10 and 6-11).

A great deal of new information has accumulated concerning Ehlers-Danlos disease in the past 4 years. The disorder has been divided into seven distinct types that are identified by collagen defects of a specific nature in four of these types. The other three, more common types, are identified by clinical and genetic study. Of the seven types, four groups have dominant inheritance, one is X-linked recessive, another is autosomal recessive, and the seventh is not yet characterized.

Each form has its own clinical characteristics related to the type of collagen and structures affected. The degree of skin stretchability is variable with the type.

In several types, the skin is smooth, very pliable, and distensible and can be pulled away from the underlying structures, especially joints, very easily; it returns to its place like rubber. It is easily damaged, develops bruises, pseudotumors, and hematomas readily, and heals very poorly.

Type 4 has fragile and inextensible tissue, but is subject to severe bleeding episodes.

Treatment is of no value. Patients should be protected from lacerations and trauma because of the poor healing.

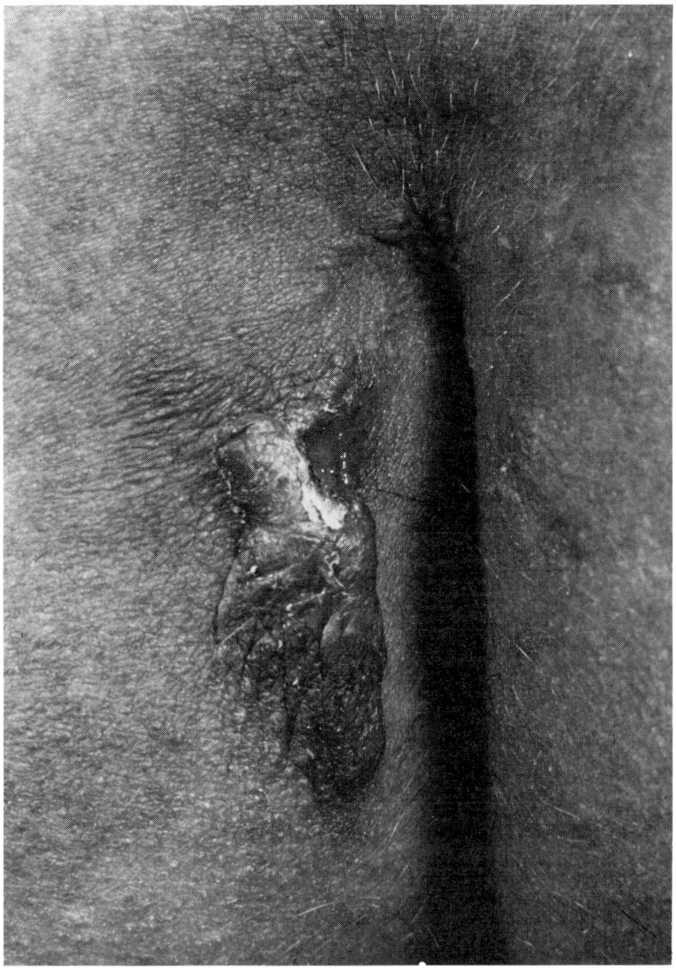

**Fig. 6-11.** Ehlers-Danlos syndrome. Pseudotumor on gluteal surface.

This entity should not be confused with cutis laxa, with its loose, pendulous skin folds and dissolution of the elastic tissue.

## AMYLOIDOSIS

Amyloid is a complex fibrillar protein. The amyloidoses are a group of disorders resulting from deposits of this abnormal protein, which consists of characteristic fibrils with a diameter of 10 to 15 μm. The material can be chemically broken down to demonstrate a variety of specific types of amyloid.

There is a frequent association of amyloid deposition with diseases of immunity, when one finds exposure to a large or prolonged antigenic load, depressed T-cell function, immunosuppressive agents, malignancy, and naturally occurring immunodeficiency states.

The following is a classification of amyloidoses (Franklin):

**primary** Associated with plasma cell and lymphoid neoplasma (Fig. 6-12).
**secondary** Result of chronic infection or inflammation.
**familial** Hereditary forms numerous.
**aging** Deposits found in aging tissues.
**endocrine-associated** Some endocrine disorders demonstrate amyloid deposits.
**localized forms** A variety of local cutaneous deposits not related to systemic disease.

***Cutaneous amyloidosis.*** Primary cuta-

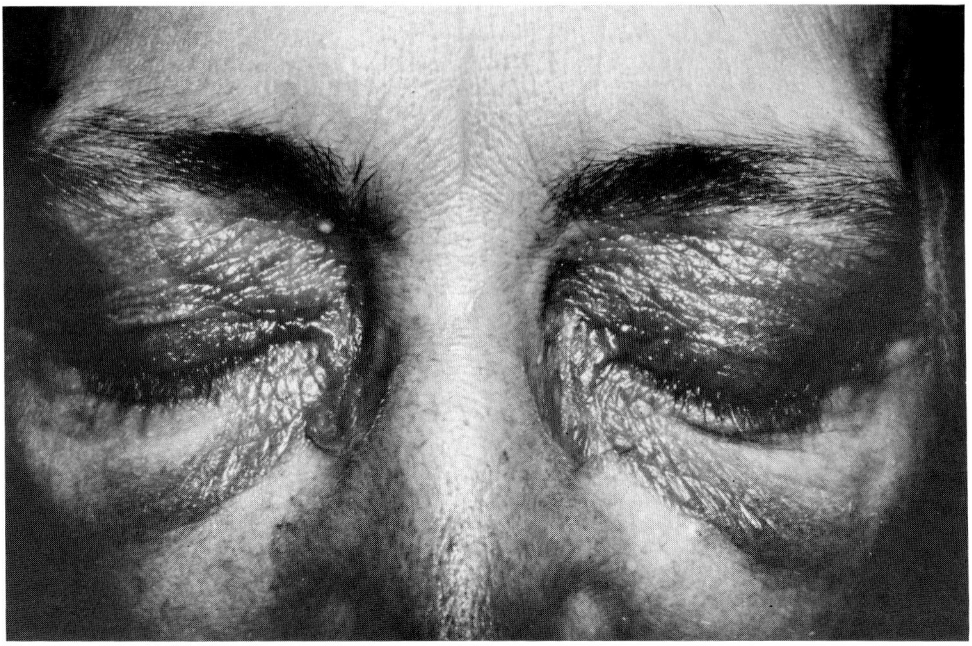

**Fig. 6-12.** Primary amyloidosis. Note shiny papules in purpuric bed.

neous amyloidosis (lichen amyloidosus) (Fig. 6-13) is not associated with systemic disease as yet known. The commonest manifestation is papular, pruritic lesions on the legs anteriorly, and over the interscapular and sacral areas, arms, and thighs. The papules are uniform and pigmented and resemble lesions of lichen simplex chronicus. They are arranged in a curious pattern described as a "ripple" effect. We see this commonly on the West Coast and in the Pacific, in people of Oriental parentage.

Macular lesions may be present as well and seem to be an earlier stage. They can progress to papules and plaques. The amyloid deposits are found in the papillary dermis and can be identified by Congo red staining and on immunofluorescence where IgM and $C_3$ are identified in a diagnostic pattern (McDonald).

*Treatment.* The pruritus is helped by corticosteroid application, but until the pathogenesis of the amyloid deposition is understood, permanent relief will be unavailable.

***Primary systemic amyloidosis.*** Primary systemic amyloidosis is now held to be always related to a plasma cell or lymphocyte dyscrasia.

Amyloid deposits are found in both voluntary and involuntary muscle, in connective tissue, and in blood vessel walls. Lesions are present most frequently in the skin, heart, liver, lungs, and gastrointestinal tract, but they can occur anywhere.

Cutaneous lesions include purpura of the eyelids, face, and neck. Papular lesions of eyelids, perioral area, perineum, flexures, or other areas may be skin colored or hemorrhagic, with a translucent waxy appearance. Scleroderma-like lesions on the face are also seen. Stroking the lesions may produce a series of small hemorrhagic points. Biopsy of a stroked purpuric area may be diagnostic.

Macroglossia is present, as is swelling of the hands, feet, ears, and nose. Ulcerations of the tongue may be present, and alopecia may occur. Carpal tunnel syndrome is frequent and alerts the clinician to the diagnosis.

Diagnosis can often be made in obscure or

A

B

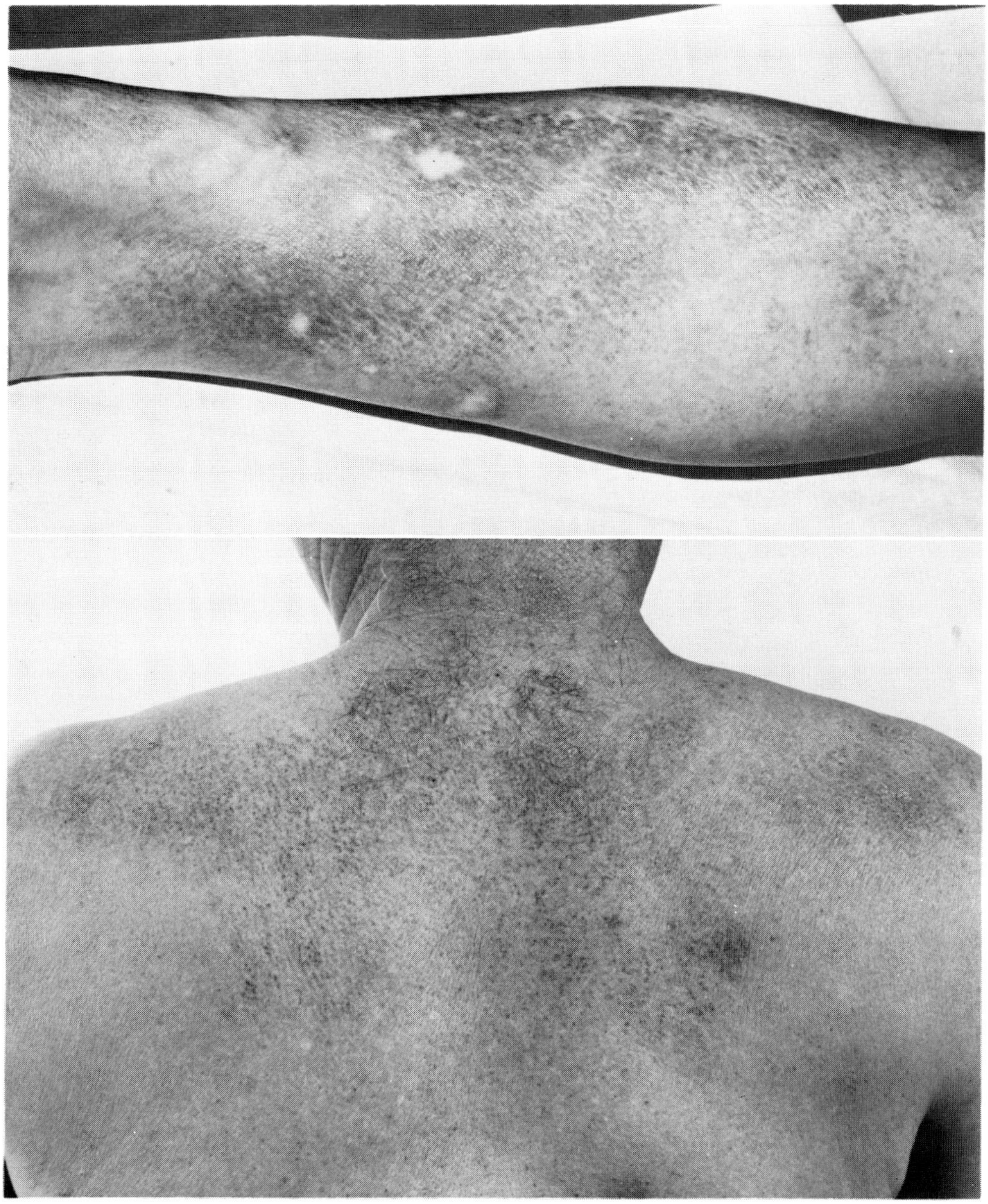

**Fig. 6-13.** Lichen amyloidosus. **A,** Note ripple effect of pigmented papules. **B,** Characteristic location of papules. Immunofluorescence positive.

difficult cases by biopsy of either gingival or rectal mucosa and staining of the specimen for amyloid. Electron microscopy is the surest identification.

The source of the amyloid is unknown although Runne has described observations that indicate fibroblasts as the source. If this is confirmed, efforts will be directed toward determining the factors that control fibroblast metabolism.

## MYXEDEMA

This diagnosis identifies a mucinous deposition in the dermis as a result of fibroblast activity that results in an increase in glycosaminoglycans and change in collagen.

Two forms of cutaneous disease occur in association with myxedema.

***Generalized myxedema.*** The skin is edematous, with a thick, viscous, mucin-containing fluid, and appears very dry with a slight fine scale. It has a distinct waxy appearance with little color. The hair is lusterless, scant, and brittle. Microscopically, there is an increase in mucin in the dermis, but little else.

***Localized myxedema.*** The lesions associated with localized myxedema are asymptomatic, circumscribed firm plaques on the anterior surface of the legs below the knees that have a yellow pallor. The follicles are prominent. There is a deposition of mucin in the dermis, accompanied by proliferation of collagen. Chemically an increase in hyaluronic acid and in glycosaminoglycans can be demonstrated. These lesions may be accompanied by exophthalmos and, less often, by clubbing of the fingernails. They have been reported to occur after treatment of hyperthyroidism with radioactive iodine. Lynch has demonstrated that long-acting thyroid stimulator (LATS) is consistently present in the sera of these patients. However, patients with this disorder may be euthyroid and have no history of thyroid disease.

Until recently, no treatment was satisfactory for these patients, and the lesions simply persisted. Success has been reported recently from the local injection of glucocorticoids or from their topical application under occlusion. Hill produced a successful result with x radiation.

## REFERENCES


Beighton, P., Price, A., Lord, J., et al.: Variants of the Ehlers-Danlos syndrome. Clinical, biochemical, hematological and chromosomal features of 100 patients, Ann. Rheum. Dis. **28**:228, 1969.
**Classified into five types.**

Dahl, M. V., Ullman, S., and Goltz, R. W.: Vasculitis in granuloma annulare, Arch. Dermatol. **113**:463, 1977.
**IgM and $C_3$ mediated vasculitis suggested.**

Franklin, E. C.: Amyloid and amyloidosis of skin, J. Invest. Dermatol. **67**:451, 1976.
**A valuable, authoritative, up-to-date review and classification.**

Gordon, S. G., Subryan, V. L., and Solomons, C. C.: In vitro uptake of calcium by dermis of patients with pseudoxanthoma elasticum, J. Lab. Clin. Med. **86**:638, 1975.
**Increased uptake of calcium might be reduced by judicious dieting.**

Hart, W. R., Norris, H. J., and Helwig, E. B.: Relation of lichen sclerosus et atrophicus of the vulva to development of carcinoma, Obstet. Gynecol. **45**:369, 1975.
**Five out of 107 cases with cancer.**

Hill, T. G., Crawford, J. N., and Rogers, C. C.: Successful management of lichen myxedematosus: report of a case, Arch. Dermatol. **112**:67, 1976.
**Radiation.**

Lang, P. G., Sisson, J. C., and Lynch, P. J.: Intralesional triamcinolone therapy for pretibial myxedema, Arch. Dermatol. **111**:197, 1975.
**One milliliter of a 5 mg./ml. solution improved a 3 cm.$^2$ area for months.**

Lynch, P. J., Maize, J. C., and Sisson, J. C.: Pretibial myxedema and nonthyrotoxic disease, Arch. Dermatol. **107**:107, 1973.
**Euthyroid patients.**

MacDonald, D. M., Black, M. M., and Ramnarain, N.: Immunofluorescence studies in primary localized cutaneous amyloid, Br. J. Dermatol. **96**:635, 1977.
**IgM and $C_3$ present in amyloid deposits in all cases.**

Martinez-Hernandez, A., and Huffer, W. E.: Pseudoxanthoma elasticum, dermal polyanions and mineralization of elastic fibers, Lab. Invest. **31**:181, 1974.
**Polyanions in elastic fibers precede calcium deposition.**

Muller, S. A., and Winkelman, R. K.: Necrobiosis lipoidica diabeticorum, Arch. Dermatol. **93**:272; **94**:1, 1966.
**NLD is a harbinger of diabetes mellitus if patients live long enough.**

Pasieczny, T. A. H.: The treatment of balanitis xerotica obliterans with testosterone propionate ointment, Acta Derm. Venereol. (Stockholm) **57**:275, 1977.
**2.5% results in good to complete clearing.**

Pope, F. M.: Autosomal dominant pseudoxanthoma elasticum, J. Med. Genet. **11**:152, 1974.
**Two separate clinical forms well documented.**

Pope, F. M.: Two types of autosomal recessive pseudoxanthoma elasticum, Ann. Intern. Med. **80**:714, 1974.
**Very significant clarification of the inheritance of pseudoxanthoma elasticum.**

Runne, W., and Orfanos, C. E.: Amyloid production by dermal fibroblasts, Br. J. Dermatol. **97**:155, 1977.
**Imaginative.**

Umbert, P., and Winkelman, R. K.: Granuloma annulare and sarcoidosis, Br. J. Dermatol. **97**:481, 1977.
**Coexistence in five patients.**

Umbert, P., and Winkelman, R. K.: Histologic ultrastructural and histochemical studies of granuloma annulare, Arch. Dermatol. **113**:1681, 1977.
**Electron microscopy shows the consistent monomorphous histiocytic and fibroblastic nature of the disease.**

Wallace, H. J.: Lichen sclerosus et atrophicus, Trans. St. John's Hosp. Dermatol. Soc. **57**:9, 1971.
**Review and discussion on 380 patients, 49 in males and 50 young girls.**

Zelle, K.: Treatment of vulvar dystrophies with topical testosterone, Am. J. Obstet. Gynecol. **109**:570, 1971.
**2% cream, with care and follow-up.**

CHAPTER 7

# Diaper dermatitis

Diaper dermatitis is an almost universal disorder of transient nature, but it is often of distressing severity. Its manifestations are usually limited to the first year of life and disappear after diapers are discontinued.

### *Natural course*

Many factors contribute to produce the disorder of diaper dermatitis. However, despite varied predisposing and causative factors, the appearance and general course of this disorder are not dissimilar.

The cutaneous lesions usually begin around the perianal area and the genitalia and tend to extend along inguinal and gluteal folds. The first lesions are erythematous; subsequent ones become moist, eroded, and crusted. Occasionally, enough maceration, heat retention, and friction take place to produce quite extensive erosions. At first the eruption is limited to the diaper area, but, if unchecked, it may quickly spread both to adjacent and to distal sites. Secondary infection is common.

The disease is made worse by friction, heat, presence of urine and fecal material, and wearing of occlusive clothing, which results in further retention of heat and moisture. It is helped by cleanliness, frequent diaper changes, dryness, coolness, and good ventilation of the area.

### *Pertinent information*

Studies by Montes and his colleagues clearly delineate the importance of bacteria and *Candida* in the etiology of diaper dermatitis. *C. albicans* was isolated from 25 out of 35 patients with diaper dermatitis and from only 3 control patients. The synergistic action between *Candida*, *Escherichia coli*, and *Staphylococcus aureus* is considered by these authors to be significant. They compare their findings with those of other authorities to confirm the significance. In the light of recent indications that atopic patients may possess a deficient immune response, these studies increase in significance for this group.

The perianal and gluteal skin of infants becomes contaminated by microorganisms after they have become established in the intestine. Heat, moisture, and organic material from fecal soiling will add to the flora of the area and produce an optimum environment for growth of bacteria and yeasts. Also, fecal material itself is irritating to the skin.

*Candida albicans* establishes itself here shortly after birth, as do *Proteus* and *Pseudomonas* organisms. The candidal organism itself may be irritating to the skin, and occlusive plastic diaper covers, rubber pants, and so forth will add to the problem. If the area is not cleansed and dried frequently, severe spreading dermatitis can result. This varies with the susceptibility of the child's skin and his inherited tendency to cutaneous disease.

### *Specific types*

***Contact dermatitis.*** Contact dermatitis is a diffuse erythema caused by a wide variety of irritants such as soaps, *fecal materials*, urine, irritating medications, and friction caused by rubbing, tight clothing, diapers, and so forth. Physical friction is a not uncommon cause of this type of dermatitis (Fig. 7-2, *A*). Allergic contact dermatitis is most unusual in infancy.

Treatment includes the general measures discussed later in this chapter, with the addition of glucocorticoid lotions or creams of effective concentration, which should be applied sparingly after compresses three times daily.

***Intertrigo.*** Intertrigo consists of a noticeable erythema of the gluteal cleft, inguinal area, and other areas where there is close apposition of skin surfaces. It is the result of poor ventilation, with resulting irritation caused by accumulation of sebum and sweat.

Treatment is discussed on p. 180; cleansing and subsequent drying procedures should be carefully performed. Neo-Medrol acne lotion is an excellent drying and anti-inflammatory lotion to be applied once or twice daily.

***Candidosis (moniliasis).*** Primary candidal lesions are common in infants, and secondary invasion by *Candida* of other dermatoses is also common. It is necessary for the humidity to be high to support growth of *Candida*. There is good evidence that the presence of *Candida* acts as a primary irritant on normal skin. The lesions are red, scaling, moist patches that possess sharply demarcated edges and are surrounded by flaccid, pustular, satellite lesions. The *C. albicans* will be found as a heavy growth on culture of material from the lesions.

Treatment of the candidal variety of dermatitis includes those general measures given later. Nystatin cream or ointment, applied sparingly three times daily after compresses, miconazole nitrate, and haloprogin, applied sparingly three times daily, are recommended in addition to the general regimen.

Again, Neo-Medrol acne lotion proves to be a satisfactory agent because of its drying and anti-inflammatory effect. It is applied daily.

***Ammonia dermatitis.*** Manifested by a diffuse erythema of the diaper area, ammonia dermatitis produces its greatest involvement in the perianal and gluteal regions. The breakdown of urea in the urine to ammonia by bacteria in the feces causes this eruption.

Treatment procedures listed on p. 180 should be effective in this type of dermatitis.

***Atopic dermatitis.*** Atopic dermatitis causes an increased intolerance of the infant's skin to the heat, moisture, and organic irritants of the diaper area. The diaper area is reddened, pruritic, and moist and may be eroded in patches. An oozing pruritic dermatitis involves the face, legs, and antecubital and popliteal areas, as well as the diaper region. There is usually a history of atopic dermatitis, asthma, or hay fever in other members of the family.

Specific treatment for infants with atopic dermatitis includes a 15-minute bath daily employing tar bath solution, 2 teaspoons to a bathinette of tepid water. It is important to avoid soap, heat, retained moisture, and contact of wool with the skin. Glucocorticoid cream or lotion should be applied three times daily.

***Seborrheic dermatitis.*** Seborrheic dermatitis in the diaper area consists of scaling and at times oozing erythematous patches (Fig. 7-1). As well as the diaper area, however, the abdomen, back, and postauricular regions may be involved. Often a "cradle cap" is present on the scalp from accumulation of sebum.

Treatment, in addition to the general measures outlined below, includes use of tar bath solution, 2 teaspoonsfuls to a bathinette of tepid water, for the infant's daily 15-minute bath. No soap is to be used.

Vioform-hydrocortisone, 1%, cream (staining) should be applied three times daily. This may be a remarkably stubborn form of diaper dermatitis to treat successfully, and a potent fluorinated steroid cream may be used, but for short intervals only.

***Dermatitis caused by sweat retention.*** Discrete and confluent pinhead-sized, erythematous vesicopapules and small pustules are present. The dermatitis is caused by obstruction of the sweat pores because of heat retention, high humidity, moisture, and inflammation. There may be secondary infection. This problem may follow any of the foregoing inflammatory dermatoses.

In addition to the basic aspects of treatment, glucocorticoid lotion such as Neo-Medrol acne lotion (for its drying as well as its glucocorticoid effects) should be applied to the affected area after each diaper change.

***Bacterial dermatitis.*** An unusual form of diaper dermatitis, bacterial dermatitis is characterized by papular, erosive, discrete lesions, suggestive of a low-grade bacterial infection, which is probably causative. It is often of more than ordinary concern because of the appearance of the lesions (Fig. 7-2, *B*), which are unusually deep, and their resistance to

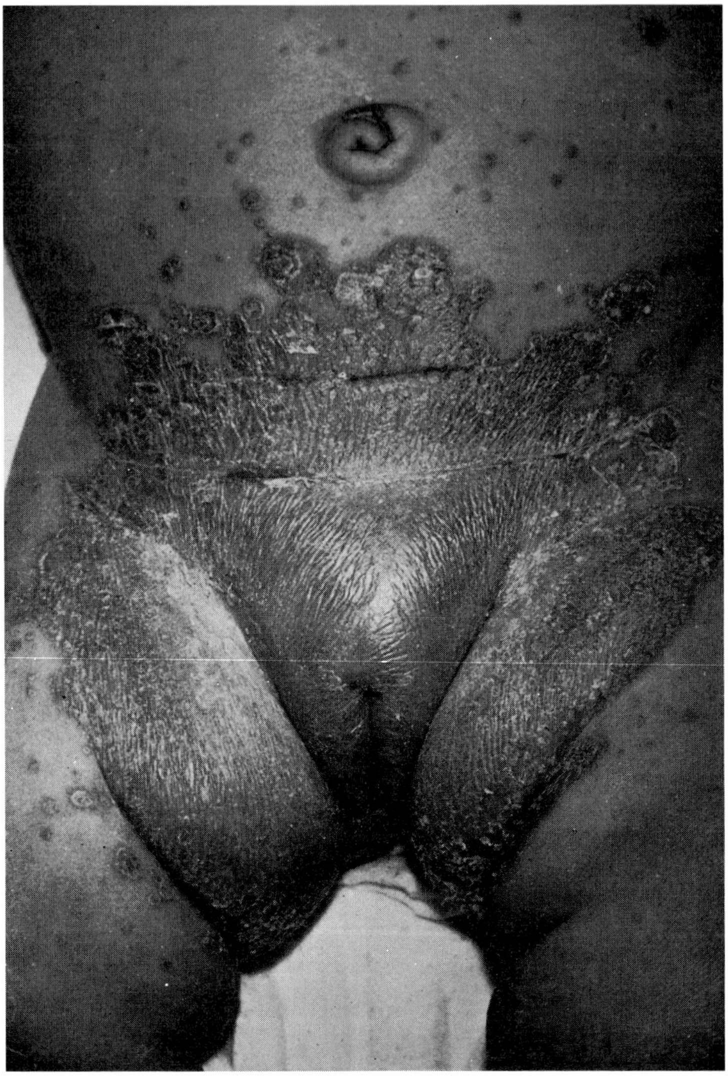

**Fig. 7-1.** Diaper dermatitis caused by seborrheic dermatitis.

therapy. They disappear without trace after topical antibacterial and steroid therapy (that is, Neo-Medrol acne lotion) combined with the general treatment measures. Keeping the surface dry is one of the important facets of treating superficial bacterial infection.

***Treatment: general rules***

The treatment of diaper dermatitis consists of certain measures generally applicable to all the foregoing types. Modifications in the treatment plan and additional measures have been mentioned in the discussion of specific entities.

Hydrocortisone, 1%, in zinc oxide ointment provides excellent anti-inflammatory action and also protection from irritants.

The area should be kept as dry and clean as possible. The diaper should be loose, well ventilated, soft, dry, and changed as quickly as possible after becoming soiled. Plastic diaper covers should be avoided, and no garments with tight-fitting, occlusive thigh or leg constrictions allowed.

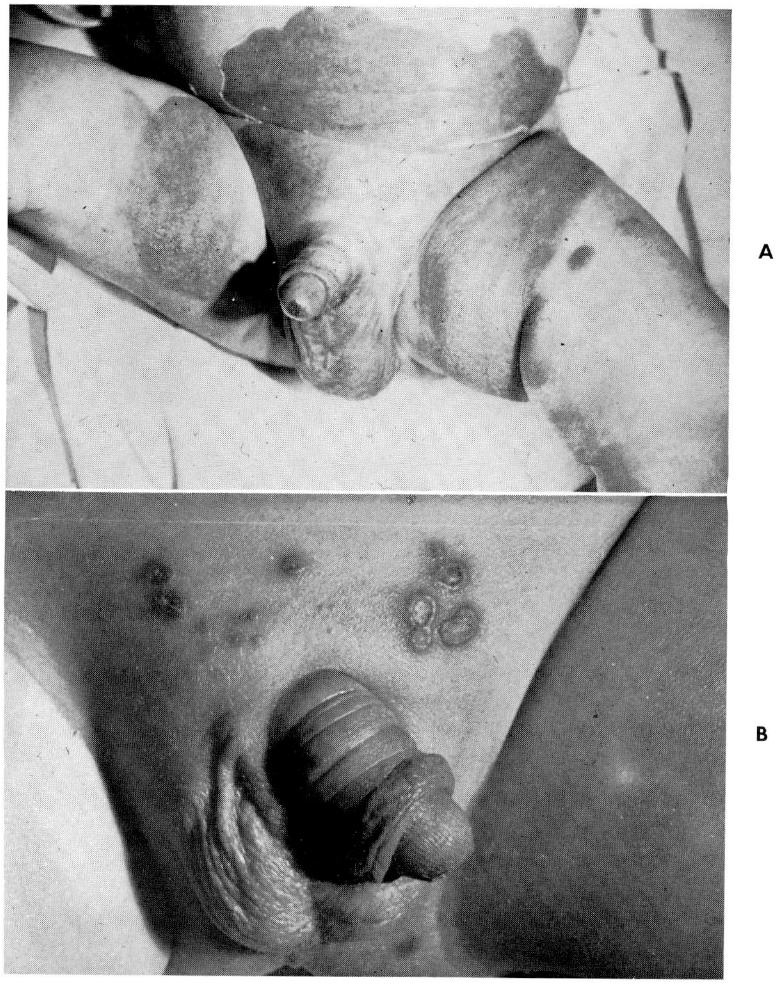

**Fig. 7-2. A,** Diaper dermatitis caused by primary irritation. **B,** Diaper dermatitis caused by secondary bacterial infection. The discrete, ulcerated lesions with rolled edges are typical of this dermatitis.

Antiseptic rinses for diapers may be irritating. Detergents should be thoroughly rinsed from diapers. Hexachlorophene should not be used.

After diapers are changed, the area should be cleansed with water particularly in the folds and creases. Minimal amounts of soap should be used and then rinsed off. Bathing is best carried out once daily, preferably in the early afternoon or evening, just before bed so that the antipruritic effect aids in sleep. The baths most used for infants are the following:

1. Tar bath solution—2 teaspoonfuls to half-full bathinette
2. Oatmeal—½ cup to bath, covered with cloth and placed in the bath; also used as a soap, to rub gently on the affected skin (Aveeno is a colloidal oatmeal preparation for this purpose.)
3. Starch bath

Dusting powder (nonmedicated, unscented talc or zinc oxide powder) can be dusted over the diaper area after bathing and drying. Powders should not be used in association with creams or in the presence of an excessively oozing dermatitis.

Compresses are used for acute weeping or moist dermatitis. Burow's solution compresses are prepared by using 1 tablet or 1 packet of powder of one of the several available aluminum subacetate preparations to 1 quart of tepid water for compressing the whole area for 10 minutes three times daily. The area is blotted dry, not rubbed. The compresses are followed by the use of a cream or lotion, the character of which depends on the chief causative factor or factors in the dermatitis. The most satisfactory anti-inflammatory cream is 1% hydrocortisone or its equivalent, applied very thinly after the compresses, three times daily. For unresponsive cases, a medium-strength glucocorticoid cream, 0.1% triamcinolone, may be used, or even a potent cream such as 0.1% betamethasone valerate will be efficacious. However, both of these latter fluorinated preparations should be used only for short intervals. They will cause systemic absorption of the compound and result in some adrenal suppression and thinning and fragility of the skin if used for prolonged intervals (Johns and Bower).

The bedroom temperature should not be excessively high. Heat and resulting perspiration are fully as irritating and maceration-producing in dermatoses of infancy as in adult dermatoses. By the same token, the infant should never be overclothed, indoors or out.

### REFERENCES

Caplan, R. M.: The irritant role of feces in the genesis of perianal itch, Gastroenterology **59:**19, 1966.
**An important observation.**

Johns, A. M., and Bower, B. D.: Wasting of napkin area after repeated use of fluorinated steroid ointment, Br. Med. J. **1:**347, 1970.
**A sobering demonstration.**

Leyden, J. J., Katz, S. I., Stewart, R., and Kligman, A. M.: Urinary ammonia and ammonia-producing microorganisms in infants with and without diaper dermatitis, Arch. Dermatol. **113:**1678, 1977.
**At last, another ghost laid to rest.**

Montes, L. F., Pittillo, R. D., Hunt, D., et al.: Microbial flora of infant's skin, Arch. Dermatol. **103:**640, 1971.
**25 to 35 patients with *Candida*.**

# CHAPTER 8

# Drug reactions

*One of the most urgent problems in medicine today lies in the accurate diagnosis and prevention of adverse reactions to drugs.* Melmon discusses this problem in depth from the point of view of a director of clinical pharmacology. He states that 18% to 30% of all hospitalized patients have a drug reaction (hospital stay is thus doubled), that 30% of patients admitted for drug reactions get a second one in the hospital, and that one seventh of all hospital days is devoted to the care of drug reaction. One in 10 admissions to Great Britain's geriatric hospitals is attributable to adverse drug reactions (Williams). Only 68.7% make a full recovery. The commonest cause is the diuretic group. Parker communicated a report that 5% of medical hospital admissions are attributable to drug reactions, and 15% of inpatients experience such a reaction. Most observers agree, however, that, even with these statistics, reporting of drug reactions is often neglected. Canadian reports generally parallel American statistics (Hoddinott and co-workers; Ogilvie and Ruedy).

Virtually any tissue or organ can be affected in drug reactions, such as in the following:

*Central nervous system*—Fever, psychoses, depression, euphoria, hallucinations.

*Hemic system*—Any cellular compound may be reduced, eliminated, or increased, sometimes with startling rapidity.

*Liver*—Parenchymal damage is often unsuspected; biliary stasis; fibrosis.

*Gastrointestinal tract*—Bleeding, ulceration, dysfunction.

*Renal system*—Hematuria, anuria, proteinuria.

*Respiratory system*—Dyspnea, spasm, cough, edema.

*Musculoskeletal system*—Arthralgias, muscle pain, and spasm.

*Cardiovascular system*—Hypotension, hypertension, arrythmias.

*Immune system*—Immune complex disease, serum sickness, urticaria.

Adverse reactions to drugs are seen more often in the skin than in any other organ. Arndt and Jick undertook to quantitate the occurrence of drug-induced *allergic skin* reactions (excluding nonallergic and noncutaneous eruptions) in 22,227 consecutive medical inpatients. Allergic skin reactions occurred in 2% to 3%. The most commonly encountered causes are in Table 3. A drug eruption can resemble almost any cutaneous disease and may be seen in any degree of severity, from a simple erythematous patch to a life-threatening, toxic, epidermal necrolysis.

Unfortunately, at present no consistently reliable and safe technique is available for identification of the causes of drug reactions. (See Diagnosis of drug reactions, p. 187.) *The prime factor in making the diagnosis of a drug reaction is clinical awareness* (Fig. 8-1).

## POLYPHARMACY

Adverse reactions to drugs are most common in patients with serious illness who receive a number of drugs. The number of reactions increases geometrically as the numbers of drugs increase. Furthermore, patients with a history of previous drug reactions appear to be more predisposed. Topical administration is more likely to induce allergy than systemic use. Allergic reactions are more common in patients with gastrointestinal diseases.

**Table 3.** Some estimated reaction rates of commonly used drugs (Arndt)

| | Rate of reactions per thousand recipients | Number of recipients in study |
|---|---|---|
| Trimethoprim-sulfamethoxazole | 59 | 169 |
| Ampicillin | 52 | 2,988 |
| Corticotropin | 28 | 106 |
| Erythromycin | 23 | 481 |
| Penicillin G | 16 | 3,286 |
| Cephalosporins | 13 | 1,308 |
| Nitrofurantoin | 9.1 | 219 |
| Barbiturates | 4.7 | 4,658 |
| Chlordiazepoxide | 4.2 | 2,161 |
| Glutethimide | 4.5 | 221 |
| Furosemide | 2.6 | 3,497 |

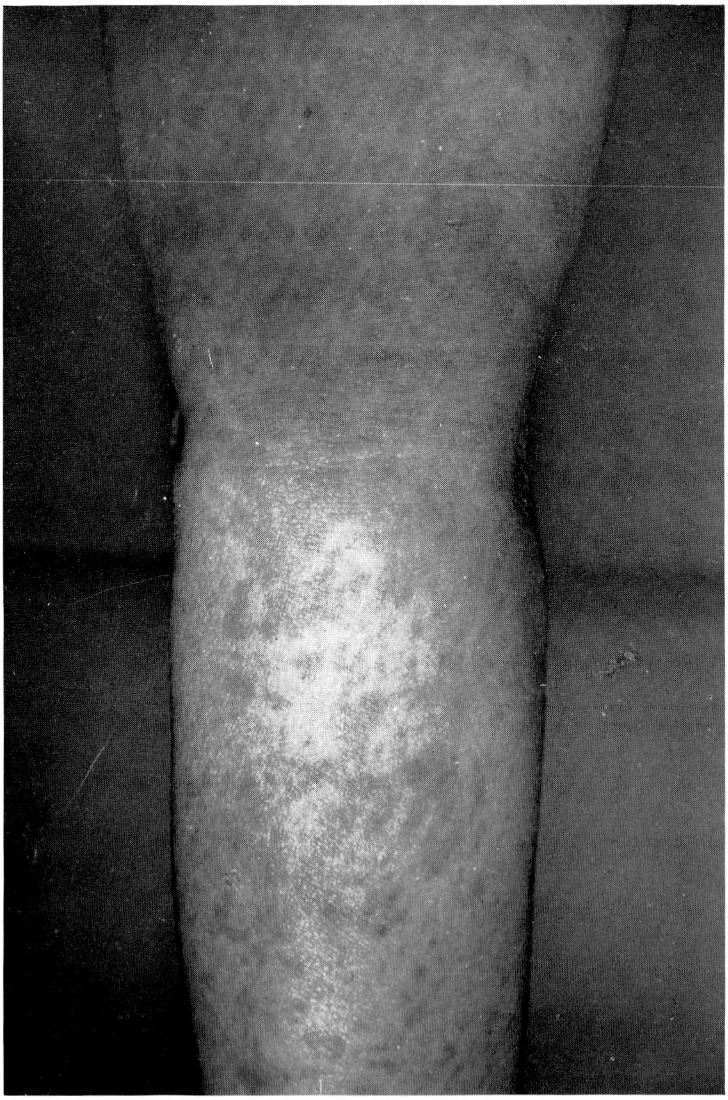

**Fig. 8-1.** Drug eruption caused by ingestion of phenobarbital.

***Coloring, flavoring, and preserving agents.*** An often neglected fact, pointed out by Mitchell, is that potentially causative chemical agents are found not only in both ethical and proprietary drugs, but also in food, in the form of coloring or flavoring agents (for example, yellow tartrazine), and preservatives. Thus the physician must be prepared to seek causes of cutaneous reactions among agents such as these, particularly when the patient denies all medications. The encyclopedia of food chemicals used in Canada is most helpful as a reference.

Kauppinen's remarkable continuing study of inpatients in Finland must be mentioned specifically, in which she reviewed 620 patients hospitalized for cutaneous drug reactions.

Two hundred seventy-four patients were observed with provocation tests with varying doses of the suspected drug. The etiological agent was identified or strongly suspected in 90% of all patients. Most common drugs were sulfonamides (in an increase over the report for the years prior to 1960), penicillin (decreasing from previous years), acetylsalicylic acid, chloramphenicol, barbiturates (decreasing from previous years), pyrazolones, antidiabetic drugs administered orally, diuretics, and antihistamines. The main types of eruptions were exanthematous (45%), urticaria and angioedema (27%), fixed (9%), and erythema multiforme (5%).

Kauppinen has demonstrated that provoking a drug eruption by readministration of suspected drugs results in a reaction at a fairly uniform time interval (less than 12 hours) regardless of the morphology of the eruption. Also, *the reaction thus produced is dose related; it does not appear when the patient is given small amounts of the drug.*

## SOME MECHANISMS OF DRUG REACTIONS—A WORKING CLASSIFICATION

1. Allergic reactions
   a. Immediate
   b. Cytotoxic
   c. Serum sickness—Arthus reaction
   d. Delayed
2. Pharmacological factors
   a. Overdosage
   b. Side effects
   c. Interaction between drugs
3. Patient variation (idiosyncrasy, intolerance, pharmacogenetic)
4. Ecological imbalance
5. Exacerbation of existing disease
6. Jarisch-Herxheimer reaction
7. Environmental influence

### Allergic reactions

Drugs producing allergic reactions usually have been administered to the patient on a previous occasion. If not, there will be a latent period of at least 5 days of sensitization before an allergic reaction occurs. Only a small proportion of patients taking the drug will react, and only small doses may be required. Closely related chemicals will sometimes be similar enough to have sensitized the patient to the drug. A drug may produce any of the forms of immune reaction.

As most drugs are chemically simple structures, they function antigenically as haptens, in combination with host proteins. Thus tightly bound drug protein complexes are more likely to be antigenic. Loosely or reversibly bound drugs are not.

***Type I.*** *Immediate allergic reactions*, including anaphylaxis occurring within minutes to hours of taking the drug, are associated with circulating antibodies. IgE forms these antibodies and is particularly capable of discharging mast cells with release of histamine, vasoactive kinins, eosinophil chemotactic factor of anaphylaxis (ECF-A), slow reactive substance of anaphylaxis (SRS-A), prostaglandins, and heparin. Systemic anaphylaxis is more likely to occur when the drug is injected.

***Type II.*** *Cytotoxic reactions* use complement and produce local cell destruction by direct affinity of the antigenic substance with the cell membrane. These may involve IgG or IgM proteins and can affect circulating peripheral blood cells, tissue cells in any organ, or basement membranes, for example, the dermoepidermal junction. They may not always result in cell death, but they may block cell surface receptors to hormones or other active agents or may even stimulate the cell's activities.

***Type III.*** *Serum sickness* reactions are the result of formation of soluble immune complexes of antigen and antibody. They also take up complement, in the deposition of these complexes, on blood vessel walls, with resulting vasculitis and systemic symptoms. IgG and IgM are involved in these dynamic, changing depositions on glomeruli, in tissues on platelets, which release vasoactive amines, and on polymorphonuclear neutrophil leukocytes, which release lysosomal enzymes. Complement is activated to produce inflammation and chemotaxis and perhaps to release further immune complexes from lymphocyte membranes.

***Type IV.*** *Delayed reactions* are cell mediated by lymphocytes; thus lymphocyte transformation occurs on exposure to these drugs. Macrophage inhibition also occurs. T-lymphocytes take part in this process and must be present in normal quantities, although abnormalities of T-helper or T-suppressor cells may enhance the reaction.

Eisner describes circulating antibody to a drug metabolite, a conjugate of an ingested drug when the drug itself was immunologically inert. Contaminants of drugs can be sensitizing, as Feinberg has demonstrated. He has also demonstrated varying degrees of sensitization potential to different forms of penicillin and cephalosporins.

### *Guidelines*

The suspected drug may have been used on many previous occasions without adverse reactions.

The drug may react quite differently in different people, for example, causing urticaria in one and a fixed reaction in another.

It may also produce different reactions at different times in the same individual.

Children are much less susceptible to immunogenic drug reactions than are adults.

## Pharmacological factors

Not infrequently, the therapeutic dose of a drug is very close to the toxic level. Symptoms of digitalis *overdosage* occur, and one can produce pigmentation in argyria because of silver in nose drops.

Expected results of drug therapy other than the main therapeutic effect are *side effects*. The drowsiness produced by antihistaminic drugs falls into this category, and alopecia from methotrexate is a good example.

In regard to *interaction between drugs*, administration of two or more drugs simultaneously often seriously alters the effect of one or both drugs. Long-continued administration of certain drugs will alter the metabolism of certain other drugs. Phenobarbital, for example, will induce enzymes metabolizing bishydroxycoumarin, diphenylhydantoin sodium, and griseofulvin to significantly alter the plasma level and lessen the therapeutic effect. Meprobamate and tolbutamide may stimulate greater production of enzymes instead of metabolizing them, which results in a decreased therapeutic effect. Aspirin may displace methotrexate from its albumin binding and also reduce its renal excretion with serious effects.

A list of drugs that are of interest to dermatologists and that react undesirably with each other follows:

| | |
|---|---|
| Acetylsalicylic acid and | alcohol<br>indomethacin<br>phenylbutazone<br>glucocorticoids<br>allopurinol<br>para-aminosalicylic acid<br>methotrexate<br>sulfonamides and sulfonylureas<br>clofibrate |
| Dicumarol and other anticoagulants and | phenylbutazone<br>indomethacin<br>acetaminophen<br>antacids<br>many other drugs |
| Methotrexate and | sulfonamides<br>phenylbutazone<br>salicylates<br>para-aminobenzoic acid |
| Phenobarbitol and | acetaminophen<br>dicumarol and anticoagulants<br>diphenylhydantoin sodium<br>griseofulvin<br>anticonvulsants<br>tranquilizers<br>alcohol |

| | |
|---|---|
| Tetracycline and | ferrous sulfate<br>antacids<br>milk and milk products<br>calcium |

## Patient variation

An unpredictable factor occurs when an individual responds in an abnormal way to a specific drug, apart from immunological or previously determined mechanisms. This is *idiosyncracy*, which is as yet unexplained. *Intolerance* describes an overreaction to a very small dose of a drug; yet the nature of the drug effect is as predicted. *Pharmacogenetics* applies to the study of inherited factors that affect the individual patient's metabolism of drugs (La Du).

Since metabolism takes place through the action of enzymes that are determined by at least one gene, a mutation of only one gene may cause a significant alteration in the metabolism of a drug in any one person. Some individuals may metabolize a drug so rapidly as to make it difficult to attain effective blood levels, whereas others may metabolize the same drug so slowly as to allow accumulation and production of toxic effects. For example, those who develop peripheral neuropathy when taking isoniazid are for the most part patients who acetylate and thus inactivate the drug more slowly than normal, allowing production of the toxic effects. Hemolytic anemia is produced by several drugs in patients whose erythrocytes lack glucose-6-phosphate dehydrogenase. These are genetically determined abnormalities.

## Ecological imbalance

Some drugs, such as tetracyclines, are capable of altering the natural balance of microorganisms in the gastrointestinal tract.

Certain drugs may activate a latent infection. Salicylates and barbiturates both can produce a flare-up of herpes simplex.

## Exacerbation of existing disease

Patients with latent porphyria may have this disorder brought to clinical manifestations by administration of griseofulvin or barbiturates.

## Jarisch-Herxheimer reaction

After the administration of a drug, new lesions may develop and existing lesions may reactivate. Furthermore, the patient may then develop a transient fever within 12 hours after therapy. With the administration of penicillin in the treatment of syphilis, this reaction is attributable to the sudden destruction of large numbers of spirochetes.

## Environmental influence

In cutaneous drug reactions, the effect of light, at least, must be included when one is classifying the mechanisms. Demethylchlortetracycline, for example, is greatly disposed to exaggerate the erythemogenic effect of sunlight, in some people more than in others.

# DIAGNOSIS OF DRUG REACTIONS

***Type I reactions.*** Mucous membrane or intradermal tests, if carefully and properly done, can give a wheal-and-flare reaction localized to the test site. Irritant reactions and nonspecific reactions (controls must be used) are confusing.

***Type II reactions.*** Antibody can be demonstrated with agglutination tests using normal cells and patient's serum.

***Type III reactions.*** Antibody may be demonstrated by sophisticated gel-precipitation techniques.

***Type IV reactions.*** Patch tests are routinely used in allergic contact dermatitis and can be tried safely in many drug reactions. Felix and Comaish found them of value and stated that they should be the first type of test. Lymphocyte transformation or macrophage inhibition tests can be used in some instances, but standardization for accurate assessment of results is a problem.

Readministration of small quantities of a drug in a carefully prepared hospital setting is the only satisfactory test with our present state of knowledge. Kauppinen's article should be studied before one attempts it. We find that this is a practical approach in the management of chronic urticaria.

## REACTIONS TO CERTAIN TYPES OF DRUGS

With each new therapeutic agent, a certain number of patients may be expected to have some form of drug reaction. Some medications are more likely than others to produce these untoward effects. An increased dosage of a drug will tend to increase the number of reactions. Thus it is wise to use any new drug alone, in a minimum dosage, after a thorough study of known side effects, and after determining the likelihood and probable nature of untoward reactions.

The number of adverse reactions increases greatly with each additional drug when several are being administered.

**ACETAMINOPHEN** (a metabolite of phenacetin)

*Cutaneous.* Gray color, purpura.

*General.* Gastrointestinal, tinnitus, hepatic, renal, hematological, hemolytic anemia.

**ACETAZOLAMIDE**

*Cutaneous.* Erythema multiforme, maculopapular.

*General.* Hematopoietic, muscular.

**ACETYLSALICYLIC ACID**

*Cutaneous.* Urticaria, maculopapular, oral ulceration, purpura, vasculitis.

*General.* Gastrointestinal (GI) bleeding, thrombocytopenia. *Interacts with* indomethacin, phenylbutazone, glucocorticoids, para-aminosalicylic acid (PAS), methotrexate, sulfonamides, sulfonylureas, alcohol.

**ALLOPURINOL**

10% show a drug reaction, a few are severe.

*Cutaneous.* Maculopapular, urticaria, alopecia, purpura, exfoliative.

*General.* Fever, gouty arthralgia, renal, abdominal pain, hepatic. IgM deposits on direct immunofluorescence.

**AMANTADINE**

*Cutaneous.* Maculopapular, urticaria, livedo reticularis.

*General.* Central nervous system (CNS) stimulation.

**AMINOPYRINE**

*Cutaneous.* Edema, maculopapular, purpura, pigmentation, toxic epidermal necrolysis (TEN).

*General.* Agranulocytosis, fever, thrombocytopenia.

**AMODIAQUIN HYDROCHLORIDE**

*Cutaneous.* Pigmentation, nail discoloration, urticaria.

*General.* Thrombocytopenia.

**AMPHOTERICIN B**

*Cutaneous.* Maculopapular, urticaria, alopecia.

*General.* Renal, liver, hematopoietic, hypotension, CNS.

**AMPICILLIN**

*Cutaneous.* Urticaria, erythematous, maculopapular (almost 100% in patients with infectious mononucleosis, hyperuricemia, or leukemia), purpura, serum sickness (see Bierman).

*General.* Interacts with allopurinol.

**AMITRIPTYLINE HYDROCHLORIDE**

*Cutaneous.* Maculopapular, urticaria, sweating, pruritus.

*General.* Hypotension, hematopoiesis, liver, CNS. *Interacts with* alcohol and CNS drugs.

**ANTIPYRINE**

*Cutaneous.* Erythema, pigmentation.

*General.* Rare.

**ARSENIC**

*Cutaneous.* Brown-gray pigmentation, keratoses, cutaneous malignancies.

*General.* GI, headache, myositis.

**AZO DYES (TARTRAZINE)**

*Cutaneous.* Urticaria, purpura, vasculitis.

**BARBITURATES**

*Cutaneous.* Maculopapular, urticaria, erythema multiforme, angiitis, fixed drug, pruritus, TEN, worsens porphyria, bullous, acne, purpura, photosensitivity, exfoliative, anaphylaxis, lupus erythematosus–like syndrome, *bullous eruptions in comatose patients.*

*General.* Withdrawal signs. *Interacts with* griseofulvin, coumarins, phenytoins.

**BENZOATES (FOOD PRESERVATIVES)**

*Cutaneous.* Urticaria, purpura, vasculitis.

**BENZOTHIADIAZINES**

*Cutaneous.* Dermatitis, urticaria, photosensitivity, cross-sensitivity to sulfonamides, lichenoid, purpura, vasculitis, erythema multiforme.

*General.* GI.

**BLEOMYCIN SULFATE**

*Cutaneous.* Vesiculobullous palms, stomatitis, alopecia, skin ulcers, nail changes, striae, bleeding.

*General.* GI, fever, fatigue, pulmonary fibrosis, renal, liver, CNS.

**BORIC ACID**

*Cutaneous.* Erythema, exfoliation, TEN.

*General.* GI, CNS, liver (from absorption).

**BROMINE AND BROMIDES**

*Cutaneous.* Acne, pustular folliculitis, eczematous, urticaria, bromoderma, bullous, vasculitis, erythema nodosum.

*General.* Psychic disturbance, blurred vision.

**CARBAMAZEPINE**

*Cutaneous.* Maculopapular, urticaria, pruritus, erythema multiforme, acne, exfoliative.

*General.* Dizziness, GI, anemia.

**CARBROMAL**

*Cutaneous.* Characteristic "cayenne pepper," purpura of legs, thighs, abdomen.

*General.* Withdrawal signs.

**CEPHALORIDINE**

*Cutaneous.* Generalized hypersensitivity reactions.

*Cross reacts* with penicillin.

*General.* Anemia, neutropenia, renal tubular necrosis in high doses.

**CHLORAL HYDRATE**

*Cutaneous.* Urticaria, photosensitivity, erythema, purpura, erythema multiforme, bullous. Reactions are uncommon.

*General.* Fever.

**CHLORDIAZEPOXIDE**

*Cutaneous.* Erythema, maculopapular, urticaria, photosensitivity, fixed drug.

*General.* Headache, worsens porphyria.

**CHLOROQUINE DIPHOSPHATE**

*Cutaneous.* Urticaria, maculopapular, photosensitivity, pigmentation, worsens psoriasis, alopecia.

*General.* A specific, irreversible retinal degeneration occurs in 40% of patients taking more than a cumulative 8 gm./kg. of this drug. Corneal opacities, optic atrophy, worsens porphyria, myopathy, blood dyscrasias.

**CLOFIBRATE**

*Cutaneous.* Reactions uncommon. Urticaria, pruritus, stomatitis, alopecia.

*General. Interacts with* anticoagulants.

**CODEINE** (Fig. 8-2)

*Cutaneous.* Urticaria, fixed drug.

*General.* Restlessness, nausea, hyperactivity, vomiting, syncope, constipation.

**COLCHICINE**

*Cutaneous.* Pruritus, alopecia, urticaria.

*General.* GI, hematopoietic, myopathy.

**CONTRACEPTIVES**

(See Progestagens).

**CORTICOTROPIN (ACTH)**

See p. 68.

**COUMARINS**

*Cutaneous.* Necrotic skin ulcers, alopecia, urticaria, maculopapular.

*General.* Altered coagulability of blood.

**DAPSONE**

*Cutaneous.* Maculopapular, lichenoid, urticaria.

*General.* Red blood cell (RBC) hemolysis, blood dyscrasias, methemoglobin. Sensory and motor neuropathy.

**DEMECLOCYCLINE HYDROCHLORIDE (DECLOMYCIN)**

*Cutaneous.* Photosensitivity, onycholysis, fingernails, pruritus ani and vulvae.

*General.* GI, teeth staining.

**DIAZEPAM**

*Cutaneous.* Maculopapular, urticaria, pruritus.

*General.* Drowsiness, impaired judgment. *Interacts with* alcohol.

**DIAZOXIDE**

*Cutaneous.* Hirsutism.

**DIGITALIS**

*Cutaneous.* Exanthems, urticaria, bullous.

*General.* GI, visual effects, gynecomastia.

**DIPHENYLHYDANTOIN SODIUM**

*Cutaneous.* Erythema, maculopapular, gingivitis, angiitis, exfoliative, acne, pseudolymphoma, erythema multiforme, TEN, alopecia, pigmentation, urticaria, hypertrichosis, fixed drug.

*General.* Lupus erythematosus, Ig abnor-

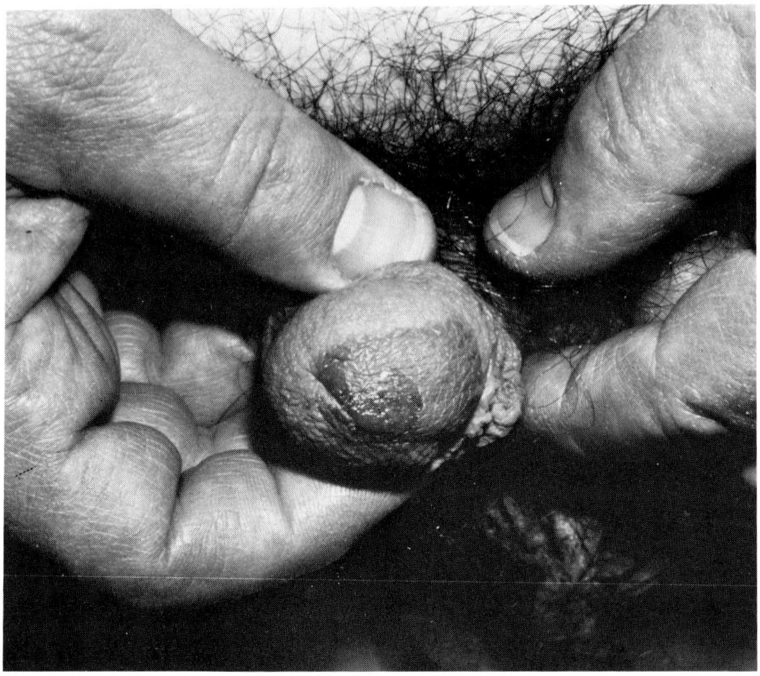

**Fig. 8-2.** Fixed drug reaction to codeine.

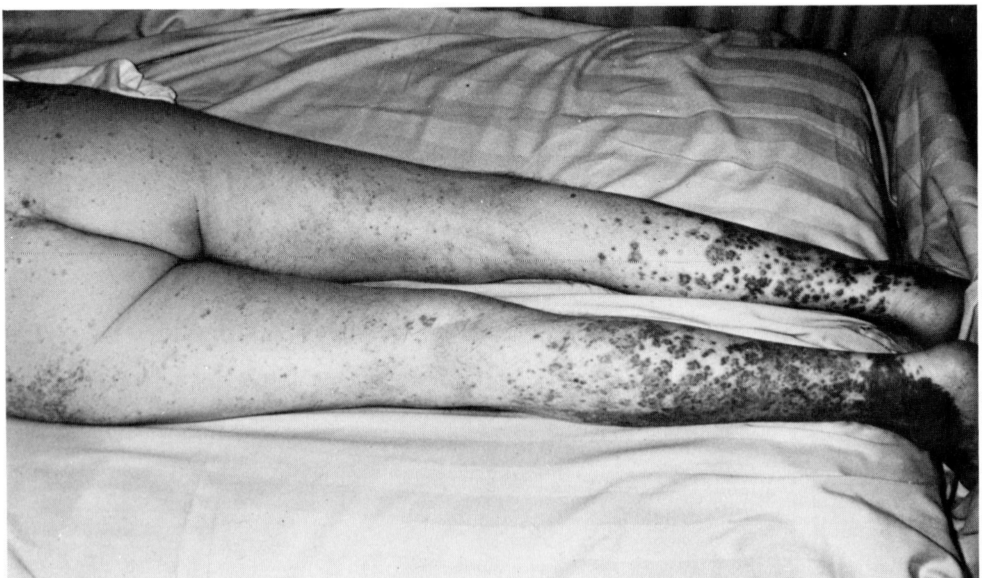

**Fig. 8-3.** Purpura of legs from furosemide.

malities, worsens porphyria, anemia, leukopenia, CNS, liver.

**DISULFIRAM**

*Cutaneous.* Fixed drug, maculopapular, urticaria, eczematous, flushing.

*General.* Dizziness, toxic symptoms with alcohol.

**ERYTHROMYCIN**

*Cutaneous.* Maculopapular, urticaria, pruritus.

*General.* Hepatitis (estolate), GI.

**ETHAMBUTOL**

*Cutaneous.* Purpura.

*General.* Visual disturbances, retrobulbar neuritis.

**ETHOSUXIMIDE**

*Cutaneous.* Maculopapular, urticaria.

*General.* GI, depression, ataxia, lupus erythematosus, blood dyscrasias.

**FLUORINE**

*Cutaneous.* Urticaria, seborrheic dermatitis, alopecia, brittle nails.

*General.* Teeth mottling, osteosclerosis. *Note:* Stannous fluoride contained in toothpastes may create erosions on the oral mucosa.

**FLUOROURACIL**

*Cutaneous.* Onycholysis, reactivation of radiation dermatitis, photosensitivity.

*General.* Stomatitis

**FUROSEMIDE** (Fig. 8-3)

*Cutaneous.* Photosensitivity, maculopapular, urticaria, erythema multiforme, purpura, bullous eruption, pruritus, lichen planus.

*General.* Weakness, dizziness, transient deafness, hyperuricemia, visual blurring, nausea, vomiting, diarrhea, anemia, leukopenia, and agranulocytosis.

**GENTAMICIN SULFATE**

*General.* Vestibular, renal.

**GLUCOCORTICOIDS**

*Cutaneous.* See p. 204. Specific compounds have produced immediate allergic reactions (Mendelson).

*Systemic.* See p. 68.

**GOLD**

*Cutaneous.* Pruritus, maculopapular, erythema, lichenoid, urticaria, exfoliative, alopecia, pigmentation, purpura, stomatitis, erythema multiforme, photosensitivity, eczema.

*General.* Albuminuria, hematopoietic, keratitis, vasculitis.

**GRISEOFULVIN**

*Cutaneous.* Maculopapular, urticaria, photosensitivity, fixed drug.

*General.* Headache, GI, worsens porphyria, lupus erythematosus. *Interacts with* anticoagulants.

**GUANETHIDINE SULFATE**

*Cutaneous.* Urticaria, maculopapular.

*General.* Diarrhea. *Interacts with* antidepressants, phenothiazines, amphetamine, cocaine.

**HEPARIN**

*Cutaneous.* Urticaria, paresthesias, alopecia. Reactions at injection site.

*General.* Altered coagulability of blood.

**HYDRALAZINE HYDROCHLORIDE**

*Cutaneous.* Erythematous, maculopapular, exfoliative, photosensitivity, purpura.

*General.* Lupus erythematosus (high percentage), renal.

**IDOXURIDINE (INTRAVENOUS)**

*Cutaneous.* Stomatitis, alopecia, purpura.

*General.* Bone marrow depression, liver, teratogenic.

**IMIPRAMINE HYDROCHLORIDE**

*Cutaneous.* Maculopapular, urticaria, increased sweating, photosensitivity, edema, pruritus, exfoliative.

*General.* Sedation, dry mouth, liver, hypotension, visual. *Interacts with* alcohol, monoamine oxidase (MAO) inhibitors, and other drugs.

**INDOMETHACIN**

*Cutaneous.* Maculopapular, urticaria, vasculitis, purpura, alopecia, pruritus, oral ulcers.

*General.* Headache, dizziness, psychic disturbance, GI, ophthalmic, and many others. *Interacts with* other drugs.

**INSULIN**

*Cutaneous.* Urticaria, pruritus, maculopapular, purpura. Dystrophy at injection site.

**IODINE (AS ORAL IODIDES)**

*Cutaneous.* Acne, pustular folliculitis, periorbital edema, bullous, urticaria, pruritus, eczematous, vasculitis, erythema nodosum, purpura.

*General.* Goiter, parotid swelling, keratitis, myxedema.

**IODINE-CONTAINING RADIOPAQUE MEDIA**

*Cutaneous.* Urticaria, pruritus.

*General.* Nausea, sneezing.

**IRON (PARENTERAL)**

*Cutaneous.* Urticaria.

*General.* Hemochromatosis, fever, liver, worsens protoporphyria. *Iron given orally* inhibits effect of tetracycline.

**ISONIAZID (INH)**

Reactions increased with dosage above 6 mg./kg. per day with INH, alcoholism and renal disease.

*Cutaneous.* Generalized erythema, maculopapular, urticaria, striae, pruritus, acne, pellagra-like, exfoliative.

*General.* GI, polyneuritis, lupus erythematosus.

**KANAMYCIN SULFATE**

*Cutaneous.* Maculopapular, urticaria, eczema, cross-sensitivity with neomycin.

*General.* Renal, proteinuria, deafness, CNS.

**LEVODOPA**

*Cutaneous.* Maculopapular, urticaria, alopecia.

*General.* Positive Coombs' test. *Interacts with* pyridoxine, MAO inhibitors, and major tranquilizers.

**LINCOMYCIN HYDROCHLORIDE**

*Cutaneous.* Maculopapular, urticaria, pruritus.

*General.* Diarrhea, liver, neutropenia.

**LITHIUM**

*Cutaneous.* Alopecia, maculopapular, urticaria, folliculitis, keratosis pilaris–like eruption of extremities and buttocks.

*General.* GI, tremor, CNS, myxedema.

**MEPHENYTOIN**

*Cutaneous.* Pigmentation, acne, angiitis.

*General.* Leukopenia, lymphocytosis, lupus erythematosus.

**MEPROBAMATE**

*Cutaneous.* Maculopapular, edema, urticaria, eczema, fixed drug, erythema multiforme, purpura.

*General.* Fever, insomnia, potentiates other drugs and alcohol.

**MERCURY**

*Cutaneous.* Dermatitis, gingivostomatitis, purpura, exfoliative, fixed drug, erythema multiforme.

*General.* Renal.

**METHOTREXATE**

*Cutaneous.* Maculopapular, urticaria, stomatitis, purpura, alopecia, reactivation of radiation dermatitis.

*General.* Hepatic fibrosis, production of cirrhosis in interaction with alcohol, oral and GI ulceration, bone marrow depression, leukopenia, thrombocytopenia.

**METHYLDOPA**

*Cutaneous.* Maculopapular, urticaria, eczematous.

*General.* Fever, diarrhea, liver, positive Coombs, sedation. *Interacts with* reserpine.

**METRONIDAZOLE**

*Cutaneous.* Urticaria, stomatitis, maculopapular, pruritus.

*General.* Headache, GI.

**MORPHINE, OPIUM ALKALOIDS**

*Cutaneous.* Urticaria, maculopapular, pruritus, fixed drug, angiitis.

*General.* Withdrawal symptoms, addiction, GI.

**NALIDIXIC ACID**

*Cutaneous.* Photosensitizing, maculopapular, urticaria.

*General.* GI, visual, convulsions.

**NIRIDAZOLE (AMBILHAR)**

*Cutaneous.* Sweating, paresthesias, urticaria, maculopapular, pruritus.

*General.* Dizziness, headaches, GI, hemolysis in G6PD deficiency. CNS, liver, bone marrow.

**NITROFURANS**

*Cutaneous.* Maculopapular, urticaria, eczema, exfoliative.

*General.* GI, hypersensitivity reactions, pulmonary, acute and chronic pulmonary disease, LE-like syndrome (nitrofurantoin), neuropathy.

**OXYPHENBUTAZONE**

See Phenylbutazone.

**PARA-AMINOSALICYLIC ACID (PAS)**

Most common antituberculous drug to produce reactions, fourth week after beginning therapy.

*Cutaneous.* Erythema, maculopapular, urticaria, pruritus, exfoliative, fixed drug, lichenoid, lupus erythematosus–like syndrome.

*General.* Fever, joint pains, conjunctivitis.

**PENICILLIN**

Most common cause of drug reaction. May produce any of all four types of reactions. Adverse reactions occur in 3% of courses. Penicilloic acid is the major determinant for type I reactions. Anaphylaxis and late (days to weeks) urticaria, both can occur. Penicilloylpolylysine and a "minor determinant mixture" are available for predictive testing for immediate and late reactions. If there is a history of immediate reactions, no tests should be done. If there is a question of late urticarial reactions, testing can be carried out carefully. *Semisynthetic penicillins all cross-react with the parent compound.*

Chiorazzi's paper gives promise for the future in the induction of tolerance to the major antigenic determinant.

Oral dose produces *least* reactions, intramuscular next, and topical most. Atopic patients likely to react.

*Cutaneous.* Generalized erythema, urticaria, exfoliative, eczematous, erythema multiforme, bullous, TEN, pruritus ani, fixed drug, maculopapular, purpura.

*General.* Fever, polyarthritis, serum sickness, anaphylaxis, GI, CNS, lupus erythematosus. *Cross reacts* with cephalosporins.

**PENICILLAMINE**

*Cutaneous.* Hemorrhagic friction blisters, yellowing and wrinkling of exposed skin, thinning of skin, digital extensor papules, stomatitis.

*General.* *Acute:* lymphadenopathy. *Chronic:* gastrointestinal irritation, optic neuritis, nephritic syndrome, neuritis.

**PHENACETIN**

*Cutaneous.* Urticaria, dermatitis, fixed drug, erythema multiforme.

*General.* CNS, nephrotoxicity, liver.

**PHENINDIONE**

*Cutaneous.* Alopecia, maculopapular, urticaria, exfoliative dermatitis, skin ulcers, purple toes.

*General.* Fever, hemorrhage, bone marrow depression, hepatic, renal. Unique allergic reaction, eleventh to forty-eighth day of treatment. Many systems involved.

**PHENOLPHTHALEIN**

*Cutaneous.* Urticaria, fixed drug, bullous, maculopapular.

**PHENOTHIAZINES**

*Cutaneous.* Urticaria, maculopapular, lichenoid, purpura, photosensitivity, unique pigmentation, eczema, seborrheic dermatitis, exfoliative, erythema multiforme. Contact dermatitis from handling.

*General.* Hypotension, liver, Parkinson's disease, emotional upset, retina, cornea, toxic psychoses, cholestatic jaundice, lupus erythematosus. *Interact with* CNS depressants, alcohol, barbiturates and narcotics.

**PHENYLBUTAZONE**

Frequent cause of drug eruptions (Plate 20) and serious side effects, particularly at higher dosages.

*Cutaneous.* Maculopapular, urticaria, exfoliative, purpura, vasculitis, erythema multiforme, bullous, TEN, alopecia, stomatitis, pruritis, edema, fixed drug.

*General.* Liver, renal, GI necrosis, agranulocytosis, sodium retention, edema, angitis, lupus erythematosus. *Interacts with* many drugs.

**PIPERAZINE**

*Cutaneous.* Purpura, urticaria, erythema multiforme.

*General.* GI, CNS, worsens epilespy, vertigo.

**POLYMYXIN**

*Cutaneous.* Flushing, pruritus, eczema, urticaria.

*General.* Nephrotoxicity, neurotoxicity.

**PRACTOLOL**

*Cutaneous.* Exfoliative, eczema, LE-like, lichen planus–like, purpura, psoriasiform. Epithelial antibody-binding positive immunofluorescence tests. Pemphigoid-like.

*General.* Ocular and corneal damage, neuropathy, renal pancreatitis, hepatitis.

**PROGESTOGENS (ORAL CONTRACEPTIVES)**

*Cutaneous.* Hyperpigmentation (chloasma), acne, urticaria, maculopapular, alopecia, hirsutism, photosensitivity, erythema nodosum, gingivitis, telangiectasia, vasculitis, urticaria, nummular eczema.

*General.* Headache, nausea, signs of preg-

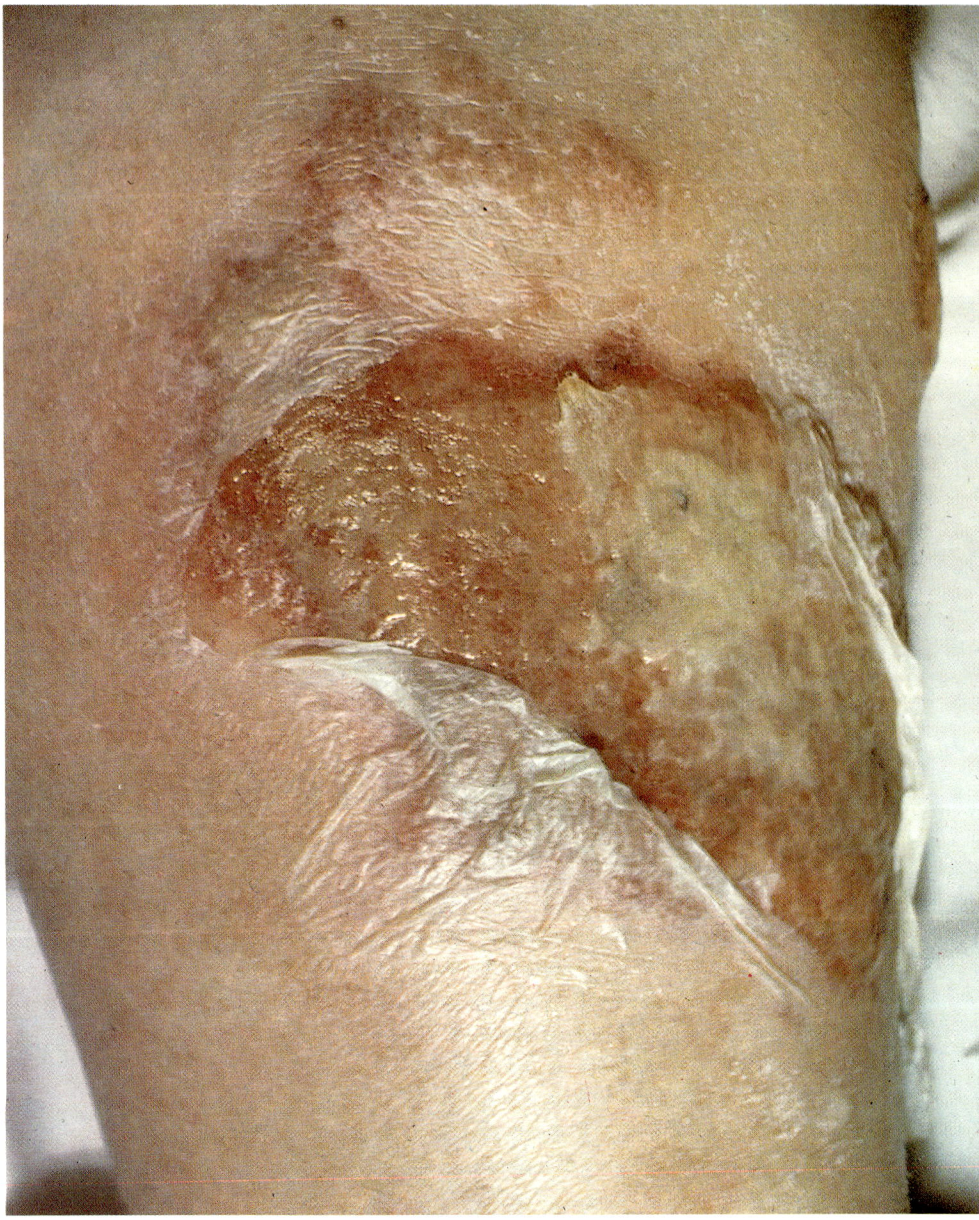

**Plate 20**

Bullous drug eruption with vasculitis caused by phenylbutazone.

nancy, lupus erythematosus, worsens porphyria, jaundice, thrombotic episodes, cerebrovascular accidents.

PROPOXYPHENE

*General.* Depressant, used in suicides, not to be mixed with alcohol or narcotics. Dizziness, drowsiness, nausea. Several hundred deaths per year.

PROPRANOLOL HYDROCHLORIDE

*Cutaneous.* Erythematous eruption, acne, urticaria, pruritus, purpura, psoriasiform.

*General.* Dizziness, fatigue, depression,

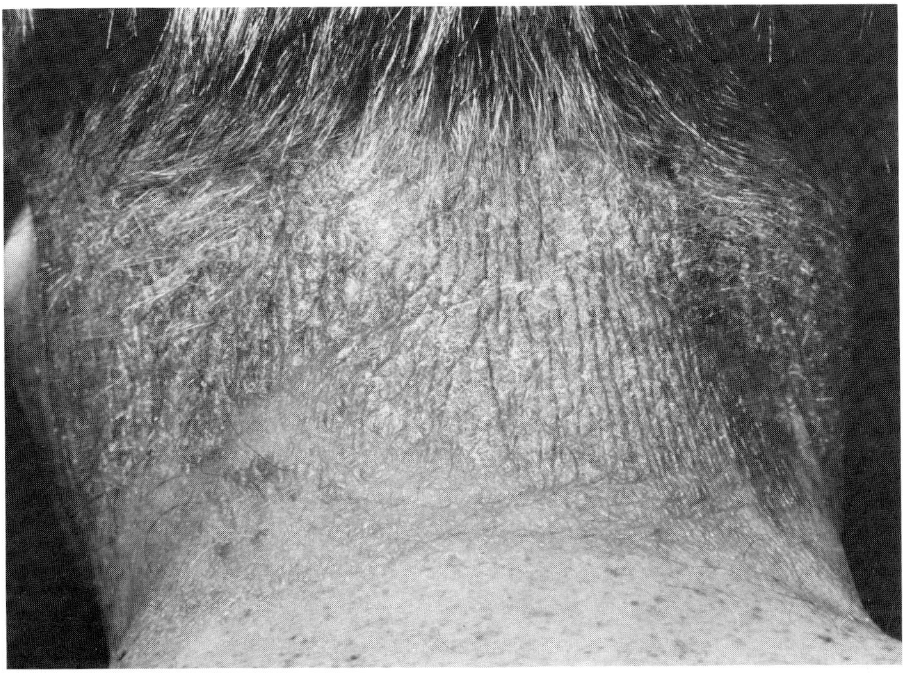

**Fig. 8-4.** Lichenoid photosensitivity eruption from quinidine.

GI, asthma, cardiac, pulmonary, corneal, ocular. *Interacts with* insulin and hypoglycemics given orally.

PYRVINIUM PAMOATE

*Cutaneous.* Photosensitivity.

*General.* GI, dizziness.

QUINACRINE (ATABRINE) HYDROCHLORIDE

*Cutaneous.* Yellow pigmentation, anhidrosis.

*General* GI, dizziness, headache.

QUININE, QUINIDINE

*Cutaneous.* Maculopapular, urticaria, photosensitivity (Fig. 8-4), pigmentation, erythema multiforme, purpura, fixed drug.

*General.* Optic neuritis, tinnitus, headache, GI.

RESERPINE

*Cutaneous.* Erythema, urticaria.

*General.* GI, lupus erythematosus, depression, psychic disturbance, nasal stuffiness.

RIFAMPIN

*Cutaneous.* Maculopapular, urticaria, roange urine and sweat.

*General.* Transient elevation of liver function tests, thrombocytopenia.

SALICYLATES

*Cutaneous.* Urticaria, purpura, vasculitis.

*General.* Gastric discomfort and irritation, bleeding, tinnitus, vertigo, asthma aggravation.

SILVER

*Cutaneous.* Pigmentation.

*General.* GI, albuminuria, amblyopia.

STREPTOMYCIN

*Cutaneous.* Maculopapular, eczematous, urticaria, purpura, pruritus, contact from handling, mouth ulcers, bullous, lichenoid, exfoliative.

*General.* Fever, vertigo, deafness, renal agranulocytosis, lupus erythematosus.

SULFAMETHOXYPYRIDAZINE

*Cutaneous.* Maculopapular, urticaria, purpura, bullous, TEN, erythema multiforme, exfoliative.

*General.* Fever, focal hepatitis, lupus erythematosus.

SULFONAMIDES

*Cutaneous.* Any variety of cutaneous reactions can occur. Pruritus, urticaria, morbilliform exanthems, allergic angiitis, photosensitivity erythema multiforme (Fig. 8-5).

*General.* Most systems, headaches, GI,

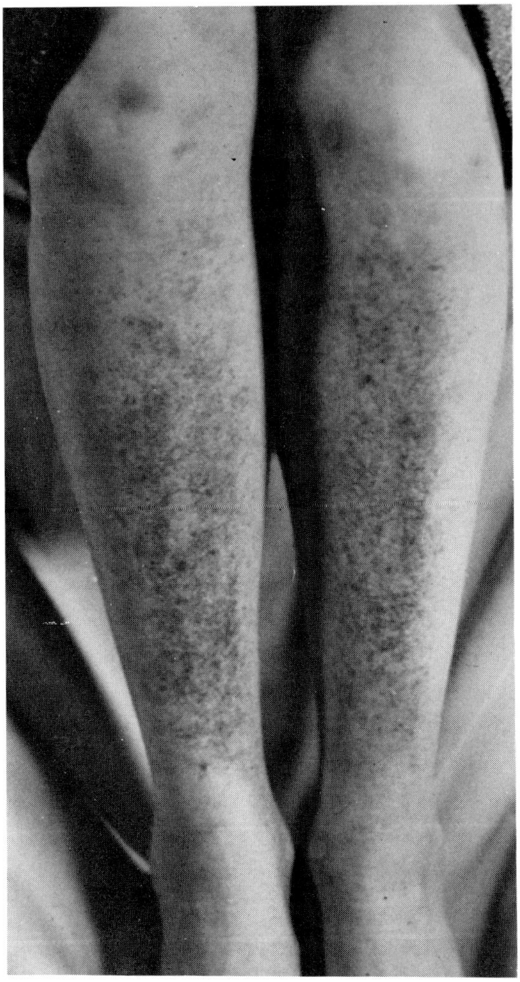

**Fig. 8-5.** Photosensitivity purpura from sulfonamides.

blood dyscrasias, renal, liver, worsens porphyria.

SULFONYLUREAS

*Cutaneous.* Maculopapular, urticaria, photosensitivity, periorbital edema, TEN, pruritus, exfoliative, erythema multiforme, bullous, flushing.

*General.* GI, hypoglycemia, hepatic, hematopoietic. *Interact with* phenylbutazone, probenecid, salicylates, sulfonamides, MAO inhibitors.

TARTRAZINE

See Azo dyes.

TETRACYCLINES

*Cutaneous.* Pruritus ani, exanthems, urticaria, black hairy tongue, photosensitivity, fixed drug, erythema multiforme, maculopapular, porphyria-like changes with scarring.

*General.* GI, malabsorption, teeth staining of fetus, infants, and children, *renal in outdated tetracyclines*, overgrowth of resistant staphylococcus, candidosis.

THIAMINE (PARENTERAL)

*Cutaneous.* Angioedema, pruritus.

*General.* Anaphylaxis.

THIAZIDE DIURETICS

*Cutaneous.* Maculopapular, eczematous, photosensitizing, urticaria, purpura, erythema multiforme, vasculitis.

*General.* Thrombocytopenia, agranulocytosis.

THIOURACIL

*Cutaneous.* Urticaria, pigmentation, alopecia, vasculitis, maculopapular.

*General.* CNS, gastritis, hematopoietic, liver, lupus erythematosus.

TRIHEXYPHENIDYL (ARTANE) HYDROCHLORIDE

*Cutaneous.* Spider angiomas.

*General.* Blurred vision, dry mouth, constipation, sedation.

TRIMETHADIONE

*Cutaneous.* Alopecia, erythema multiforme, angiitis, exfoliative, acne.

*General.* Visual effects, hepatitis, leukopenia, lupus erythematosus, nephrotic syndrome.

TRIMETHOPRIM-SULFAMETHOXAZOLE

Reactions are caused by either trimethoprim or sulfonamide component.

*Cutaneous.* Morbilliform, vesicular, vasculitis, erythema multiforme, toxic epidermal necrolysis, exfoliative dermatitis, photosensitivity.

*General.* Anorexia, abdominal pain, vomiting in 5%. Diminution of limited renal function, anemia.

VACCINES AND SERUMS

*Cutaneous.* Anaphylactic reactions, urticaria, serum sickness.

*General.* Malaise, fever, headache, myalgia.

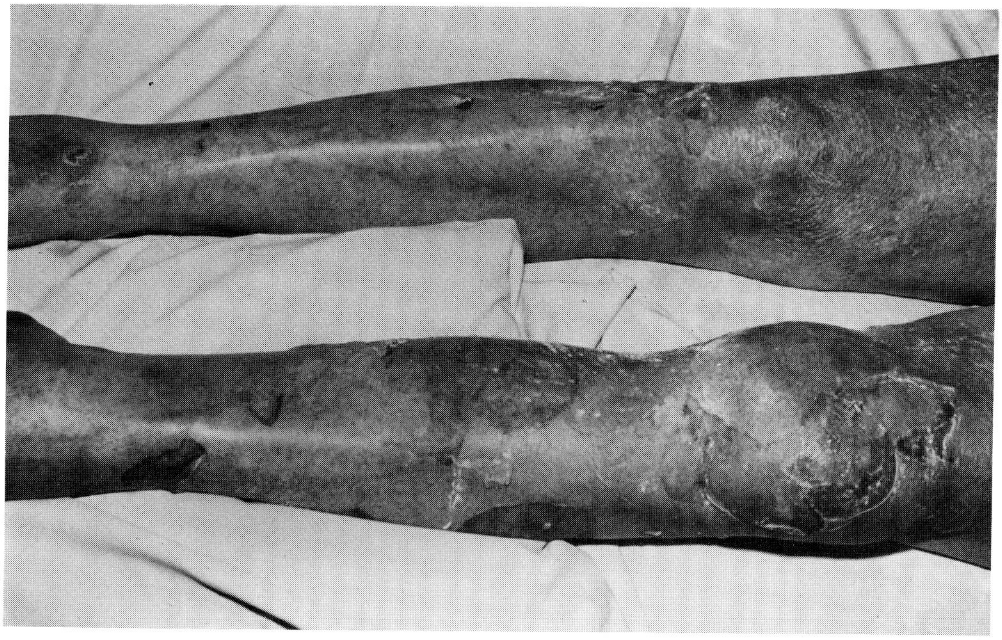

**Fig. 8-6.** Toxic epidermal necrolysis. Fatal in 80-year-old male.

VANCOMYCIN

*Cutaneous.* Urticaria, maculopapular.

*General.* Neuropathy, eighth nerve damage, renal, thrombophlebitis.

VITAMIN A

*Cutaneous.* Dry, scaly skin, alopecia.

*General.* Headache, irritability, anorexia.

## SPECIFIC TYPES OF CUTANEOUS LESIONS AND DRUGS MOST LIKELY TO PRODUCE THEM

### *Life-threatening drug eruptions*

STEVENS-JOHNSON SYNDROME. The most common of the severe eruptions, with bullous cutaneous target lesions, mucous membrane erosions, fever, CNS symptoms, prostration, myalgias.

Carbamazepine*
Chlorpropamide*
Diphenylhydantoin*
Penicillin
Phenobarbital*
Phenylbutazone and other pyrazolones*
Sulfamethoxypyridazine
Sulfonamides
Trimethadione

TOXIC EPIDERMAL NECROLYSIS (Fig. 8-6). Erythema, tenderness, and massive peeling off of extensive areas of nonhairy skin, preceded by confusion, fever, and periorbital edema.

Boric acid
Chloramphenicol
Chlorpropamide*
Diphenylhydantoin*
Phenolphthalein
Phenylbutazone and other pyrazolones*
Sulfamethoxypyridazine*
Sulfonamides

LUPUS ERYTHEMATOSUS–LIKE SYNDROME. May produce all of the findings present in idiopathic systemic lupus erythematosus.

Diphenylhydantoin and related drugs*
Griseofulvin
Hydralazine*
Isoniazid
Nitrofurans
Para-aminosalicylic acid
Penicillin
Phenylbutazone
Practolol
Procaine amide hydrochloride*
Progestogens

* Asterisks in this section indicate the drugs most likely to be the causes of the eruptions

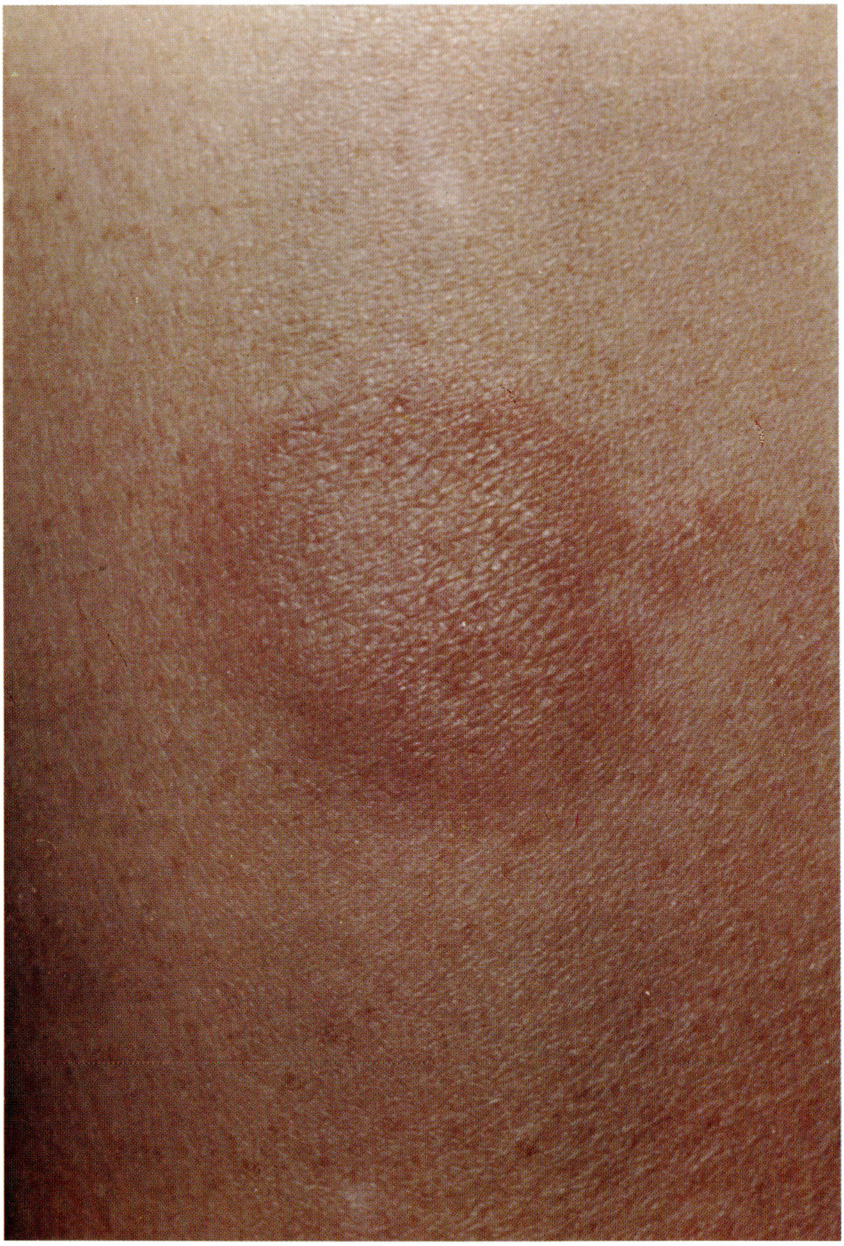

**Plate 21**

Fixed drug eruption caused by phenacetin. Note varying shades of color.

Reserpine
Streptomycin
Sulfamethoxypyridazine
Sulfonamides
Thiouracils

**EXFOLIATIVE DERMATITIS OR ERYTHRODERMA.** Generalized erythroderma and skin surface exfoliation.

Barbiturates*
Carbamazepine*
Chloroquine* (in patients with psoriasis)
Diphenylhydantoin*
Isoniazid
Mercurials
Nitrofurans
Para-aminosalicylic acid*
Phenindione*
Phenothiazines
Phenurone
Phenylbutazone, other pyrazolones*
Practolol
Streptomycin
Sulfamethoxypyridazine
Sulfonylureas

### *Other drug eruptions*

**FIXED DRUG ERUPTIONS.** Recurrent eruptions, macular to bullous, at the same site with each readministration of the drug. Disappears slowly. Purplish red, round or oval plaque with sharp border (Plate 21), or urticarial, nodular, eczematous, bullous. Pigmentation deepens with each episode, leaving varying shades of color. Skin tests of no practical value. More common on extremities, rare on buccal mucous membranes.

Antipyrine
Barbiturates*
Chlordiazepoxide hydrochloride
Codeine (Fig. 8-2)
Dapsone
Griseofulvin
Morphine
Pentazocine
Phenacetin
Phenolphthalein*
Phenylbutazone, other pyrazolones*
Progestagens
Sulfonamides*
Tetracyclines

**URTICARIAL REACTIONS** (Plate 22)

Acetylsalicylic acid*
Azo dyes (note tartrazine)
Barbiturates
Benzoic acid
Bromides
Chloramphenicol
Codeine*
Erythromycin
Griseofulvin
Imipramine hydrochloride
Meprobamate
Morphine*
Penicillin*
Phenolphthalein
Salicylates*
Serums*
Streptomycin
Sulfonamides*
Tartrazine*

**BULLOUS ERUPTIONS** (Plate 20)

Barbiturates*
Bromides, iodides*
Phenolphthalein
Phenylbutazone and pyrazolones
Sulfonamides*

**PHOTOSENSITIVITY REACTIONS.** Erythematous, vesicobullous, papular, pigmentary cutaneous reactions to light.

Certain drugs produce an inflammatory reaction in the skin when light is present. These are photochemically active and able to absorb light. They produce inflammation (1) by emitting the absorbed light energy as fluorescent light or as a phosphorescence, resulting in other photochemical reactions, or (2) by causing dissociation of the molecule, which is then chemically reactive and may exert *allergic* or direct *toxic* actions.

Antimalarials
Bithionol
Chlordiazepoxide
Chlorothiazide*
Cyclamates
Demethylchlortetracycline*
Gold
Griseofulvin
Isoniazid
Nalidixic acid
Phenothiazines*
Protriptyline hydrochloride
Psoralens
Quinine, quinidine (Fig. 8-4)
Sulfonamides*
Sulfonylureas*
Tetracyclines

**ACNEIFORM ERUPTIONS.** Papules and pustules in acne areas, with or without comedones (Fig. 8-7).

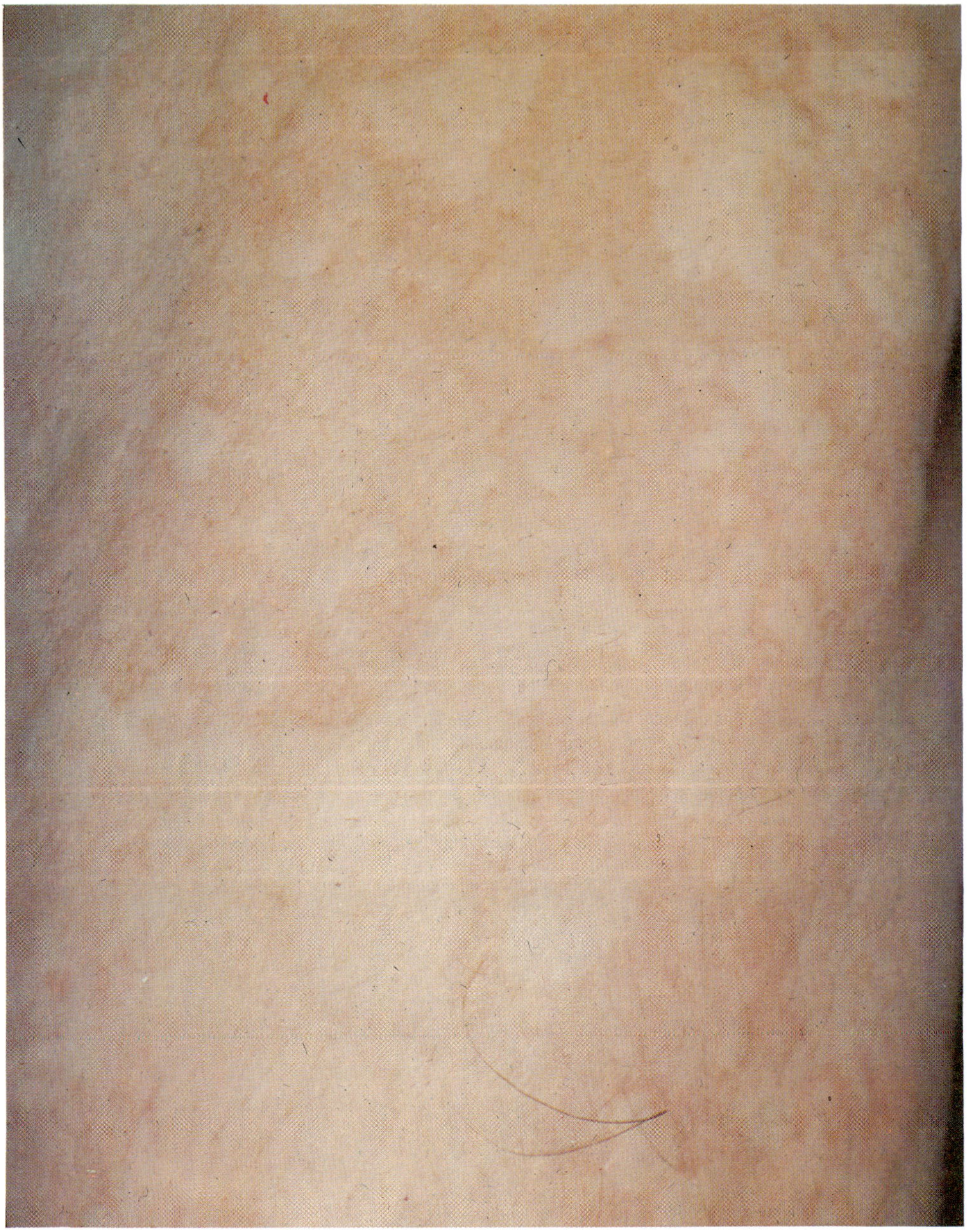

**Plate 22**

Urticaria.

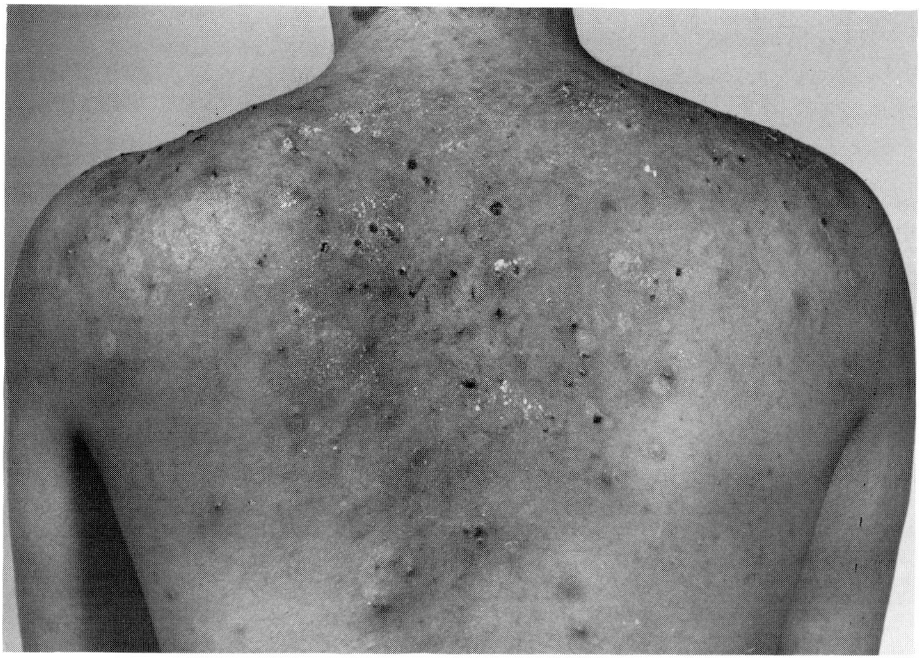

**Fig. 8-7.** Severe acne occurring after androgenic drug therapy.

Adrenocorticotropic hormone*
Androgenic hormones*
Bromides, iodides
Diphenylhydantoin*
Glucocorticoids*
Isoniazid
Phenobarbital
Progestogens
Trimethadione

ALOPECIA. Hair loss, usually most notable in scalp, beginning within 1 day and up to 3 months after initiation of therapy.

Coumarins*
Cytotoxics*
Dextran
Heparin
Phenindione*
Quinacrine
Thiouracil
Trimethadione
Triparanol

PORPHYRIA. May refer to first onset of symptoms of any of the porphyrias, or exacerbation of existing disease.

Alcohol*
Barbiturates*
Chloroquine phosphate*
Estrogens
Griseofulvin*
Hexochlorobenzene
Phenylhydrazine
Progestogens
Sulfonamides*
Sulfonmethane
Tetracycline

MACULOPAPULAR ERUPTIONS

Acetylsalicylic acid
Allopurinol*
Carbamazepine*
Chloramphenicol
Gold*
Hydantoin derivatives
Isoniazid
Nitrofurans
Para-aminosalicylic acid*
Penicillin, ampicillin*
Phenothiazines
Phenylbutazone and pyrazolones*
Sulfonamides*
Sulfonylureas
Tetracyclines*
Thiazide derivatives

PURPURA

Acetylsalicylic acid
Azo dyes

Barbiturates
Benzoates
Carbromal
Chlorpromazine hydrochloride
Furosemide (Fig. 8-3)
Glucocorticoids
Gold*
Indomethacin*
Iodides
Meprobamate
Penicillin
Phenothiazines
Phenylbutazone and pyrazolones*
Practolol
Propranolol
Quinine, quinidine*
Sulfonamides

## PREVENTION OF DRUG REACTIONS

1. *Make a correct diagnosis* so that the effects of the prescribed medication can be effectively monitored against reduction in symptoms.
2. *Give a drug only when a positive indication exists* and be alert for secondary or unwanted pharmacologic effects.
3. *Give as few drugs as possible* and discontinue any that have completed their usefulness.
4. *Review all drugs* a patient is receiving at stated intervals.
5. *Be sure patients understand the prescribed intentions for the drug.* Family or nurses should be apprised in some instances.

## TREATMENT OF DRUG REACTIONS

### *Acute immediate allergic reactions (anaphylaxis, acute urticaria)*

1. Tourniquet around limb proximal to site of injection, is possible
2. Epinephrine, 0.5 to 1 ml. of 1:1,000 solution subcutaneously, repeated every 5 to 10 minutes if necessary (direct histamine antagonist)
3. Intravenous or intramuscular antihistaminics
4. Soluble glucocorticoids such as Solu-Cortef and prednisolone sodium hemisuccinate intravenously
5. Intravenous drip with norepinephrine (noradrenaline) in case of circulatory collapse

### *Delayed cutaneous reactions*

1. First, discontinue all possible prescribed and proprietary medications. Substitute if necessary for essential drugs.
2. Withdrawal of the suspected drug usually results in prompt improvement. However, in the case of some drugs, such as penicillin, the eruption may persist for months.
3. If an urticarial component is prominent, use of antihistamines in adequate dosage is the treatment of choice. Hydroxyzine (Atarax), 10 to 25 mg. three times a day, has been shown to be effective in the control of pruritus and the more chronic urticarial reactions associated with drugs.
4. If the lesions are widespread and severe, the use of glucocorticoids is indicated. Steroids may also be used to hasten the clearing of the dermatitis in less severe cases.
5. In cases of toxicity to heavy metals such as arsenic, mercury, and gold, one may use dimercaprol (BAL) to eliminate accumulated metal. It is given according to a precise schedule, which may be found in more detailed texts on this subject.
6. If an iodide or a bromide eruption is suspected, ingestion of more than usual amounts of table salt will promote excretion of the accumulated bromide salts.
7. The patient should be advised of the drug or group of drugs responsible for the allergic reaction and of the potential seriousness if the drug is again administered.
8. Consider patch testing to suspected drugs (Felix and Comaish).
9. Hyposensitization is not without risk, and the results do not usually justify employing the technique.
10. Some drug reactions, such as those to ampicillin, may unaccountably fade, and disappear while the patient continues to take the drug. The mechanism, perhaps because of the formation of blocking antibodies, is as yet unexplained and cannot be depended on.

## REFERENCES


Almeyda, J.: Cutaneous reactions to imipramine and chlordiazepoxide, Br. J. Dermatol. **84**:298, 1971.
**Infrequent and nonspecific.**

Almeyda, J., and Baker, H.: Cutaneous reactions to antirheumatic drugs, Br. J. Dermatol. **83**:707, 1970.
**(1) Anti-inflammatory, (2) immunosuppressive, and (3) gold and chloroquine.**

Almeyda, J., and Levantine, A.: Lichenoid drug eruptions, Br. J. Dermatol. **85**:604, 1971.
**Eleven drugs or groups of drugs.**

Almeyda, J., and Levantine, A.: Adverse cutaneous reactions to the penicillins-ampicillin rashes, Br. J. Dermatol. **87**:293, 1972.
**Penicillin—nonspecific; ampicillin—nonallergic.**

Almeyda, J., and Levantine, A.: Cutaneous reactions to anticonvulsants, Br. J. Dermatol. **87**:646, 1972.
**Hydantoin, oxazolidine, and succinimide derivatives.**

Almeyda, J., and Levantine, A.: Cutaneous reactions to barbiturates, chloral hydrate and its derivatives, Br. J. Dermatol. **86**:313, 1972.
**Chiefly allergic.**

Almeyda, J., and Levantine, A.: Cutaneous reactions to cardiovascular drugs, Br. J. Dermatol. **88**:313, 1973.
**Diuretics, hypotensives, and anti-arrhythmic and anti-anginal drugs.**

Arndt, K. A., and Jick, H.: Rates of cutaneous reactions to drugs, J.A.M.A. **235**:918, 1976.
**Rash itching and hives in medical inpatients is about 3 per 1,000.**

Baker, H., and Moore-Robinson, M.: Cutaneous responses to aspirin and its derivatives, Br. J. Dermatol. **82**:319, 1970.
**An initiation into the now better known side effects of aspirin.**

Bierman, C. W., Pierson, W. E., Zertz, S. J., et al.: Reactions associated with ampicillin therapy. J.A.M.A. **220**:1098, 1972.
**Two thirds of cases maculopapular, one third urticarial. Patients should be skin tested.**

Brigden, W. D., and Almeyda, J.: Adverse reaction to the beta-adrenergic blocking drugs, Br. J. Dermatol. **93**:335, 1976.
**There is an unclear effect on the immunological response. A chemical grouping to watch out for.**

Bruinsma, W.: A guide to drug eruptions, Amsterdam, 1973, Excerpta Medica Foundation.
**From the international drug monitoring center of the WHO.**

Chiorazzi, N., Eshlar, Z., and Katz, D. H.: Induction of immunologic tolerance to major antigenic determinant of penicillin: therapeutic approach to penicillin allergy, Proc. Natl. Acad. Sci. USA **73**:3091, 1976.
**Tolerance to benzylpenicilloyl hapten in mice produced that was specific, lasted at least 6 months, and might be applicable to man.**

Coskey, R. J.: Eruption due to oral contraceptives, Arch. Dermatol. **113**:333, 1977.
**Fixed drug, lichen simplex, and nummular eczema.**

Cram, D. L.: Life-threatening dermatoses, Calif. Med. **118**:5, 1973.
**Stevens-Johnson, TEN, purpura fulminans, Kaposi's varicelliform eruption.**

Eisner, E. V., and Shahidi, N. T.: Immunothrombocytopenia due to a drug metabolite, N. Engl. J. Med. **287**:376, 1972.
**An acetaminophen fragment.**

Encylopedia of Food Chemicals in Food in Canada, Toronto, 1971, MacLean-Hunter, Ltd., vol. 31, pp. 31-34.

Epstein, J. H., Tuffanelli, D. L., Seibert, J. S., and Epstein, W. L.: Porphyria-like changes induced by tetracycline HCl photosensitization, Arch. Dermatol. **112**:661, 1976.
**Subepidermal blisters, scarring, 2 to 4 months after sun exposure.**

Felix, R. H., and Comaish, J. S.: Value of patch and other skin tests in drug eruptions, Lancet **1**:1017, 1974.
**Patch tests positive in some eczematous eruptions.**

Gordon, H. H: Untoward reactions to saccharin, Cutis **10**:77, 1972.
**Photosensitivity included.**

Hagermark, O., Goran, W., and Almeyda, J.: Cutaneous side effects of phenothiazines, Br. J. Dermatol. **84**:605, 1971.
**Allergic, photosensitive, and pigmentary.**

Hart, R.: Autoimmune progesterone dermatitis, Arch. Dermatol. **113**:426, 1977.
**Seven patients with premenstrually recurrent eruptions with the cause confirmed by intradermal tests.**

Jensen, A. E., Mikkelson, H. I., Wadskov, S., and Sondergard, J.: Cutaneous reactions to propanolol (Inderal), Acta Med. Scand. **199**:363, 1976.
**Related to practolol.**

Kauppinen, K.: Cutaneous reactions to drugs, Acta Derm. Venereol. **68**(suppl.):1, 1972.
**A valuable and courageous study of 620 patients and 274 challenges.**

La Du, B. N.: Pharmacogenetics: defective enzymes in relation to reactions to drugs, Annu. Rev. Med. **23**:453, 1972.
**A review of mechanisms involved.**

Levantine, A., and Almeyda, J.: Cutaneous reactions to antituberculous drugs, Br. J. Dermatol. **86**:651, 1972.
**Streptomycin, PAS, and isoniazid.**

Levantine, A., and Almeyda, J.: Cutaneous reactions to

food and drug additives, Br. J. Dermatol. **91**:359, 1974.
**Cyclamate, quinine, cinnamon, vanilla, salicylates, tartrazine, and phenolphthalein.**

Melmon, K. L.: Preventable drug reactions: causes and cures, N. Engl. J. Med. **284**:1361, 1971.
**We are a pill-taking society.**

Mendelson, L. M., Meltzer, E. O., and Hamburger, R. N.: Anaphylaxis-like reactions to corticosteroid therapy, J. Allergy Clin. Immunol. **54**:125, 1974.
**Proved by positive skin reactions to hydrocortisone and methylprednisolone.**

Meyers, F. H., Jametz, E., and Goldfein, A.: Review of medical pharmacology, ed. 4, Los Altos, Calif., 1974, Lange Medical Publications.

Michaëlsson, G., and Juhlin, L.: Urticaria induced by preservatives and dye additives to food and drugs, Br. J. Dermatol. **88**:525, 1973.
**A significant cause of chronic urticaria revealed.**

Michaëlsson, G., Pettersson, L., and Juhlin, L.: Purpura caused by food and drug additives, Arch. Dermatol. **109**:49, 1974.
**Seven patients with vasculitis all responded to provocation tests.**

Mitchell, J. C.: The skin and chemical additives to food, Arch. Dermatol. **104**:329, 1971.
**A perspicacious letter.**

Montgomery, D. C., and Jackson, R.: One hundred consecutive patients with drug reactions, Can. Med. Assoc. J. **99**:712, 1968.
**Barbiturates well in front.**

Ogilvie, R. J., and Ruedy, J.: Adverse drug reactions during hospitalization, Can. Med. Assoc. J. **97**:1450, 1967.
**Most from old and known medications.**

Parker, C. W.: Drug allergy. Medical intelligence, N. Engl. J. Med. **292**:511, 732, 957, 1975.
**A discussion of the clinical spectrum of drug allergy.**

Rostenberg, A., Jr., and Fagelson, H.J.: Life-threatening drug eruptions, J.A.M.A. **194**:660, 1965.
**Stevens-Johnson, TEN, SLE, exfoliative dermatitis.**

Skokan, J. D., Hewlett, J. S., and Hoffman, E. C.: Thrombocytopenia purpura associated with ingestion of acetaminophen (Tylenol), Cleveland Clin. Q. **40**:89, 1973.
**A prognosis of things to come?**

Sturner, W. Q., and Garriott, J. C.: Deaths involving propoxyphene, J.A.M.A. **223**:1125, 1973.
**41 deaths in 2 years. Depressant, particularly with alcohol.**

Terr, A. I.: Drug allergy; penicillin allergy. In Fudenberg, H. H., Stites, D. P., Caldwell, J. L., and Wells, J. V., editors: Basic and clinical immunology, Los Altos, Calif., 1976, Lange Medical Publications, pp. 442, 444.

Williams, J.: More than 1 in 10 of United Kingdom's aged admitted to hospital due to adverse drug reaction, The Medical Post, Oct 11, 1977.
**1998 patients with 248 experiencing reactions caused by 312 drugs.**

Wyatt, E., Greaves, M., and Sondergaard, J.: Fixed drug eruption (phenolphthalein) evidence for a blood borne mediator, Arch. Dermatol. **106**:671, 1972.
**Serum reinjected produced the eruption because of a thermolabile substance that was not the drug.**

## ADVERSE EFFECTS OF TOPICAL GLUCOCORTICOIDS

Topically applied glucocorticoids have become more and more effective with the continued development of new compounds. Refinements in substitution by fluorine, chlorine, and methyl molecules on the steroid nucleus and addition of various side chains have made the compounds more potent, have increased their speed of skin penetration, and have probably lengthened their retention in the tissue at the site of action. In addition, more sophisticated vehicles increase delivery of the therapeutic compound to the skin for absorption.

We assist this trend to increasing therapeutic potency and promote skin absorption by prescribing these compounds to be used under plastic occlusive dressings. This macerates the skin and makes it more amenable to penetration by selected potent glucocorticoids.

Since the Epsteins' report in 1963, which identified topical corticosteroid therapy as a possible cause of stria formation, further observations and investigations have accumulated from many countries on the subject of side effects of topical glucocorticoids. A list of adverse effects associated with the use of these compounds follows.

STRIAE (Figs. 8-8 and 8-9). Inguinal, axillary, and inner thigh areas in adolescence are most vulnerable; permanent. May occur at sites distal to the application.

EPIDERMAL THINNING (Fig. 8-10). Exposed areas most vulnerable. Winter and Burton demonstrated epidermal thinning measured by histologic methods. Wilson-Jones, a highly

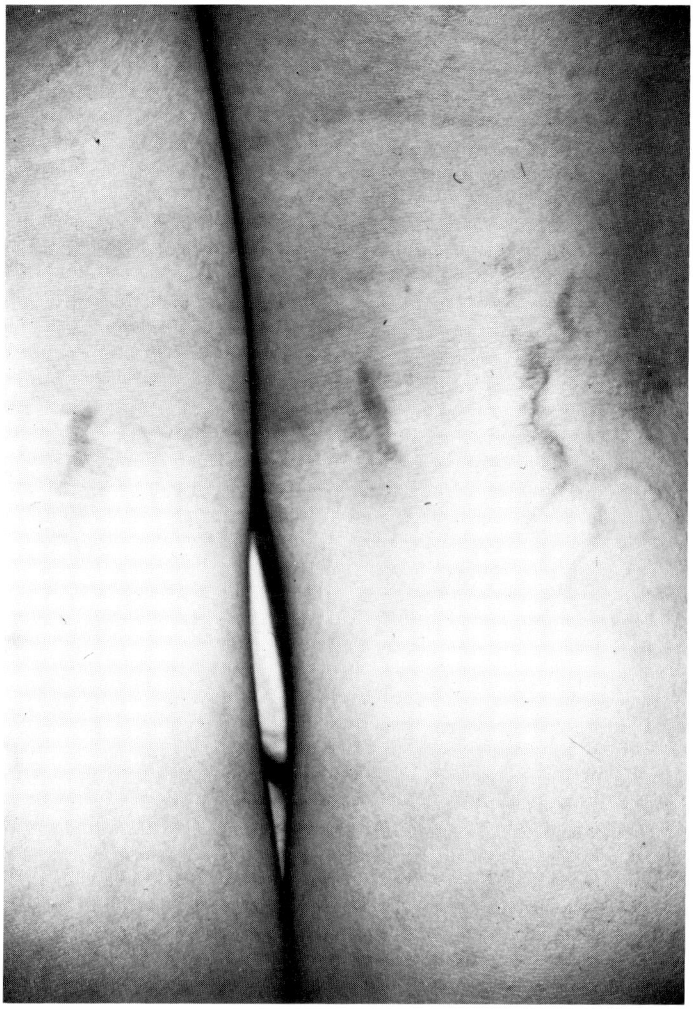

**Fig. 8-8.** Striae. Subsequent to topical nonoccluded, fluorinated steroids.

regarded dermatopathologist, believes that dermal effects may be secondary to epidermal thinning. This thinning of the epidermis reduces a tough, hardened horny efficient barrier to the appearance of a film of plastic wrap. The subepidermal vessels are easily visible, and purpura is induced with minimal or no trauma. The skin can be torn in a triangular flap pattern as a piece of paper is torn and tends to heal slowly.

ERYTHEMA. Diffuse erythema may appear over the site of application. Erythema also appears very quickly with minimal sun exposure. Patients recognize that they cannot take as long an exposure as before the use of steroids.

TELANGIECTASIA (Fig. 8-11). Face, neck, and upper anterior chest above midsternum most vulnerable. Appears to be associated with epidermal atrophy.

PURPURA (Fig. 8-12). Senile and posttraumatic purpura occurs with increased frequency.

DERMAL THINNING (Fig. 8-10). The thinning of the dermis, attributed classically to inhibition of fibroblasts and collagen synthesis, is more complicated. Snyder demonstrated dermal thinning within a week, which is too rapid

A

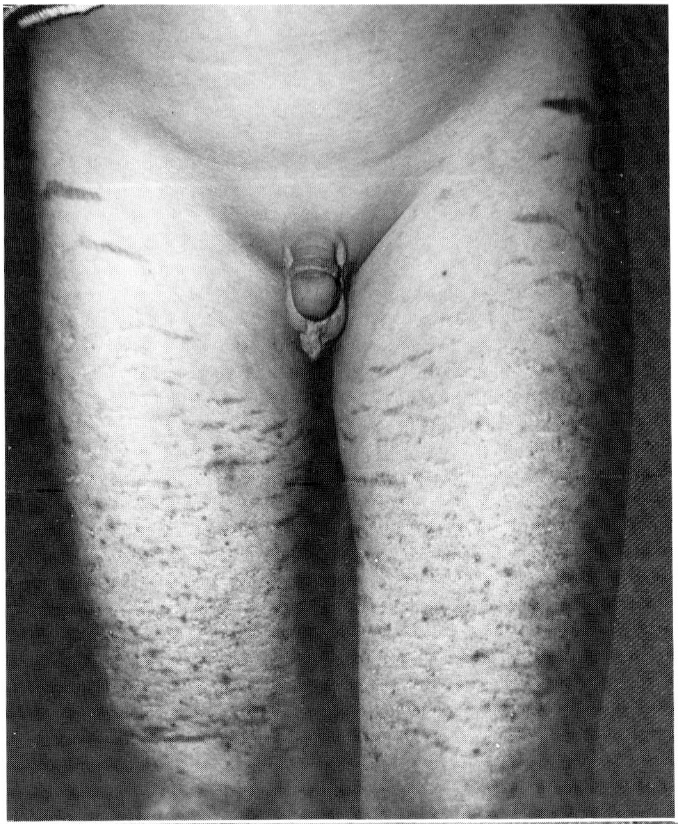

B

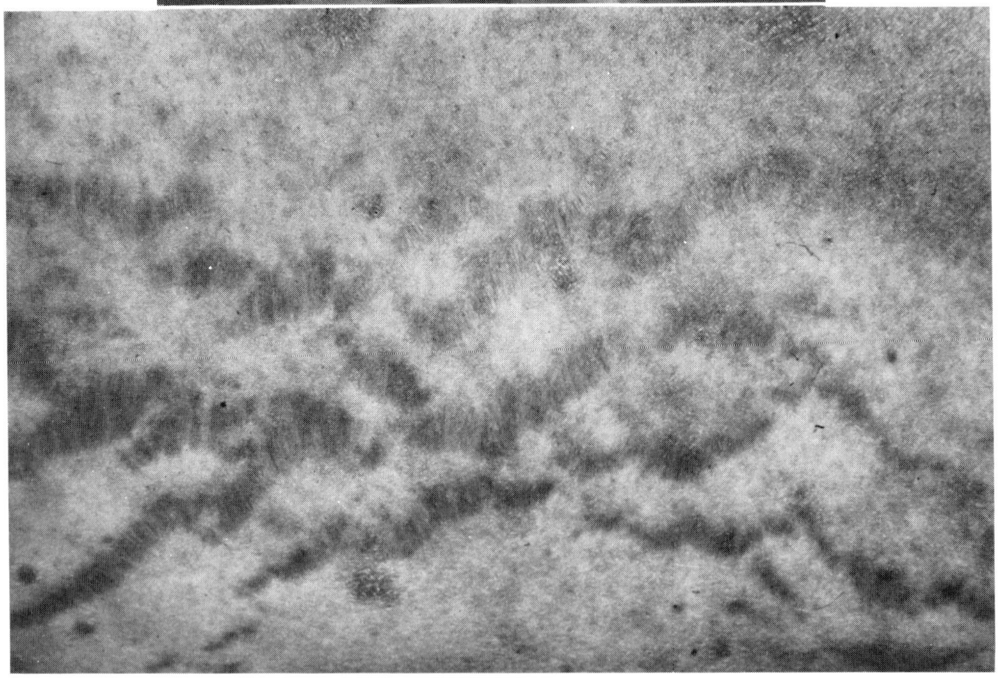

**Fig. 8-9. A,** Transverse striae resulting from topical betamethasone valerate, 0.1%, q.i.d. for 1 year. **B,** Closeup of striae.

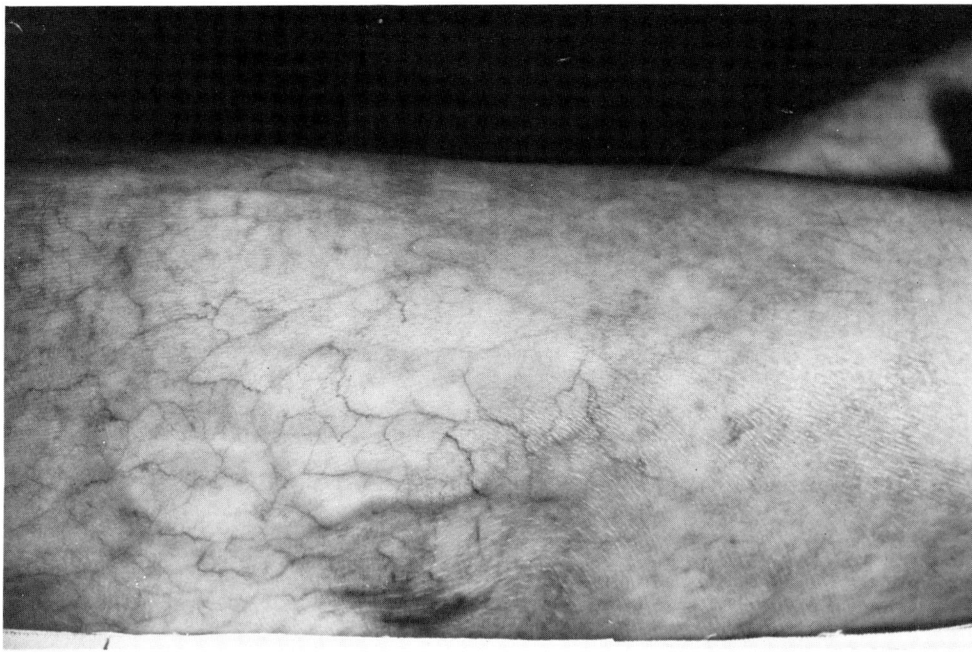

**Fig. 8-10.** Atrophy. Note translucency of dermis and finely wrinkled epidermis.

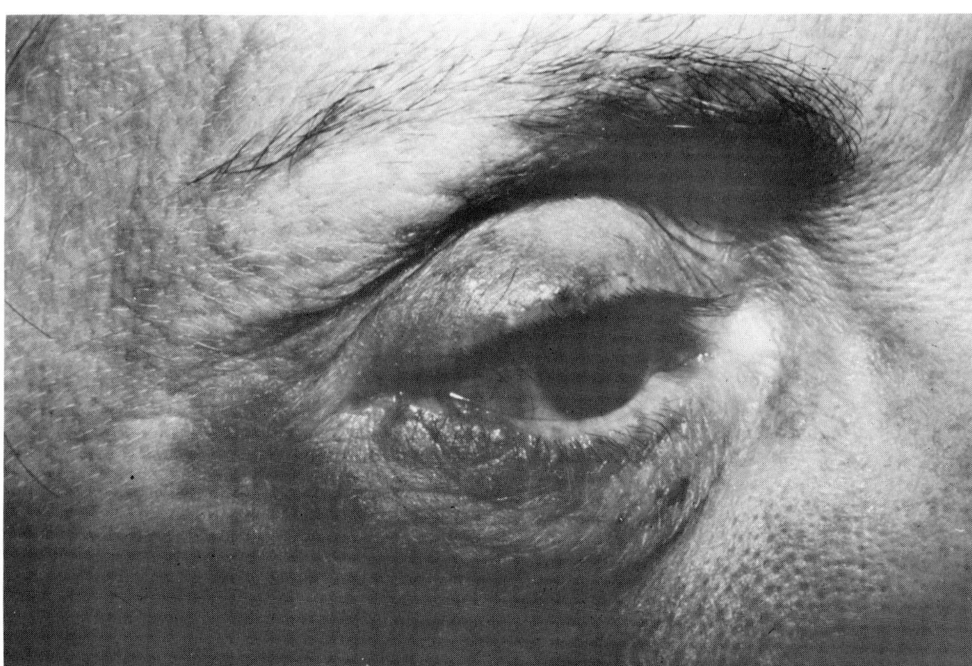

**Fig. 8-11.** Telangiectasia of eyelid and papule formation from fluorinated steroids.

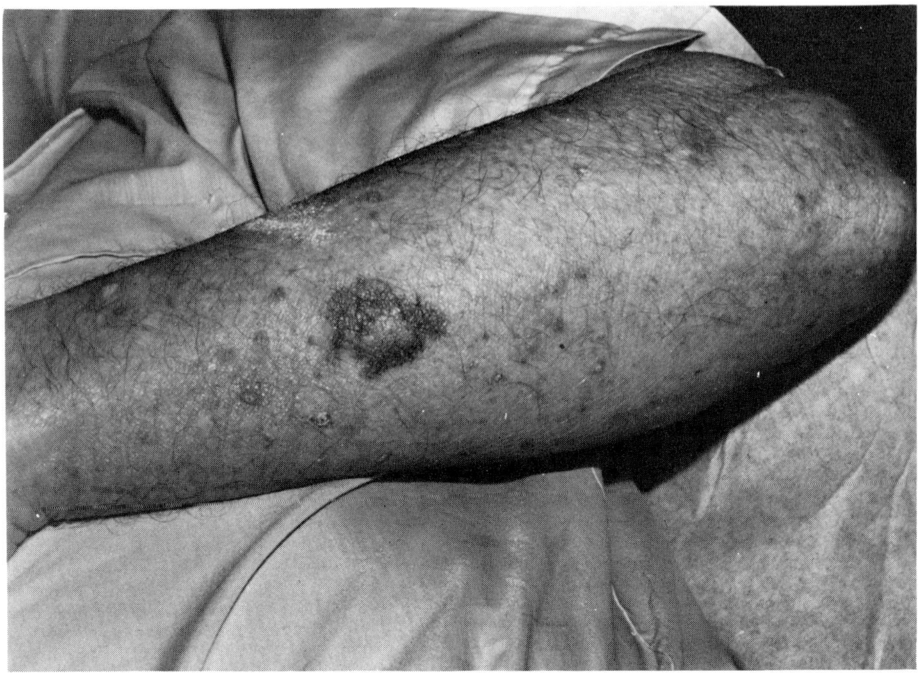

**Fig. 8-12.** Purpura. Similar to senile purpura.

to result from decreased synthesis. Collagenase may be stimulated to destroy collagen more rapidly by the glucocorticoids. Runikis and Kirk have both demonstrated increased activity in human fibroblasts in culture produced by glucocorticoids. However, the thinning lasts for a very long time, an unlikely effect of collagenases. It might be an effect on the glycosaminoglycans.

A striking report of subcutaneous atrophy in a finger has been received (Tanenbaum), as well as dermal atrophy of the diaper area.

It may be that some areas are more affected than others, for example, the inguinal, genital, and perianal areas. James measured the relative dermal thinning effect of several topical glucocorticoids over 3 months and found that it varied with the compound used and also in individuals. Hydrocortisone did not produce thinning over this time. The response did not appear to be a steady, consistent thinning, but varied even with the control, fluocinolone acetonide, from month to month.

LOCAL HAIR GROWTH. Appears associated with topical steroid therapy. We have observed unilateral upper lip hair growth on an Oriental child treated with topical glucocorticoids. Paradoxically, hair loss is also reported.

## CUTANEOUS DISEASES WORSENED BY POTENT STEROIDS

Glucocorticoids overlap in some of their effects with other steroid hormones that have androgenic, progestational, estrogenic effects (Snell), and the cutaneous end organ response may be variable as well.

ACNE VULGARIS. Although the inflammatory response is reduced, topical glucocorticoids allow an increased intensity to occur on stopping of the drug.

We were first warned by Sneddon that *rosacea, rosacea-like dermatitis* (Weber), and *perioral dermatitis* (Fig. 8-13) (Hjorth and coworkers) may be temporarily suppressed by topical potent glucocorticoids only to show noticeable exacerbations when they are discontinued. Also, with long-term use, these dermatoses will escape the glucocorticoid effect and show refractoriness to therapy.

LEG ULCERS. Ulcerated areas caused by ve-

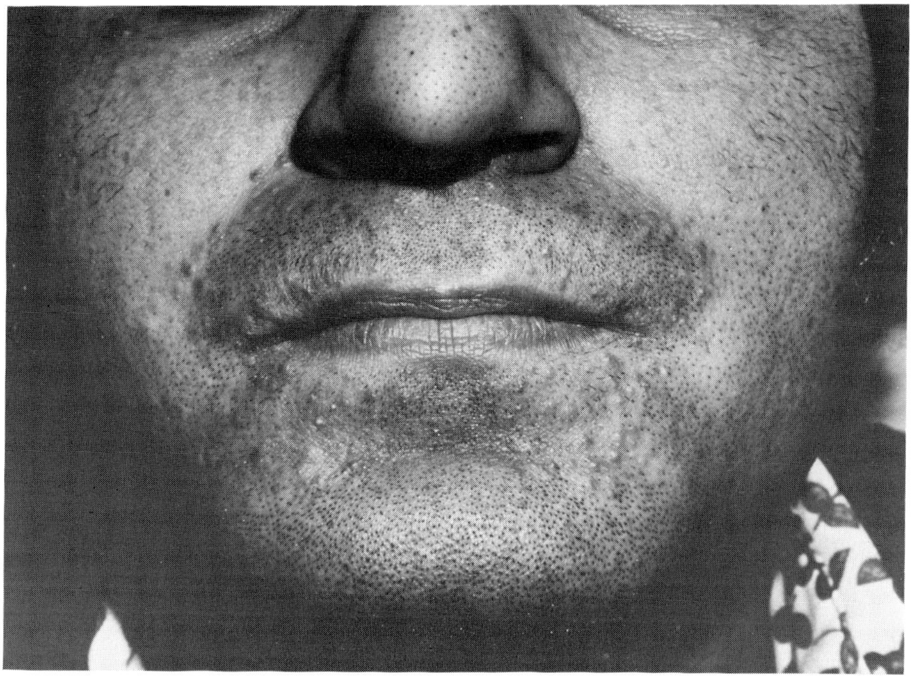

**Fig. 8-13.** Perioral dermatitis in male. Bearded sites spared.

nous stasis, rheumatoid arthritis, and ischemia from other causes widen, deepen, and demonstrate a disclination to healing under glucocorticoid influence.

SCABIES. Suppression of the pruritus and inflammatory reaction in scabies is produced by topical glucocorticoids as well as systemic steroids. Unfortunately, the parasite continues to spread under the anti-inflammatory protection.

WARTS. Clinical evidence indicates that condylomata acuminata flourish in a glucocorticoid environment.

MOLLUSCUM CONTAGIOSUM. As with warts, clinicians see a spread of these lesions in areas under treatment with topical glucocorticoids, not apparent otherwise.

FUNGAL INFECTION. Dermatophytosis is not discouraged by topical steroids, although the inflammatory reaction is suppressed and recognition of the process if thus made difficult.

BALANITIS. Inflammation of the glans penis from nonspecific causes is often suppressed and then worsened by the use of potent topical steroids. This is an area particularly susceptible to effects of fluorinated corticosteroids. They should be used only for short intervals.

OTHER CUTANEOUS EFFECTS. Topical glucocorticoids are absorbed through the skin and can produce depression of adrenocortical steroid output as recorded for two currently used products by Gomez. One had more suppressive effect than the other. Sparkes' review is reassuring for moderate rational use of topical steroids in controlled amounts, but patients must be followed. Glaucoma has been produced from regular application of fluorinated steroids to the lids (Cubey). It is reasonable to use only hydrocortisone-containing preparations for eyelid dermatitis.

Children are unusually susceptible to corticosteroid effects, topical and systemic. For this reason, fluorinated corticosteroids should be used only in localized areas, and hydrocortisone or desonide (Tridesilon) for larger areas. If potent corticosteroids are required in larger areas, they must be changed to less potent compounds within a month. Weston and others have shown complete adrenal suppression over a short term in children, from topical potent topical steroids. It probably is not the fluorination per se, but the potency of the compounds in use today that produces the suppression.

For adults, a rule of thumb indicates that 60 Gm. or 2 oz. of an average potent fluorinated steroid is acceptable per week, and for preadolescent children, 15 to 30 Gm. per week depending on size.

Stevanovic demonstrated electron microscopic changes in tissues of volunteers receiving glucocorticoid therapy after 3 to 4 months of treatment. He felt the first changes were in the ground substance, and he may well yet be proved to be right.

**SECONDARY EFFECTS.** Furunculosis as a result of occlusive plastic film therapy, from staphylococci developing in the area occluded has been reported many times. It is not clear whether this would occur equally as often without the steroids, but with only the plastic film. We do not subscribe to the generally held belief that corticosteroids encourage the spread of bacterial infections.

Glaucoma was reported to be produced from application of a fluorinated steroid cream to the eyelids. Glaucoma from installation of glucocorticoids into the conjunctival sac and from systemic glucocorticoids is known.

## REFERENCES


Bond, W. S.: Toxic reactions and side effects of glucocorticoids in man, Am. J. Hosp. Pharm. **34**:479, 1977.
**Cutaneous and systemic glucocorticoids, a thorough review.**

Carruthers, J. A., August, P. J., and Staughton, R. C. D.: Observations on the systemic effect of topical clobetasol propionate (Dermovate), Br. Med. J. **4**:203, 1975.
**"Safe" dose less than 50 Gm. per week to prevent profound pituitary-adrenal axis suppression.**

Cubey, E. B.: Glaucoma following application of corticosteroid to skin of eyelids, Br. J. Dermatol. **95**:207, 1976.
**Intractable glaucoma with 0.01% fluocinolone acetonide to face for 7 years.**

Epstein, N. N., Epstein, W. L., and Epstein, J. H.: Atrophic striae in patients with inguinal intertrigo, Arch. Dermatol. **87**:450, 1963.
**The first report.**

Fiewel, M.: Percutaneous absorption of topical steroids in children, Br. J. Dermatol. **81**(suppl. 4):113, 1969.
**Noticeable atrophy of diaper area.**

Goldman, L., and Kitzmiller, K. W.: Perianal atrophoderma from topical corticosteroids, Arch. Dermatol. **107**:611, 1973.
**Still a major problem because of necessity for potent steroids and long-term use.**

Gomez, E. C., Kaminster, L., and Frost, P.: Topical halcinonide and betamethasone valerate effects on plasma cortisol, Arch. Dermatol. **113**:1196, 1977.
**A 5-day trial and a 6-week trial compared.**

Hjorth, N., Osmundsen, P., Rook, A. J., et al.: Perioral dermatitis, Br. J. Dermatol. **80**:307, 1968.
**The commonest patient complaint of steroid side effects.**

James, D. M., Black, M. M., and Sparkes, C. G.: Measurement of dermal atrophy induced by topical steroids using a radiographic technique, Br. J. Dermatol. **96**:303, 1977.
**Unpredictable variation.**

Jones, E. W.: Steroid atrophy. A histological appraisal, Dermatologica **152**(suppl. 1):107, 1976.
**Epidermal thinning apparent, but no dermal effect in 1 month.**

Kirk, D., and Mittwoch, W.: Effects of topically potent glucocorticoids on human diploid fibroblasts in vitro, Br. J. Dermatol. **97**:69, 1977.
**Not inhibition, but stimulation.**

Ricciatti, D., and Lester, R. S.: Topical corticosteroid therapy, Mod. Med. Can. **32**:546, 1977.
**Good balanced brief review.**

Runikis, J. O., McLean, D. I., and Stewart, W. D.: Glucocorticoid stimulation of human and inhibition of mouse L929 skin fibroblasts in cell culture, J. Invest. Dermatol. **70**:348, 1978.
**Opposite effects in mice and men.**

Sneddon, I.: Adverse effect of topical fluorinated corticosteroids in rosacea, Br. Med. J. **1**:671, 1969.
**Rebound phenomenon after the drug was stopped.**

Snyder, D. S., and Greenberg, R. A.: Evaluation of atrophy production and vasoconstrictor potency in humans following intradermally injected corticoids, J. Invest. Dermatol. **63**:461, 1974.
**Atrophy within 1 week.**

Sparkes, C. G.: Measuring adrenal function in patients using topical corticosteroids, Br. J. Dermatol. **94**(suppl. 12):77, 1976.
**Adrenal function will not be affected by thoughtful use of topical corticosteroids.**

Stevanovic, D. V.: Corticosteroid induced atrophy of the skin with telangiectasia, Br. J. Dermatol. **87**:548, 1972.
**The first good look at steroid effects.**

Tanenbaum, M. H.: Topical steroid atrophy: "a disappearing digit." Letter to the editor, J.A.M.A. **220**:125, 1972.
**Startling.**

Weber, G.: Rosacea-like dermatitis: contraindication or intolerance reaction to strong steroids, Br. J. Dermatol. **86**:253, 1972.
**A forerunner of things to come.**

Winter, G. D., and Burton, J. L.: Experimentally induced steroid atrophy in the domestic pig and man, Br. J. Dermatol. **94**(suppl. 12):107, 1976.
**Epidermal thinning measured as a function of glucocorticoid effect.**

Zugerman, C., Sanders, D., and Levit, F.: Glaucoma from topically applied steroids, Arch. Dermatol. **112**:1326, 1976.
**Not the most potent topical glucocorticoid either!**

## CHAPTER 9

# Erythema multiforme

A symptom complex rather than a well-defined disease entity, erythema multiforme (Plate 23) is produced by a variety of causes.

### *Natural course*

The usual course of the disease begins with small papular lesions of the dorsa of the hands and feet. The lesions grow larger and more numerous, extending proximally and often becoming vesicular. The onset is sometimes sudden and may be associated with a fever, upper respiratory tract symptoms of infection, and muscular aches and pains. The idiopathic self-limited variety of the disease lasts from 4 to 6 weeks before disappearing completely. It may, however, recur many times. It is most often seen in the spring or fall and may be an annual occurrence for years. It may follow an upper respiratory tract infection or more commonly, an episode of herpes simplex of the lips each time.

The lesions are pathognomonic, with elevated circular borders, a depressed inner ring, and a central erythema or fluid-filled bulla. They are referred to as *target* or *iris* lesions (Fig. 9-1, *B*) and are quite unmistakable when fully developed. It may be that following Orfanos' observation of two distinct pathologic lesions, clinicians will separate an epidermal vesicular type from a more clearly bullous type. We believe that this is likely.

Mucous membrane lesions are not uncommonly associated with this disorder and include vesicles or bullae of the lips and white patches or erosions of the buccal cavity, tongue, or other mucous membranes. When bullae or mucous membrane lesions are present, the condition is referred to as *erythema multiforme bullosum* (Fig. 9-2).

Erythema multiforme, then, varies from the mild form, involving a few papular lesions without symptoms, to a completely generalized, serious bullous disorder with a febrile course, malaise, toxicity, and prostration (Fig. 9-3). Acute tubular necrosis has been reported by Bluefarb and several others. Erythema nodosum has been described in association with erythema multiforme in a number of cases.

***Stevens-Johnson syndrome.*** In children and young adults this serious, sometimes fatal variation of erythema multiforme begins with a sudden, febrile onset and involvement by vesicles and later ulcerations of the mucous membranes of the lips (Fig. 9-1, *A*), buccal cavity, nasal passages, eyes, and genitalia. Involvement of mucous membranes may or may not be accompanied by the characteristic cutaneous lesions. The conjunctival and corneal signs present in 90% of cases may rarely produce blindness. A patchy pneumonia is often present, and there may be symptoms of joint inflammation and general prostration.

This type of erythema multiforme, as with the others, may result from an allergic drug reaction. The following have been recorded: sulfa compounds, anticonvulsants, barbiturates, and phenylbutazone.

### *Pertinent information*

Etiology and pathogenesis of erythema multiforme are unknown, although the disease is believed to be of allergic origin. It may follow any of six general causes.

1. Idiopathic, self-limited.
2. Immediately occurring after herpes simplex, oral or genital, infection. Shelley reproduced the lesions in a generalized flare by intradermal injection of killed herpesvirus.
3. Drug eruption, occurring after ingestion

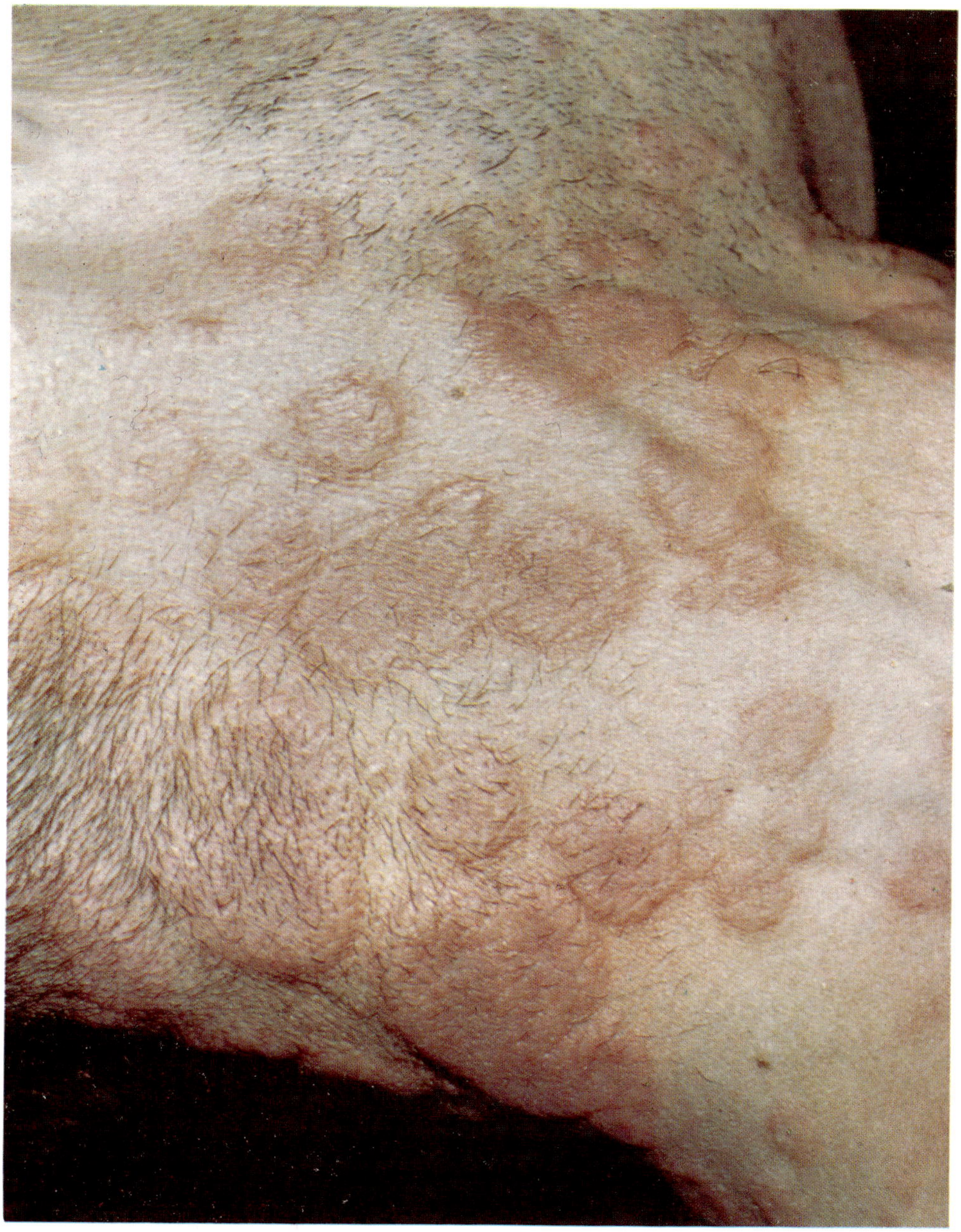

**Plate 23**

Erythema multiforme.

A

B

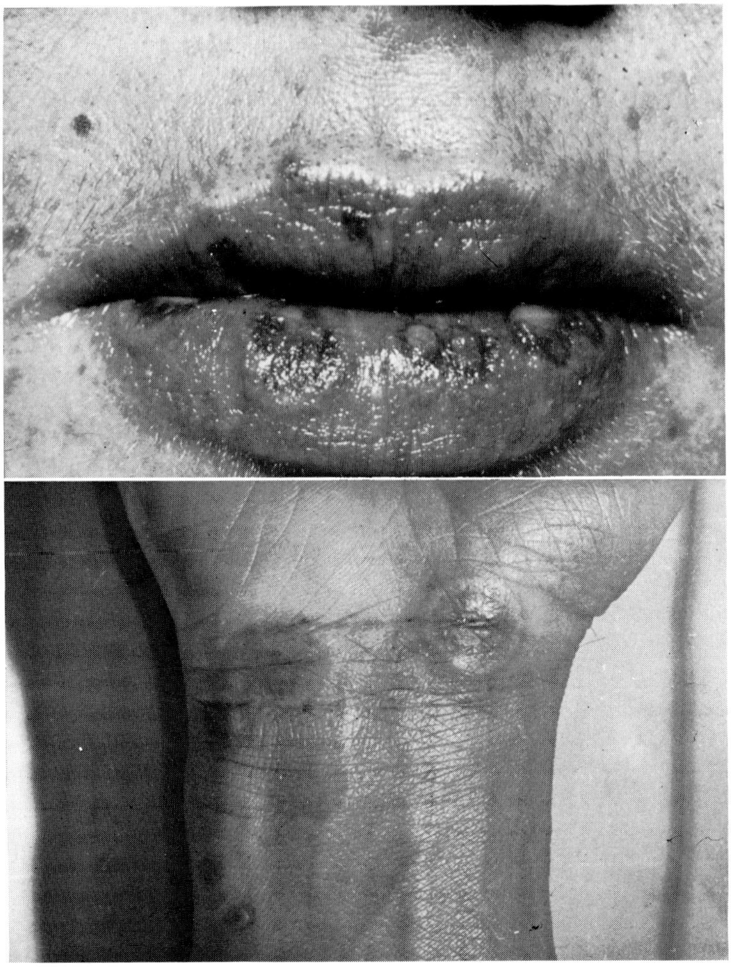

**Fig. 9-1. A,** Erythema multiforme involving lips in Stevens-Johnson syndrome. **B,** Iris lesion in erythema multiforme.

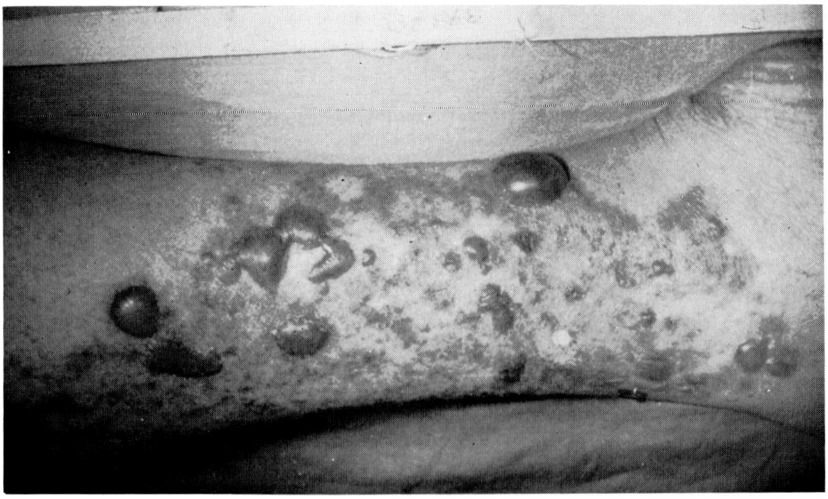

**Fig. 9-2.** Erythema multiforme bullosum.

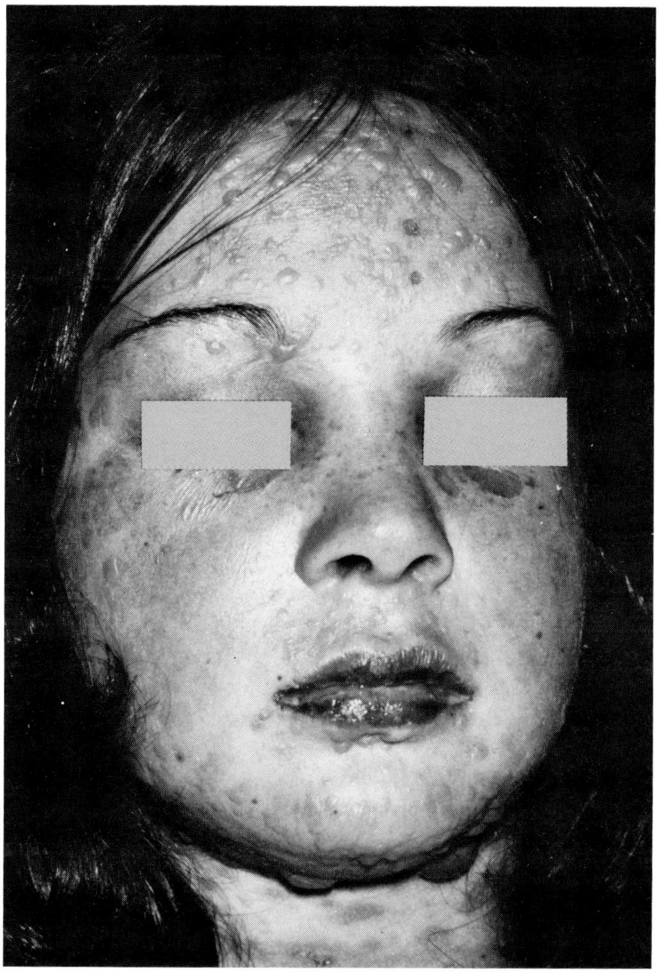

**Fig. 9-3.** Stevens-Johnson syndrome. Drug reaction.

of penicillin, salicylates, barbiturates, long-acting sulfonamides, bromides, quinine, and many others.

4. Associated with pregnancy, occurring usually in the latter half of pregnancy and ending with successful termination of pregnancy.
5. Associated with internal infections (rheumatic fever, streptococcal or other bacterial infection, mycoplasma infection, coccidioidomycosis, histoplasmosis, or viral infection such as primary atypical pneumonia, vaccinia, infectious mononucleosis, mumps, zoster, echovirus or coxsackievirus).
6. Associated rarely with various kinds of malignancy or radiation therapy for malignancy.

Any of the forms of erythema multiforme may present a leukocytosis and an elevation of the sedimentation rate. Albuminuria and occasionally hematuria are found in increasing numbers of patients, and renal lesions can develop. There will be an elevation of the antistreptolysin titer if the disease occurs after a streptococcal infection.

### *Microscopic findings*

Orfanos describes two types of histologic changes. Papular lesions with dermal infiltrate and epidermal vesiculation and bulla formation. Blood vessel involvement was more apparent in dermal lesions.

### Differential diagnosis—nonbullous form

***Urticaria.*** Urticaria may resemble erythema multiforme closely, and careful observation is sometimes necessary to confirm the transient nature of the wheals of urticaria, which last for only a day or so in any one place.

***Granuloma annulare.*** Absence of associated symptoms, and skin-colored, usually torpid lesions distinguish granuloma annulare.

***Nummular eczema.*** Individual symmetrical lesions with a moist, vesicular surface typify nummular eczema.

### Differential diagnosis—bullous form

***Pemphigus.*** In pemphigus, large bullae rapidly appear on normal skin, without macular or papular lesions.

***Dermatitis herpetiformis.*** Lesions in dermatitis herpetiformis are variable—some vesicular, macular, or papular—and extremely pruritic, healing with pigmentation.

### Differential diagnosis—Stevens-Johnson syndrome

***Reiter's disease.*** A syndrome of arthritis, urethritis, and conjunctivitis, Reiter's disease is similar to Stevens-Johnson syndrome, but distinguished by a definite urethritis of nonspecific etiology and the frequent finding of hard, crusted lesions on the feet, hands, and occasionally elsewhere (keratoderma blennorrhagica).

***Aphthous stomatitis.*** Aphthous stomatitis is limited to the lips and mouth, is an afebrile disease lasting 2 to 3 weeks, and exhibits a tendency to recurrence and chronicity.

***Behçet's syndrome.*** A triad of symptoms including aphthous lesions of the mouth, ulcerations of the genital mucous membranes, and uveitis or iridocyclitis comprises Behçet's syndrome. The ulcerations are small, but deep and chronic.

### Investigation

History and physical examination are directed toward recent drugs, including contact medications or chemicals, recent infections, particularly herpes simplex and possible mycoplasma, joint disease, and debilitation.

Antistreptolysin titer, peripheral blood count, and sedimentation rate are taken.

Urinalysis, with observation for developing renal disease, is done.

Studies are made for presence of *Trichomonas*, *Candida*, and fungal infection.

If lesions are atypical, biopsy of a fresh bulla is taken.

### Treatment

In patients with febrile illness, those with urinary abnormalities, and those with generally severe cases, bed rest is indicated; hospitalization may be desirable until all abnormal findings return to normal. Frequent urinalysis should be performed.

Antibiotic therapy may be indicated in the presence of infection or pneumonitis. There is some controversy about whether systemic glucocorticoids will relieve the symptoms and shorten the course. If no infection or underlying disease is found, however, we believe they make the patient more comfortable. These drugs also seem to be indicated in Stevens-Johnson syndrome of children, together with analgesic agents, mouthwashes, antibiotics if indicated, and sedatives, if no contraindication for their use can be identified.

For sore, tender mouths, particularly prior to meals, the following is recommended:

| | |
|---|---|
| Soluble betamethasone tables (0.5 mg.) | 28 |
| Zephiran hydrochloride (21.3%) | 1 drop |
| Peppermint oil | 1 drop |
| Lidocaine hydrochloride | 3% |
| Tragacanth | 4.8 Gm. |
| Distilled water | to make 4 oz. |

¼ tsp. to be swirled around mouth q.3h. (gives 0.1 mg. of betamethasone per dose).

Ophthalmic consultation is required in the presence of eye involvement in cases of Stevens-Johnson syndrome, because of the danger of irreversible complications.

#### REFERENCES

Bluefarb, S. M., and Szanto, P.: Erythema multiforme associated with acute renal necrosis, Arch. Dermatol. **92**:367, 1965.
**Worth remembering.**

Gordon, A. M., and Lyell, A.: Mycoplasmas and their association with skin disease, Br. J. Dermatol. **82**:414, 1970.

**In two of 13 cases of EM plus antibody titer.**

Orfanos, C. E., Schaumburg-Lever, G., and Lever, W. F.: Dermal and epidermal types of erythema multiforme. Histopathologic study of 24 cases, Arch. Dermatol. **109**:682, 1974.

**One type is dermal and the other, epidermomembrane.**

Pearson, R. W.: Advances in the diagnosis and treatment of blistering diseases. A selective review, In Malkinson, F. W., and Pearson, R. W., editors: The year book of dermatology, Chicago, 1977, Year Book Medical Publishers, Inc., p. 39.

**Concise overview.**

Rasmussen, J. E.: Erythema multiforme in children. Response to treatment with systemic corticosteroids, Br. J. Dermatol. **95**:181, 1976.

**Steroid effectiveness in question.**

Shelley, W. B.: Herpes simplex virus as a cause of erythema multiforme, J.A.M.A. **201**:153, 1967.

**Our most common cause.**

## CHAPTER 10

# Erythema nodosum

Erythema nodosum is a deep, nodular, inflammatory reaction, chiefly of the legs, thighs, and buttocks, attributable to a number of different causes.

### *Natural course*

The classic form of the disease begins with a small, tender, erythematous nodule that enlarges fairly rapidly to develop the appearance of a bruise (Plate 24). It occurs on the legs and thighs, usually anteriorly, and may also be seen on the forearms. It usually varies in size from 6 to 8 cm., but may be much larger. These developing nodules are usually bilaterally symmetrical. There may be very few lesions in the course of the disease, or as many as 30 to 50 may be seen at one time. The lesions each progress individually through a cycle of an acute, tender, erythematous nodule, to a less acute, dark purple lesion, and finally to a brown, flat pigmentation that slowly fades completely. The course ordinarily takes from 3 to 7 weeks. The course in some instances, however, may be shorter or more prolonged, and recurrences are not unusual. There is often an associated musculoskeletal discomfort, without specific joint redness or swelling. There also may be minimal temperature elevation. Many cases are associated with a symmetrical pulmonary hilar lymphadenopathy, usually sarcoid.

It is now proposed that the spectrum of clinical disease identified as erythema nodosum can be broadened to include nodulovascular lesions of varying sizes, that have a wider and more variable distribution and a more chronic course.

The disorder is seen in children and in adults, but more frequently in the latter. In children, both sexes are equally involved; in adults, the disorder predominates in women.

### *Pertinent information*

A number of systemic vascular nodular pathologic processes with more or less localized lesions have been identified and maintained as separate entities because of apparent differences in etiology, clinical course, or pathologic changes. These include the angiitides, nodular vasculitis, erythema induratum, erythema nodosum, superficial thrombophlebitis, pernio, panniculitis of various kinds, and the like.

There has been a desire expressed to bring these various disorders together, because of similar clinical and histological appearances despite the wide variety of etiologic factors. Wilkinson helped unify the mechanism of nodular leg lesions, and there has been a growing clinical tendency to emphasize the similarities between these different nodular lesions, rather than the differences. Förström and Winkelmann have recently shown the similarities in the pathological processes.

Ryan has taken a courageous approach to erythema nodosum and other diseases with a vascular inflammatory process of this nature. He considers them part of a continuum of vascular injury from purpura to intravascular coagulation and thrombosis, in which fibrin and fibrinolytic mechanisms are the significant end point of the process that initiates the vascular disorder. He brings together diseases caused by multiple etiologies, such as, stasis, hypertension, immune mechanisms, allergy, cold, bacterial infection, and drugs. He emphasizes erythema, effusion (edema), purpura, and necrosis as basic initial lesions,

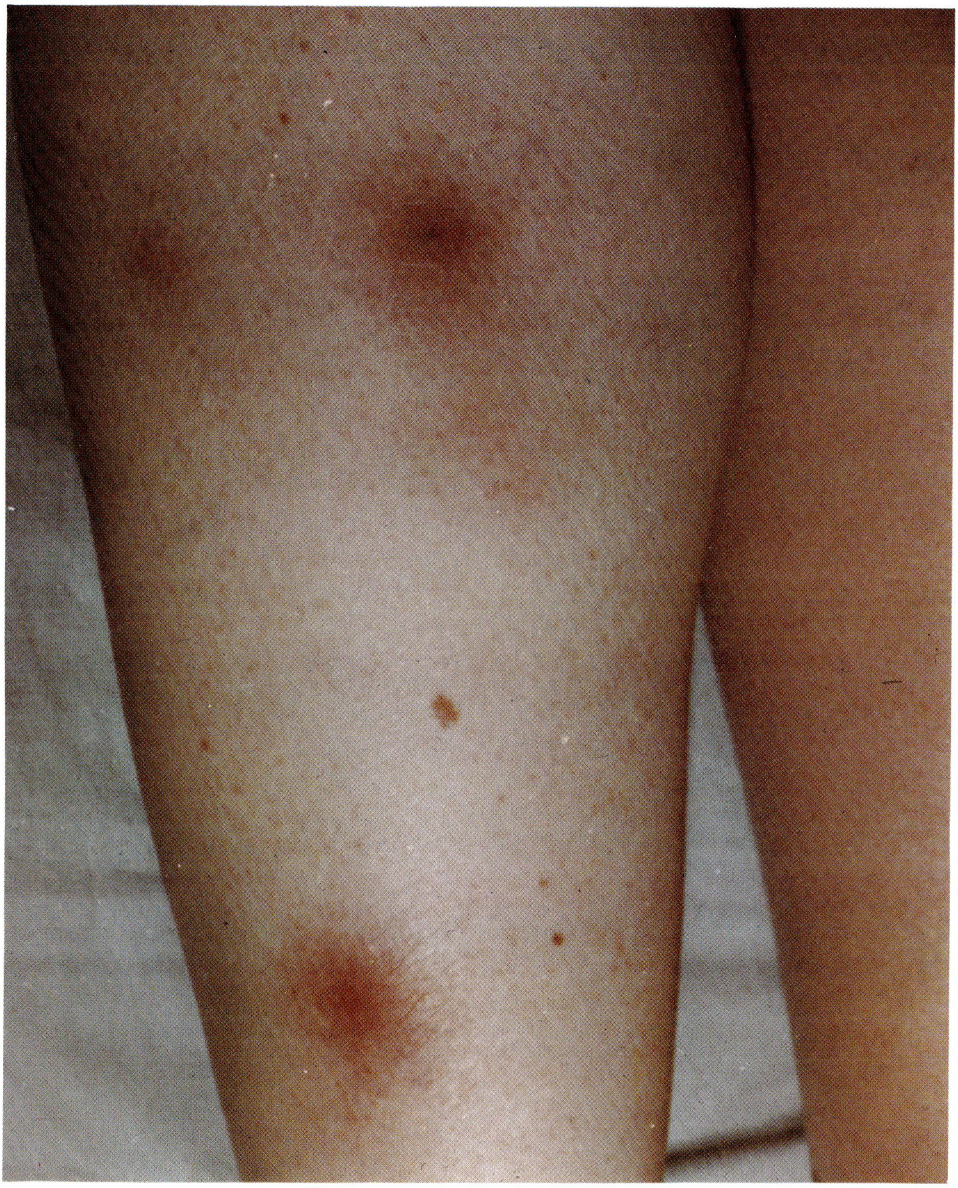

**Plate 24**

Erythema nodosum.

followed by bullae, papules, nodules, and ulcers as manifestations of the fibrinogen-fibrin, fibrinolytic-antifibrinolytic mechanisms of vascular injury. He decries rigid adherence to specific clinical entities that are all part of the same overall process.

There is an identifiable underlying systemic cause in more than 50% of cases. The remaining cases occur in otherwise apparently healthy young adults. The causative agent, which may be related to the geographical location, varies in those cases associated with an underlying systemic disease. In North America the most common causative agent is *Streptococcus*, with signs and symptoms of an acute upper respiratory tract infection occurring 14 to 21 days prior to the onset of the lesions.

In areas of California where *coccidioidomycosis* is endemic, erythema nodosum is associated with a primary infection by *Coccidioides immitis*. It is important as the initial cutaneous sign of *sarcoidosis*, particularly in Finland, occurring in some 30% of cases of that disease, and it is apparently associated with a reversion of a positive tuberculin test to an anergic state (Scadding).

In parts of Europe *tuberculosis* was, and appears still to be, a leading cause of erythema nodosum, and the appearance of the nodules is synchronous with the development of a positive tuberculin test.

Causes of erythema nodosum can be listed as follows:

**INFECTIONS**

Coccidioidomycosis, blastomycosis, histoplasmosis
Tuberculosis
Streptococcus
Lymphogranuloma venereum
Psittacosis
Cat-scratch disease
*Yersinia (Pasteurella) pseudotuberculosis*

**DRUGS**

Progestogens (progesterone)
Salicylates
Sulfonamides
Iodides
Bromides
Gold

**DISEASES**

Sarcoidosis
Leprosy
Behçet's disease
Leukemia, Hodgkin's disease
Chronic ulcerative colitis and regional enteritis

**PREGNANCY**

Pregnancy may predispose to this disorder.

Sams and Winkelmann believed that active ulcerative colitis may be closely related to erythema nodosum and that questioning toward symptoms of chronic ulcerative colitis in any patient with erythema nodosum in whom no other cause is apparent may prove fruitful.

Ryan asks the interesting question why it occurs both in disease, with good T-cell function and a high degree of sensitivity (tuberculosis and deep fungal disorder), as well as in leprosy and sarcoidosis, in which T-cell activity is impaired.

Erythema nodosum has also been described by several authors, as noted by Elias, in association with oral contraceptives. He hypothesizes a predisposing role of female hormones. If this disease is related to progestogens, there should have been an increased incidence with wide use of these drugs, which, however, may not have been seen by dermatologists.

Fibrinolytic activity is lower in the legs than in the arms, but transient stasis elevates this activity to levels found in the arms.

Erythema nodosum leprosum, as a reaction in leprosy under therapy, is ordinarily considered a separate entity, not to be confused with nonleprotic erythema nodosum.

### *Microscopic findings*

The microscopic changes are characteristic, with an early acute polymorphonuclear inflammatory reaction deep in the dermis, extending down into the fat and fibrous septa, with giant cells producing a true acute panniculitis, and is followed within 1 or 2 days by a mononuclear cellular infiltrate. Small blood vessels show a mild vasculitis and proliferation producing minimal obstruction of the flow. Necrosis may be present but is not severe enough to produce ulceration.

Some suggest that a cell-mediated immunity may explain the process. A variety of clinical observations support this.

Förström and Winkelmann have made a significant unifying step in identifying similarities in pathologic changes in several of these similar disorders.

### *Differential diagnosis*

***Insect bites.*** Insect bites, although not large, can mimic erythema nodosum, but they are characteristically pruritic.

***Thrombophlebitis.*** Tenderness, positive Homan's sign, edema, increased sedimentation rate, fever.

***Cellulitis.*** Ordinarily caused by streptococcal infection, a diffuse cellulitis extends until treated adequately, and produces constitutional symptoms out of proportion to those in erythema nodosum.

Until there is a clearer concept of the differences in etiology between these disorders, the following are included in this group:

- Erythema induratum (tends to ulcerate)
- Nodular vasculitis
- Weber-Christian disease
- Lipogranulomatosis
- Pernio
- Superficial thrombophlebitis
- Vilanova's panniculitis

### *Investigation*

***Initial.*** History and physical examination directed toward recent infection, areas of travel, febrile illness, gastrointestinal or joint disease, extremes of temperature, sunburn, known chronic illness, recent surgery or pregnancy:

- Complete blood count, sedimentation rate, and urinalysis
- Platelet estimation
- Chest x-ray study
- Antistreptolysin titer and throat culture
- Tuberculin test
- Biopsy if diagnosis is in doubt
- Rheumatoid and antinuclear factors
- Review of foods and drugs

***Secondary.*** As indicated by results from initial investigation:

- Lymph node biopsy and Kveim test
- Histoplasmin and coccidioidin skin testing
- Barium enema
- Serum protein electrophoresis

### *Treatment*

Bed rest may be indicated while a thorough search for underlying systemic disease is undertaken. Analgesics and antibiotics may be necessary, depending on the signs and symptoms. Schulz reported an impressive response to potassium iodide 400 to 900 mg./day, orally for a few days to 8 weeks. It suppresses granuloma reactions by releasing heparin. Whether this is most effective at a certain stage of these lesions is not shown.

Ryan states that heparin is an effective fibrinolytic agent in vasculitis and intravascular coagulation.

Glucocorticoids may be used if infection can be excluded, but they are seldom indicated, unless they are used early in the disease at the acute polymorphonuclear leukocyte stage.

#### REFERENCES


Darlington, L. G.: Erythema nodosum and oral contraceptives, Br. J. Dermatol. **90**:209, 1974.
**These hormones may influence the milieu so that erythema nodosum may occur from other causes.**

Elias, P. M.: Erythema nodosum and serological lupus erythematosus: simultaneous occurrence in a patient using oral contraceptives, Arch. Dermatol. **108**:716, 1973.
**The hormone may have prepared the vessels.**

Förström, L., and Winkelmann, R. K.: Acute panniculitis. A clinical and histopathologic study of 34 cases, Arch. Dermatol. **113**:909, 1977.
**The histologic process of erythema nodosum is polymorphous, but includes a true polymorphonuclear panniculitis.**

Hannuksela, M.: Erythema nodosum with special reference to sarcoidosis: a clinical study of 343 Finnish adult patients, Ann. Clin. Res. **3**(suppl. 7):1, 1971.
**Erythema nodosum is a special event in the clinical course of sarcoidosis.**

Michelson, H. E.: Erythema nodosum, Arch. Dermatol. **77**:546, 1958.
**The strict morphologic criteria for diagnosis.**

Ryan, T. J.: Microvascular injury, Philadelphia, 1976, W. B. Saunders Co., p. 175.
**Erythema nodosum becomes a part of the big picture of fibrinogen-fibrin and fibrinolysin concept.**

Sams, M., and Winkelmann, R. K.: The association of erythema nodosum with ulcerative colitis, South. Med. J. **61**:676, 1968.
**48 of 679 patients.**

Scadding, J. G.: Sarcoidosis, London, 1967, Eyre & Spottiswoode (Publishers) Ltd., p. 360.

Schulz, E. J., and Whiting, D. A.: Treatment of erythema nodosum and nodular vasculitis with potassium iodide, Br. J. Dermatol. **94**:75, 1976.
**45 patients with nodular lesions. Of 28 patients with erythema nodosum, 25 responded quickly.**

Wilkinson, D. S.: The vascular basis for some nodular eruptions of the legs, Br. J. Dermatol. **66**:201, 1974.
**A unification of etiologies about the central pathologic problem.**

CHAPTER 11

# Exfoliative dermatitis

The rare generalized cutaneous syndrome of exfoliative dermatitis is one of the most challenging diagnostic and therapeutic problems in dermatology.

### *Natural course*

This syndrome follows a previously diagnosed generalized dermatitis in 33% of cases and is a part of a drug reaction in an additional 20%. An important few cases are attributable to lymphomas and leukemias, but the disease occurs for unknown reasons in approximately half the cases.

It is ushered in by an elevated temperature in some patients, particularly those in whom the syndrome results from a drug reaction. An erythema, first patchy then generalized, appears.

The course then consists of a more or less sudden episode of generalized exfoliation, in which there is a striking erythema followed by a remarkable scaling off of the cutaneous surface, either in fine scales or in larger sheets. Frequently, hair loss and nail shedding accompany the disorder. The palms and soles may be spared. There is often a generalized persistent pruritus (Fig. 11-1).

The moist warm skin is receptive to infection and quickly becomes colonized with large numbers of pathogenic *Staphylococcus aureus*, which produce crusts and further inflammation. They disseminate widely to adjacent areas and to other patients.

The symptoms associated with an acute exfoliation include malaise, a characteristic feeling of chilliness and shaking, and a fore-

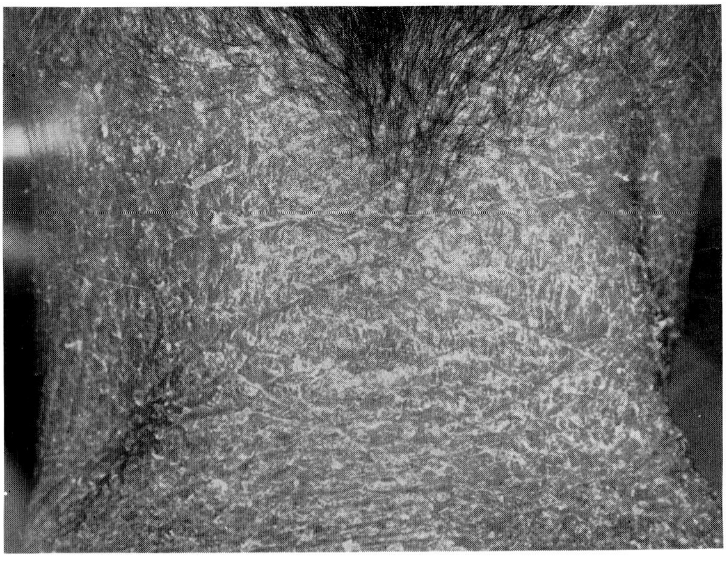

**Fig. 11-1.** Exfoliative dermatitis involving posterior aspect of neck.

boding sensation. In all forms there is considerable water and protein loss from the skin surface. Control of heat regulation is poor, and the patient is very susceptible to infection. Generalized lymphadenopathy (dermatopathic lymphadenopathy) may be expected to be present, although Nicolis and Helwig describe it as occurring in only 62% of their 135 cases. Hepatomegaly or splenomegaly or both may occur in patients without underlying malignancies and without generalized lymphoadenopathy.

This disease is by no means always acute; indeed, the average duration of the idiopathic variety is approximately 5 years. It occurs at all ages from childhood to old age. Although the syndrome chiefly involves males 45 years of age and older, a significant group involves young children with generalized infection (Ritter's disease) and generalized seborrheic dermatitis (Leiner's disease).

Death, when it occurs, is most frequently caused by intercurrent infection, such as bronchopneumonia, or circulatory collapse from the universal cutaneous vasodilatation and fluid loss. The hyperemia and increased cutaneous blood flow that result can produce a *cardiac failure of high output origin*, capable of causing death in elderly individuals or those with decreased cardiac reserve. A fatal outcome can occur in such benign diseases as psoriasis, as well as in malignancies.

In Nicolis and Helwig's series the most common causes of death in order of frequency included pneumonia (undetermined, but assumed to be caused by exfoliative dermatitis), liver degeneration, Hodgkin's disease, septicemia, myocardial infarction, myocarditis, leukemia-lymphoma, and vascular collapse. This was a clinicopathologic study. In Adams and Abrahams' series, approximately 20% of the patients died of causes related to their disease.

### *Pertinent information*

The preexisting generalized dermatitis is usually psoriasis, which may be irritated into an exfoliative dermatitis by overtreatment. Hypostatic dermatitis and a generalized eczematous process may become exfoliative. Atopic dermatitis, allergic contact dermatitis, seborrheic dermatitis, pemphigus, lichen planus, and pityriasis rubra pilaris may also lead to exfoliative dermatitis.

Sudden onset of this syndrome is seen in drug reactions, in which the development may be explosive with such drugs as phenylbutazone. Other drugs incriminated, although not all have been proved, are sulfonamides, antimalarials, penicillin, mercurials, arsenicals, barbiturates, streptomycin, and gold.

Laboratory findings are often not helpful in determining the severity or therapeutic direction. Anemia is usually present, leukocytosis is often strong, and sedimentation rate is moderately elevated. Serum albumin level is often low, which Shuster has calculated to be attributable to dilution factors rather than protein loss. There is, however, a low serum folate level caused by loss of folate from skin.

### *Etiology*

- Idiopathic
- Secondary to known dermatoses, such as:
  - Psoriasis
  - Pemphigus
  - Seborrheic dermatitis
  - Atopic dermatitis
  - Stasis dermatitis with eczematization
  - Other eczemas
  - Toxic epidermal necrolysis
  - Lichen planus
  - Pityriasis rubra pilaris
- Drug reactions
- Contact dermatitis
- Senile xerosis and primary irritation dermatitis
- Mycosis fungoides and Sézary syndrome
- Lymphomas and leukemia or internal malignancy
- Bacterial infection and seborrheic dermatitis (infants only)

### *Microscopic findings*

Biopsy is of distinct diagnostic help in those conditions secondary to a lymphoma or to a specific cutaneous disease. It is of little help and may be misleading in the others

### *Investigation*

***Initial.*** The most helpful aspect of patient assessment in this disorder is a good clinical history and bedside assessment by thorough examination.

Skin biopsies, skin culture
Lymph node biopsies (Neither is likely to be helpful except in the case of specific malignant infiltrations)
White blood count
Liver function tests
Electrocardiograph and assessment of cardiac status
Chest x-ray examination
Bone marrow studies

***Secondary.*** Further studies are indicated in individual cases.

### *Treatment*

Careful attentive daily nursing care is essential, and isolation is usually wise to prevent bacterial dissemination. If infection is present and is producing clinical signs, antibiotics as chosen by culture and sensitivity results are indicated.

Bland, nonsensitizing topical oily lotions and daily baths are welcomed and helpful.

Treatment in such a disorder as this must, of course, be individualized, supportive, and dependent on the underlying disease. Important aspects in treating all patients are the following: maintenance of fluid balance; prevention of intercurrent or cutaneous infection; avoidance of all possible irritants and potential drug causes; and externally applied anti-inflammatory agents. Consultative management is essential in all cases of this type.

The systemic administration of glucocorticoid compounds may be a lifesaving procedure. They are not ordinarily required in massive doses.

In carefully selected cases of exfoliative psoriasis, immunosuppressives are effective but must be administered by one familiar with the use of these toxic drugs and only with carefully monitored testing of kidney, liver, and hematological function.

#### REFERENCES

Abrahams, I., McCarthy, J. T., and Sanders, S. L.: One hundred one cases of exfoliative dermatitis, Arch. Dermatol. **87**:96, 1963.
**Almost 50% etiology undetermined.**

Adam, J. E.: Exfoliative dermatitis, Can. Med. Assoc. J. **99**:661, 1968.
**176 patients reviewed, 37% idiopathic.**

Nicolis, G. D., and Helwig, E. B.: Exfoliative dermatitis: a clinicopathological study of 135 cases, Arch. Dermatol. **108**:788, 1973.
**12% undetermined; 40% cases caused by drugs.**

Shuster, S.: High output cardiac failure from skin disease, Lancet **1**:1338, 1963.
**The hemodynamic skin vasculitis changes may cause failure in compromised patients.**

Winkelmann, R. K., and Linman, J. W.: Erythroderma with atypical lymphocytes (Sézary syndrome), Am. J. Med. **55**:192, 1973.
**Clinical details well presented on 19 patients.**

## CHAPTER 12

# Diseases of the hair

Human hair is a curiosity. No one seems quite sure why it has retained the vestigial erratic distribution that it has in comparison to other mammals. At man's present evolutionary stage, his hair retains significant social and protective importance, but it has lost the insulating and temperature-retaining qualities it possesses in furred animals. It screens orifices, such as the nose, and may have value as a sensory warning system in ears.

Pilosebaceous units are comprised of the hair, hair sheath or follicle, attached sebaceous glands, dermal papilla, and attached blood vessels and nerves. It is immediately perceived as a complex of unrelated tissues and structures integrated for the single purpose of hair production. Since hair growth is a cyclic phenomenon, the production of hair is a repetitive process, and the pilosebaceous apparatus is at any time, either proliferating actively, regressing, or resting.

### Embryology

Hair growth provides the most impressive evidence for the close dermoepidermal interrelationship that apparently is essential for many of the functions of both. Normal regional functioning tissue of *both* epidermis and dermis is essential for the normal development of the final mutual product.

The hair follicles develop from both ectoderm and mesoderm, appearing first in the third intrauterine month and continuing to appear through the next 3 months. The first follicles appear on the eyebrows, then on the upper lip, chin, and scalp, and caudally over the torso and extremities. Indicative of the future asynchronous behavior of individual mature hair units, pilosebaceous follicles tend to develop asynchronously and individually in the embryo. Buds of epithelial cells push downward into the dermis to partially surround and isolate a collection of dermal cells that progress to form the *papilla* of the hair root. Hair begins to form by multiplication of the epidermal cells that cap the hair papilla, and the tip of the new hair shaft pushes upward, emerging above the skin surface at about the fourth or fifth month.

Just before this, two small epithelial cell bulges on the posterior side of the follicle develop. These are the sebaceous glands and the site of attachment of the *arrector pili* muscle, which itself now forms from a linear collection of mesenchymal cells (Fig. 3-1, *A*).

### Anatomy

The mature hair shaft rests in a deep pocket of epidermal cells, the *hair follicle* (Fig. 12-1, *A*). Each follicle is directly associated with a sebaceous gland. At a point immediately beneath the sebaceous gland are one or more bundles of smooth muscle fibers, called the *arrector pili* muscle (plural, arrectores pilorum). This muscle, innervated by adrenergic fibers, pulls the hair follicle, which in turn wrinkles the skin surface, causing "goose flesh."

**Hair bulb** (Fig. 12-2). The projecting tongue of tissue at the base of the hair follicle that is seen in longitudinal section dividing it like a cloven hoof, is called the papilla. It is the part of the pilosebaceous unit that is derived from mesenchyme. The actively proliferating, undifferentiated epidermal cells holding the papilla form part of the *hair bulb* and are called the *matrix* (Fig. 12-1, *B*). This is the site of hair shaft formation, and these active cells give rise to all cells of the hair shaft and inner root sheath. The papilla contains fibroblast-

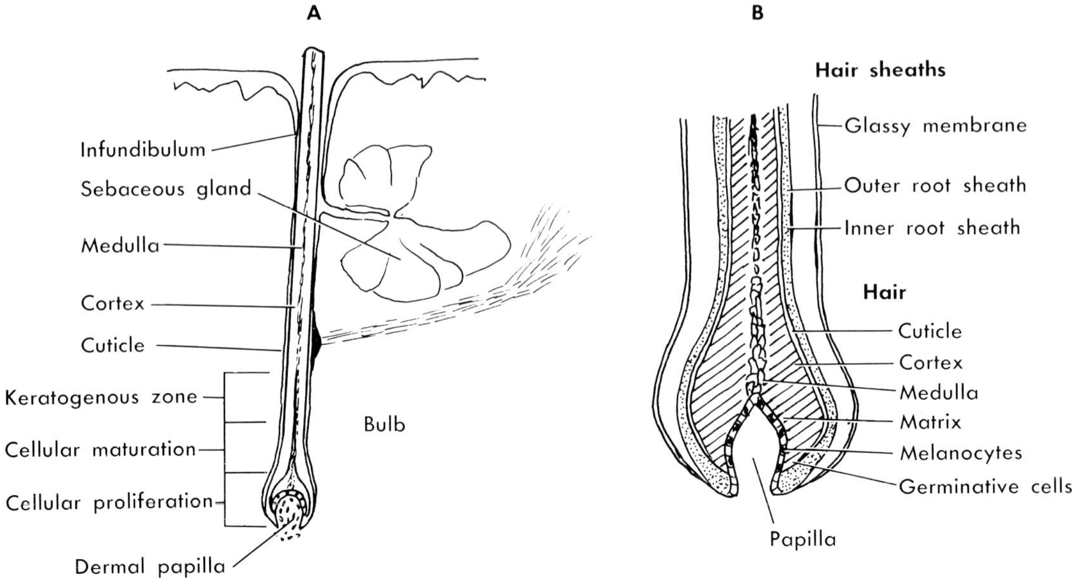


**Fig. 12-1. A,** Hair and its follicle. **B,** Hair bulb.

like cells, wispy collagen microfibrils, and amorphous material. The mesenchymal cells at the papilla tip retain embryonic characteristics. Melanocytes provide pigment that is transferred to the hair cortex. The developing hair shaft becomes completely keratinized in the upper bulb and in the *keratogenous zone.* No living cells remain in the hair shaft above this level. It is a lifeless, cornified end product of the rapid cellular activity of the pilosebaceous unit. The scalp hair shaft reaches its maximum diameter by 10 to 12 years of age, but beard-hair maximum comes later.

***Hair follicle.*** The epidermal pocket of cells that holds the hair and guides it obliquely to the surface, arises from the matrix. It is called the *inner root sheath.* This structure is layered and forms part of the permanent covering or cuticle of the hair, as well as the lining that keratinizes and remains behind as the hair is pushed out of the follicular opening. The *outer root sheath* becomes continuous with the epidermis of the adjacent skin.

***Hair shaft.*** The outside layer of the hair shaft, the cuticle, is made up of a single layer of overlapping scales and is tough, translucent, and free of pigment. These scales interlock with those of the cuticle of the inner root sheath and anchor the hair in the follicle. A thin layer of lipid and carbohydrate surrounds the cuticle and affords physical protection.

Pigmentation of the hair shaft arises from melanocytes in the upper portion of the hair bulb adjacent to the matrix. Some are also present in the outer root sheath. The melanin is passed on to the cortex and medulla, but the cuticle and inner sheath remain nonpigmented. White hair shafts are produced in follicles possessing no active melanocytes. Graying or whitening of hair is an irreversible process for that hair shaft, although subsequent hair growth may repair pigment.

The *cortex* is made up of keratinized cells cemented together to create the major bulk of the hair shaft. Pigment (melanin) and air spaces are both ordinarily present.

The medulla, which makes up the central part of the hair, is composed of loosely connected keratinized cells. In small hairs, it may be absent.

Most hair is round or oval, and occasionally is quite flattened. It varies greatly in thickness, length, and color.

Each hair follicle is abundantly served by a

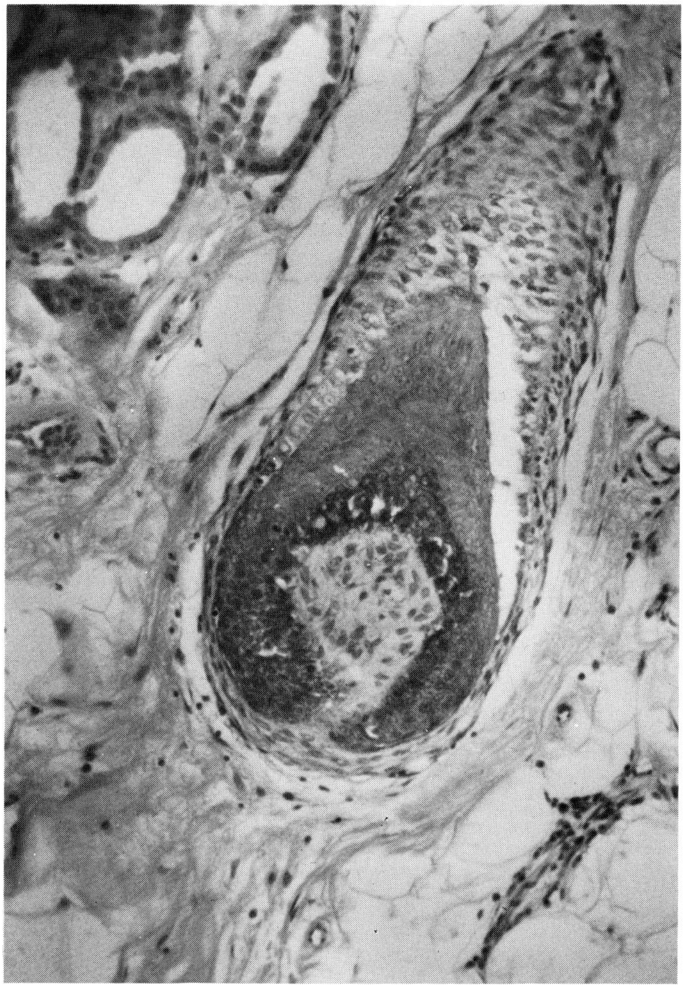

**Fig. 12-2.** Photomicrograph of human hair bulb, showing papilla and germinative cells around it.

dense collar of both vessels and sensory nerves. These nerves surrounding the follicle are highly organized in similar complex patterns for all follicles and are most important in supplying touch perception for the organism as a whole. The vascular network that surrounds each follicle includes the sebaceous gland of that follicle and forms a continuous unit. During the active growing phase, there is an abundant lattice work of vessels chiefly disposed in the area of the keratogenous zone. With involution, these capillaries and arterioles degenerate and collapse. When anagen causes the rejuvenation of the hair bulb, a vascular proliferation recommences.

## Keratinization

Keratinization of the hair shaft varies both as to the layer being studied and from the same process in the epidermis. Hard hair keratin found in the cortex of the hair contains more sulfur-rich amino acids, largely placed between tough protein filaments as a kind of cement. The end product is rigid and resistant to external destructive factors. Proteins in the medulla of the hair are quite different from other keratinized tissues (Montagna and Parakkal). The cuticles are relatively nonfilamentous, and the inner root sheath is resistant and as difficult to dissolve as the medulla.

Granules called *trichohyaline* granules,

similar in ways to keratohyaline granules elsewhere in the epidermis, are formed in the inner root sheath, but keratinization of the cortex occurs without these structures.

## Growth

The first fine hairs that form in the embyro and are present as a dense fine growth over the entire skin surface are called *lanugo* hairs. These are ordinarily lost during fetal life. *Vellus* hairs are fine nonpigmented hairs that are present on apparently "hairless" areas of the human. *Terminal* hair is longer and coarser than lanugo and vellus hair, is pigmented, and is found in several varieties in hairy areas. Most male body hair is terminal, whereas most female body hair is vellus. Most terminal hairs grow in groups of two or three. Hair follicle activity is cyclic, and each follicle is independent of other follicles. The cyclic period of hair growth varies with area and with individuals, but for scalp hair the active growing period appears to last several years, or long enough for the hair to grow to average scalp hair length, at a rate of 1 mm. every 3 days, or about 2.5 mm. a week. After reaching the end of the active growth cycle, the hair forms a *club hair*, recognizable in plucked hairs as having a small, hard, inconspicuous white bulb with no sheath or covering, such as is seen with plucked growing hairs. Growing hairs are fully pigmented, with a less abrupt expansion at the follicular end, and possess a soft covering sheath of tissue, the *root sheath*.

The actively growing phase of hair is referred to as the *anagen stage*, whereas the resting or club hair is in the *telogen stage*. A transition from the end of anagen to the beginning of telogen is the short, actively involuting *catagen stage* (Fig. 12-3). At any time in a normal scalp, the active growing hairs constitute more than 80% (85% in women and 80% in men) of the total 100,000 to 150,000 hairs. The most actively growing hair is in the vertex. The normal range of hair loss in adults is from 20 to 100 hairs daily. Body hair goes through a 3- to 4-month growing period; beard hair, 3 to 4 years; axillary hair, a year or so, and eyelash hair, a month. The impressive metabolic activity of the hair matrix, unique in the body, attains a production of 100 feet of protein-rich hair daily in health (Pillsbury, quoted by Reeves and Maibach).

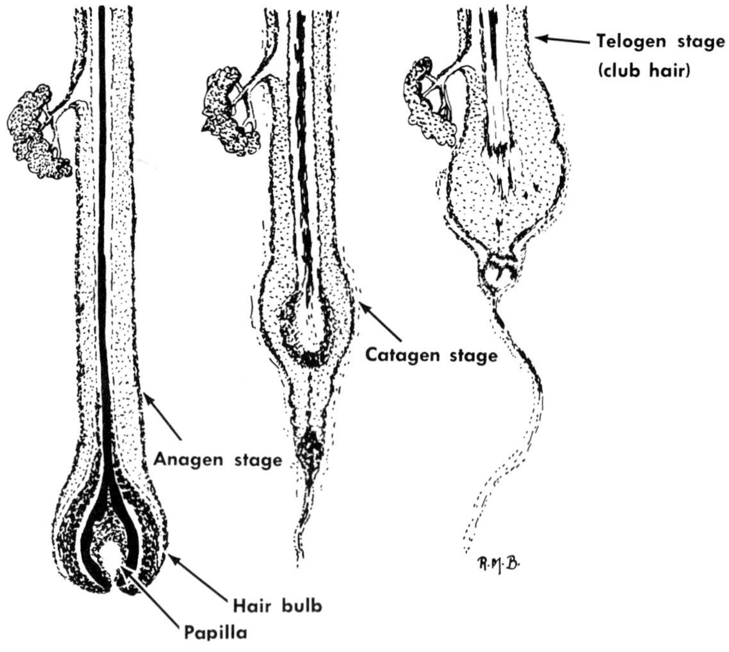


**Fig. 12-3.** Hair growth cycle: anagen—active growing stage; catagen—very short transitional stage; telogen—resting, or club, stage, identifiable by small, firm, white bulb at hair end.

Hair plucking does not seem to permanently damage the hair follicle, which, as with many active tissues, has a remarkable re-formative ability and can recover from considerable trauma. Plucking shortens the resting phase of hair growth. However, destruction of the hair papilla permanently destroys the hair follicle.

Hair growth reflects the state of health to a considerable degree. The formation of hair is a result of rapid cellular activity that appears to become expendable to the body economy under certain circumstances. Febrile illness, severe anemia, iron deficiency, inadequate dietary protein, and generally debilitating disorders produce cessation or slowing of hair growth. Malnutrition can be assayed, as shown by Crounse, with an assessment of hair follicles.

Hair roots are ideal protein-rich structures for the study of early protein deprivation, not only because they accurately reflect protein depletion, but because they can be transported easily and examined in hot, humid, and backward countries with minimal facilities. Synthesis of nuclear DNA parallels protein synthesis. The protein equivalent of one matrix cell is added to each of the cells in the keratogenous zone every hour. With this degree of anabolic activity, measurements of hair root diameter and other bulb parameters allow assessment of protein-calorie malnutrition in children or adults. The method is primarily intended for groups rather than individuals because of the range of variations.

Among other advances, the examination of the hair has become a significant part of the search for markers of genetic disease. Many aspects of hair, such as its rapid metabolic rate, the availability of chromosomes easily determined from plucked hair, and accurate knowledge of several chemical processes taking place in hair, represent its usefulness in identifying hereditary patterns.

## Effect of hormones on hair

***Androgens.*** Androgen excess produces hirsutism. The response of target organs to testosterone is dependent on its conversion to its metabolites that are more potent than the parent hormone. Among these metabolites, dihydrotestosterone appears most potent (Price), although potency may depend on stages of the cycle, geographic area in question, the tissue involved, the receptors available in the target cell, or the protein binding of the hormone. Hay has shown a difference in sensitivity to specific selected androgens by scalp, axillary, and pubic skin. The ability of the hair roots to produce estrogen may afford a means of blocking the androgen effect on the hair.

Testosterone paradoxically produces large pigmented terminal hairs from vellus hairs in most areas, but it also causes regression of terminal hairs to nonpigmented fine vellus hairs on the scalp of genetically predisposed males. Also, inexplicably, androgens cause increased sebaceous gland activity and inhibition of hair growth simultaneously in the balding scalp. Androgen incubation studies on human hair roots indicate a divergence from the metabolites found in other androgen-sensitive tissues and the ability to convert androgens to estrogen. Scalp hair roots vary from pubic hair roots in their metabolites.

***Glucocorticoids.*** Glucocorticoids appear to prolong the telogen stage and may shorten the active growing stage. Deficiency produces no recognizable effect.

***Thyroid.*** Thyroid hormone favors the anagen, or growing, phase and acts to maintain this phase. Deficiency produces loss of hair, poorly formed coarse hair, and generally sparse hair everywhere.

***Estrogens.*** Estrogens seem to produce no consistent effect on hair growth during pregnancy.

After pregnancy, a postpartum shortening of the active growing cycle commonly occurs, and many hairs revert to the resting phase. This results in an increased hair fall and temporary thinning of the scalp hair. Oral contraceptive agents may produce similar scalp hair thinning.

## Endocrinological classification

It is helpful to categorize hair as nonsexual (that is, not under control of the sex hormones), ambosexual (controlled by the normal level of sex hormones in the female), or male sexual (controlled by male levels of hormones).

It must be noted here that some forms of androgens are produced in both sexes by the adrenal glands and that the normal ovary produces an androgenic hormone. LH (luteinizing hormone) stimulates ovarian androgen production.

*Scalp*, *eyebrow*, and *eyelash* hair is nonsexual. It is however, dependent on pituitary function, without which it becomes thin and dry.

*Aural* and *nasal* hair is dependent on adequate levels of androgens from any source.

*Beard* and *mustache* hair is dependent on male levels of androgens, which in normal individuals are of testicular origin. This hair is increased in hirsute women, presumably from increased adrenal or ovarian androgenic hormones.

*Body* hair of chest, shoulders, back, and abdomen is male sexual and androgen dependent, although breast hair is common in women and increases with age.

*Pubic* hair is divided into upper and lower areas. The characteristic male upper pubic triangle or the upper border of pubic hair is male sexual—thus androgen dependent. In women with increased levels of androgens, the area may assume a male appearance.

Axillary hair is ambosexual, that is, of postpubertal origin. It is scant or absent in men or women with hypoadrenalism. Adrenal androgens probably control its growth and maintenance.

*Extremity* hair is of mixed control. Some is undoubtedly nonsexual, some is ambosexual, and some seems to be male sexual. Heredity plays an important part in the amount of extremity hirsutism.

### REFERENCES


Bradfield, R. B.: Effects of malnutrition on the morphology of hair roots. In Montagna, W., and Parakkal, P. F., editors: Structure and function of the skin, New York, 1974, Academic Press, Inc., Chapter 8.
**Identifies even moderately malnourished children.**

Breathnach, A. S., and Smith, J.: Fine structure of the early hair germ and dermal papilla in the human foetus, J. Anat. **102**:511, 1968.
**At 11 to 16 weeks the hair buds are forming in association with dermal changes.**

Crounse, R. G., Bollet, A. J., and Owens, S.: Quantitative assay of human malnutrition using scalp hair roots, Nature (London) **228**:465, 1970.
**Hair root protein content reflects the state of nutrition accurately.**

Hay, J. B.: A study of the in vitro metabolism of androgens by human scalp and pubic skin, Br. J. Dermatol. **97**:237, 1977.
**Difference in direction of operation of androgenic dehydrogenase enzymes in different skin sites.**

Kirschner, M. A., Zucker, I. F., and Jesperson, D.: Idiopathic hirsutism: an ovarian abnormality, N. Engl. J. Med. **294**:637, 1976.
**Ovarian androgens cause hirsutism and may be suppressed by glucocorticoids, surgical intervention, and LH suppression.**

Montagna, W., and Parakkal, P. F.: The structure and function of skin, ed. 3, New York, 1974, Academic Press, Inc.
**Unique personal encyclopedic source. Eminently readable.**

Pinkus, H.: Embryology of hair. In Montagna, W., and Ellis, R. A., editors: The biology of hair growth, New York, 1958, Academic Press, Inc., pp. 1-32.
**Detailed chronology of the development of follicles and associated structures.**

Price, V. H.: Testosterone metabolism in the skin: review of its function in androgenetic alopecia, acne vulgaris, and idiopathic hirsutism including recent studies with antiandrogens, Arch. Dermatol. **111**:1496, 1975.
**Testosterone metabolism and DHT production in the skin reviewed and their relation to acne, alopecia, and hirsutism proposed.**

Schweikert, H. U., Milewich, L., and Wilson, J. D.: Aromatization of androstenedione by isolated human hairs, J. Clin. Endrocrinol. Metab. **40**:413, 1975.
**Hair roots contain the complex enzymes necessary for estrogen formation from an androgen.**

Schweikert, H. U., and Wilson, J. D.: Regulation of human hair growth by steroid hormones. I. Testosterone metabolism in isolated hairs, J. Clin. Endrocrinol. Metab. **39**:1012, 1974.
**Pathways of androgen metabolism in anagen and telogen hair roots were studied. Hormone relationship to hair growth or hair loss is confusing. Differential androgen response by individual hairs may be present.**


## DIFFUSE ALOPECIA

### Androgenetic alopecia (physiological alopecia, diffuse alopecia of women (Fig. 12-4), male pattern baldness, and common baldness)

Hair regression over the anterior portion of the scalp, followed by similar changes over the vertex, may become apparent in normal

A

B

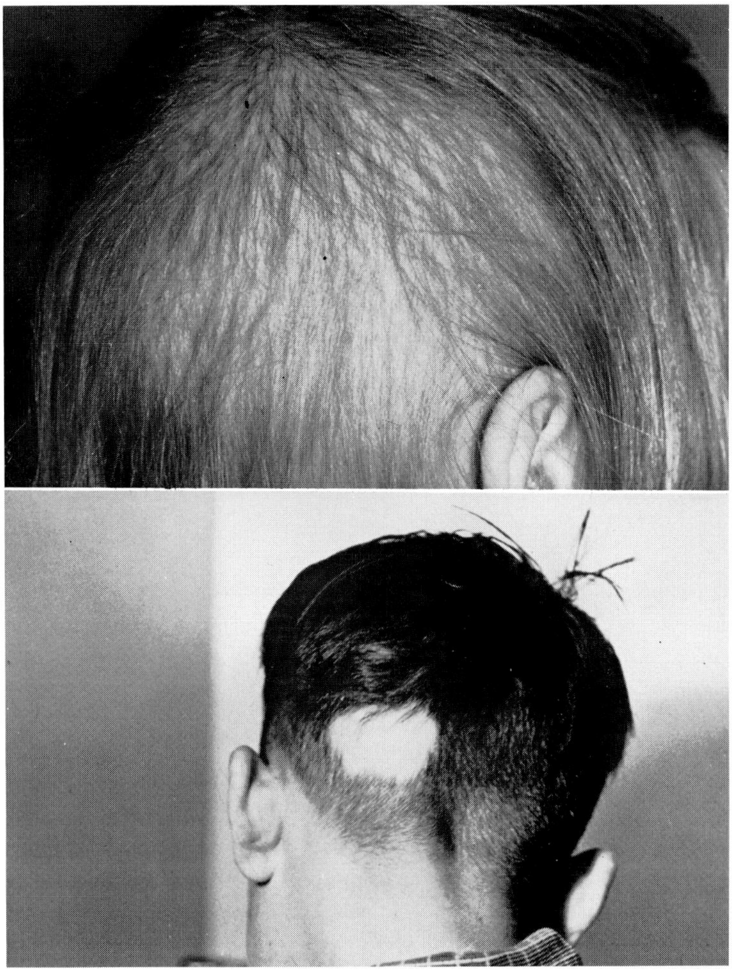

**Fig. 12-4. A,** Diffuse alopecia in young woman. **B,** Alopecia areata.

males in the late teens or early twenties. The presence of androgenic hormone and a genetic predisposition are the causative factors and thus the label *androgenetic.* It should be emphasized that hair is not lost, instead it regresses to a vellus form, but its presence in fine nonpigmented follicles is easily demonstrable microscopically. This condition also occurs in women in whom mild forms are not unusual (Fig. 12-4, *A*). The balding process in the female begins with thinning over the vertex. In opposition to the pattern in the male, there is a well-preserved fringe in the frontal hairline. There may be early frontotemporal recession in females as well. The vertex thinning may become severe, approaching baldness by menopause. Hereditary patterns must be differentiated from early virilizing syndromes. Castrated men do not develop this type of baldness, and castration prevents extension of the process. Administration of testosterone, however, does not produce extension.

Family histories must be obtained to confirm or reject a hereditary etiology. The degree of baldness of parents, grandparents, siblings, aunts, and uncles should be established. The disorder is inherited, but the mode of transmission is uncertain. Both hair follicles and sebaceous glands decrease. Pigmented coarse hairs are replaced by finer ones, which are eventually small and nonpigmented. Excessive shedding of hair is not a feature, although a concerned individual will be cognizant of every lost one, being unaware of the amount of the usual previous daily loss.

### *Treatment*

Other forms of alopecia, syphilitic alopecia, and alopecia areata must be recognized. The young man in his late teens or early twenties is deeply concerned if he notes hair loss, or if his family has some history of early baldness. The problem should be discussed sympathetically and convincingly with him. There are multitudinous "hair restorers" where he can spend a great deal of money for unconfirmed and questionable practices to regrow hair, and if he is not informed, an attempt to save his hair is hard for him to resist.

Hair transplantation, for those who are disabled by their baldness, results in an acceptable appearance.

In young women with severe baldness, who do not have amenorrhea or clitoral hypertrophy, there is a likelihood that antiandrogens, such as cyproterone acetate, may offer some help. Antiandrogen treatment is not established in North America although reports of successful cessation of hair loss in women from antiandrogens, such as cyproterone acetate, are available in the European literature (Ludwig). Virilizing syndromes in women must be considered, even in women with a family history of alopecia, because they may represent a generally androgen-sensitive group. Amenorrhea and clitoral enlargement may help to differentiate them.

## Hair loss occurring after high fever (telogen effluvium)

Hair loss after high fever is now quite uncommon, but in those clinical instances in which a temperature of about 39° C. continues for a number of days, a diffuse form of hair loss may become apparent up to several weeks after the febrile episodes. The hair usually grows back immediately, but it may take up to 4 to 6 months. The nails in such cases may also form ridges. Other forms of stress, such as accidents, surgical shock, hemorrhage, and other traumatic episodes may produce similar findings.

## Hair loss from endocrine causes

***Postpartum hair loss.*** During pregnancy less than one third of the normal number of hairs are resting, and after pregnancy more than twice the normal numbers are resting in preparation for being shed. Diffuse alopecia may occur from the first to the twelfth week after delivery and last for months. Regrowth is complete. This may be a glucocorticoid-produced phenomenon. A certain number of women who have been taking contraceptive pills report hair loss on discontinuation of the drug. The mechanism is not clear, and the pattern of hair regrowth is more prolonged than that occurring post partum.

***Hypothyroidism, hypoparathyroidism, diabetes mellitus, hyperthyroidism, and hypopituitarism.*** These disorders may result in reversible thinning of the scalp hair.

## Hair loss caused by malnutrition

"Crash" diets have been shown to cause hair loss by slowed growth rates in anagen, or by hairs turning into the resting or telogen phase. Protein deficiency will result in dry, brittle, fine sparse hair that is easily shed, although a severe, continued nutritional problem must exist to effect these changes (p. 229). Iron deficiency as well may result in a diffuse scalp hair thinning. Serum iron determinations are more valuable in assessing this problem than other indices (Hard).

## Hair loss caused by drugs

The anticoagulant drugs such as heparin, the folic acid antagonists, and thallium (pesticides) are the drugs most often responsible for diffuse hair loss. Coumarins, antimetabolites, quinacrine, arsenic, dextran, boric acid, clofibrate, triparanol, vitamin A excess, thiouracil, carbimazole, potassium thiocyanate, bismuth, amphetamines, androgens, and trimethadione have all been associated with a temporary alopecia. Salicylates have also been suggested as a cause.

Reeves and Maibach review the mechanisms in drug- and chemical-induced hair loss. They differentiate between anagen hair loss (antimitotic agents), telogen hair loss (oral contraceptives, anticoagulants, propranolol, triparanol, and thallium), and the unknown type of hair loss (antithyroids, clofibrate, boric acid, vitamin A).

## Hair loss caused by genetic defect

Muller records 48 such syndromes in which hair loss is a feature. The complete absence of hair over the scalp and body from birth is recorded. Some sparsity of the hair of the scalp and elsewhere is a common accompaniment of many hereditary syndromes. Often the hair in these states is scattered, thin, brittle, and hypopigmented. When associated with abnormal dentition, nail defects, and sweat gland aplasia, the condition may be included with congenital ectodermal defect. Some congenital alopecias are circumscribed, that is, small areas of hair loss that remain fixed.

## Genetic structural defects of hair

Poorly formed hairs are inherited in monilethrix (beaded hair), trichorrhexis invaginata (telescoped hairs), trichorrhexis nodosa (fractured, frayed hair), pili torti (twisted hair). The hair in these disorders may look sparse and abnormal grossly. Microscopic examination clarifies the disorders that may have other than genetic significance.

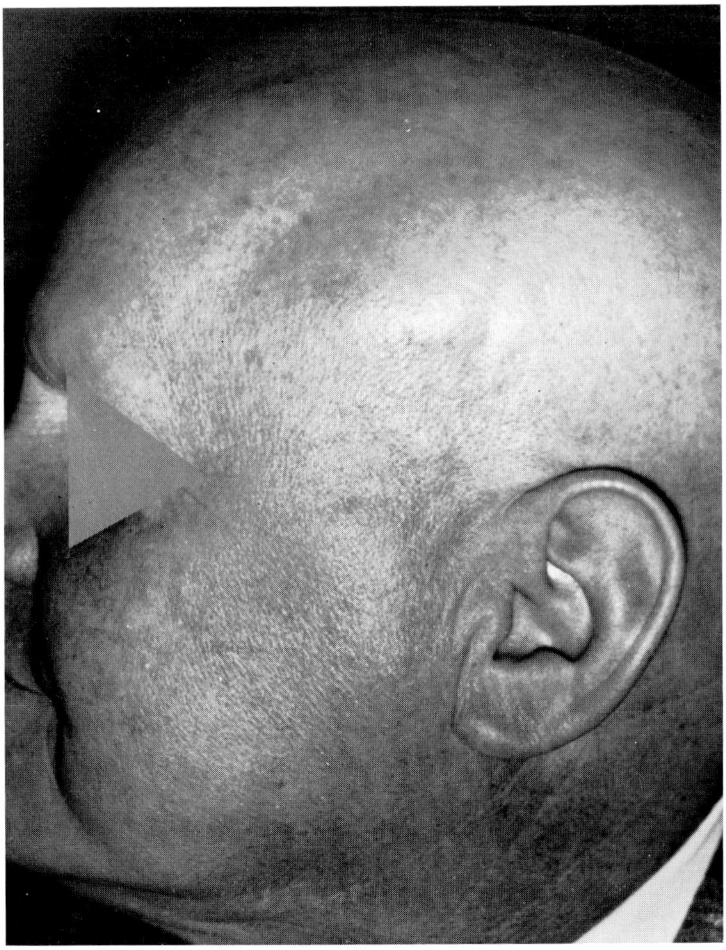

**Fig. 12-5.** Alopecia universalis. Hair was lost from all body and extremity areas as well.

## LOCALIZED ALOPECIA

### Alopecia areata

A common form of patchy hair loss, alopecia areata appears suddenly and is without symptoms. The involved areas may be one or all of the following sites—scalp, eyebrows, eyelashes, or beard. In the case of a generalized alopecia, all areas of hair growth on the body may be affected. Apart from the absence of hair from one or more circumscribed areas (Fig. 12-4, *B*), there are no other major accompanying clinical signs. Such an occurrence may be followed by other areas of baldness. One patch may show evidence of regrowth while another new area of hair loss makes its appearance. Nail changes, including pitting and ridging, even shedding, occur in about one tenth to one third of the cases. With the regrowth of hair, the new hair shafts may be initially white or gray, but with maturity, the hairs take on the normal pigmentation.

*Alopecia totalis* is a more severe form of alopecia areata, resulting in total loss of scalp hair.

*Alopecia universalis*, an unusual form of hair loss, results in total or near total loss of hair from all areas of the body (Fig 12-5).

Alopecia areata is about equally distributed between the sexes. It is found from infancy to old age, with most cases occurring before 40 years of age.

There is evidence of an association with autoimmune disorders, with atopic dermatitis, perhaps with some stressful initiator and a familial incidence.

There is a significant association with vitiligo (4%), thyroid disease (8%), and emotional stress prior to an episode of partial loss. There is no evidence of psychological disorder in most cases. Alopecia areata has been demonstrated by Kern and colleagues to be associated with circulating antibodies against thyroglobulin and the cytoplasm of parietal, thyroid, hair follicle, and adrenal cells.

In Stankler's review of 42 patients with chronic mucocutaneous candidosis, 44% had alopecia areata. This finding encourages the concept of association with immune deficiency and endocrine abnormality in some cases. Alopecia areata is frequent in the Down syndrome, which, itself, has immunological deficits.

Although an impressive number of patients report a traumatic or stressful episode prior to the onset of their alopecia, Whitlock, in reviewing the data, does not find the case proved to confirm psychologic causes in this disease.

A familial incidence of 10% rises to 18% if the disorder is alopecia totalis (Muller). Identical twins have been affected and there are reports of involvement affecting three generations in a family. Ikeda classifies patients with alopecia areata into four groups, on the basis of records of 1989 patients.

Her classification is important for prognosis and treatment:

1. *Common type:* 83% of all cases between 20 and 40 years of age with a 6-month duration of individual patches and total clearing in 3 years. Chance of total alopecia, 6%. Some psychosocial stress is present.
2. *Atopic type:* 10% of all cases, children chiefly; patches last more than 1 year. The disease lasts more than 10 years, and the chance of total alopecia is 75%.
3. *Prehypertensive:* Less than 7% of all cases. 20 years of age or older, and 39% chance of total alopecia.
4. *Endocrine-autonomic:* Less than 7% of all cases. 40 years and above. Chance of total alopecia 10%.

Rook has reclassified Ikeda's grouping for his own 200 patients. It should be mentioned that recognition of Ikeda's perspicacity belongs to Rook. He classifies the patients with alopecia areata as follows:

| | |
|---|---|
| 1. Personal atopic history; persistent in children | Chance of total alopecia 32% |
| 2. Personal autoimmune history; all older women | Chance of total alopecia 58% |
| 3. Family atopic history | Intermediate features |
| 4. Family autoimmune history | Intermediate features |

| | |
|---|---|
| 5. No personal or family history of either form; short attacks, young adults | Chance of total alopecia 14% |

This appears to be a valuable predictive grouping, and results of therapy should be based on classification such as this rather than be lumped together.

### *Diagnosis*

Examination of the affected area reveals a smooth, virtually hair-free surface, with notably smooth, soft skin. Follicles are present, but no individual hairs are likely. At the periphery of the patch, which may be sharp or which may blend in with growing scalp hairs, one finds many hairs easily tugged from the scalp. On examination of their shafts, it is apparent that the diameter lessens to a constriction, a spear point, or a small bulb, denoting some decrease in hair size prior to shedding. There may or may not be a clear bulb. There are also tapering, but short (3 to 5 mm.), broken-off hairs apparent in the scalp. These are referred to as exclamation-point hairs. Biopsy may be used to confirm diagnosis. Affected hairs possess a lymphocytic inflammation around hair sheaths and atrophic anagen hairs.

### *Differential diagnosis*

The complete absence of scaling, scarring, inflammation, or crusting differentiates alopecia areata from most other patchy alopecias of fungal, bacterial, or inflammatory origin.

*Syphilitic alopecia* is more ragged, and the hair loss within the patch is incomplete. It tends to involve the posterior scalp.

*Trichotillomania*, produced by habitual pulling of small groups of hairs, demonstrates broken hairs of various sizes in the irregular patches.

### *Treatment*

The uneveness of treatment results cannot be judged until the natural course is known. If Ikeda's, Mali's, and Rook's (and others) concept that some forms will regrow within 6 months and some never completely is correct, all claims for therapy are meaningless until these groups are defined.

We do not believe, in most instances, that it is justifiable to start an individual on systemic glucocorticoids until we can tell them how this therapy will benefit their form of the disease.

Topical or intralesional use of glucocorticoids such as triamcinolone acetonide or betamethasone valerate may be of benefit. This is especially the case in the treatment of a single patch of alopecia where glucocorticoid ointments under occlusion can be used in concentrations such as 0.1% betamethasone, 0.025% fluocinolone, or 0.05% flurandrenolone, or where a sublesional injection of 1 to 2 ml. of triamcinolone in a concentration of 10 mg./ml. can be given. Neither is effective in the more severe or extensive forms of alopecia areata.

Oral steroid therapy is not dependable or predictable in regrowing hair.

Interestingly, Happle and Enternacht, after Rosenberg's successful initiation, have recently demonstrated regrowth of scalp hair in 33 patients with alopecia areata. Twenty-six of 31 patients with a history of the disorder for 5 years or less, and 7 of 12 patients with a history of the disorder for 5 or more years, were successful in regrowing hair at the site of treatment. Therapy consisted of sensitizing the patient to dinitrochlorobenzene, a very potent sensitizer dissolved in acetone, and then applying a dilute solution capable of producing a mild inflammatory reaction only, daily. It would seem wise before exposing patients irresponsibly to the hazards of this very potent sensitizer, to be thoroughly aware of the type of alopecia areata that responds to this therapy and the chance of success.

Abell and Munro found the use of the jet injector disappointing except in recent, small areas of involvement.

Many forms of local vasodilators have been used in an effort to stimulate hair growth. They must be applied over small areas only, with care to avoid excessive use.

## Localized alopecia with scar formation

In patients with *discoid lupus erythematosus*, alopecia with scar formation is not uncommon. Initially, the affected area becomes

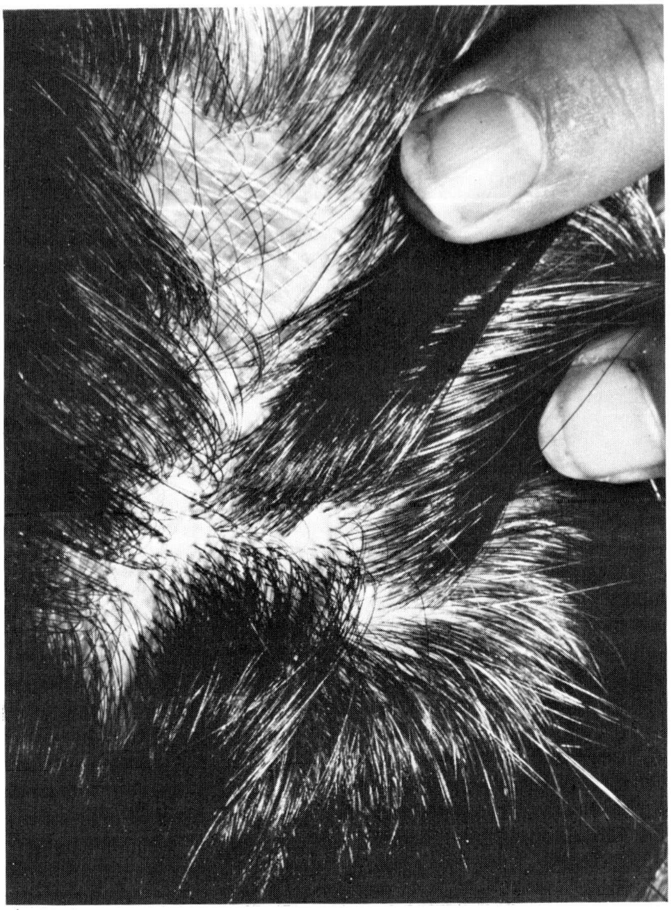

**Fig. 12-6.** Cicatricial alopecia. Idiopathic, progressive, permanent hair loss, unassociated with systemic disease.

red and slightly scaly. This condition is followed by alopecia and scar formation. Biopsy may be necessary to establish the diagnosis.

There are two rather rare skin disorders producing hair loss that result in patchy, scarred, residual lesions. Referred to as the cicatricial alopecias (Fig. 12-6), they include *pseudopelade,* with round or oval, smooth, nonregenerating, scarred areas that result from a folliculitis process, and *folliculitis decalvans,* a pustular alopecia.

Other forms of scarring alopecia include localized scleroderma, burns and scalds, radiation effect, lichen planus, furunculosis, and some forms of tinea capitis.

Tuberculosis of the skin, leprosy, leishmaniasis, zoster, and syphilis can demonstrate scarring when involving the scalp. Sarcoid, necrobiosis, pemphigoid, and cutaneous neoplasma produce scarring and permanent hair loss.

## Trichotillomania

See p. 478.

### REFERENCES

Abell, E., and Monro, P. D.: Intralesional treatment of alopecia areata with triamcinolone acetonide by jet injector, Br. J. Dermatol. 88:55, 1973.
**Usefulness limited to localized areas.**

Carter, D. M., and Jegasothy, B. V.: Alopecia areata and Down syndrome, Arch. Dermatol. 112:1347, 1976.
**19 of 214 cases had alopecia areata.**

Editorial: Alopecia areata, Br. Med. J. 1:335, 1977.
**Conclusion: no satisfactory explanation.**

Goette, D. K., and Odom, R. B.: Alopecia in crash dieters, J.A.M.A. **235**:2622, 1976.
**Nine patients, 2 to 5 months after initiating a stringent diet.**

Griffiths, W. A. D.: Diffuse hair loss and oral contraceptives, Br. J. Dermatol. **88**:31, 1973.
**Occurs 2 to 3 months after use because of a mechanism different from that in pregnancy.**

Hard, S.: Nonanemic iron deficiency as an etiologic factor in diffuse loss of hair of the scalp of woman, Acta Derm. Venereol. **43**:562, 1963.
**Of 96 cases, 18% showed iron deficiency corrected by oral iron.**

Ikeda, T.: A new classification for alopecia areata, Dermatologica **131**:421, 1965.
**1,989 patients reviewed and a natural history of the disease emerged that she grouped into four significant types.**

Kligman, A. M.: Pathologic dynamics of human hair loss. I. Telogen effluvium, Arch Dermatol. **83**:175, 1961.
**More than 25% telogen hairs comprise effluvium.**

Ludwig, E.: Classification of the types of androgenetic alopecia (common baldness) occurring in the female sex, Br. J. Dermatol. **97**:247, 1977.
**Grades I, II and III, based on 468 cases, illustrated.**

Mali, J.W.H.: Alopecia areata, Br. J. Dermatol. **93**:605, 1975.
**Confirmation of Ikeda's classification.**

Muller, S. A.: Alopecia: syndromes of genetic significance, J. Invest. Dermatol. **60**:475, 1973
**Most cases of alopecia are not related to hormonal factors directly.**

Norwood, O.T.: Male pattern baldness. Classification and incidence, South. Med. J. **68**:1359, 1975.
**Patterns in 1,000 white adult males.**

Orentreich, N.: Hair transplant. In Maddin, S., editor: Current dermatologic management, St. Louis, 1975, The C. V. Mosby Co., p. 26.
**Methodology and patient reaction.**

Reeves, J. R. T., and Maibach, H. I.: Drug and chemical induced hair loss. In Marzulli, F. N., and Maibach, H. I., editors: Advances in modern toxicology. Vol. 4, Dermatotoxicology and pharmacology, New York, 1977, John Wiley & Sons, p. 487.
**A practical approach to identifying the etiologic agent.**

Rook, A.: Common baldness and alopecia areata. In Rook, A., editor: Recent advances in dermatology, Edinburgh, 1977, Churchill Livingstone, p. 223.
**The distillation of humanity, observation, acumen, and reflection.**

Rosenberg, W. E.: Alopecia areata (case report), Arch. Dermatol. **112**:256, 1976.
**The initial report of successful growth by nonempiric therapy.**

Saitoh, M., Uzuka, M., and Sakamoto, M.: Human hair cycle, J. Invest. Dermatol. **54**:65, 1970.
**An exact photographic record.**

Stankler, L., and Bewsher, P. D.: Chronic mucocutaneous candidiasis, endocrine deficiency and alopecia areata, Br. J. Dermatol. **86**:238, 1972.
**An association of immune deficits.**

Whitlock, F. A.: Psychophysiological aspects of skin disease. London, 1976, W. B. Saunders Co., Ltd., p. 183.
**Although there is a frequent history of intense trauma preceding hair loss, the case for psychologic causation has not been proved beyond reasonable doubt.**

Winter, R. J., Kern, F., and Blizzard, R. M.: Prednisone therapy for alopecia areata, Arch. Dermatol. **112**:1549, 1976.
**Discouraging.**

## HYPERTRICHOSIS AND HIRSUTISM

*Hypertrichosis* identifies nonspecified excessive hair growth of all types. *Hirsutism* applies to excessive hair growth of androgen-induced origin in the female of a type and distribution to simulate the male.

To establish a base line of hair distribution in a normal young female population, a Welsh study examined 400 university students. Almost one tenth were clinically hirsute, showing a male pattern of hair quantity and distribution of sufficient extent to cause concern to themselves. From this study, a concept of the degree of hirsutism in a group of young white women may be obtained from the following figures:

Face—26% of subjects had hair on upper lip. In 10% the condition was easily apparent.
Chest—17% had periareolar breast hair.
Abdomen—35% had linea alba–located midabdominal hair; 10% had a masculine type of upper border to the pubic hair.
Lumbosacral region—16% had coarse hair in this area.
Arms and legs—84% had coarse hair on the extremities.

Genetic effects are important in determining amount and, to some extent, distribution of hair. Muller points out the differences in the reported degree and distribution of hair in various races. Near Eastern women are more hirsute and Oriental women much less so than the average white North American. The hormone levels to which an individual's hair follicles will respond are probably genetically determined. A greatly hirsute young woman may be one member of a line of hairy ancestors and yet be an endocrinologically normal individual. Great individual variation is apparent in the amount of hairiness possessed by normal men and women. Also, factors of illness, end-organ responsiveness, other endocrine glands, and many unknown factors play significant roles in abnormal hair growth. According to Muller, 1% of women complaining of excessive hair growth will have an endocrinological abnormality affecting the pituitary gland, adrenal glands, or ovaries.

The causes of hirsutism are the following:

1. Adrenal disorders
   a. Hyperplasia
   b. Tumor
   c. Cushing's syndrome
2. Ovarian disorders
   a. Dysfunction polycystic (Stein-Leventhal)
   b. Tumor (arrhenoblastoma, other)
3. Drugs
4. Nonendocrine diseases—porphyria, anorexia nervosa

Kirschner et al. have clearly demonstrated that hirsute women may have elevated testosterone production rates and high androstenedione plasma levels. These androgens were ovarian in origin in virtually all of their 44 patients despite normal-sized ovaries. Dexamethasone suppressed the androgen levels. Luteinizing hormone (LH) stimulates androgen production and inhibition of LH by depomedroxyprogesterone acetate has been shown to benefit hirsute females.

Because adrenal and ovarian tumors are not primarily dermatological problems, they will not be discussed here.

*The female with a distinctly masculine type of hair distribution pattern attributable to endocrinological androgen-producing abnormalities* is likely to have coarse, pigmented hair on face, breasts, lumbosacral area, and shoulders or upper back. Clitoral hypertrophy is the most significant physical finding. She will tend to have persistent menstrual disorders, acne, obesity, and possibly hypertension, although recently it has been shown that there are cases of virilization by excessive androgens *with normal menses*.

With increasing knowledge of the limits of normal female hormone levels and excretion, more knowledge will be forthcoming concerning the hirsute adult woman and the details of her endocrinological disorder. *Testosterone* is by far the most potent cause of female hirsutism, and estimation of plasma levels of this hormone is the most significant laboratory investigation in many cases, although normal levels may overlap into the pathological range.

Blair and Reuter described the use of adrenal venography in 50 women with virilization. Thirty-six had normal patterns, 11 had adrenal hypertrophy, and three had patterns suggestive of adrenal tumors, two confirmed by surgery.

## Drug-induced hirsutism

Drugs are an increasingly common cause of excessive hair growth. Androgens, such as testosterone, progesterone, and norethindrone, and anabolic compounds can cause virilization and hirsutism, although individual susceptibility is an important factor.

Phenytoin (diphenylhydantoin sodium, Dilantin) causes hirsutism affecting the face, trunk, and extremities. Corticotropin (ACTH) produces hirsutism to a variable and unpredictable degree. Diazoxide causes hypertrichosis in children and less commonly in adults.

### *Investigation*

History
- Details of onset
- Progression
- Menstrual history
- Physical development
- Mental achievement
- Drug history
- Family history of hirsutism (confirmed)
- Genetic background

Examination
- Description of hairiness, type, distribution
- Blood pressure
- Examination of bodily status, male or female habits

Genitals
- Clitoral enlargement
- Pelvic examination
- Size of ovaries
- Uterus development

Signs of virilization
- Amenorrhea, mammary atrophy, temporal scalp alopecia, voice deepening, masculine body contours, and clitoral hypertrophy

Laboratory examination at this date is placed in the hands of a competent internist-endocrinologist.

### *Treatment*

Surgery is required for treatment of adrenal tumor, and treatment with glucocorticoids is required for adrenal hyperplasia.

Luteinizing hormone suppressors may be applicable and safe in individual cases.

Cyproterone acetate has been used to reduce idiopathic hirsutism successfully with decreased hairiness over limbs, face, and torso within 2 months. Its topical use indicates a promising field for the future.

Since women are concerned about the appearance of facial hair, those with apparent upper lip or chin hair will seek aid in removing it. *If there is no endocrinological basis for the hair growth*, they can be advised of the following methods of hair removal:

1. Diathermy is the quickest method, but carries the greatest risk of scarring by a careless or inexperienced operator.
2. Electrolysis, using a galvanic (direct) current, is tedious but effective. With care it is relatively painless.
3. Depilatories consist of easily available commercial creams that contain barium or calcium sulfide or calcium thiosulfate. They may be locally irritating. Most women use this method for temporary removal of facial hair.
4. Shaving, either with electric or safety razors, does not to our knowledge increase or thicken subsequent hair growth but is not looked on with favor by most women.
5. Gently rubbing the area with a pumice stone is a long-established and satisfactory method, but may enhance the hair growth through hyperemia and continued irritation.
6. Plucking, although commonly used in small areas, may lead to infection and distorted follicles, either of which can result in further complications of hair growth.
7. Wax or tape and glue depilatories are moulded on the skin and then are pulled suddenly while still soft and pliable. The hair that returns is not blunt or bristly.
8. Bleaching of multiple, fine, pigmented hairs may be the most satisfactory method for some individuals. A solution of hydrogen peroxide and ammonia is used. This is easy to apply and simply depigments the hair, rendering it less conspicuous.

#### REFERENCES


Blair, A. J., and Reuter, S. R.: Adrenal venography in virilized women, J.A.M.A. **213**:1623, 1970.
**Three of 50 probably tumors.**

Ebling, F. J., Thomas, A. K., Cooke, I. D., et al.: Effect of cyproterone acetate on hair growth, sebaceous secretion and endocrine parameters in a hirsute subject, Br. J. Dermatol. **97**:371, 1977.
**Hair growth, size, and sebum were reduced in 2 months.**

Kirschner, M. A., Zucker, I. R., and Jesperson, D.: Idiopathic hirsutism: an ovarian abnormality, N. Engl. J. Med. **294**:637, 1976.
**Establishes the ovary as the source of excessive androgen production, primarily testosterone.**

MacKnight, E.: The prevalence of hirsutism in young women, Lancet **1**:410, 1964.
**Distribution of body hair in 400 consecutive women students at the University of Wales.**

Muller, S.: Hirsutism, Am. J. Med. **46**:803, 1969.
**Often quoted.**

Price, V. H.: Testosterone metabolism in the skin. A review of its function in androgenetic alopecia, acne vulgaris and idiopathic hirsutism including recent studies with antiandrogens, Arch. Dermatol. **111**:1496, 1975.
**A review leading up to the use of antiandrogens.**

CHAPTER **13**

# Bacterial infections

## SKIN ECOLOGY

Immense numbers of bacteria reside on the human skin, described in terms of millions of organisms (for example, 4 million on the hands). They appear to live on the skin in microcolonies rather than as individuals, with a range of 1,400 to 10,000 cells per colony (aerobes) in one study (Noble and Somerville). After use of antibacterial soaps, completely different results can be obtained by bacteria counts versus colony counts. It is concluded that the effect may be to reduce the size but not the number of colonies. The colonies, seen on scanning electron microscopy, are on the skin surface and in follicle openings. Some bacteria reside under the outer few cell layers, but, of these, the majority are found in the first 0.3 mm. depth of skin.

The normal bacterial flora of the human skin includes the following: coagulase-negative staphylococci (which have become important because of their propensity to colonize sites of cardiovascular and orthopedic prostheses and to cause infective endocarditis), coagulase-positive staphylococci (*Staphylococcus aureus*, when present, seems related to contamination from nasal carriage or in the navel of infants), nonhemolytic streptococci, diphtheroids, corynebacteria (including *Corynebacterium acnes*), gram-negative bacilli (including *Mima, Escherichia coli*, and *Proteus*), and *Pseudomonas* organisms.

The major pathogenic bacterium is the staphylococcus, followed closely by the streptococcus. Degrees of pathogenicity depend on the organism's invasiveness and toxicogenicity; the host skin, in which dryness and integrity act as barriers; and the immune and cellular defenses of the host.

Interaction between bacteria, competitive mechanisms, antibacterial substances produced by one strain against others of its species (bacteriocins) and substances harmful to other strains have been investigated and appear to be important in determining the flora present in a geographic site. Aly reviews the effects of systemic and topical antibacterial agents on the skin flora. Systemic antibiotics only affect the cutaneous resident bacteria if they are concentrated in sweat, diffuse through epidermis, or are incorporated into epidermal or sebaceous cells. Tetracycline profoundly affects cutaneous populations and multiple or mixed antibiotic therapy increases gram-negative infections and candidosis. Topical antimicrobials in soaps and deodorants seem to produce few complications or problems.

No short summary or list can give significant information, and the reader is referred to the many excellent reference works available on this topic.

Marples' *Ecology of the Human Skin* has carefully detailed, factual material on all aspects of normal and abnormal skin bacteria populations. Considerable insight into the ways of the staphylococcus, as well as other pathogenic cutaneous bacteria, is to be found in the book edited by Maibach and Hildick-Smith. The *Microbiology of the Skin* by Noble and Somerville is in the tradition of Marples with a global view of the importance of their subject but an intimate knowledge of the organisms they deal with. The impressive volume on *Infectious Diseases* edited by Paul Hoeprich is recommended highly for its up-to-date detail, although references are not extensive.

## ANTIBACTERIAL THERAPY

In a recent review of antimicrobials in the *Mayo Clinic Proceedings* (**52**:601, 1977), Hermans presents a concise rational basis for the use of these drugs. It is recommended for reading by all who treat infectious disease. The particulars of each are found in the following:

| | | |
|---|---|---|
| Hermans | General principles of antimicrobial therapy, | p. 603 |
| Wilkowske | The penicillins, | p. 616 |
| Thompson | The cephalosporins, | p. 625 |
| Geraci | Vancomycin, | p. 631 |
| Wilson | Tetracyclines, chloramphenicol, erythromycin, clindamycin, | p. 635 |
| Brewer | The aminoglycosides | p. 675 |

## STAPHYLOCOCCI

Staphylococci invade through the pilosebaceous apparatus, become localized, and are difficult to attack with antimicrobial agents because of the "walling-off" process of the inflammatory reaction. A local area of infection is associated with an almost immediate increase in numbers of bacteria all over the skin surface, which serve as a source of continuing infections. Furuncles, carbuncles, impetigo, and abscesses are the usual lesions produced.

The incidence of staphylococcal infections decreases with increasing age. The location of lesions varies with the sex of the individual. In males the most frequent sites of staphylococcal lesions are the upper extremities, buttocks, upper thighs, neck, and chest. Females are more likely to develop lesions in the axillae, the pubic area, and, in lactating women, the breasts.

Most staphylococci cultured from infected lesions of outpatients are sensitive to routinely used antibiotics. Hospital infections, however, are frequently penicillin resistant. Recurrent pyogenic infections, both dermatological and internal, may be the presenting sign of gamma globulin deficiencies, as reported by Schur and his colleagues.

***Carriers of staphylococci.*** More than half the general population harbor staphylococci in the external nares, and in many individuals these organisms can also be cultured from the perineum (22%) and in some cases the toe webs (23% in children). Hair is a surprisingly common source (10% in adults and 50% in eczema patients). Also, a damaged area of skin quickly becomes a focus of staphylococci.

Staphylococci readily colonize in moist cutaneous lesions, which may prove a prolific source of dissemination, yet give little clinical sign of their presence. Isolation of disseminators and patients particularly prone to infection in hospitals significantly reduces the colonization rate with resistant strains (Nystrom and Molin).

Areas of skin that have healed after an active staphylococcal lesion can become a residence of the bacteria for months and even years afterward, in the deeper layers of the stratum corneum. Most infants quickly become carriers of *Staphylococcus aureus*, with the nostrils, axillae, groin, and particularly the umbilicus being the areas from which the organism can be most frequently cultured.

Certain strains of staphylococci are dermotropic and colonize and flourish in the layers of the corneum. *Phage type 71* is one of these strains and can be isolated in most cases of impetigo. *Phage type 80/81*, the hospital infection strain, is also dermotropic and readily transmissible. It may be more virulent than other strains. Once the skin is colonized, it can be shown that the incidence of pyodermas in the individual and his contacts rises measurably.

## STREPTOCOCCI

The following is a classification of streptococci (Noble and Somerville)

- Alpha hemolytic—present in most mouths and on hands
  - *Streptococcus viridans*, *S. mitis*, *S. mutans*
- Beta-hemolytic groups (Lancefield) causing disease
  - A. *Streptococcus pyogenes*
  - B. Human pathogen
  - C. Animal strain
  - D. Enterococci
  - G. Human pathogen
- Gamma-hemolytic "indifferent" streptococci

Beta-hemolytic streptococci multiply beneath the stratum corneum under semianaerobic conditions, after entry has been gained by some injury to the skin. They may be rapidly destroyed on the surface of the skin by the fatty acids. Some 10% or less of group A beta-hemolytic streptococci are considered to be resistant to tetracycline.

Streptococci readily colonize cutaneous infections, although not so frequently as staphylococci. It is interesting to note that clinical observations indicating far-reaching effects of streptococcal infection have not been clarified, despite considerable good investigative study. Striking cutaneous complications of streptococcal pharyngitis include vasculitis, erythema nodosum, guttate psoriasis, and a unique nodular reaction on the elbows and knees. Levene has reviewed current knowledge of these disorders, pointing out that such mechanisms as decreased antibody response to specific streptococcal antigens, cross-reaction of streptococcal antigens, cross-reaction of streptococcal antibodies with skin antigens, and abnormalities of individual host responses may be operative.

***Carriers of streptococci.*** Some streptococci can be harbored in the nostrils. They have been found in 10% of normal individuals in mouths, on hands, and in toe webs. In patients with pyoderma, 50% of skins sampled were carrying beta-hemolytic streptococci. This leads to a wide dissemination of streptococci to other hosts. Streptococci have as their main human headquarters the throat and respiratory passages.

## Impetigo

Impetigo is a highly contagious, rapidly spreading cutaneous infection that begins as an erythema and quickly develops eroded vesicles with an oozing, sticky fluid. It is exceptionally pruritic at this stage. Shortly, crusts begin to form from the fluid, and the lesion enlarges peripherally, as well as spreading by satellite lesions. It usually appears first in the central facial area adjacent to the nose and mouth and, depending on its severity, may spread widely or remain localized (Fig. 13-1, *A*). The disorder may occur at any site.

### *Pertinent information*

*Impetigo is produced by coagulase-positive staphylococci and by beta-hemolytic streptococci.* It is possible that under certain circumstances each genus mutually promotes the growth of the other, thus producing the rapid spread that is characteristic of some of these lesions. Because of the much more significant role of the streptococcus in these infections, impetigo should be considered a streptococcal disorder. Acute glomerulonephritis may develop in 2% to 5% of patients, because of the nephritogenic strain of beta-hemolytic streptococci that causes the disorder. Impetigo in an adult may have a more serious prognosis than impetigo occurring in childhood. Geographic factors are also important here, and streptococci seem more likely to participate actively in impetigo in tropical and semitropical areas. Also, biting insects, mosquitoes, and flies appear to be important in transmission of these infections.

*Bullous impetigo* is a similar malady, but is characterized by bullous lesions containing turbid fluid. The thin bullae soon rupture, leaving thin crusts. It is usually attributable to phage group II staphylococci alone.

### *Microscopic findings*

Microscopic studies of impetigo reveal an acute inflammatory exudate throughout the epidermis, with early vesicle and bulla formation immediately beneath the stratum corneum. There are large numbers of neutrophils, which, together with fibrin, form the characteristic crust.

### *Investigation*

Culture of the lesion with antibiotic sensitivity tests for both staphylococci and streptococci should be performed. Urinalysis for microscopic hematuria may be performed, both during the episode and again about 6 weeks afterwards.

### *Treatment*

Erythromycin and phenoxymethyl penicillin orally in weight-regulated doses should be given at the onset of extensive, rapidly spreading, or unusual cases of impetigo or where there are other cases among contacts. Cloxacillin should be used if the organism is penicillinase-producing, and cephalexin if the patient is sensitive to penicillin. One should

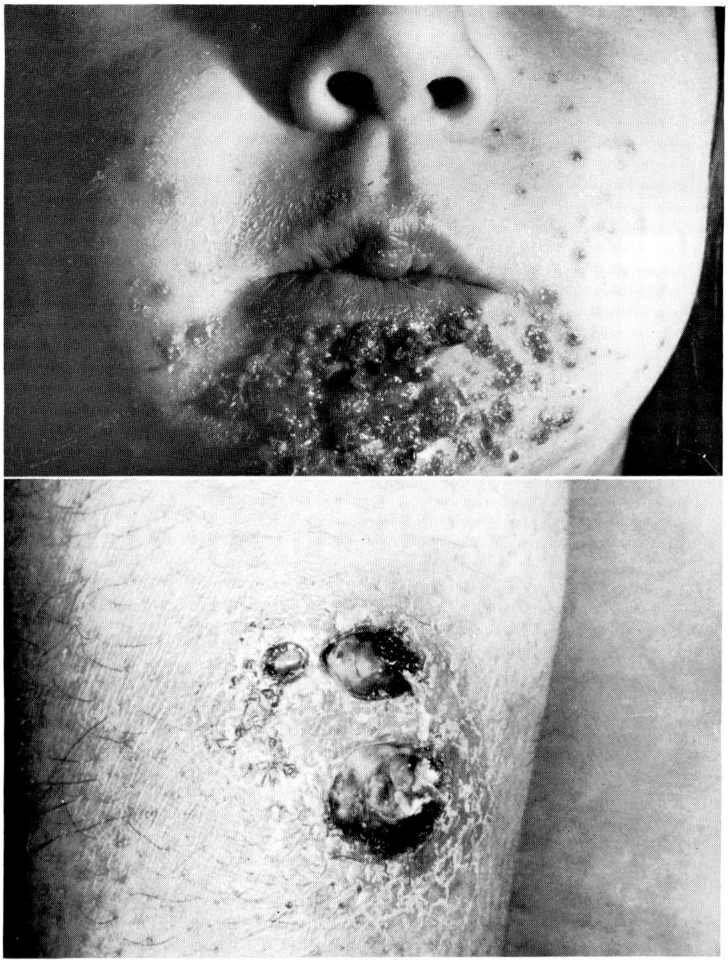

A

B

**Fig. 13-1.** Bacterial infections. **A,** Impetigo contagiosa. **B,** Ecthyma of leg. One crust is in place on lower lesion. Crust on upper lesion has been removed.

note that it is not proved that this therapy prevents development of nephritis though prophylactic.

If bacteremia is threatening, or the patient is seriously ill, nafcillin 150 to 200 mg./kg./day I.V. in 4 doses or cefazolin 75 to 100 mg./kg./ day I.V., q.i.d., should be prescribed. Penicillin G can be used if the staphylococcus is penicillinase-negative.

Thorough cleansing of the area with soap and water will help prevent the condition from spreading. All family members should avoid unessential direct contact with the patient during the disorder and until danger of infection is over.

Burow's solution, prepackaged tablets or powders of aluminum acetate (1 tablet or package of powder to 1 pint of cool water), is used as a compress on the crusts. After the area is thoroughly softened (about 20 to 25 minutes), crusts are usually easily removed. Neomycin, preferably in combination with an antiseptic such as chlorhexidine, should be applied three times daily, after the compresses. These may well be applied to the nostrils also (Williams).

## Ecthyma

Ecthyma (Fig. 13-1, *B*) is a deeper infection than impetigo, often developing because of neglect or lack of appropriate treatment measures for the initial infection. It occurs most often on the legs and develops as an erythematous, moist, then eroded and crusted lesion, going through these stages rather rapidly. It does not spread peripherally, as does facial impetigo, but burrows more deeply into the tissues. Bandaging with an occlusive and infrequently changed dressing leads to the deep, ulcerated, bowl-shaped lesions of ecthyma.

Bacteriological studies of ecthyma reveal essentially the same pattern of causative organisms as in impetigo.

### *Treatment*

As for impetigo, after culture.

Compresses of Burow's solution in cool water, along with the prepackaged medication, will soften the crusts, which should be removed. Hexachlorophene-, povidone-iodine-, or chlorhexidine-containing soaps can be used in bathing to reduce contamination in adults.

## Folliculitis

Folliculitis is a variable disease, with lesions ranging from minute, white-topped pustules in the newborn infant to large, yellow, pus-containing tender lesions in the adult scalp or beard (Fig. 13-2). The staphylococci rapidly take advantage of hair-damaged or blocked pilosebaceous units and sweat glands to colonize in these areas. If they are blocked for any reason, a staphylococcal folliculitis may quickly follow.

Newborn infants may demonstrate multiple lesions of forehead, face, and neck that are nonerythematous but reveal staphylococcal organisms on culture. These lesions ordinarily respond quite satisfactorily to therapy.

In adults the lesion of folliculitis is a discrete, reddened, indurated, tender papule with a developing central pustule, often pierced by a hair or located over a follicular orifice. These lesions are found in hairy areas, such as thigh, face, scalp, groin, or axilla. In the bearded area of males there may be a collection of these minute abscesses, which are closely adjacent and produce a rather wide, reddened, tender induration of the area around them. If they persist, the condition can become chronic and difficult to eradicate. In these chronic cases histopathological examination reveals an infiltrate largely composed of lymphocytes, rather than polymorphs and an inflammatory process that tends to involve the deeper layers of the dermis.

Differential diagnosis includes an oil or grease folliculitis, pustular folliculitis from occlusive tape dressings or hot, humid environment.

### *Treatment*

All lesions suspected of being bacterial should be cultured.

***Facial folliculitis of infants.*** Thorough cleansing with soap, povidone-iodine, or chlorhexidine cleansers, followed by a neomycin-containing drying lotion is ordinarily curative. The nose should be treated with applications of the lotion as well.

***Adult folliculitis.*** More extensive treatment is necessary for folliculitis in adults.

1. Culture and sensitivity studies may be required to determine antibiotic resistance. Antibiotics chosen on the basis of these studies should be given systemically, supplemented by the topical therapy described below.
2. Hexachlorophene-, povidone-iodine-, or chlorhexidine-containing soap should be used for thorough cleansing of the area in adults.
3. Topical neomycin or bacitracin lotion or cream in combinations to reduce resistance is helpful when applied three times daily. The nostrils should be thoroughly treated with the topical medication in an attempt to eliminate carrier infections. Gentamicin 0.3% is most effective, but to avoid resistance developing, neomycin plus chlorhexidine is a good combination.

Many peeling and drying acne lotions provide a drying and antibacterial effect that is most salutary in preventing recurrence (benzoyl peroxide gel, lotions). Drying and peeling of the epidermis, as opposed to macera-

A

B

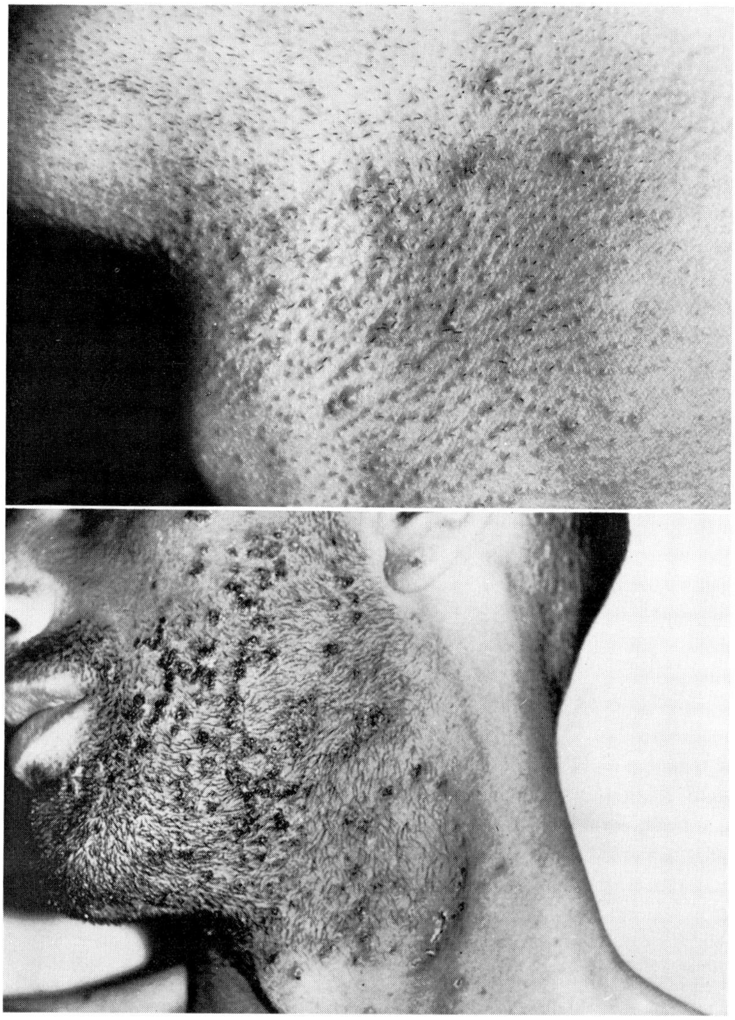

**Fig. 13-2. A,** Early stage of folliculitis. **B,** Folliculitis with crusted lesions.

tion by creams and ointments, is essential to aid the natural defenses.

## Recurrent staphylococcal infections

***Impetigo (atopic dermatitis).*** Atopic patients have recently been demonstrated to show recurrent very superficial bacterial infections, chiefly staphylococcal (p. 122) as a result of their variable immune defect. This is more pronounced with active atopic dermatitis and less apparent during remissions. These are usually localized, erythematous plaques and patches, crusted and excoriated, moist and very pruritic. Culture and sensitivity tests reveal the cause, and a course of oral antibiotics selected on the basis of the tests will prove satisfactory. The patient appears to suffer a temporary derangement of host-bacterial resistance that may include deficits in cellular phagocytosis, chemotaxis, and even humorocellular immune mechanisms.

***Furuncle and carbuncle.*** A furuncle develops as a small perifollicular abscess that ordinarily destroys the hair and the follicle during its early stages. It is a deep inflammation and produces residual scarring.

A carbuncle involves more than one pilosebaceous unit and may involve many. There may be regional lymphadenopathy.

Characteristically, because of the increase

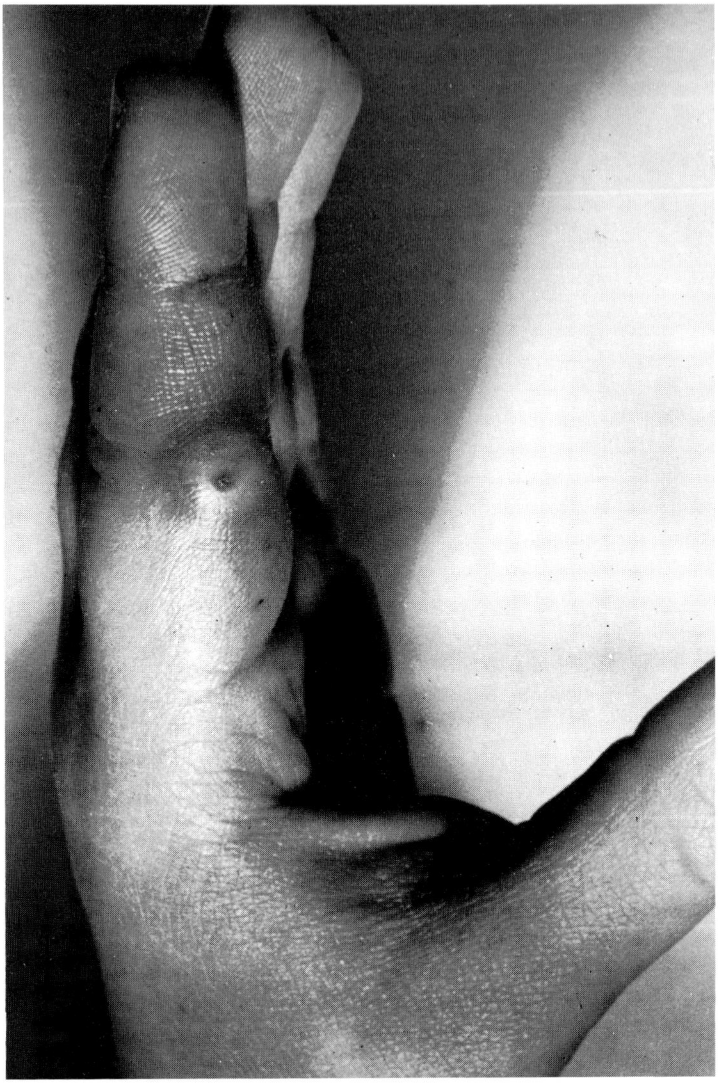

**Fig. 13-3.** Staphylococcal pyoderma.

in numbers of staphylococci generally on the remainder of the skin surface, new lesions follow, and a recurrence even in a healed initial lesion is common. Other members of the patient's family are likely to develop cutaneous lesions. Trauma, friction, retained moisture, and macerated or bruised skin all predispose to recurrences of staphylococcal cutaneous infection. This is often a recurrent and persistant problem in a family environment, and its eradication requires much care and patience (Fig. 13-3).

***Hidradenitis suppurativa.*** A dysfunction of the apocrine glands, hidradenitis suppurativa results in recurrent staphylococcal (ordinarily not coagulase-positive) invasion of the duct and secretory portion of the gland (see p. 90).

### *Differential diagnosis*

***Acne vulgaris.*** Acne vulgaris is a pustular dermatitis affecting adolescents and consisting of essentially *sterile* lesions developing from comedones.

***Sebaceous cysts.*** Sebaceous cysts are smooth, globular lesions that may become infected and simulate a boil.

***Actinomycosis.*** Actinomycosis causes painful pustular swelling of the face, neck, or sinus tracts, with purulent discharge. Culture reveals the organism.

### *Management*

Patients with recurrent staphylococcal skin and respiratory infections must be surveyed for evidence of immune deficiency. This may rest in the leukocyte function, humoral or cellular immune mechanisms, or elsewhere. Such patients may not be severely compromised, and the defect may be variable. Atopic patients may demonstrate this immune defect (Dahl). Also diabetes must be ruled out in recurrent staphylococcal disease.

No simple remedy exists for the treatment of otherwise normal patients with chronic lesions caused by recurrent and persistent cutaneous staphylococcal infection. A clearly explained program for the general hygiene and care of the patient and his family must be instituted. Culture and sensitivity tests are performed on the patient, but similar tests from nasal and potential carrier sites in each member of the family are a wise and often very helpful measure in these difficult and recurrent infections. Hair is often overlooked as a source of pathogens. Summers and colleagues have demonstrated its importance. All towels, linen, and articles of clothing used by the patient should be kept separate until thoroughly laundered. The patient's hands and face should be cleansed thoroughly several times daily with hexachlorophene-, povidone-iodine-, or chlorhexidine-containing liquid soap. Full baths or showers should be taken daily.

The patient should be effectually isolated from close contact with other family members, all of whom should bathe daily with hexachlorophene, povidone-iodine, or chlorhexidine-containing liquid soap. Infants and young children should not use hexachlorophene.

All moist skin areas should be kept dry with antiperspirants or alcohol-containing shake lotions, since *dryness inhibits growth of bacteria on the skin.*

Draining or moist lesions should be kept covered with a thin dressing, which should be changed when contaminated. All used dressings, bandages, and so forth must be burned.

*Culture and sensitivity tests must be performed to determine the antibiotic of choice,* and full doses of this drug should be given for at least a week. The choices are as follows:

Penicillin V, 15 to 20 mg./kg./day in four equal doses every 6 hours. (Cloxacillin, dicloxacillin, or amoxicillin are also relatively gastric acid–resistant and may be used in penicillinase-producing infections.)

Cephalexin, 20 to 30 mg./kg./day, every 6 hours for patients allergic to penicillin

Neomycin or bacitracin lotion or ointment treatment of the nostrils and probable carrier sites should be performed at least twice daily. Rest, immobilization, and antibiotic therapy usually render surgery unnecessary. An exception to this is *breast abscess* occurring in lactating women, which is almost always staphylococcal in origin. This must be cultured and treated with the appropriate antibiotic, but it rarely heals without surgical intervention. Extension of the process occurs easily and is a frequent complication. *The skin of the nursing infant, and particularly the navel, may be the source of the mastitis in the mother.*

Other lesions that should be treated surgically with an antibiotic cover are *tendon sheath infections* of the hand, *palmar space infections*, and some *pulp space infections.*

## Erysipelas

Erysipelas is a superficial form of streptococcal cellulitis. The organisms, group A beta-hemolytic streptococci, invade the dermis, usually through a break in the skin, and incite a spreading erythematous, acute inflammatory response. The area of involvement is red, raised, hot, and painful and has a characteristically well-defined advancing border. Although the face is usually considered in one's clinical memory of erysipelas, the condition does involve the limbs, abdominal wall, or other areas. With subsidence, there is pronounced exfoliation of the overlying skin. There is local lymphadenopathy, with other quite noticeable constitutional symptoms. There may be repeated infections in the same site, a situation that not infrequently results in chronic lymphedema of the area.

## Cellulitis

Invasion of the dermis and subcutaneous tissue by streptococci results in an infection that is similar to erysipelas, but deeper and more serious. Red streaks indicate extending lymphangitis, and there are associated enlarged regional nodes. Subsequent septicemia is seen, and deep suppuration may occur. Profound constitutional symptoms are common in association with streptococcal cellulitis. If the infection is recurrent, permanent lymphedema results.

## Pyoderma

Although pustules and cutaneous abscesses are considered traditionally to be staphylococ-

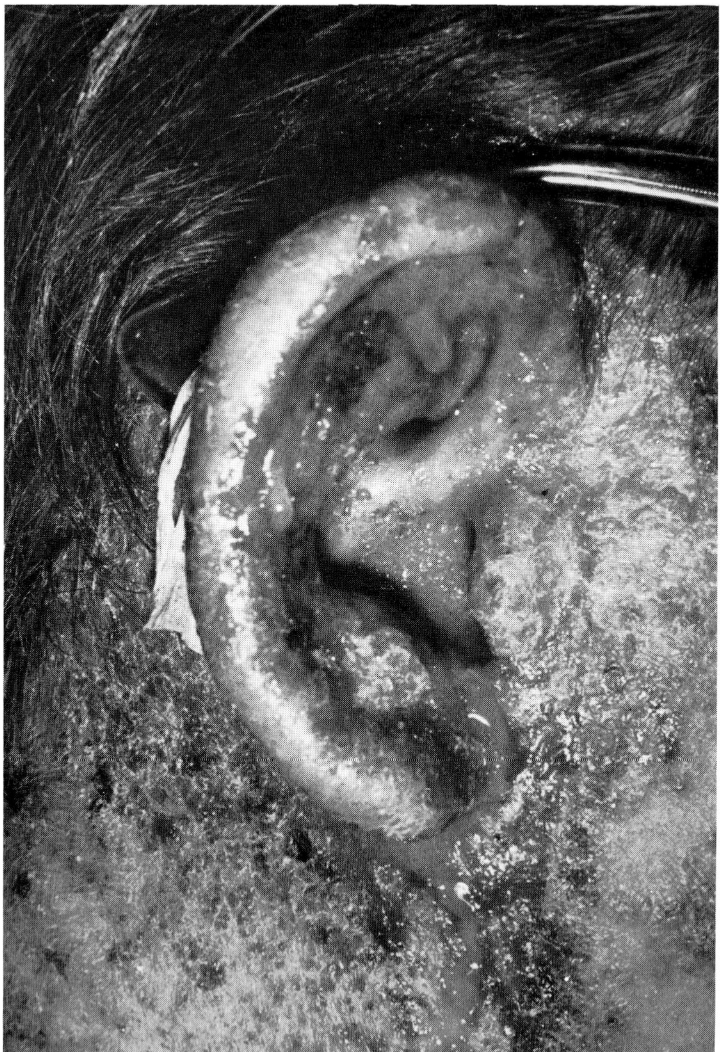

**Fig. 13-4.** Infectious eczematoid dermatitis. Occurrence is secondary to presence of pus from inner ear.

cal, they may be primary streptococcal lesions as well. Pustules, boils, punched-out ulcers, and necrotic lesions are described by Noble and Somerville as caused by identifiable antigenic types of streptococci particularly in patients in the 10- to 20-years-of-age group.

### *Treatment*

Rest and immobilization, both of the area and of the patient, are essential. Hospitalization is wise for the patient showing constitutional symptoms.

The dosage is one intramuscular injection of benzathine penicillin G of 1.2 million units in adults, but half that for children. Oral penicillin is acceptable, with penicillin V, 15 mg./kg./day in four doses for 10 days. Erythromycin 500 mg. four times daily for a week is generally satisfactory.

## Paronychia

See p. 285.

## Infectious eczematoid dermatitis

This localized, acute, inflammatory dermatitis develops adjacent to a suppurative process in the ear, such as a draining sinus or a boil. It appears in conjunction with both staphylococcal and streptococcal infections, arising in an area over which the pus tends to flow.

The lesion is moist, crusted, and brightly erythematous (Fig. 13-4) and is resistant to therapy while the original infectious focus persists.

### *Treatment*

Culture and determination of the antibiotic sensitivity of the causative organism and administration of the antibiotic are necessary for the treatment of this infection.

Compresses of Burow's solution, employing prepared tablets or powders, 1 tablet to 1 pint of cool water, are used on the affected area in 15-minute periods three times daily.

After air drying, a steroid-antibiotic combination should be applied sparingly:

| | |
|---|---|
| Neomycin | 1% |
| Hydrocortisone (or equivalent) | 1% |
| Hydrophilic ointment | 30 Gm. |

A betamethasone-neomycin combination is also effective.

### REFERENCES


Aly R: Effects of drugs in cutaneous microbial flora. In Marzulli, F. N., and Maibach, H. I., editors: Advances in modern toxicology. Vol. 4, Dermatotoxicology and pharmacology, New York, 1977, John Wiley & Son, p. 50.

Dahl, M. V., Greene, W. H., and Quie, P. G.: Infection, dermatitis, increased IgE, and impaired neutrophil chemotaxis, Arch. Dermatol. **112**:1387, 1976.
**Eleven patients with eczema, staphylococcal, and candidal infections, and defective immune-mediated defenses.**

Dillon, H. C., and Reeves, M. S. A.: Streptococcal immune response in nephritis after skin infection, Am. J. Med. **56**:333, 1974.
**Precise mechanism is still lacking.**

Hoeprich, P. D., editor: Infectious diseases, New York, 1977, Harper & Row, Publishers.

Kelly, C., Taplin, D., and Allen, A. M.: Streptococcal ecthyma, Arch. Dermatol. **103**:306, 1971.
**Benzathine penicillin 600,000 units successful.**

Levene, G. M.: Immunology of streptococcal infection, Br. J. Dermatol. **86**(suppl. 8):62, 1972.
**Selective decreased antibody responses.**

Leyden, J. J., Marples, R. R., and Kligman, A. M.: *Staphylococcus aureus* in the lesions of atopic dermatitis, Br. J. Dermatol. **90**:525, 1974.
**This confirms the known clinical response to a course of oral antibiotics.**

Maibach, H. I., and Hildick-Smith, G., editors: Skin bacteria and their role in infection, New York, 1965, McGraw-Hill Book Co.

Marples, M. J.: The ecology of the human skin, Springfield, Ill., 1965, Charles C Thomas, Publisher.

Noble, W. C., and Somerville, D. A.: Microbiology of human skin, Philadelphia, 1974, W. B. Saunders Co.

Nystrom, B., and Molin, L.: Colonization with staphylococci in dermatology wards with different designs and practices, Br. J. Dermatol. **86**(suppl. 8):21, 1972.
**Protective isolation of susceptible persons is effective.**

Parish, W. E.: Studies on vasculitis. III. Decreased formation of antibody to *M. proteus*, group A polysaccharide, and to some exotoxins in persons with cutaneous vasculitis after streptococcal infection, Clin. Allergy **1**:295, 1971.
**Selective decrease in antibody formation.**

Peter, G., and Smith, A. L.: Group A streptococcal infections of the skin and pharynx, N. Engl. J. Med. **297**:311, 365, 1977.
**Constitute 10% of pediatric practice.**

Schur, P. H., Borel, H., Gelfand, E. W., et al.: Selective gamma globulin deficiencies in patients with recurrent pyogenic infections, N. Engl. J. Med. **283**:631, 1970.
**Three patients with highly selective globulin deficiencies.**

Williams, J. D., Waltho, C. A., Ayliffe, J. A. G., et al.: Trials of five antibacterial creams in the control of nasal carriage of *Staphylococcus aureus*, Lancet **2**:390, 1967.
**Gentamicin 0.3% best followed by neomycin-chlorhexidine combination.**

## DIPHTHERIA

*Corynebacterium diphtheriae*, the cause of diphtheria, is primarily an inhabitant of the mucous membranes and probably occurs only as a transient on human skin. It does, however, establish itself on damaged skin and may become a more or less permanent inhabitant of superficial cutaneous lesions. It may be a primary pathogen in skin ulcers, or a fortuitous colonizer. Jellard found the organism common in western Canada in the Indian population, and it is found in neglected superficial ulcers in the U.S. Northwest and in the Canadian West. Immunity has been linked to a high incidence elsewhere.

The lesions are nonspecific, often nonexudative, dry, scaling, undramatic, ulcerated, and abraded areas in a variety of sites.

They respond promptly to erythromycin, 30 to 40 mg./kg./day for 2 weeks.

### REFERENCE

Jellard, C. H.: Diphtheria infection in North West Canada, 1969, 1970, and 1971, J. Hyg. (Camb.) **70**:503, 1972.
**Transmission by air and contact.**

## PITTED KERATOLYSIS (Fig. 1-15)

A common, superficial infection of the keratin of the soles that produces pits and larger erosions of the outer layers. Most cases are asymptomatic, but occasionally the lesions become tender and painful. A peripheral erythema and mild swelling is seen in such cases. Hydrated, macerated keratin seems to be a predisposing factor. The causative organism may be a *Corynebacterium*.

Drying and application of 1% to 10% aqueous solutions of glutaraldehyde daily or weekly are ordinarily curative.

### REFERENCE

Noble, W. C., and Somerville, D. A.: Microbiology of human skin, Philadelphia, 1974, W. B. Saunders Co., p. 110.

## ERYTHRASMA

Although erythrasma was first described as a fungal infection 100 years ago, it was not until 1961 that Sarkany, Taplin, and Blank at the University of Miami successfully cultured the gram-positive bacillus *Corynebacterium minutissimum* from the lesions of erythrasma.

This bacterial infection occurs most often in persons living in hot and humid tropical and subtropical climates. However, recent culture studies reveal a surprising frequency of asymptomatic erythrasma in the intertriginous areas of otherwise normal individuals in temperate climates.

The individual lesions consist of a scaly, mildly erythematous patch that becomes brown or yellow (Fig. 13-5). Pruritus is not a feature. The intertriginous sites most often involved are the groin, axillae, and toe webs. Infrequently the extremities and the trunk are affected. The occurrence of a bright red fluorescence with Wood's light is characteristic and believed to be attributable to the presence of porphyrins produced by the bacteria. The typical organisms may be found on direct microscopic examination of Gram- or Giemsa-stained preparations.

*A significant number of patients with erythrasma have been shown to have diabetes mellitus.*

### *Differential diagnosis*

Erythrasma must be differentiated from superficial fungal infections, candidosis, intertrigo, and seborrheic dermatitis.

### *Treatment*

Erythrasma responds promptly to erythromycin, 15 mg./kg./day given four times daily for up to 3 weeks. The tetracyclines are also effective.

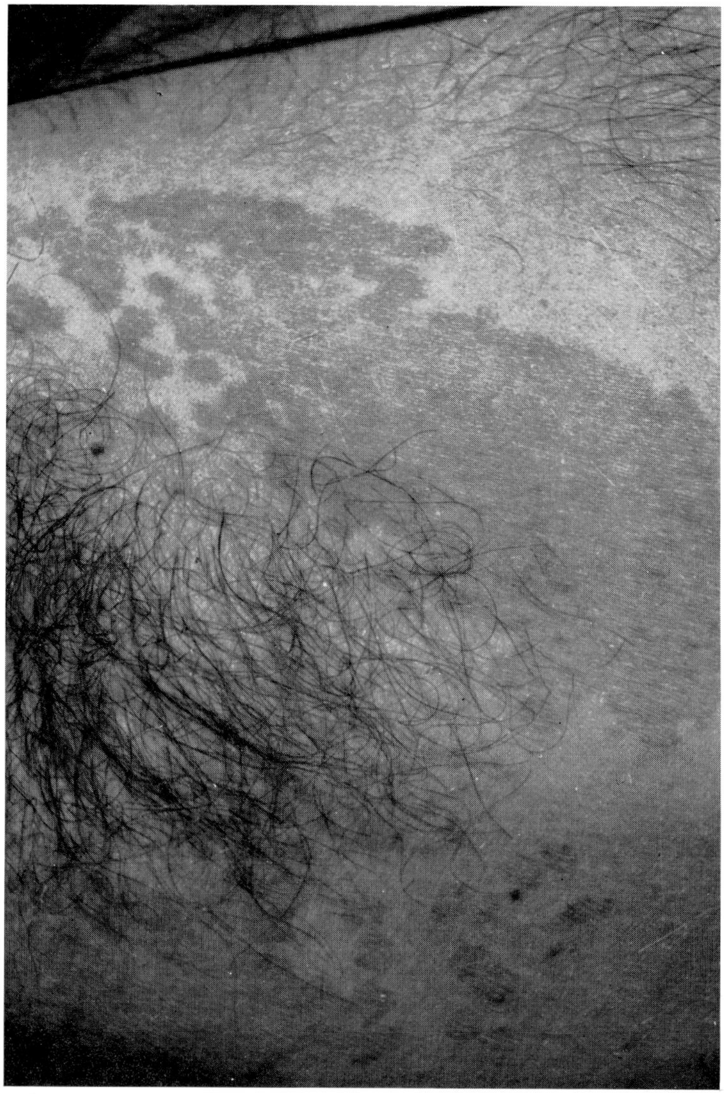

**Fig. 13-5.** Erythrasma involving axilla.

It will also respond to the application of a saturated solution of sodium hyposulfite after a hot soapy bath, nightly for 2 weeks or longer. Simple mild cases may respond to the use of bactericidal soaps alone.

#### REFERENCE

Sarkany, I., Taplin, D., and Blank, H.: The etiology and treatment of erythrasma, J. Invest. Dermatol. **37**:382, 1961.

## GONORRHEA

Gonorrhea has become one of today's major public health problems. It has reached epidemic proportions, is the most prevalent bacterial infection of adults in the United States, and the number of known cases is probably smaller than the number unreported. Its incredible increase in incidence since 1963 is in teenagers and young adults. Its increasing incidence has stopped in the United Kingdom and is falling in northern Europe. The incidence in Canada, like the United Kingdom, has leveled off. In the United States, the incidence continues to rise.

Within a week or at most 2 weeks after sexual intercourse, acute gonorrhea produces in the male a painful periurethral balanitis, purulent urethral discharge, and burning dysuria. The female may experience one or all of the following: an acute membranous inflammation of the vulvar mucous membrane, purulent vaginal discharge, abnormal menstrual bleeding, unilateral labial pain, anorectal discomfort, lower abdominal pain, frequency, and dysuria. Rectal disease is associated with pain, bleeding, tenesmus, and purulent discharge. Erosions may occur in any area contacted by the purulent discharge. Local abscess and lymphadenopathy occur in all types of the disease. Women can develop a chronic pelvic inflammation, which may be subclinical. Men may harbor an asymptomatic urethral or prostatic infection; thus an unknown percent of males never develop symptoms but retain the organism to serve as the main source of spread of infection to women.

Less than 3% of patients with gonorrhea develop disseminated gonococcal infection with hematogenous spread. If bacteremia occurs, there is associated fever and a transient asymmetric arthritis that affects the extensor tendons of wrists, fingers, knees, and ankles most often. Cutaneous lesions of papular, petechial, or hemorrhagic vesicopustules with a red halo develop usually on the extremities. They are few and often overlooked (Plate 25). Menstruation appears to facilitate spread to the upper genital tract, and there is bacteremic spread as well.

### *Diagnosis*

Identification of the organism is essential. Cultures taken from the endocervix are more diagnostic than are vaginal swabs. Cervical

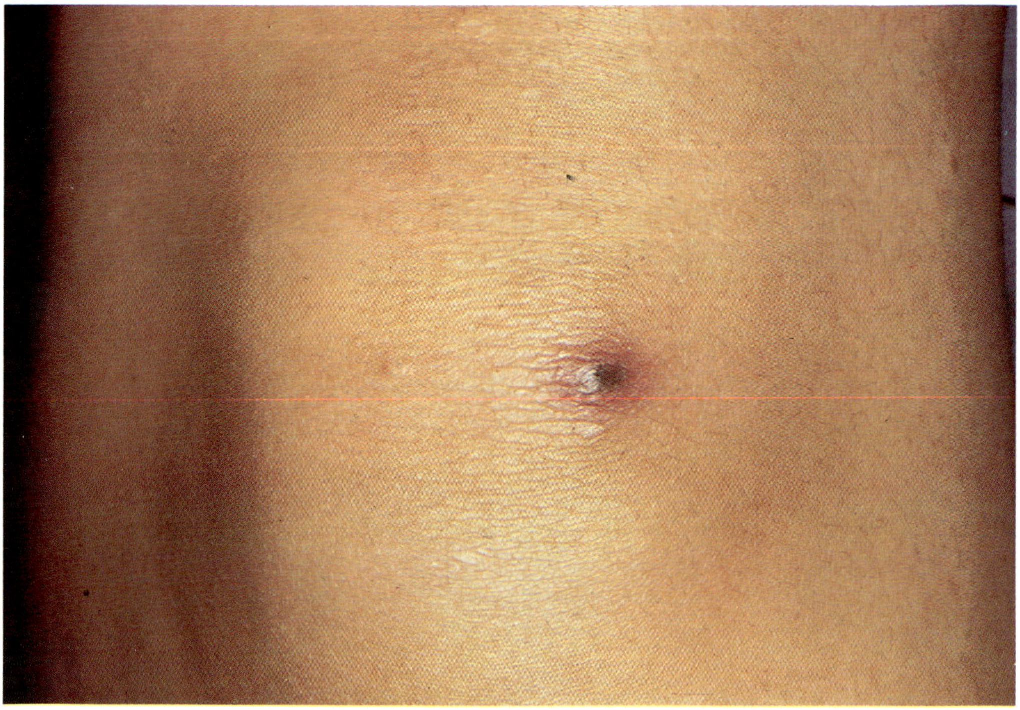

**Plate 25**

Gonorrhea. Hemorrhagic pustule. May be the only cutaneous manifestation.

compression may reveal an exudate otherwise not noted. Blood cultures should be attempted repeatedly if signs of bacteremia are found. Cutaneous lesions do not ordinarily yield positive cultures, but organisms may be identified with proper immunofluorescent technique. In males, a thin swab or wire loop is passed 2 cm. into the anterior urethra. Anal and pharyngeal swabs should be taken from females and homosexual males. Special media must be used (Thayer-Martin), and immediate planting of the swab is essential, because the organism dies within 1 to 2 hours on drying and requires a narrow range of temperature. At least five different colony forms are seen. The organism has an intrinsic resistance to antimicrobials that is variable in different geographic areas. A strain was isolated in the United States and others elsewhere in 1976 that were resistant to penicillin.

### *Treatment*

Inadequate treatment must be avoided. Aqueous procaine penicillin G is the drug of choice, 4.8 million units in two injections, in one visit. A second swab is taken if there is a second visit. Tetracycline, 30 mg./kg./day in 4 doses for 4 days is an alternate therapy for patients who are penicillin sensitive. Spectinomycin, 2 Gm., as a single intramuscular injection is a second alternate.

Patients with gonococcal pelvic inflammatory disease or disseminated gonococcal infection are best hospitalized for treatment.

Cultures are taken 1 week after completion of therapy and again at 6 weeks.

#### REFERENCES

Holmes, K. K., and Stilwell, G. H.: Gonococcal infection. In Hoeprich, P. D., editor: Infectious diseases, Hagerstown, Md., 1977, Harper & Row, Publishers, p. 491.

Morton, R. S.: Gonorrhea, Philadelphia, 1977, W. B. Saunders Co.
**Encyclopedic: including public health aspects.**

## TUBERCULOSIS

Cutaneous tuberculosis demonstrates a variety of immunological reactions of the skin to the tubercle bacillus.

### *Natural course*

Primary infection resulting from the first contact with the organism usually occurs in childhood. It almost always involves the lungs and produces a degree of immunity or disseminates rapidly and produces a miliary picture.

If tuberculosis occurs first in the skin, rather than the lungs, a lesion of primary inoculation, or chancre, is produced. This is a nodule that develops into an ulcer, with regional lymphadenopathy, and tubercle bacilli are present in the lesion.

Secondary, or reinfection, tuberculosis occurs after a degree of immunity is produced by the primary infection. Tubercle bacilli may be very difficult to demonstrate in the lesions, depending on the amount of immunity. The greater the degree of immunity, the fewer the bacilli.

### *Classification of cutaneous tuberculosis*

***Cutaneous primary tuberculosis.*** Cutaneous primary tuberculosis is an initial skin infection in a previously uninfected individual. At the site of inoculation there is a papule that develops into a painful ulcer. There is regional adenopathy.

Diagnosis may be made by culture for acid-fast bacilli. Tissue sections from biopsy material can be stained for these organisms. The disease may remain localized to the skin, show secondary effects deeper in the adjoining tissues, or spread systemically, depending on the patient's immunity.

***Cutaneous secondary tuberculosis.*** Cutaneous secondary tuberculosis is an infection secondary to tuberculosis elsewhere and occurs in several forms. The course of the infection and the host response depend on the number of organisms in the original exposure, the host's immune responses, both humeral and cellular, and the host's degree of sensitivity to the mycobacterium.

***Lupus vulgaris.*** In lupus vulgaris, small, multiple, amber-colored plaques or nodules enlarge and form a roughly circular lesion, in which atrophy and scarring occur in the center (Fig. 13-6, *A*). The condition occurs on the face, most often on the nose, cheek, or lip,

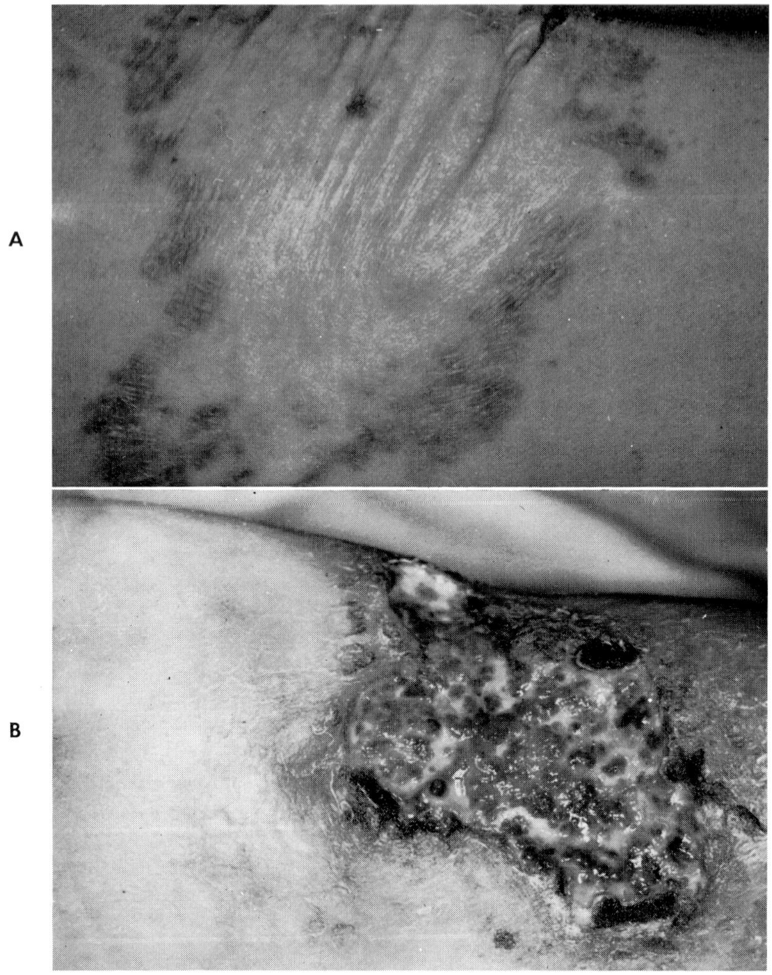

Fig. 13-6. A, Lupus vulgaris. B, Erythema induratum with extensive ulceration.

but may occur on the arms. Long-term lesions may be quite disfiguring as a result of scarring. This occurs in individuals with a significant immunological response to the acid-fast organisms.

***Verrucous tuberculosis.*** Verrucous tuberculosis occurs as warty lesions that result from cutaneous inoculation in a strongly immune patient. It occurs as a result of walking barefoot on sidewalks contaminated by the mycobacterium.

Although relatively rare in Western countries, this form of the disease is the commonest form seen in Hong Kong, comprising 46% of cases of skin tuberculosis. Cutaneous tuberculosis is also relatively common there.

***Scrofuloderma.*** In scrofuloderma, sinus tracts lead to the cutaneous surface from infected bone or lymph nodes. The disease begins in the larynx, usually from tubercle bacilli in milk from infected cows. It classically occurs in children and follows a chronic course.

***Tuberculosis orificial ulcers.*** Mucous membrane lesions near orifices, resulting from *extension* of an infection to the skin, are known as tuberculosus orificial ulcers. They occur in patients with minimal immune response.

***Tuberculids.*** Tuberculids are cutaneous lesions that occur in association with active tuberculosis, but bacteria are rarely found in the lesions.

PAPULAR TUBERCULID. The papular form of tuberculid consists of varying types of scarring papular and necrotic lesions that appear on the face, neck, and trunk in individuals with positive tuberculin tests.

ERYTHEMA INDURATUM. In erythema induratum, the lesion is an ulcerated form of cutaneous tuberculosis, occurring in a hyperimmune individual. The large, blue-red, painless nodules that form are found on the posterior aspect of both legs and have a tendency to ulcerate (Fig. 13-6, *B*). The lesions are bilaterally symmetrical, recurrent, and seen usually in young females. Erythema induratum is often unassociated with demonstrable active tuberculosis elsewhere. The tuberculin test is always positive, however.

### *Diagnosis*

This entity is differentiated from nodose leg lesions by its tendency to ulcerate.

Diagnosis is achieved by interpretation of adequate biopsy material and, as in a study by Förström and Hannuksela (1970), by response to antituberculous therapy.

### *Differential diagnosis of erythema induratum*

*Erythema nodosum* is characterized by tender and painful erythematous nodules that do not ulcerate.

*Varicose ulcers* are associated with venous varicosities and ankle edema.

*Nodular vasculitis* may clinically resemble erythema induratum, but is rarely limited to the legs.

See also leg ulcers, p. 585.

### *Treatment*

Treatment of patients with cutaneous forms of tuberculosis is now the same as that for systemic tuberculosis. This requires the use of isoniazid, with either ethambutol (Myambutol), or streptomycin, or both, given over a 2-year period. Alternatively, isoniazid (INH) plus rifampin for 1½ to 2 years. Rifampin, however, has a potential for producing hepatitis.

An important report by Förström and colleagues on the effectiveness of isoniazid in patients who inactivate the drug more rapidly than others reveals significantly different therapeutic results in tuberculosis of the skin between these groups. The study indicates that serum levels are higher in slow inactivators, which bears importantly on the length of treatment.

Rifampin is now one of the most useful new antituberculous drugs, but its initial reputation for being free of side effects has been disproved because 20% to 30% of patients on combined therapy with rifampin develop hepatitis.

#### REFERENCES


Förström, L., and Hannuksela, M.: Antituberculous treatment of erythema induratum basin, Acta Derm. Venereol. **50**:143, 1970.
**May be the only way to differentiate from nodose leg lesions.**

Förström, L., Mattila, M. J., and Tiitinen, H.: Correlation between INH inactivation and therapeutic result in skin tuberculosis (lupus vulgaris), Ann. Clin. Res. **4**:165, 1972.
**Significant.**

Rees, R. J. W., and Meade, T. W.: Comparison of modes of spread and incidence of tuberculosis and leprosy, Lancet **1**:47, 1974.
**The same sort in both diseases.**

Vall-Spinosa, A., Lester, W., Moulding, T., et al.: Rifampicin in the treatment of drug-resistant *Mycobacterium tuberculosis* infections, N. Engl. J. Med. **283**:616, 1970.
**21 of 30 patients with far advanced disease developed culture conversion in average of 40 days.**

Van Scoy, R. E.: Antituberculous agents, isoniazid, rifampin, streptomycin, ethambutol, Mayo Clin. Proc. **52**:694, 1977.
**The latest information and combinations of these effective drugs.**

Wong, K. O., Lee K. P., and Chu, S. F.: Tuberculosis of the skin in Hong Kong, Br. J. Dermatol. **80**:429, 1968.
**160 cases with 46% showing verrucous tuberculosis.**


## LEPROSY

Leprosy is a historical cutaneous and neurological disease caused by *Mycobacterium leprae*, whose most disabling symptoms can be prevented by proper therapy.

The discovery that *M. leprae* can be grown in the armadillo in 40% of animals inoculated was a major breakthrough in the study of this crippling disease (Storrs).

### *Natural course*

Leprosy produces its widely recognized damaging clinical effects at the site of the major concentration of the bacilli in cool, superficial tissues, predominantly the skin and superficial sensory nerves (Plate 26).

Leprosy is endemic to certain southern states on the North American continent and may be seen sporadically in Canada. Canadian cases are usually seen in immigrants, although in 1973 one patient was identified who had never left Canada and had not to his knowledge been in contact with anyone who had the disease.

The incubation period is measured in years, probably an average of 3 years. There are two main types of leprosy: tuberculoid, in which the patient has a degree of immunity to the organism, and lepromatous, in which the patient appears to have little resistance to the bacterium. These are at the two ends of the spectrum of the disease, and varying proportions of the two types provide most of the clinical cases seen.

Children are most susceptible and contract the disease more easily than adults. However, they may become adults before full signs of the disease are apparent. Some 2% of the general adult population are susceptible to the infection. Arnold and Fasal inimitably share their profound knowledge of this disease in a 1973 publication.

***Tuberculoid type.*** A patient with tuberculoid leprosy presents more involvement of the peripheral nerves than of the skin. The peripheral nerves such as the ulnar nerve are thickened and tender and can be felt easily. Areas of anesthesia are apparent.

Cutaneous lesions are pink or light brown, annular, macular lesions or plaques, with well-defined borders. They may form large irregular lesions or small pinhead-sized papules. There may be peripheral erythema around a large, scaling plaque.

Neurological lesions include anesthetic areas and trophic changes distal to damaged nerves, including ulcerations and bullae. Motor changes are late and result in contractures.

***Lepromatous type.*** Tan to pink macules become infiltrated and nodular, yellowish in color, and possibly ulcerated. They develop on the face, hands, extensor surfaces, and earlobes. Mucous membranes are affected and may be the most reliable source of bacilli in early cases. Bleeding from the nose and swelling of the submucous tissue are common, leading to ulceration. Liver, spleen, kidneys, testicles, and lymph nodes are involved.

The *lepromin test* is performed by the infection of killed lepra bacilli from an active lesion and subsequent evaluation of the reaction. It is helpful in determining the patient's response to the organism. It is not essentially a diagnostic test. It is negative in the lepromatous form and positive in the tuberculoid form.

The leprosy bacillus is probably the most successful human parasite known. Drutz, Chen, and Lu have recently demonstrated that $10^5$ lepra bacilli may be present per milliliter of blood of patients with untreated lepromatous leprosy. This occurs with minimal signs of disorder in the host. Symptoms appear, however, with increasing resistance.

Leprologists have long recognized that patients with leprosy have varying degrees of resistance to the lepra bacillus and that as signs of increased resistance to the infection appear, the disease is more violent and chances of recovery increase. Patients with lepromatous leprosy have little or no cell-mediated immunity, and the bacteria abound, present in nerve sheaths and peripheral tissues, with little cellular response. As Dwyer has shown, this is a result of depression of the *T lymphocytes*, and the paracortical areas of these patients' lymph nodes show a pronounced depletion of these important purveyors of immunity against the organism. These patients also show a depressed delayed allergic response to other antigens. Interestingly, Bullock has shown a progression toward normalcy of this mechanism in patients under treatment for their leprosy. Patients with tuberculoid leprosy have more active delayed allergic responses than those with lepromatous leprosy and clinically demonstrate greater inflammatory responses to the bacillus. Pettit believes that the erythema nodosum leprosum response reflects an increase

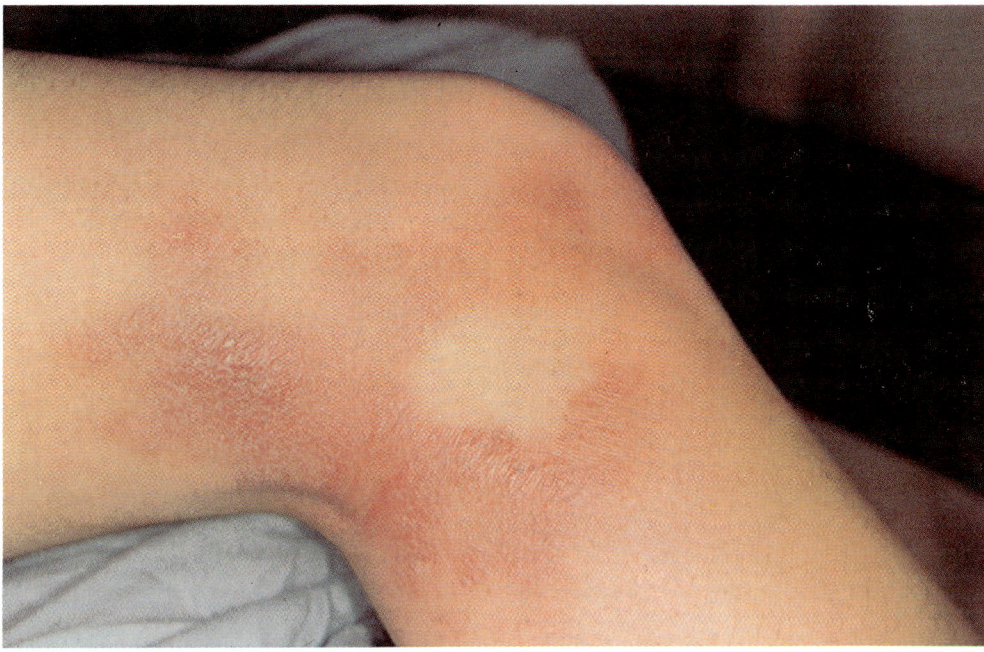

**Plate 26**

Leprosy. "Swiss cheese" appearance with central analgesic area that lacks a flare on stroking.

in host aggression toward the organism and is a salutary sign. Iveson warns of the true immunologic significance of this sign. The disease is not a simple failure of cellular immunity, however. Bullock describes abnormalities of circulating antibodies as well. Convit reviewed the current knowledge of immune mechanisms in this disease and some possible reasons for them.

### *Treatment*

The treatment of leprosy poses many problems in an ordinarily leprosy-free society. Supposedly, a rather fixed percentage of the adult population, estimated at around 2%, is susceptible to invasion by the bacillus and, on exposure, stand a risk of infection. Children are particularly at risk. Other members of the population may develop varying degrees of resistance, depending on their immune defenses and degree of exposure. In a virgin country, however, where the population has developed no degree of immunity, lepromatous leprosy patients, some with incredible numbers of bacteria in their systems and no longer spreading bacilli from skin and nose secretions, should be guarded from contact with susceptible friends and relatives (Rao).

Multiple dapsone-resistant strains have been identified that may result from low intermittent dosage. High dose therapy is thus now more common. Fifty milligrams per day or 500 mg. once weekly are acceptable.

After 3 months of dapsone therapy, these patients are no longer shedding bacilli and bacteremia has ceased. They are safely able to carry on a more normal life. With present medication, they should be given therapy for years and perhaps for life. Children in the family should receive prophylactic dapsone, 50 mg. once daily for 1 to 2 years. Therapeutic achievement is followed by bacteriological examinations and experienced estimates of killed or viable bacilli or the bacterial index.

If too large numbers of bacteria are killed

abruptly, reactions damaging to the patient occur. Skilled therapy may be necessary to prevent permanent disability from nerve paralysis or loss of function.

Rifampin is now accepted as the most rapid and active antileprosy agent now available. It is bactericidal, binding strongly to the bacterial transcription process for multiplication. Relatively low doses are necessary, and tolerance by the patient is good; side effects are rare, although it has a definite hazard of producing hepatitis. It is quite widely used where its expense is not a major factor in determining therapy. Some leprosy programs employ dapsone and rifampin for the early months of therapy.

#### REFERENCES

Arnold, H. L., and Fasal, P.: Leprosy. Diagnosis and management, ed. 2, Springfield, Ill., 1973, Charles C Thomas, Publisher.
**A clinician's prize.**

Bullock, W. E., Fields, J. P., and Brandriss, M. W.: An evaluation of transfer factor as immunotherapy for patients with lepromatous leprosy, N. Engl. J. Med. **287**:1053, 1972.
**Reversal of anergy and appearance of erythema nodosum leprosum.**

Convit, J., and Ulrich, M.: Recent advances in the immunology of leprosy, Int. J. Dermatol. **15**:157, 1976.
**A review.**

Drutz, D. J., Chen, T. S. N., and Lu, W. H.: The continuous bacteremia of lepromatous leprosy, N. Engl. J. Med. **287**:159, 1972.
**$10^5$ bacilli per milliliter!**

Dwyer, J. M., Bullock, W. E., and Fields, J. P.: Disturbance of the blood T:B lymphocyte ratio in lepromatous leprosy, N. Engl. J. Med. **288**:1036, 1973.
**T-cell decrease.**

Hudson, A. L.: A comment on leprosy, Mod. Med. Canada **30**:1076, 1975.
**Its status in Canada.**

Iveson, J. M. I., McDougall, A. L., Leathem, A. J., et al.: Lepromatous leprosy presenting with polyarthritis, myositis and immune complex glomerulonephritis, Br. Med. J. **3**:619, 1975.
**Erythema nodosum leprosum as an important serious immune complex reaction.**

Leiker, D. L.: Chemotherapy in leprosy, Int. J. Dermatol. **14**:254, 1975.
**Eight drugs and combined therapy discussed.**

Pettit, J. H. S., and Waters, M. F. R.: The etiology of erythema nodosum leprosum, Int. J. Lepr. **35**:1, 1967.
**A promising sign for the patient.**

Rao, P. S. S., Karat, A. B. A., Kaliaperumal, V. G., et al.: Transmission of leprosy within households, Int. J. Lepr. **43**:45, 1975.
**Borderline cases did not increase the attack rate, which peaked at 5 to 9 years.**

Storrs, E. E., Walsh, G. P., Walsh, H. P., et al.: Leprosy in the armadillo: new model for biomedical research, Science **183**:851, 1974.
**The search for a receptor host successfully ended.**

## TREPONEMAL INFECTIONS

### Syphilis

Caused by *Treponema pallidum,* syphilis is transmitted essentially by sexual intercourse, with the primary lesion appearing at the site of first contact with the disease organism.

#### Early primary syphilis

From 2 to 10 weeks after the initial contact, the primary lesion (chancre) will appear. It is not always on the genitalia, but may be found on the anus, lip, tongue, or elsewhere, at the site of first contact with the spirochete. It is easily seen on the penis, but may be missed in females when it is present on the cervix. There is noticeable local lymphadenopathy in the nearest lymph node draining the chancre area.

The *chancre* (Plate 27, *A*) is a moist ulceration that usually develops from a small papule or erosion. It exudes fluid, has an elevated firm edge, and may be painless. There is, however, such a variety of appearances that a detailed description is misleading. Any suspected ulceration or moist patch in a likely area should be examined by dark-field microscopy.

At this stage of the disease, the serological test for syphilis may not be positive, and *the diagnosis must be made on dark-field examination, with identification of the organism.*

If left untreated, the chancre will disappear spontaneously in 1 to 2 months, and further stages in the disease process follow in due course.

Serological tests for syphilis become positive 4 to 6 weeks after first contact with the spirochete.

A

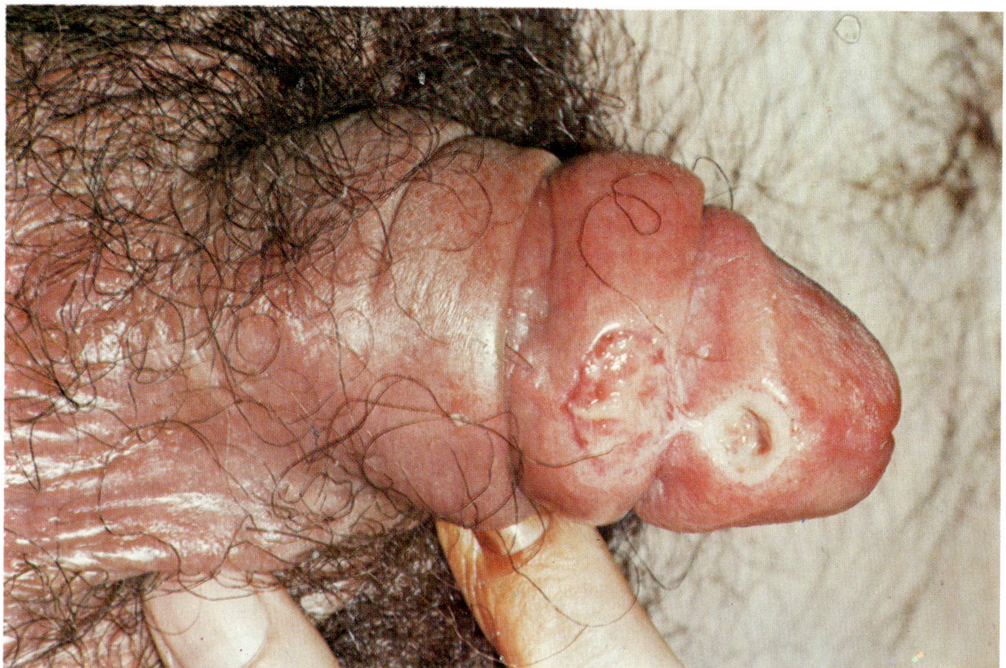

B

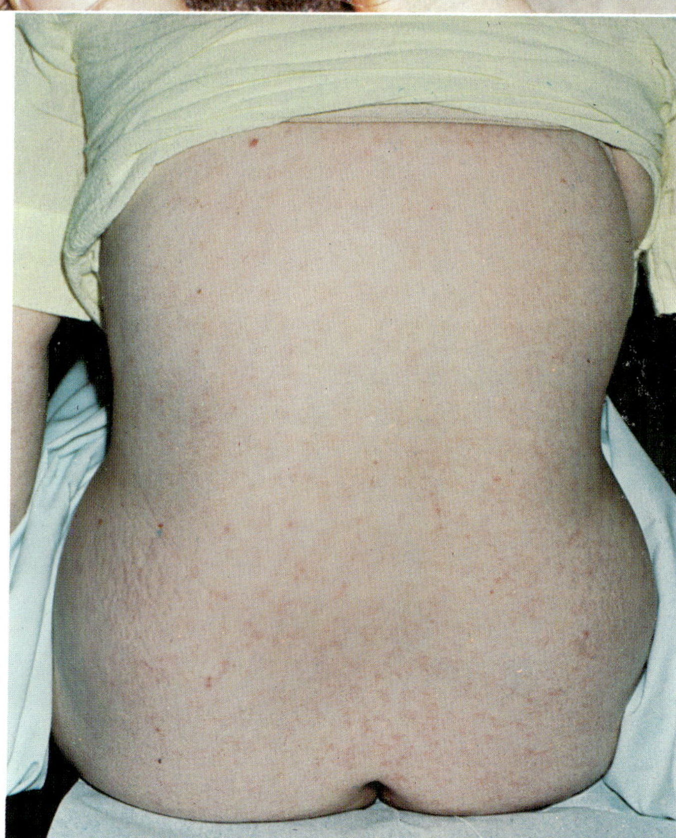

**Plate 27**

**A,** Syphilitic chancre mimicking chancroid. **B,** Secondary syphilis. Characteristic pale, unobtrusive eruption.

*Microscopic findings*

The chancre demonstrates an inflammatory reaction composed chiefly of lymphocytes and plasma cells in a perivascular pattern. Fibrosis and endarteritis are seen. There is nothing characteristic about the lesion, and although it indicates the diagnosis, it is not specific.

*Differential diagnosis*

***Herpes progenitalis.*** Recurrent vesicles in a small cluster are seen, with crusting, through a duration of 8 to 10 days before fading. All tests for syphilis are negative.

***Carcinoma.*** Carcinoma of the penis presents a slowly developing, steadily enlarging ulceration. Biopsy establishes the diagnosis.

***Bacterial ulcers.*** Common infections can produce erosions that, however, are usually painful.

*Treatment*

Benzathine penicillin, 2.4 million units (1.2 million in each buttock), is given intramuscularly; or aqueous penicillin G, 600,000 units daily for 8 days to total 4.8 million units, is administered intramuscularly; or erythromycin, 30 Gm., is given orally in a dose of 2 Gm. daily for 15 days.

Tetracycline may also be used to a total of 30 or 40 Gm. over 15 days. Repeat serological

A

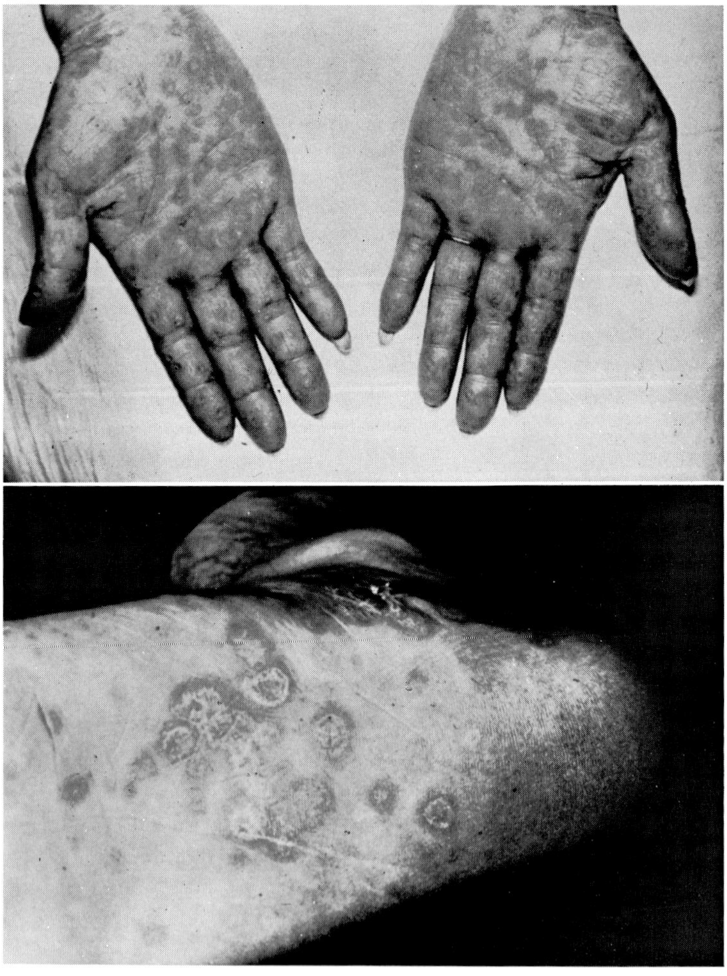

B

**Fig. 13-7. A,** Lesions of secondary syphilis of palms. **B,** Lesions of secondary syphilis of soles.

tests for syphilis should be done at 1-, 6-, and 12-month intervals, or until the titer is lower than original.

## Early secondary syphilis

The clinical appearance of the lesions of secondary syphilis is extremely varied. The diagnosis is based on a history of chancre, the cutaneous lesions, and the serological test for syphilis, which is positive at this stage.

The cutaneous lesions of secondary syphilis appear 6 weeks to 6 months after the chancre. There are associated constitutional symptoms of malaise, fever, and mild headache, which are usually present for most of the duration of the eruption. The lesions may follow different patterns of distribution and may be macular, papular, scaling, or pustular, but are rarely pruritic. A characteristic feature is their presence on the palms and soles (Fig. 13-7). Any suddenly appearing, generalized eruption should cause one to entertain the possibility of secondary syphilis (Plate 27, *B*).

Other manifestations of secondary syphilis are gray mucous patches; or dull, erythematous erosions of the tongue, lips, throat, or any mucous membrane; patchy alopecia of the scalp; wide-based warty condylomas of the genital or perianal area; retinitis; iritis; and a papule at the corner of the mouth, "split" by the angle of the lips. All these lesions are teeming with spirochetes and are highly infectious.

### *Microscopic findings*

Varying degrees of infiltration by round cells and plasma cells are seen. Some larger multinucleated cells are also sometimes present. The picture is indicative, but not diagnostic.

### *Differential diagnosis*

***Pityriasis rosea.*** A characteristic history of a herald patch reveals pityriasis rosea, but the lesions may appear identical to those of syphilis. Serological tests for syphilis are negative.

***Drug eruption.*** Both drug eruptions and syphilis are "great imitators." Serological tests for syphilis are negative.

***Acute exanthems.*** Although rarer in adults than children, these febrile conditions may present many features in common with secondary syphilis, including palm and sole lesions. Serological tests for syphilis are negative.

***Lichen planus.*** The angular, flat-topped, shiny lesions and gray surface lines identify the disease. Serological tests for syphilis are negative.

***Psoriasis.*** Psoriasis, particularly the guttate form, may resemble secondary syphilis.

***Other diseases.*** Seborrheic dermatitis, crusted pyodermas, and many other diseases may be considered in the differential diagnosis of secondary syphilis. Therefore, *the importance of a high index of suspicion and the performance of the serological tests for syphilis cannot be overstated.*

### *Treatment*

Treatment and follow-up are the same as for early primary syphilis, described previously. The serological reaction should be followed up at 1- or 2-month intervals for 1 year after treatment.

*It is of vital importance to report each case of syphilis and to see that all sexual contacts are followed up, examined, and treated. Assistance from the local, state, or provincial health department is required for this purpose. Because of the increased incidence of this disease apparent in teen-aged patients and in homosexual patients, the index of suspicion must be broadened to include these individuals.*

## Latent syphilis (late asymptomatic syphilis)

After the disappearance of signs of early syphilis, the latent stage and then the late stage may appear. There may be no symptoms, signs, or positive findings on examination. The serological test for syphilis is positive, and if a definite medical history of a chancre is unavailable, the confirmatory tests (described later) should be considered.

Women with latent syphilis can pass it on in pregnancy to their fetus, and it can be transmitted by blood donors.

*Treatment*

Benzathine penicillin, 7.2 million units, given on three occasions (2.4 million units each time, with 1.2 million units given in each buttock), or aqueous penicillin G, 600,000 units daily for 15 days to a total 9 million units, is the treatment of choice.

After treatment, the serological test for syphilis may remain positive at this stage. However, serological tests should be repeated at 6-month intervals for 2 years.

## Late symptomatic syphilis

Late syphilis involves the central nervous system, cardiovascular system, skin, and bone and may involve other organs. It is not infectious. *Treponema pallidum* is not demonstrable in the lesions by dark-field examination.

The diffuse granulomatous or gummatous lesions are slowly progressive and destructive.

*Treatment*

Benzathine penicillin, 7.2 million to 9 million units total, is given in doses of 2.4 million units (1.2 million in each buttock) at 7-day intervals for 3 weeks, or aqueous penicillin G, 600,000 units daily, is given for 15 days to a total of 9 million units. Alternatively erythromycin or tetracycline, 500 mg. four times daily for 30 days, may be given.

## Syphilis in pregnancy

Drug dosage in syphilis occurring during pregnancy is dependent on the stage of the disease. No additional therapy is required because of the pregnancy.

## Early and late congenital syphilis

Early congenital syphilis in an infant ordinarily causes maculopapular lesions, bullous cutaneous lesions, rhinitis, lymphadenopathy, bone lesions, and visceral lesions. These are not often apparent at birth, but begin to appear after 2 to 3 months or later. Late hereditary lesions of syphilis are chronic, destructive, and gummatous.

Treated patients who have had congenital syphilis can acquire early infectious syphilis even in the presence of a positive VDRL test (Fiumara).

The mother and child should be methodically followed with serological tests to determine whether the titer of the tests is rising or falling, since antibodies can be passed from mother to child prior to birth.

Late congenital syphilis demonstrates a positive serological test for syphilis in only 60% of cases.

*Treatment*

Aqueous penicillin, 100,000 units/kg., is given in daily injections for 10 days, or benzathine penicillin, 50,000 units/kg., is given in one injection.

## Laboratory tests for syphilis

***Dark-field examination.*** Direct examination of the organism from an early lesion, when done by one familiar with the technique, is a highly accurate test, except in oral lesions. It is positive in primary, secondary, and early congenital syphilis.

***Routine serological tests.*** The most frequently performed serological tests for syphilis remain the Kahn, Kolmer, and VDRL tests. These are generally considered screening tests, to be confirmed by further studies in doubtful cases. In the usual case, however, the results of these tests give all the information necessary. The ART, or automated reagin test, if properly done, is equivalent to the VDRL. It is now widely used.

Some false-positive reactions and some negative reactions in syphilitic infections are obtained by these tests. The VDRL and ART become positive 1 to 3 weeks after the chancre appears. In secondary syphilis they are most accurate. In general, routine serological tests become nonreactive after 1 year in adequately treated early syphilis and after 1½ years in adequately treated secondary syphilis.

***Treponemal tests.*** Treponemal tests such as *Treponema pallidum* immobilization (TPI) use the spirochete as the antigen and are specific tests. However, the TPI is difficult to perform and expensive, although it is the best available test for syphilis—its accuracy being almost 100%. It becomes positive slightly *later* than the routine serological tests for syphilis, so it is of less value in early syphilis than in the later stages. *It is of extreme value in differentiating between biological false-positive reactions, such as occur in lupus erythematosus, and true positive tests.*

The fluorescent treponemal antibody absorption test (FTA-ABS) is less expensive, just as specific, and more sensitive. It may give a false-positive test in a few cases of lupus erythematosus (almost one sixth of patients with lupus erythematosus in Kraus and Haserick's series) or similar disorders, but when there is doubt, recourse to the TPI may be had. If negative, it may be assumed that the TPI test is also negative.

Atwood and Miller have demonstrated that early in syphilis the FTA-ABS is attributable to IgM accumulation, but later IgG is responsible.

***Biological false-positive reactions.*** Acute infectious diseases caused by bacteria, viruses, rickettsiae, protozoa, or vaccinations may produce a transient (less than 6 months) false-positive reaction for syphilis. Chronic (more than 6 months) false-positive reactions may be found in persons with lupus erythematosus, rheumatoid arthritis, leprosy, or rheumatic fever. As mentioned previously, the TPI finds its greatest use in these situations, in which it is negative in the face of a positive routine serological test for syphilis. Catterall discusses the various disorders and clinical circumstances associated with biological false-positive reactions in a very worthwhile review. They are much commoner in women than in men.

### Persistent spirochetes in treated patients

Persistent treponema-like viable forms have been repeatedly recovered from lymph nodes, aqueous humor, cerebrospinal fluid, brain, and bone of patients after adequate penicillin therapy for both late and early syphilis. The significance and pathogenicity of these forms is as yet unclear. They may reflect inadequacy of the modern shorter but accepted methods of penicillin therapy. Benzathine penicillin and tetracycline are brought into question in Tramont's report.

## Yaws

*Treponema pertenue* is the etiological agent responsible for yaws. The extensive campaigns that have been mounted in areas where yaws is endemic have been so successful that some authorities believe this disease may be eradicated eventually, although victims still number in the millions. Yaws mainly affects children. The secondary cutaneous lesions, which are infectious, occur before 15 years of age in more than 80% of cases. Minor trauma, flies, and poor personal hygiene are all factors that assist in the spread of this treponemal disease. Heat, humidity, and poor drainage of the geographical area contribute to this problem. It is largely limited to Africa, Asia, India, and the Caribbean.

The initial lesion is a papule that becomes crusted and ulcerated (mother yaw); the secondary frambesiform lesions are widespread. Papules and areas of plantar hyperkeratosis are also present. The bones and joints may be involved, and large areas of ulceration may occur.

### *Treatment*

Penicillin is effective. Procaine penicillin G, 1.2 million units daily, is given intramuscularly for 10 days, and half this dose to individuals under 15.

## Pinta (carate)

*Treponema carateum* is the causative agent of pinta. It is likely that this form of treponemal infection requires both prolonged and intimate contact for it to be transmitted. Pinta is found for the most part in South and Central America. Trauma, such as an insect bite, is responsible for providing a portal of entry for the infecting organisms. The primary lesion may take the form of an erythematous squamous plaque, with peripheral lesions appearing. The secondary or pintid lesions are scattered plaques, which appear in crops. Lesions demonstrate color changes and are achromic, red, or blue. The early lesions are erythematous or violaceous; later lesions are gray to blue or black. The tertiary stages are depigmented, particularly in flexures. The depigmented areas show an absence of melanocytes and an increase in Langerhans cells.

### *Treatment*

Penicillin, as used for primary syphilis, is the treatment of choice.

#### REFERENCES

Catterall, F. D.: Systemic disease and biological false-positive reactions, Br. J. Vener. Dis. **48**:1, 1972.
**Causes of acute and chronic biological false-positive reactions in 200 patient records.**

Fiumara, N. J.: Acquired syphilis in three patients with congenital syphilis, N. Engl. J. Med. **290**:1119, 1974.
**Early infectious syphilis occurring in the presence of an already positive VDRL test.**

Kraus, S. J., Haserick, J. R., and Lautz, M. A.: Fluorescent treponemal antibody absorption test reactions in lupus erythematosus: atypical beading pattern and probably false-positive reactions, N. Engl. J. Med. **282**:1287, 1970.
**10% to 15%.**

Levene, G. M., Wright, D. J. M., and Turk, J. L.: Cell-mediated immunity and lymphocyte transformation in syphilis, Proc. Roy. Soc. Med. **64**:426, 1971.
**Deficiency in cell-mediated mechanisms.**

Musher, D. M., Schell, R. F., and Knox, J. M.: The immunology of syphilis, Int. J. Dermatol. **8**:566, 1976.
**A review of current knowledge.**

Rudolph, A. H.: Syphilis. In Hoeprich, P. D., editor: Infectious diseases, ed. 2, Hagerstown, Md., 1977, Harper & Row, Publishers, p. 517.
**Therapy specifically set down.**

Tramont, E. C.: Resistence of *Treponema pallidum* following penicillin G therapy. Report of 2 cases, J.A.M.A. **236**:2206, 1976.
**Very disturbing: 100 patients like these now described.**

CHAPTER **14**

# Fungal infections

## SUPERFICIAL FUNGAL INFECTIONS

A fungus is a saprophytic or parasitic plant that possesses cells lacking true chlorophyll. It may exist as a single cell or a compact mass (such as a mushroom) or form septate hyphae disposed in a soft mycelium or in complex fruiting bodies.

The fungi causing dermatophytoses (ringworm) include *Microsporum, Epidermophyton,* and *Trichophyton* species, which are referred to as superficial pathogens because they live on the keratin of the skin, hair, and nails and cannot exist in the deeper layers of the skin. Since the keratin is being constantly desquamated, the rate of multiplication of the fungus must equal the rate of production of the keratin; otherwise, the infection would be discarded. However, superficial fungal infections in the human (ringworm) can be produced experimentally by the introduction of only one spore.

Superficial fungal infections may be transmitted to man from infected animals or from one person to another. Animals are the preferred hosts of some of these pathogenic fungi *(zoophilic),* whereas other fungi prefer man *(anthropophilic).* Children are most commonly infected with the superficial zoophilic fungi.

The first response to fungal colonies in the stratum corneum appears to be a cell-mediated immune reaction with erythema, spongiosis, vesicle formation, oozing, weeping, etc. Whether this is damaging to the fungus is not clear, but it does disrupt the epidermis, produces symptoms, and, if violent, seems to shorten the course of the infection. Without cell-mediated immunity, the skin is only slightly inflamed, with scaling, erythema, and pruritus. Unsaturated transferrin has been identified as a part of the defense against fungal invasion because of its avidity for iron. Moisture, either external as with wet feet, or self-produced as in hyperhidrosis, predisposes to colonization by fungi. Immune deficiencies, atopy, glucocorticoid therapy, immunosuppressive drugs, and diabetes lead to superficial dermatophytosis.

### *Immunology of superficial fungal infections*

For years dermatologists have puzzled over the responses of patients to dermatophyte infections. Some clinical infections are abrupt, inflammatory, self-limited, and transmissible, whereas others are notable for their chronicity, recurrences, and essential nontransmissibility. Our present knowledge of immune reactions to disease has helped to clarify some of these paradoxes, but some are still unclear. Acute inflammatory reactions with polymorphonuclear leukocytes, mononuclear cells, and tissue destruction occur with zoophilic fungi such as *Microsporum canis* and *Trichophyton verrucosum* (in faviform group) (Fig. 14-1) (Birt and Wieb). These are self-limited infections. Sulzberger noted the curing effect of inflammatory fungal infections and reported that artificially induced inflammation did not hasten cure. Sulzberger recorded the unexplained chronicity and problems in therapy caused by relatively noninflammatory fungi such as *Trichophyton rubrum* and *M. audouini.*

Sulzberger also noted that only certain individuals contracted these infections, including patients with lymphomas and leukemias, and that massive exposure to fungal elements did not produce disease in most individuals. Finally he reported the decreased incidence of immediate hypersensitivity responses to trichophyton extract in patients with clinical *T. rubrum* infections.

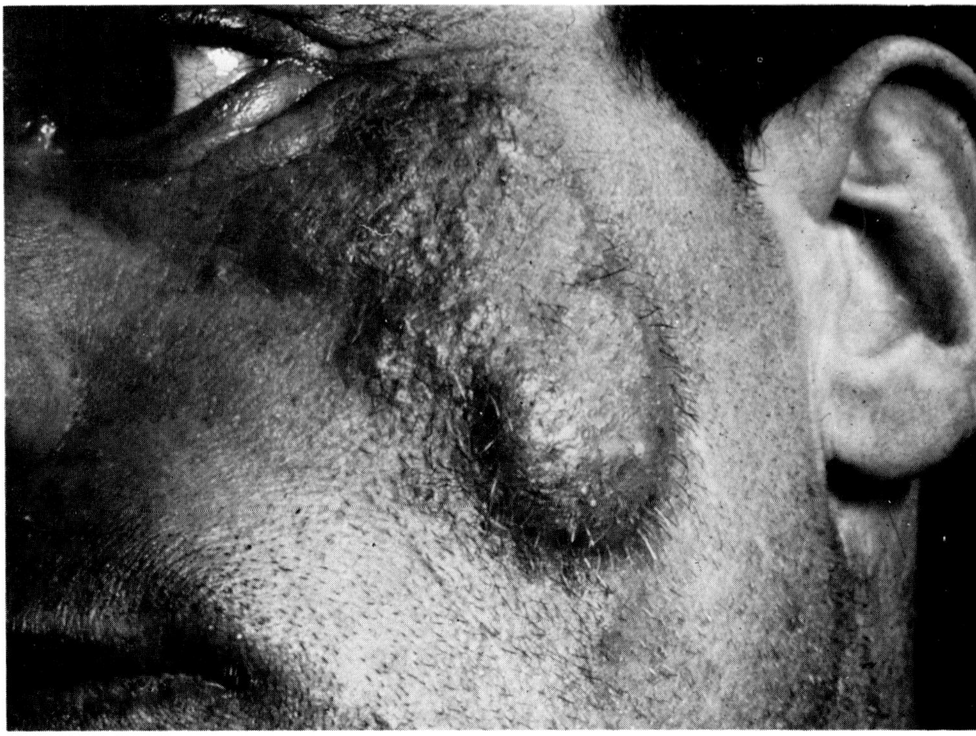

**Fig. 14-1.** Faviform tinea. Beard fungus seen in central Canada with acute inflammatory, pustular reaction. (Courtesy Dr. Arthur R. Birt, Winnipeg, Manitoba.)

Jones, Reinhardt, and Rinaldi studied 180 male prisoners and determined that patients with chronic or recurrent superficial fungal infection were likely to have reduction in delayed hypersensitivity to trichophyton extract. Some 20% of the population studied were subject to chronic ringworm infection.

Hanifin, Ray, and Lobitz have shown that most patients with naturally acquired *T. rubrum* infections have a selective anergy to trichophyton extract, as measured by lymphocyte transformation. *At least 40%* of these individuals are atopic.

Jones and co-workers in 1974 also demonstrated an interesting relationship between immediate and delayed hypersensitivity to dermatophyte infections in patients with atopy. A local antagonism of immune processes seems to develop. If immediate type I hypersensitivity is high, cell-mediated immunity seems likely to be defective and a dermatophyte infection may become chronic. The degree and type of immunity vary with the antigenic load. The greater the load in some patients with atopy, the weaker the immune response.

In those with no atopy who were experimentally infected, cell-mediated immunity developed, and they were resistant to inoculations of fungal spores. In patients who were experimentally infected and developed chronic tinea pedis, corporis, or cruris (19% of the study population), one fourth had developed cell-mediated immunity, one third had cell-mediated and immediate immunity, one fifth had immediate reactions only, and one fifth had no immune response to *Trichophyton*. It is apparent then that the factors determining resistance to fungal infections are complex and unclear as yet. We do know, however, that atopic patients are unduly susceptible.

Ringworm infections from *T. rubrum* often are unilateral and remain localized for years. An involvement of one foot, or one or two toe webs, or one hand, is a common observation.

Despite the fact that there is a deficit in delayed hypersensitivity, there is some factor of local resistance that prevents spread.

Attempts at immunization of animals and man have resulted only in increased inflammatory response to the presence of the fungus, and no lasting protective immunity. Although it must be emphasized that there is a variety of fungi and, obviously therefore, a multitude of antigens.

### *Diagnostic techniques*

Diagnosis is established by one of the following methods:

1. Examination of infected hairs for fluorescence under *Wood's light*. This is an ultraviolet lamp with a filter that cuts out all but those wavelengths that are responsible for the fluorescence. When the beam of light strikes the infected hairs, the fungus alters the wavelength of the beam, thus producing a fluorescence. This establishes the presence of a fungus, but not the species of the fungus. Sebum, ointment, or scales at the site of examination are confusing because they may also fluoresce, although with a different color; thus the scalp should be thoroughly shampooed prior to examination.

2. *Microscopic examination* of skin scrapings, hair, and nails for the presence of fungal elements. The area to be examined microscopically is first cleansed with 70% alcohol. Scales from the site of infection are gently but firmly scraped from the skin onto a clean glass slide, a hair is plucked from the infected site, or clippings are taken from the nail. A drop of 10% potassium hydroxide is applied to the material thus obtained to dissolve the keratin. A cover glass is gently placed over this area, and it is left for a period of 20 minutes. The slide is then examined for the presence of branching mycelia or spores, under high dry magnification and low illumination. Direct examination of scraped material by an experienced observer yields the highest percent of positive results.

3. Appearance of the *culture* produced on an artificial medium. The purpose of this procedure is to further identify the causative fungus. After the scales, nail clippings, or hair samples are obtained, the specimen is placed on a sterile tube slant or plate of Sabouraud's medium. This is then incubated at room temperature for a period of 2 to 6 weeks. Colonies become visible within 5 days. The diagnosis is established by gross and microscopic examination of the culture growth.

## Dermatophytes

### Tinea capitis (ringworm of the scalp)

Patchy loss of scalp hair in children, with or without inflammation, may be produced by a fungal infection (Fig. 14-2, *A*).

*M. canis* and *M. audouini* cause the majority of these scalp infections. *M. canis* is usually contracted from pets and *M. audouini* is transmitted from one human being to another. Suppurative tinea capitis is chiefly attributable to the cattle fungus, *T. verrucosum*. Tinea capitis is uncommon in adults. (History and clinical and laboratory findings are given in Table 4.)

#### *Differential diagnosis*

***Alopecia areata.*** Noninflamed patches of alopecia, with neither scaling nor evidence of broken hairs, are found in this disorder.

***Traumatic alopecia.*** Small areas of alopecia may result from prolonged traction of ponytail, curlers, braids, and so forth.

***Trichotillomania.*** Ragged areas of broken-off hairs are found in persons with trichotillomania, a habit or compulsion to pull out hairs.

***Lupus erythematosus.*** Uncommon inflammatory alopecia, producing scarring and often associated with facial lesions, is caused by lupus erythematosus.

***Seborrheic dermatitis.*** Seborrheic dermatitis may produce discrete, crusted, multiple, pruritic scalp lesions without loss of scalp hair.

#### *Treatment*

***Systemic.*** Griseofulvin is the most effective treatment for all forms of dermatophytosis except tinea pedis. It is excreted in sweat and probably attains much of its effect by this route. It is also effective by deposition in epidermis. Resistant strains that require in-

A

B

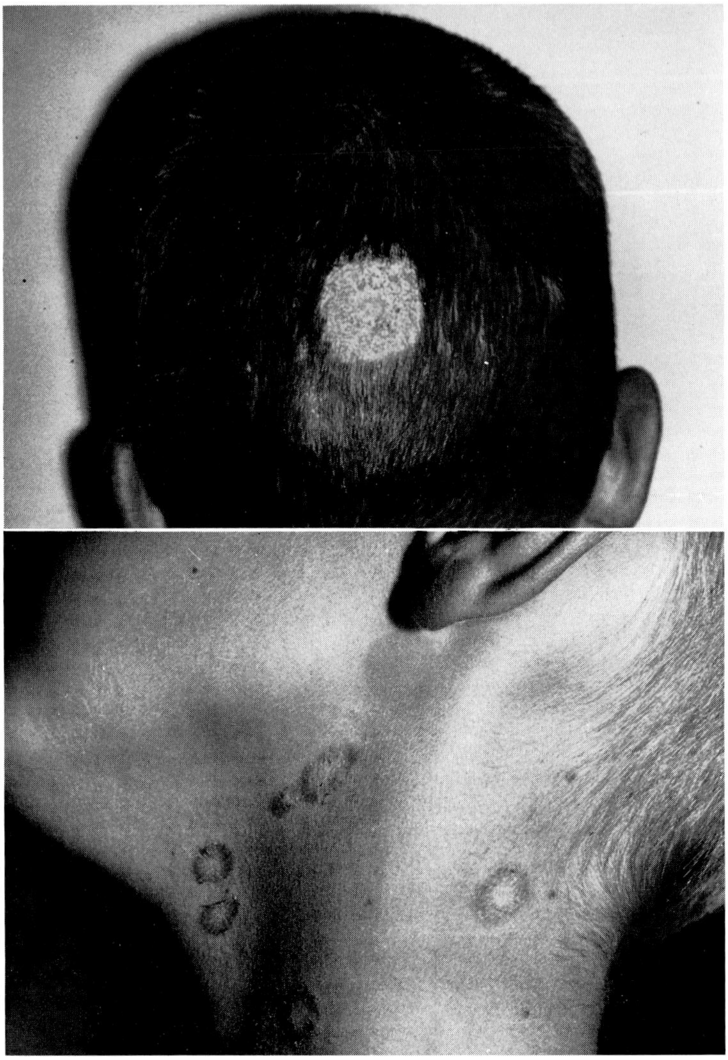

**Fig. 14-2. A,** Tinea capitis. **B,** Tinea corporis. Both infections caused by *Microsporum canis,* the "kitten" or "puppy" fungus.

creased concentrations of drug for inhibition are appearing. It is not locally effective.

Griseofulvin should be used in its micronized form and given with a fat-containing meal, thus producing better absorption and a higher blood level. *Headaches*, which are not an infrequent effect of griseofulvin ingestion, can be avoided if the drug is taken with meals. It may also cause *phototoxicity*, *urticaria*, and *nausea*. It can produce *exacerbation of porphyria* and *antagonizes warfarin*, necessitating an increased dose of that anticoagulant if given concurrently. *Phenobarbital will reduce the efficacy of griseofulvin and should not be taken concurrently.*

For children weighing 30 to 50 pounds, dosage is 0.5 Gm. daily in divided doses; for those weighing 50 pounds or over, 0.75 Gm. daily in divided doses. Dosage for adults is 1 Gm. daily (micronized) for a minimum of 4 weeks. Treatment with griseofulvin should be continued for a minimum of 2 weeks after the last sign of clinical activity or of positive cultures, usually a total of 4 weeks.

| Fungus | History | Clinical findings | Wood's light examination | Microscopic examination of hair | Culture growth on Sabouraud's medium |
|---|---|---|---|---|---|
| *Microsporum canis* | Common in North America generally; causes self-limited, moderately contagious infection, often contracted from kitten or puppy, but also transmitted from child to child (Fig. 14-2) | Hairless patches, with scalp inflammation; nonhairy skin surfaces may be similarly infected | Bright green fluorescence of infected hair; no fluorescence on infected smooth skin | Spores present about the outside of hair shaft only (ectothrix) | White fluffy growth with diagnostic bright yellow color change in underlying medium; large (80 to 200 μm.) spindle-shaped structures with tapering ends (fuseaux), seen on microscopic examination of culture |
| *Microsporum audouini* | Common in eastern and southern North America, but uncommonly seen in western areas; infection transmitted from man to man, frequently has a chronic course, and ends by puberty | Hairless, noninflamed patches with hair broken off at level of skin surface, giving a gray appearance; nonhairy skin surfaces may be similarly involved | Bright green fluorescence of infected hair; no fluorescence on infected smooth skin | Spores present about the outside of hair shaft only (ectothrix) | White fluffy growth with pink or tan color change in underlying medium; no diagnostic features revealed by microscopic examination of culture |
| *Trichophyton tonsurans* comprised of *T. violaceum, T. sulfureum, T. crateriforme* | Increase in epidemic tinea capitis from *T. tonsurans* reported in New York and Texas; not a common fungal infection | Clinical picture varying from dry scaling patches with short broken hairs (black dot appearance) to inflamed, yellow, crusted areas of alopecia | No fluorescence | Fungal elements present within hair shaft (endothrix) | *T. violaceum,* violet convoluted growth; *T. sulfureum,* yellow growth; *T. crateriforme,* pure white growth with depressed center |
| *Trichophyton schoenleini* (member of faviform group) | Causes favus, rare infection limited to man, chiefly European and Asian in distribution, but occasionally seen in North America; occurs chiefly in children, but may persist into adult life | Scalp involvement, with thick, yellow, crusted lesions, often suppurative, that lead to scarring and permanent alopecia; distinctive odor described as "mousy" | Dull green fluorescence (inconstant finding) | Spores in chain formation within the hair (endothrix) | Convoluted, smooth, waxy growth that extends into medium; antlerlike structures (favic chandeliers) seen on microscopic examination |
| *Trichophyton verrucosum* | Causes suppurative ringworm in central and western Canada, northeastern United States, and England | Nodular, tender inflamed lesions that become boggy and dotted with perifollicular abscesses in the scalp; beard and smooth skin may also be affected | No fluorescence. | Spores seen within the hair shaft | Yellow, waxy subsurface colonies with radial folds |

The hairs over the affected site should be kept clipped to prevent spread by infected hairs to other children.

Adjuvant topical treatment may be used in addition to systemic treatment with griseofulvin to help prevent spread of the infected scales and hairs while the systemic drug takes effect.

***Antifungal topical agents.*** In controlled trials, where placebo preparations were used as comparisons, available antifungal topical agents compared approximately as follows:

| | | |
|---|---|---|
| Miconazole 2% cream and powder | (75%-95% of patients cleared) | Effective against both dermatophytes and yeasts |
| Clotrimazole cream, ointment, and liquid | (30%-88%) | Effective against dermatophytes and yeasts |
| Haloprogin 1% cream and alcohol | (60%-80%) | Suppresses yeasts; effective against dermatophytes; tends to produce burning |
| Sodium omadine 1% cream | — | Very effective against dermatophytes and has prolonged action |
| Tolnaftate 1% cream, powder, and solution | (60%-70%) | Ineffective in yeast infections; less effective in scaling, red palm, and sole problems than any of the above; effective in tinea pedis; good in powder form |
| Thiabendazole 5% | — | Very effective against dermatophytes with prolonged action |
| Whitfield's ointment (salicylic acid 3% and benzoic acid 6% in zinc oxide ointment) | (57%) | Effective in one half or more of fungal infections |
| Undecylenic acid | (27%-68%) | Reasonably effective in tinea pedis |

In *M. canis* infections, household pets, particularly puppies or kittens, should be examined carefully under Wood's light and, if necessary, treated for fungi. In *M. audouini* infections, it is important to examine all contacts with Wood's light in order to halt the spread of the infection and to treat those asymptomatic individuals harboring the infection.

### Tinea corporis (ringworm of the nonhairy skin)

Tinea corporis is an infection of the keratin layer of the smooth skin caused by species of *Microsporum* and *Trichophyton*. It is more common in hot and humid climates than in temperate ones and more prevalent in rural than in urban areas.

*M. canis* and *M. audouini* account for the majority of infections occurring in children. They cause pruritic, red, scaling, circular patches with a pale center and a finely vesicular border (Fig. 14-2, *B*). They are usually fairly uniform in size and less than 3 inches in diameter. Lesions are found on the face, neck, and extremities. The scalp may also be infected, particularly in children. An infected pet is the common source of infection with *M. canis* (Fig. 14-3).

*T. rubrum (T. purpureum)* infection causes larger, more irregularly shaped, dull red, chronic, pruritic, scaling plaques on the trunk or the extremities. This is the most common West Coast fungal infection in adults. *T. mentagrophytes* causes similar lesions. The palms, soles, and fingernails or toenails may also be involved in both infections.

*T. verrucosum* (Fig. 14-4) is seen in areas of Canada east of the Coast Mountains, where it is present in cattle and is carried on hides to men working with cattle, who carry it on their hair and clothes, thereby spreading it to their families. It is the most common fungal infection of central Canada. It produces an inflammatory crusted, vesicopustular, circular lesion on smooth skin.

### *Differential diagnosis*

Diagnosis of fungal infections is established by clinical findings, by microscopic evidence

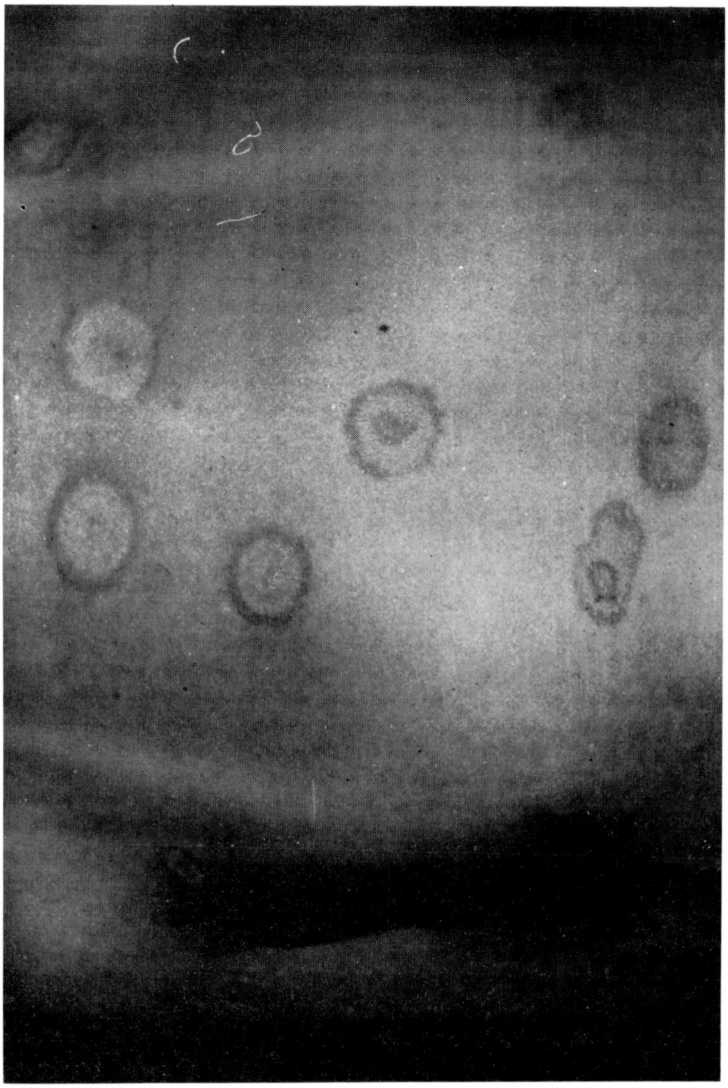

**Fig. 14-3.** Tinea corporis (ringworm) caused by *Microsporum canis.*

of fungi in skin scrapings, and by demonstration of fungi on culture examination.

***Pityriasis rosea.*** The oval-shaped, scaling, erythematous lesions of pityriasis rosea involve the thorax and extremities but not the face or scalp. The herald plaque and following course are characteristic.

***Psoriasis.*** The dull red, erythematous patches have a heavy scale, and elbows and knees are primarily involved.

***Nummular eczema.*** The vesicular, moist surface of the lesions in nummular eczema is usually more pruritic than the surface of tinea corporis lesions. Nummular eczema does not involve face or scalp.

***Lichen simplex chronicus.*** Patches of lichenified, pruritic, and pigmented dermatitis that are usually slightly elevated characterize lichen simplex chronicus.

***Seborrheic dermatitis.*** The distribution of lesions in seborrheic dermatitis (in the postauricular, paranasal, and anterior hairline areas and on the midsternum) is characteristic.

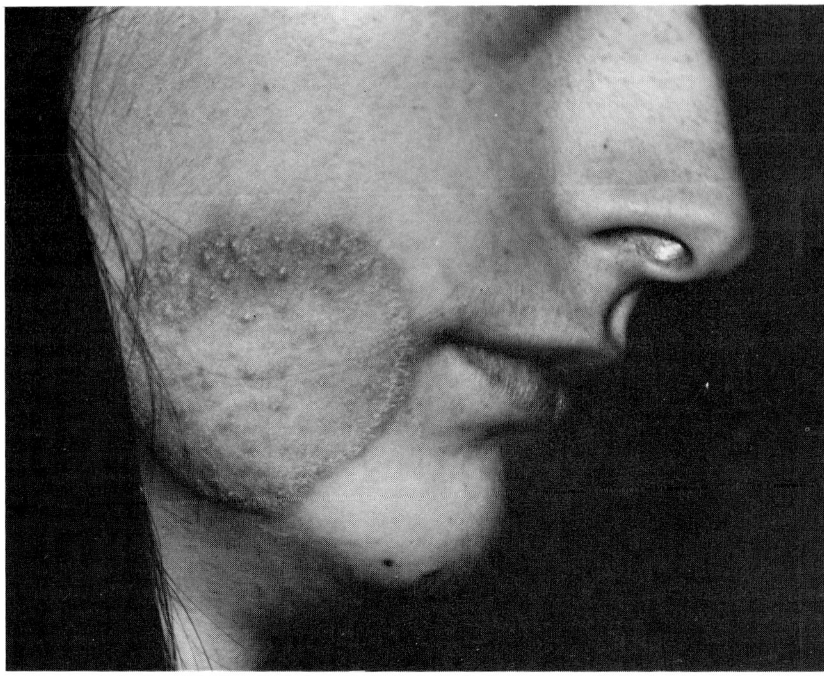

**Fig. 14-4.** Tinea of the face. *Trichophyton verrucosum* from animal hides. Note less reaction than that in Fig. 14-1. (Courtesy Dr. J. Barrie Ross, Halifax, Nova Scotia.)

### *Treatment*

***Systemic.*** See also p. 267.

Griseofulvin (micronized), 1 Gm. daily in adults, is given for a minimum of 4 weeks and up to 3 months for *T. rubrum* infections. Dosage for children weighing 30 to 50 pounds is 0.5 Gm. daily in divided doses; for children 50 pounds or over, 0.75 Gm. daily in divided doses.

Griseofulvin may cause *phototoxicity, urticaria, headaches,* and *nausea.* It can produce *exacerbation of porphyria* and *antagonizes warfarin,* necessitating an increased dose of that anticoagulant if given concurrently. *Phenobarbital will reduce the efficacy of griseofulvin* and should not be taken concurrently.

***Topical.*** See p. 270.

### *Prophylaxis*

After clearing a cutaneous fungal infection, the problem of preventing recurrences necessitates consideration. General measures of cleanliness, thorough drying after washing, prevention of sweat accumulation and moisture from other sources, and wearing of well-ventilated clothing and shoes is essential. In addition, topical antifungal powders (tolnaftate, miconazole) may be used. As stated above, several new agents may prove superior for this use, among them sodium omadine or thiabendazole, but tolnaftate, with all of its deficiencies as reported by Knight, is the best available at this time.

## Tinea cruris

Tinea cruris most frequently affects adult males. The infection begins as a small but slowly enlarging patch of scaling erythematous dermatitis in the inguinal fold, on the scrotum, and on the upper inner thigh. Both the axillae and the feet may also be sites of fungal infection. There is usually an active erythematous border that may show vesiculation. The central area is pale and scaling, and the lesion is pruritic (Plate 28). Heat, perspi-

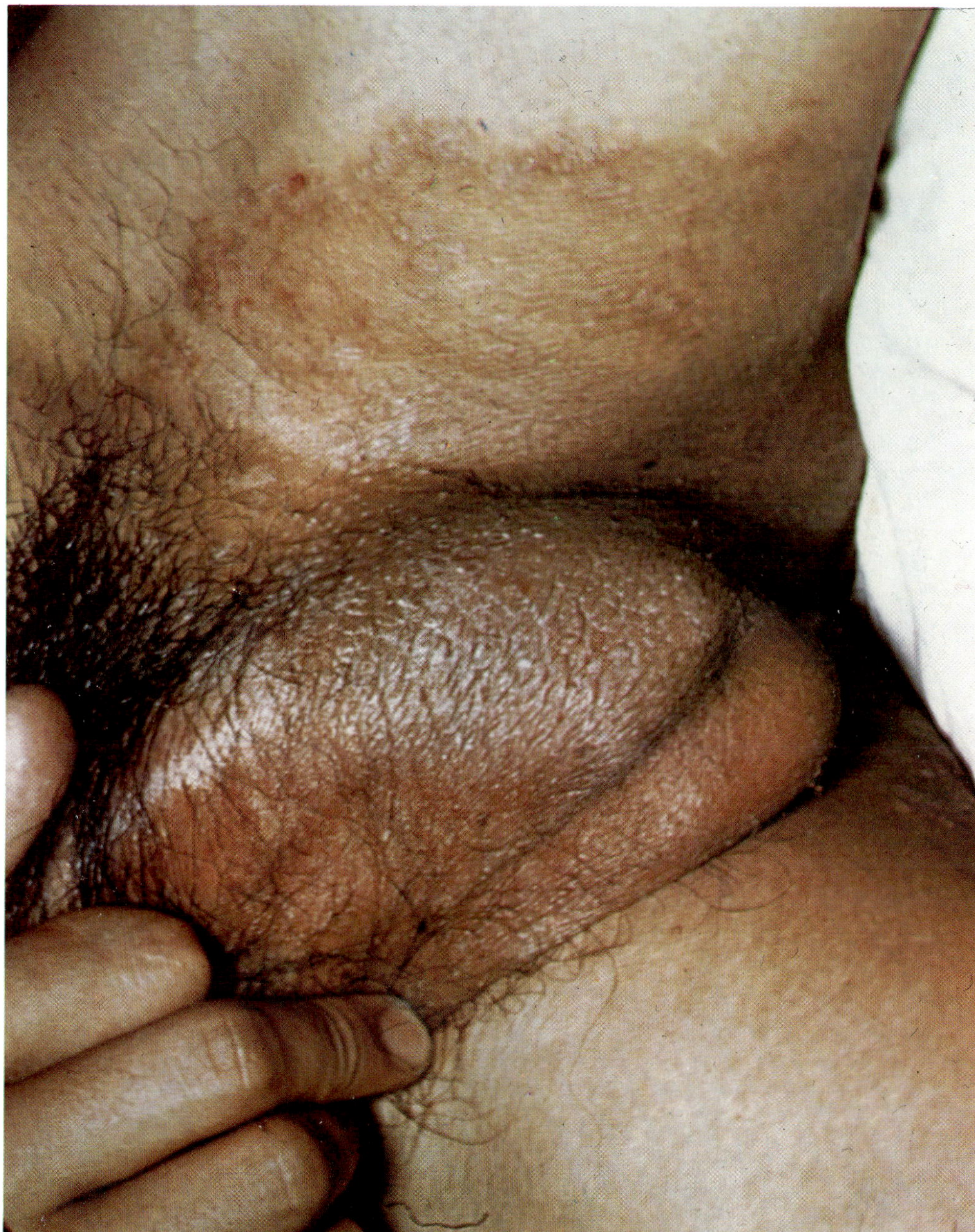

**Plate 28**

Fungal infection; tinea cruris caused by *Trichophyton rubrum.*

ration, and physical activity tend to aggravate the pruritus. Initially the lesion may be unilateral, but it almost always spreads to involve the opposite side as well.

The disease tends to be recurrent, and dermatophyte infection is usually present in the intertoe spaces or on the soles of the feet as well. Nails may be involved. These areas should be examined for signs of disease.

The organisms most commonly producing tinea cruris are *T. rubrum, Epidermophyton floccosum*, and *T. mentagrophytes*.

### *Differential diagnosis*

***Intertrigo.*** Sweat, heat, and maceration associated with chafing and trauma can produce an uncomfortable but less pruritic inguinal inflammation. Cultures from the site are negative.

***Candidosis (moniliasis).*** Candidal lesions are erythematous and moist, with pustular satellite lesions. There are often similar lesions in other intertriginous areas. Culture will reveal the characteristic organism.

***Psoriasis and seborrheic dermatitis.*** Sharply demarcated, shiny, erythematous lesions of apposing skin surfaces of inguinal folds, with scaling lesions apparent elsewhere on the cutaneous surface, occur in both psoriasis and seborreic dermatitis. Skin scrapings are negative on examination for the fungus.

***Erythrasma.*** Erythrasma is a bacterial infection producing a well-demarcated erythematous, wrinkled, finely scaling dermatitis of the inner thighs and scrotum. The lesion fluoresces bright red under Wood's light.

### *Treatment*

Griseofulvin (micronized) is given in a dose of 1 Gm. daily and continued for 2 to 3-month periods. We strongly advise that this drug be used *only after culture identification* of a causative fungus is made. It should be taken with meals.

Topical therapy consists of application of tolnaftate liquid (Tinactin) sparingly three times daily. Because of the frequency of recurrences, it seems advisable to use both topical and systemic therapy, as well as altering the moist, warm environment that encourages fungal growth.

Thus elimination of predisposing factors (for example, moisture retention, heat, and friction in this area) and avoidance of tight or restrictive underclothing and excessive perspiration are important aspects of treatment and prophylaxis against future infection.

Because certain individuals seem predisposed to these infections, prophylaxis is important. Continued use of tolnaftate, miconazole,or other antifungal preparations after regular bathing seems indicated. (See therapy of tinea corporis.)

## Tinea pedis (fungal infection of the foot, athlete's foot)

Tinea pedis can be diagnosed with certainty only by a fungal culture or direct examination of the skin scrapings.

The clinical manifestations vary between acute, weeping, severe inflammation and mild scaling only.

*T. rubrum* and *T. mentagrophytes* are the most common causes of the infection. In the intertriginous type, pruritus is the most troublesome complaint. It is intensified by heat and sweating. White macerated tissue and fissuring are found between the toes and on the flexural surface. This occurs in most males at some age period and is a persistent and recurrent condition. On the soles, particularly along the instep, the involvement of the smooth skin is vesicular, scaling, and erythematous. There may also be pruritic scaling or vesiculation, or both, extending up the sides of the feet (Fig. 14-5). One or more nails are commonly involved, with thickening and discoloration.

It has been demonstrated that this fungal infection is not transmitted by simple extensive exposure to fungal elemants. Baer has shown that trauma, and often blistering trauma, plus exposure to fungus may be necessary to produce clinical infection in some individuals. It appears that there are many degrees of susceptibility, from instantaneous "takes" of infection by as little as a single spore to the necessity of severe trauma plus massive exposure, to produce a clinical infection. The

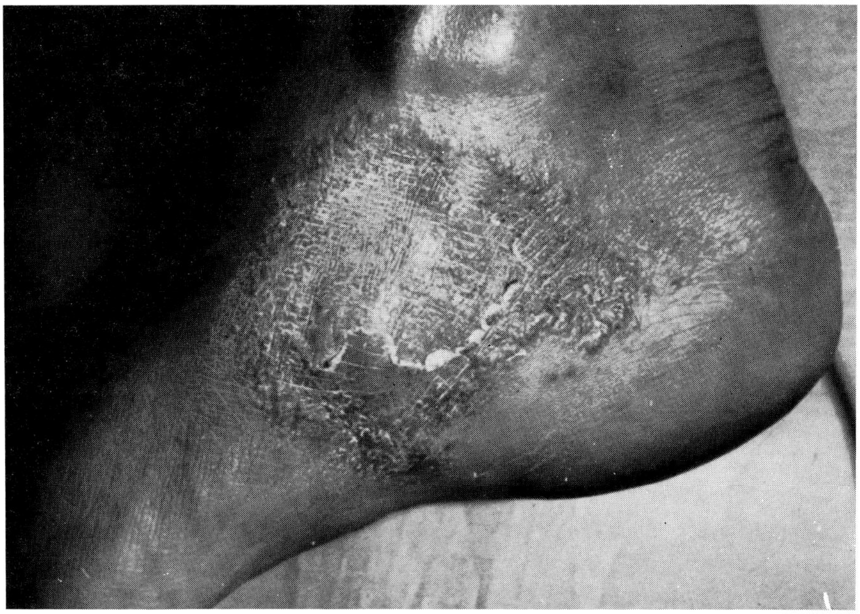

**Fig. 14-5.** Fungal infection, tinea pedis, caused by *Trichophyton rubrum.*

relationship of fungi to bacterial infection is a factor in susceptibility. *T. mentagrophytes* produces penicillin, for example.

In our experience, tinea pedis is rare in children. However, a review of this problem in English schoolchildren shows 20% infected with fungus. *Culture of skin scrapings does not yield as high a percentage of positive results as direct examination of the material with a KOH preparation.*

### *Differential diagnosis*

***Sweat retention.*** The dermatosis caused by sweat retention consists of deep-seated, tender vesicles on the sole of the foot and over the toes, made worse by occlusive footwear. These findings in prepubertal children suggest sweat retention rather than tinea pedis. Scrapings from the affected area show no fungal elements.

***Atopic dermatitis.*** Atopic dermatitis produces a dry pruritic scaling of the toes and dorsum of the foot.

***Allergic contact dermatitis.*** Allergic contact dermatitis causes a pruritic scaling erythema with vesiculation that involves chiefly the dorsum of the foot or toes and usually results from contact with shoe leather, dyes, or ointments. The sole is less likely to be involved. Skin scrapings are negative for fungal elements.

### *Treatment*

Elimination of the predisposing factors of heat and perspiration is important. Shoes and light socks that allow ventilation should be worn. Occlusive footwear, canvas rubber-soled running shoes, and plastic shoes are to be avoided. The patient should be cautioned against overzealous cleansing with soap and vigorous drying between the toes, which tend to irritate the area.

Transmission of the infection to other individuals is rare, despite general opinion to the contrary. Foot baths are of little or no value in prevention of tinea pedis.

Topical therapy with ointments is not generally successful, since the vehicle tends to retain sweat and moisture. Liquids and powders are more desirable.

One of the topical antifungal agents should be applied twice daily to the affected areas, and one of the antifungal powders containing tolnaftate or one of the newer, more effective agents should be dusted between the toes and into the socks daily. The powder is more effective as a prophylactic measure than as a treatment for acute conditions.

Griseofulvin (micronized), 1 Gm. daily, will eliminate the condition, but there may be recurrences, and clinical evidence suggests topicalagents are preferable. The medication should be continued until affected nails have completely grown out normally. In some patients this may take many months and, indeed, may be impractical, since 1½ years may be required to grow a complete nail and an infected nail can act as a reservoir for the fungus. (See p. 272 for complications of griseofulvin therapy.)

In acute inflammatory tinea pedis, an erythematous, weeping condition, general measures to counteract the inflammation must be used before antifungal therapy is begun. Bacterial cultures are a good precaution, since most of these acute processes are caused by bacterial infection and antibiotics given systemically may be the most efficacious therapy. Rest is essential; the patient should be off his feet. Burow's solution (utilizing the prepared tablets or powders, 1 packet to a pint of cool water) is used for compresses, which are applied twice daily in 15-minute periods. Compressing is followed by the application of an effective glucocorticoid cream. Therapy is continued until relief is obtained; then antifungal therapy may be begun if the acute inflammation has not caused a sloughing off of the epidermis and is thus cleared of fungal elements as well.

### Tinea of the hand (fungal infection of the hand)

Tinea of the hand is the least common of the superficial fungal infections. The clinical findings consist of an asymptomatic, dry, scaling hyperkeratosis of the palm, which may be associated with a dry scaling lesion having an active, vesicular, extending periphery.

Usually only one hand is involved, and one or more nails on the same hand may show evidence of fungal infection. Interestingly enough, both feet of the same individual may demonstrate intertoe infection or even fungal elements on the soles of the feet. The causative fungus is usually *T. rubrum*. The infection is often of long duration and is very rare in children. Orientals, at least in southwest Canada, seem to be particularly susceptible to this infection and to tinea pedis. However, tinea cruris is less common in this segment of the population.

#### *Differential diagnosis*

***Psoriasis.*** Psoriasis may present an appearance similar to that in fungal infection, including nail involvement. Elbows, knees, and other characteristic sites of involvement should be examined.

***Atopic dermatitis.*** Dryness, fissuring, erythema, and noticeable pruritus may be present in atopic dermatitis. The skin generally is dry, and there is a characteristic family and personal history of infantile eczema, asthma, and hay fever.

***Primary irritant dermatitis.*** In primary irritant dermatitis there is a history of contact with soap, hot water, and external irritants, either of recent or long-standing orgin.

***Allergic contact dermatitis.*** Allergic contact dermatitis ordinarily has a sudden onset, with lesions displaying some weeping and vesiculation. Examinations for fungi are negative (as in all the foregoing dermatoses).

#### *Treatment*

Griseofulvin (micronized), 1 Gm. daily with meals for a 3-month period, is the treatment of choice. If nails are involved, it will be necessary to continue therapy until the nail has completely grown out normally.

Topical treatment (see discussion of tinea corporis), or use Whitfield's ointment: salicylic acid 3%, benzoic acid 6%, hydrophilic ointment U.S.P. q.s. Apply sparingly three times daily.

### Tinea of the nails (fungal infection of the nails, onychomycosis)

Tinea of the nails begins as a fungal infection of the soft keratin of the nail bed, which secondarily extends upward into the hard keratin of the nail itself. The most common causative fungi are *T. rubrum*, *T. mentagrophytes*, and *E. floccosum*.

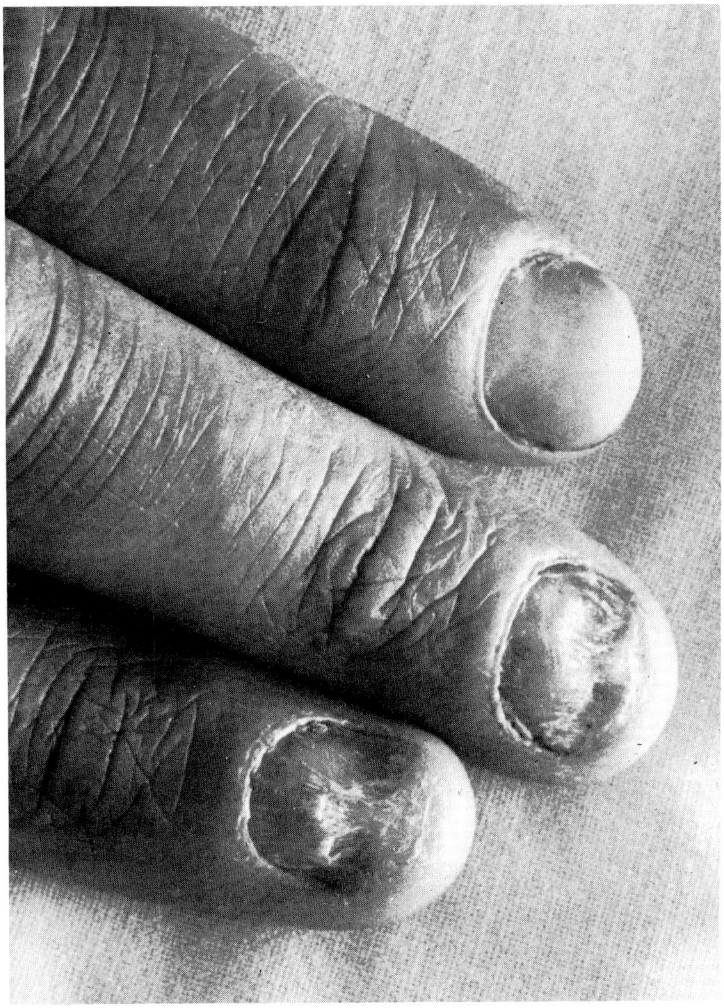

**Fig. 14-6.** Fungal infection of nails. Note noninvolvement of one nail, characteristic of fungal infection.

The infection begins at the lateral distal edge of the nail, causing the nail to become brittle and yellow. The process then spreads to involve the whole nail, producing a distorted, opaque, and discolored nail plate (Fig. 14-6). The distal portion of the nail tends to separate from the nail bed, and a crumbling hyperkeratosis forms beneath the nail (subungual keratosis). This is the chief source of fungal elements. The matrix beneath the cuticle remains uninvolved.

Once established, the process continues and may spread to unaffected nails and to adjacent skin. Toenails are much more frequently involved than fingernails.

### *Differential diagnosis*

Differential diagnosis includes conditions that produce distortion and discoloration of the nails, such as psoriasis and simple trauma, congenital disorders, some keratinizing disorders, and chronic inflammation (paronychia). No fungus is found on examination of nail clippings in these conditions.

Candidosis of the nails is also to be considered and is now regarded as more common than previously allowed. It produces a longitudinal shredding or ridging or a green-black discoloration.

### *Treatment*

The only even partially satisfactory treatment consists of administration of griseofulvin (micronized), 1 Gm. daily for 6 to 8 months for fingernail infection, and 12 to 24 months for toenail infections. The drug should be taken until repeated nail clippings are negative. Griseofulvin is best absorbed along with a fatty meal. Even with this duration of therapy, attempts at successful eradication of a toenail infection are usually disappointing. Avulsion of the affected nail does not improve the prognosis. Studies indicate chances of lasting healing of toenail infection in the range of 15%.

## Dermatophytid

Dermatophytid is an eruption occurring secondary to a fungal infection. It results from sensitization to the fungi or their breakdown products and presumably from an absorption and hematogenous spread of these products to distant sites, with production of local eruption at those sites. The most common clinical finding is vesiculation on the sides of the fingers and at times on the palms. No fungi are found in these lesions. The active fungal infection is almost always on the toes or foot. Dermatophytid on the hand tends to clear quickly with eradication of the active infection.

The most common precursor of this eruption is irritation and aggravation of the primary focus of infection.

### *Differential diagnosis*

***Sweat retention (dyshidrosis).*** A vesicular, pruritic dermatitis of the hands and feet resulting from sweat retention, dyshidrosis is worsened by heat and perspiration.

***Contact dermatitis.*** Both allergic and primary forms of contact dermatitis of the hands and fingers can produce vesiculation.

### *Treatment*

Treatment consists of eliminating the primary focus of fungal infection. Compresses of Burow's solution 1:20 for 15-minute periods should be applied to the fingers once or twice daily, followed by an adequate glucocorticoid cream applied sparingly at least three times daily. Thorough investigation of the primary fungal infection must be performed and its elimination achieved.

## Tinea versicolor

Tinea versicolor is a very superficial fungal infection of the skin, caused by *Malassezia furfur* (Plate 29).

### *Pertinent information*

Clinical and laboratory investigations reveal that this disease occurs in association with the transition of a benign component of the normal skin flora, *Pityrosporon orbiculare*, into a filamentous aggressive pathogen for the outer layers of the stratum corneum. Roberts writes an interesting account of this transformation. Although conjugal or other intimate associations do not ordinarily result in spread from one to another individual, there are susceptible persons who will develop the disease from such contacts. Cushing's disease and malnutrition produce patients liable to contract the disease. Experimental inoculations of *P. orbiculare* in these persons will result in clinical lesions of tinea versicolor. Also, patients on long-term systemic corticosteroids and some of those on continued topical glucocorticoid applications seem to be susceptible to this disorder.

### *Natural course*

The lesions consist of asymptomatic, fawn to dark brown pigmented patches with a fine scale. The back, chest, and upper arms are the most commonly involved sites. The affected areas filter out the tanning rays of the sun, producing nonpigmented patches on an otherwise tanned skin; hence the name versicolor. The course is chronic, with gradual extension. Marinaro's scanning electron micrographs demonstrate why recurrences after treatment are common. The disease is universal. The fungal elements, which may be seen on microscopic examination of skin scrapings, are found only in the horny layers of the skin and do not extend deeper. They consist of

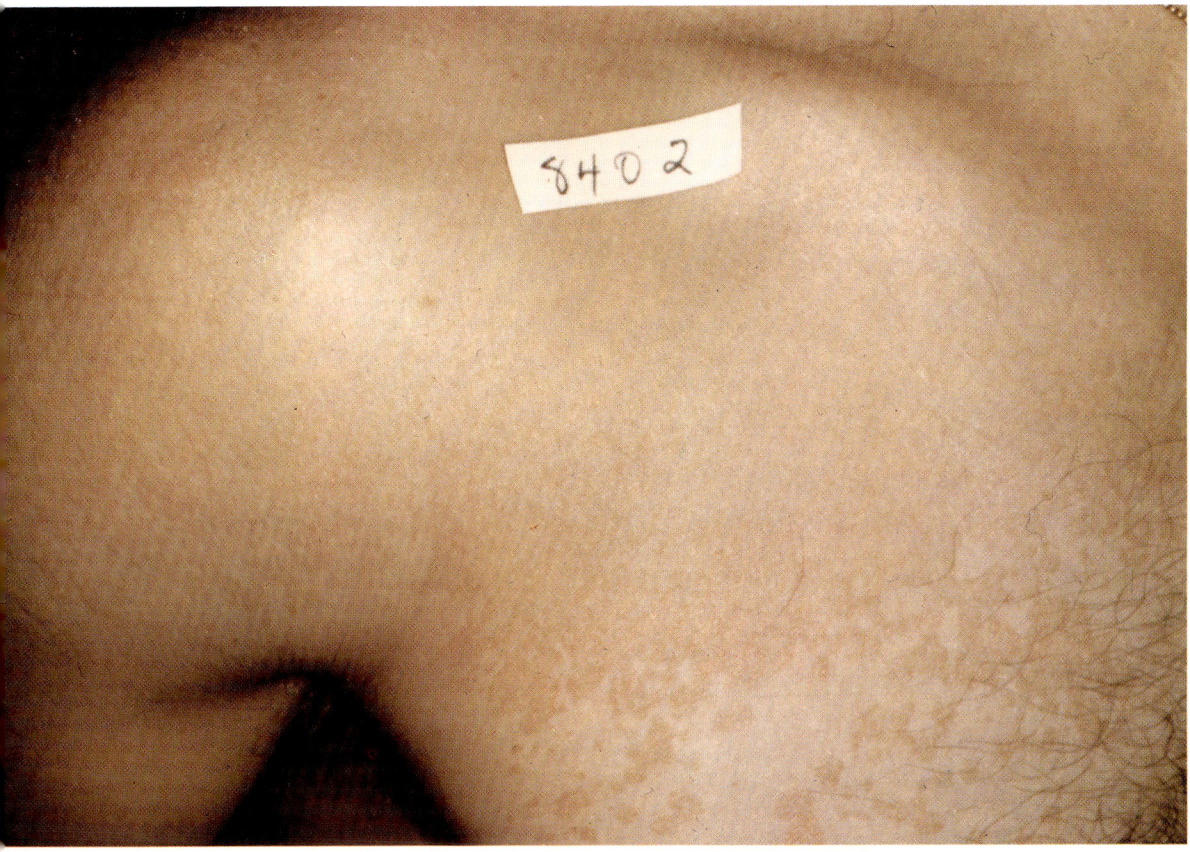


**Plate 29**

Tinea versicolor. Involved areas are brown on untanned skin, pale on tanned skin.

minute hyphal elements associated with spore clusters. The causative organism cannot be cultured. Examination under Wood's filtered ultraviolet light demonstrates a coral fluorescence of the involved areas. If this is done thoroughly, one will be suprised at the number of times infection is seen in pubic areas, thighs, popliteal spaces, and other unexpected sites.

### *Differential diagnosis*

***Vitiligo.*** Vitiligo is a disorder of pigmentation resulting in depigmented white patches on a normal skin. There is no superficial scale.

***Seborrheic dermatitis.*** Erythematous, scaling, pruritic patches of dermatitis are usually present on the midsternal and midscapular areas.

***Pityriasis rosea.*** Pityriasis rosea is a self-limited, scaling dermatitis consisting of small, discrete oval patches, originating with a characteristic herald patch.

### *Treatment*

Application of selenium sulfide suspension (Selsun), *once a week* sparingly with fingers, then left on overnight only and washed off in the morning, is done four times, or for 1 month. Miconazole is more agreeable to use and is as effective. The affected area should be viewed with Wood's light before and after treatment, for assurance that all residual areas of fluorescence have been eliminated.

**REFERENCES**

Baer, R. L., and Rosenthal, S. A.: The biology of fungous infections of the feet, J.A.M.A. **197**:1017, 1966.
**The disease categorized in three groups of 150 volunteers.**

Birt, A. R., and Wilt, J. C.: Mycology, bacteriology, and histopathology of suppurative ringworm, Arch. Dermatol. Syph. **69**:441, 1954.
**30 patients revealed an abacterial, purulent, allergic response to the fungus.**

Epstein, W. L., Shah, V. P., Jones, H. E., et al.: Topically applied griseofulvin in prevention and treatment of *Trichophyton mentagrophytes*, Arch. Dermatol. **111**:1293, 1975.
**No clinical effect despite very high surface concentrations.**

Gentles, J. C., Evans, E. G. V., and Jones, C. R.: Control of tinea pedis in a swimming bath, Br. Med. J. **2**:577, 1974.
**Tolnaftate powder selectively reduced *T. mentagrophytes* infections.**

Gentles, J. C., Jones, G. R., and Roberts, D. T.: Efficacy of miconazole in the topical treatment of tinea pedis in sportsmen, Br. J. Dermatol. **93**:79, 1975.
**60% effective in double-blind home-use active-participant trial.**

Hanifin, J. M., Ray, L. F., and Lobitz, W. C.: Immunological reactivity in dermatophytosis, Br. J. Dermatol. **90**:1, 1974.
**Variable immediate and delayed responses depending on organism.**

Jones, H. E., Reinhardt, J. H., and Rinaldi, M. G.: A clinical mycological and immunological survey for dermatophytosis, Arch. Dermatol. **108**:61, 1973.
**The first series associating immune mechanisms and chronicity of the disease.**

Jones, H. E., Reinhardt, J. A., and Rinaldi, M. G.: Immunologic susceptibility to dermatophytosis, Arch. Dermatol. **110**:213, 1974.
**Relationship between cell-mediated and humoral immune mechanisms.**

Jones, H. E., Reinhardt, J. H., and Rinaldi, M. G.: Model dermatophytosis in naturally infected subjects, Arch. Dermatol. **110**:369, 1974.
**Delineation of the types of response to fungal infection.**

King, R. D., Khan, H. A., and Toye, J. C.: Transferrin iron and dermatophytes. I. Serum dermatophyte inhibitory component definitively identified as unsaturated transferrin, J. Lab. Clin. Med. **86**:204, 1975.
**Dermatophytes require iron, and transferrin binds it too firmly for their use.**

Knight, A. G.: Human models for in vivo and in vitro assessment of topical antifungal compounds, Br. J. Dermatol. **89**:509, 1973.
**Thiabendazole and sodium omadine are the most effective of four.**

Marinaro, R. E., Gershenbaum, M. R., Roisen, F. J., et al.: Tinea versicolor. A scanning electron microscopic view, J. Cutan. Pathol. **5**:15, 1978.
**Deep follicular location possibly explains recurrences.**

Roberts, S. O. B.: Pityriasis versicolor: a mycological investigation, Br. J. Dermatol. **81**:315, 1969.
**Now a saprophyte and now a pathogen. The same organism.**

Smith, E. B.: New topical agents for dermatophytosis, Cutis **17**:54, 1976.
**A good controlled evaluation.**

Sulzberger, M. B., and Baer, R. L.: Some recent advances in dermatologic mycology. In Sulzberger, M. B., and Baer, R. L., editors: Yearbook of dermatology and syphilology, 1954-55, Chicago, 1954, Year Book Medical Publishers, Inc., p. 7.
**Important and valid observations.**

## CANDIDOSIS (MONILIASIS)

*Candida albicans* is the species of candidal (monilial) organisms most frequently isolated from human candidal infections. Other species of *Candida* cause infections, but more rarely. The important point to remember here is that in any patient the presence of other species of *Candida* must not be taken lightly, because any of seven other species can cause superficial and systemic or fatal disease.

*Candida* can be recovered from 50% of normal oral cavities and from the vagina, gastrointestinal tract, and perianal skin folds. It appears to live in these areas, as Marples says, as an opportunist pathogen in uneasy balance with its host. A large percentage of the general population show delayed cellular hypersensitivity to *Candida*.

*C. albicans* has been shown to appear as a colonizer within 2 weeks after the development of a chronically moist area on the skin. It has also been shown to produce inflammation and pustular lesions when applied in adequate concentrations under a completely occlusive adhesive tape. Pustular lesions develop within 72 hours under these circumstances. This pus-producing ability is ascribed by Ray and Wuepper to activation of complement by *Candida*. This leads to chemotaxis and leukocyte aggregation. Although the organism can be persuaded experimentally to colonize on skin of all types (damaged, inflamed, stripped, and so forth), the skin reverts to normal, and the infection disappears when the experimental consitions are discontinued. Culture of *C. albicans* from a dermatitis denotes a true pathogenic state of the organism.

*C. albicans* exists in yeastlike (budding) and filamentous (mycelial) forms. These are antigenically distinct. In certain conditions it is pathogenic, invades, and produces inflammation, related to the development and growth of mycelia.

This microorganism grows in the keratin layer of the skin, as the foregoing experiments indicate, where softening and maceration are necessary for the acquisition of the infection and for production of inflammation. Increased supplies of glucose allow the organism to proliferate. Living epidermis appears to have anticandidal properties that limit invasion of the keratin layer. Serum anticandidal factors are not well defined, and serous exudate from stripped skin does not seem to inhibit growth of *Candida*. However, *Candida* can activate complement and polymorphonuclear neutrophil leukocytes, as well as tissue macrophages, and can kill and phagocytose yeast cells. Transferrin, the iron-binding globulin in human plasma, has anticandidal properties when unsaturated with iron, but loses these properties when fully saturated. Its effect may result from its ability to bind iron; thus an essential nutrient is kept away from the invading yeast.

Although development of pathogenicity has been considered an alteration in the candidal organism, it is also held that the pathogenicity results because of a change in the host and host susceptibility to which *C. albicans* is remarkably sensitive. As a result, the presence of *C. albicans* in a lesion requires a research for the weakness in body defenses that induced its pathogenicity. *It is a clinical aphorism that C. albicans can recognize systemic abnormalities before the laboratory can.*

Predisposing factors to candidal infection are diabetes mellitus, idiopathic hypoparathyroidism, hypoadrenalism, hypothyroidism, pernicious anemia, thymus abnormalities, and defects in cellular immunity, which are often associated with chemotactic impairment as well. Old age, infancy, pregnancy, obesity, profuse sweating, and malnutrition, will support *Candida*. People occupied with wet work, such as housewives, bartenders, and dairy workers, have an increased incidence of paronychia.

Administration of antibiotics causes an increase in incidence of gastrointestinal candidosis, from 7% before treatment to 71% after tetracycline therapy. This is probably not attributable to decreased competition by other organisms but to a change in immunological defenses and to local tissue damage. Patients taking systemic glucocorticoids, topical glucocorticoids under occlusion, and most significant of all, immunosuppressive agents are prone to develop cutaneous and systemic candidosis. Recognition of candidal organisms in the blood and other specimens may or may not be significant, as reported by Toala and his co-workers.

### Disseminated candidosis

Rarely, the entire skin surface may become infected, or systemic involvement may occur with candidal septicemia, meningitis, or endocarditis, any of which can have a fatal outcome. In desseminated candidosis, Bodey described 10% to 15% of ill patients showing discrete, red yeast-containing nodules in the dermis, which can be diagnostic. The symptoms of systemic candidosis are similar to those of a severe bacterial infection. Chills, spiking fever, hypotension and prostration, dysphagia, orbital pain, blurred vision, symptoms related to renal involvement and failure or headache, neck rigidity, hemoptysis, or embolic phenomena may be presented.

Failure to demonstrate *candida* is common. Absence of the almost universal immune response of cell-mediated immunity to *Candida* antigen is suggestive of the anergy seen in disseminate candidosis.

There is considerable concern regarding the increasing incidence of candidal infections. Part of the growing incidence of these infections results from the wider use of *immunosuppressive agents* in organ transplant

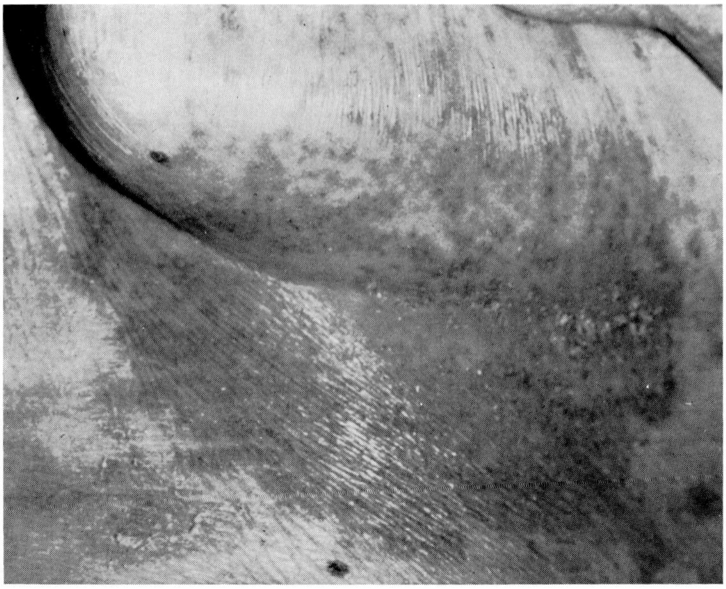

**Fig. 14-7.** Inframammary candidosis (moniliasis).

cases, in collagen diseases and autoallergies, and with use of such drugs as methotrexate in psoriasis.

Another group of patients with candidosis are those who develop a chronic form of the disease in childhood, without the help of drugs or other disease states. Many of these patients demonstrate selective immune deficiency states and an inability to produce delayed hypersensitivity to *Candida*. They also may demonstrate iron-deficiency anemia and susceptibility to *some* viral and bacterial infections. Remarkably, therapy of the candidal infection and correction of the anemic state may produce a normal individual with normal delayed-hypersensitivity reactions, including that to *Candida*.

### Intertrigo

In areas where apposed skin surfaces prevent adequate ventilation and keep the site warm and moist, there is a predisposition to candidal infection. These include the inguinal fold, submammary area (Fig. 14-7), gluteal fold, axillae, interdigital spaces, umbilicus, and abdominal fold of obese individuals. *C. albicans* is the primary agent in at least a small percentage of cases of diaper dermatitis.

The lesions of candidosis on a cutaneous surface are erythematous, moist, macerated, well-demarcated areas with irregular borders. These are probably originally vesicopustules from which the soft moist skin is rubbed off. They characteristically have small satellite pustular lesions, which also become denuded, around the primary lesions. All lesions are pruritic and tender. They tend to remain limited to the intertriginous areas.

These lesions are aggravated by heat, activity, perspiration, tight or occlusive clothing, and friction. As with other forms of candidosis, intertrigo is more frequent in persons with diabetes mellitus.

### Interdigital candidosis (erosio interdigitalis)

Candidosis may occur as an erosive, chronic inflammation, appearing with white macerated tissue, fissures, and denuded areas between the fingers, usually the ring and middle fingers (Fig. 14-8). It occurs chiefly in individuals who are engaged in wet work (for example, housewives and launderers).

#### *Treatment*

First and most important is keeping the area dry. Clotrimazole lotion may be used

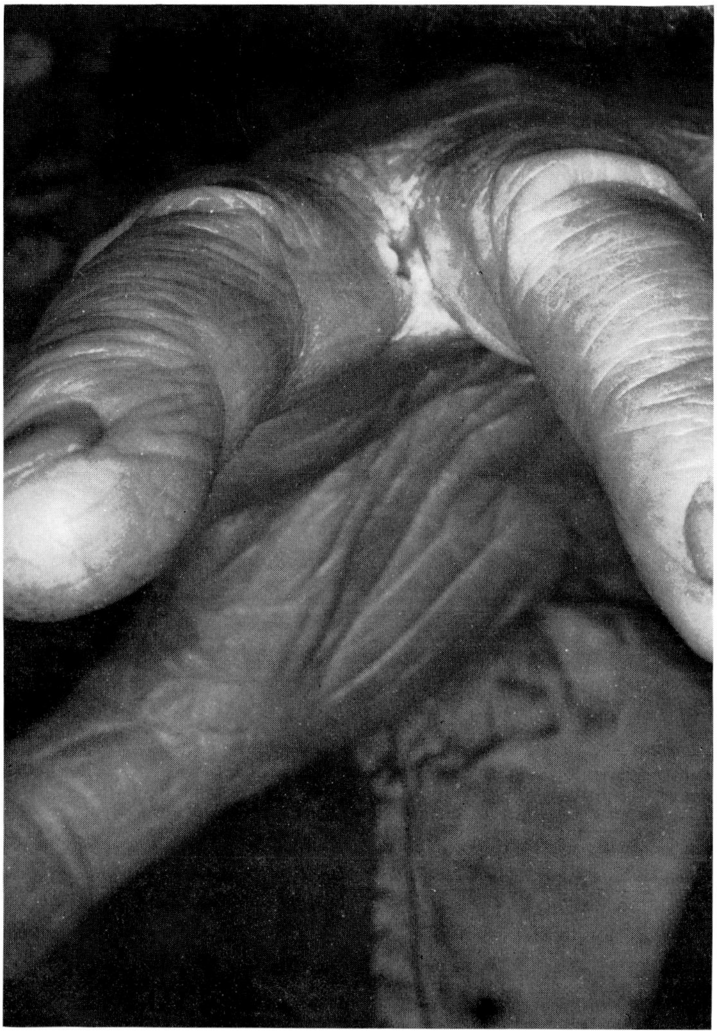

**Fig. 14-8.** Interdigital candidosis (moniliasis).

with benefit to dry the area and reduce pruritus. If indicated, weight reduction should be effected. To reduce the irritation produced by the *Candida* organism, Burow's solution 1:20 compresses or packaged tablets or powders, 1 to a pint of cool water, should be applied for 10 minutes twice daily. One of the anticandidal agents (amphotericin B [Fungizone], nystatin [Mycostatin], miconazole [Micatin], clotrimazole [Canestin]) in the form of cream, ointment, or lotion is applied after compresses. After the dermatitis is cleared satisfactorily, the area is kept dry with a bland application of talcum powder to which 1% to 2% nystatin may be added.

### Candidal vaginitis

Although *C. albicans* inhabits the vaginal vault as a nonpathogen in 20% or more of normal women, and considerably more in pregnancy, under certain poorly understood circumstances it becomes capable of producing inflammation. Pruritic candidal vaginitis is a not infrequent result. The incidence of symptomatic candidal vaginitis increases with pregnancy, diabetes mellitus, and antibiotic therapy. The increased incidence in pregnancy may be related to systemic factors (reduced cell-mediated immunity) rather than local.

The vaginitis begins with a thin, white, lumpy vaginal discharge and may produce no further symptoms. Often, however, itching and burning associated with labial edema and inflammation accompany the discharge. Dysuria and dyspareunia may be present, but are less frequent. The mucous membrane of the vaginal orifice is reddened diffusely, with the characteristic white plaques of friable cheesy material adherent to the surface; the vulva is almost always affected with erythema and itching.

The cutaneous inflammation of the vulva may extend to the perianal area and, in obese individuals, along apposed skin surfaces, exhibiting a course similar to the process in intertrigo.

Male sexual partners may contract a temporary, uncomfortable, reddened glans penis. This ordinarily subsides in 2 or 3 days *if it is not overtreated.*

#### *Differential diagnosis*

Differential diagnosis includes vaginitis caused by *Trichomonas vaginalis*, which produces a thick, foul, vaginal discharge. The organism is identified microscopically by the hanging drop technique on a glass slide. Concurrent infection with both *Trichomonas* and *Candida* is not uncommon.

#### *Treatment*

A thorough examination for underlying diabetes or local gynecological disease is indicated. Treatment consists of local applications of miconazole (Monistat) by a vaginal applicator or clotrimazole (Lotrimin) as tablets, or nystatin (Mycostatin) as vaginal tablets.

### Thrush

Oral candidosis (thrush) is not an uncommon finding in newborn infants. It is probably contracted from the maternal vaginal canal, where *C. albicans* flourishes during pregnancy.

The lesions, occurring on the buccal mucosa, gums, pharynx, and tongue, consist of creamy white plaques on the mucosal surface that leave a red, eroded surface when removed. It is usually a self-limited condition in infants unless there are complications of systemic debilitating disease.

#### *Treatment*

Nystatin (Mycostatin) suspension, in a dosage of 100,000 units/ml., is administered four times daily for 2 weeks, or a nystatin tablet, allowed to dissolve in the mouth, is given once daily. Amphotericin B lotion (Fungizone) is applied four times daily for 4 weeks. In older children, these suspensions can be gargled and swirled in the mouth. It is too early to determine the safety of the newer anticandidal agents in the infant.

### Perlèche (angular cheilitis)

Perlèche is a fissuring inflammation of the corners of the mouth, associated with maceration and softening of the cutaneous surface. It is usually seen in elderly persons and is associated with an edentulous mouth. Dentures leave a space beneath the palate, where *Candida* grows, produces palatal inflammation, and provides increasing numbers of candidal organisms. Iron deficiency anemia predisposes one to this infection, whereas iron therapy improves the quality of the oral epithelium and the clinical state benefits (Fig. 14-9). The edentulous condition causes bone absorption of the jaw, with resulting overlapping of the corners of the mouth. In this warm moist area candidal organisms may be found in most cases. Perlèche is seen in debilitated children and in individuals susceptible to candidal infection (for example, those with diabetes mellitus).

Cheilitis caused by deficiency of vitamin B must be ruled out. A smooth tongue, glossitis, and stomatitis are associated in these cases.

#### *Treatment*

Temporary nonuse of dentures and *correction of the iron-deficiency anemia* are both important. Mycostatin may be applied to the palate.

Overlapping of the corners of the mouth

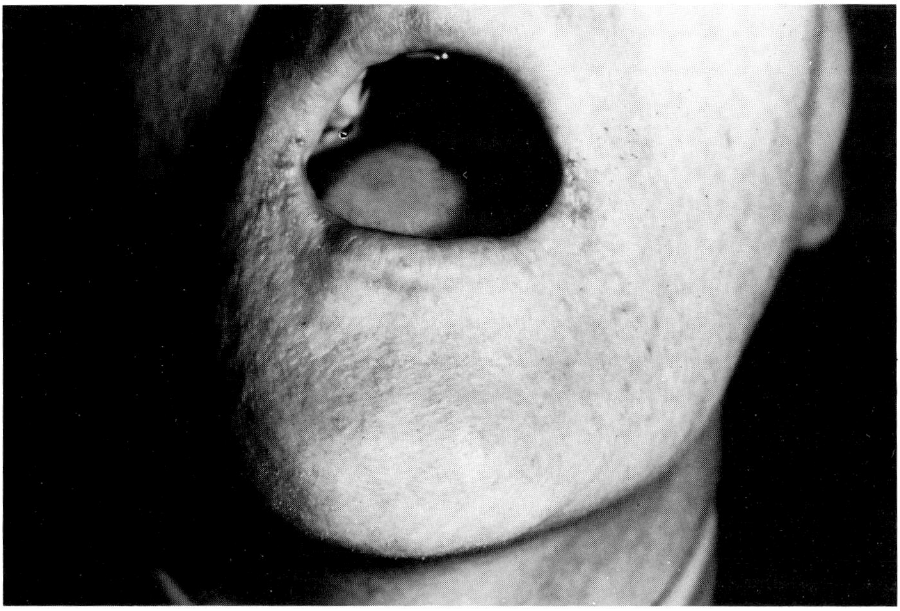

**Fig. 14-9.** Angular cheilitis. Associated with palatal candidosis.

may be corrected by opening the bite (building up the vertical dimensions of the dentures); dental consultation should be obtained when this is necessary.

In the presence of *Candida*, nystatin (Mycostatin) ointment is applied to the carefully dried surface three times daily. The palate and buccal mucosa should be examined for evidence of involvement.

In the absence of *Candida* or bacterial infection, glucocorticoid cream may be applied before and after meals. Trauma must be carefully avoided.

## Chronic hyperplastic cheilitis

Candidal infection may also produce persistent thickened white plaques of the lips, the buccal mucosa, or the tongue. Cawson and others have described a leukoplakia-like lesion with epithelial hyperplasia that may be related to eventual malignant changes. The yeast elements are hard to see on microscopic sections if they are not stained specially.

### *Treatment*

Therapy is difficult. Cawson's patients apply a nystatin tablet to the lesion four times daily, with some success. We are not aware of reports on the effect of the more potent new anticandidal agents on this entity.

## Paronychia

Paronychia is an inflammation and edema of the tissue at the base of the fingernail (Fig. 14-10), which is caused by *Candida* in only half the cases usually seen.

### *Natural course*

The tissue adjacent to and including the nail fold becomes red, swollen, and tender. The process may be acute or chronic, and the nails of the involved finger develop transverse ridges and become opaque. *C. albicans* can be cultured from the nail fold in approximately half the patients. The organism is not cultured from this area under normal conditions. Other organisms found are staphylococci, micrococci, and streptococci; often there is a mixture of these.

Paronychia is most frequently found in middle-aged people, especially women who are engaged in wet work, such as cleaning women, kitchen workers, and nurses. It is approximately three times more common in patients with diabetes than in the general population. The disease is persistent and

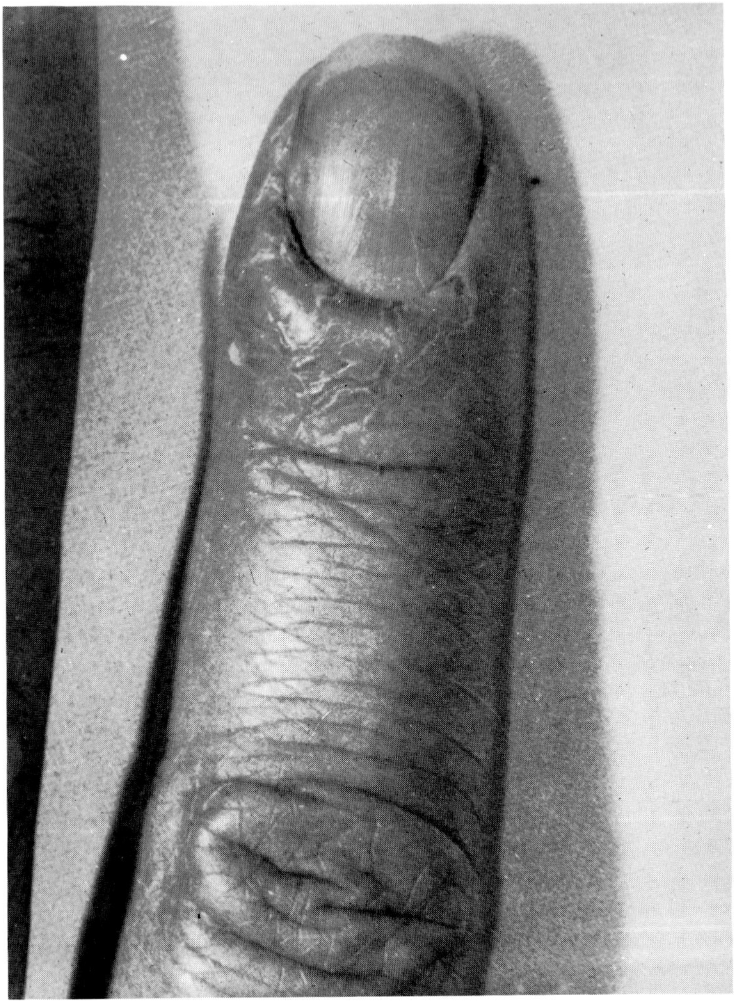

**Fig. 14-10.** Paronychia. Almost invariably associated with "wet work."

chronic so long as the contributing factors exist.

A mild form of this disease has been experimentally produced in normal individuals by simple watertight occlusion of the nail and nail fold with sticky plaster tape. *C. albicans* appears in the area after less than 2 weeks of occlusion.

The fingernail itself may be involved, with greenish gray discolorations, some surface irregularities, but not destruction as seen in onychomycosis. The lateral edges are chiefly involved.

### *Differential diagnosis*

***Tinea of the nails.*** Superficial fungal infections of the nails involve only the nail tissue and not the surrounding folds at the base of the nail.

***Psoriasis.*** Erythema and scaling of the tissue at the base of the nail, as well as dystrophic nail changes, may occur in psoriasis.

### *Treatment*

Oral antibacterial antibiotics are administered when indicated by culture of the discharge. The most important factor in therapy of this disorder, and one without which no treatment will succeed, is to *keep the affected site scrupulously dry*. Squeezing of the affected area will aggravate the situation.

When culture reveals *Candida*, treatment includes amphotericin B lotion (Fungizone), 1 drop three times daily, miconazole (Micatin), clotrimazole (Canestin, Lotrimin), or nystatin (Mycostatin) ointment, cream, or lotion applied three times daily. (See also general treatment for candidosis, below.)

For those cases caused by a mixed low-grade infection, a lotion consisting of resorcin and alcohol is applied to the affected area:

| | |
|---|---|
| Resorcin | 2% |
| Alcohol | q.s. |

Apply 1 drop to affected area three times daily.

If the nail is involved, it will respond to the above therapy, but will take some weeks to clear completely.

### Chronic mucocutaneous candidosis

There is a group of individuals who have chronic *oral*, *skin*, and *nail* candidal infections, often from childhood, sometimes clearing slowly with age, and sometimes beginning in adult life. These infections are unresponsive to topical anticandidal agents. Associated endocrine abnormalities are hypoparathyroidism and hypoadrenocorticism. Higgs and Wells classify these patients as type I, linked with primary immunodeficiencies, and type II, having four groups:

1. Susceptibility to candidal invasion of the epithelium inherited as a dominant trait
2. Diffuse generalized cutaneous candidosis from childhood
3. Endocrine disorders in association
4. Late-onset chronic oral candidosis.

Transfer factor may offer some hope to many of these patients (Mackie).

## General treatment of candidosis

*Disseminated candidosis* is treated by the methylester of amphotericin B, 5-fluorocytosine, or intravenous miconazole. Each of these agents carries its own adverse effects and danger/benefit risk. Only the first two are fungicidal. The methylester of amphotericin B is less toxic to the kidneys than its parent compound. The agent 5-fluorocytosine converts to 5-fluorouracil for its anticandidal effect within the invading organism's cell.

Cutaneous lesions are often red, irritated, and burning, because of the presence of the organism itself. Burow's solution compresses for 15 minutes each, two or three times daily, are very soothing. The area is air dried after application of compresses, and an anticandidal agent, usually in lotion or cream form, is applied. If the irritation is severe, a glucocorticoid component may be added to the cream. Hydrocortisone 1% or 2%, triamcinolone 0.1%, or one of the more potent glucocorticoids might be required.

The topical anticandidal preparations include miconazole, clotrimazole, haloprogin, amphotericin B, and nystatin (see pp. 270 and 283). Drying the area is important in producing an unfriendly environment for *Candida*, which likes warmth and moisture. Intertriginous areas benefit from anticandidal powders (miconazole, nystatin).

A search for diabetes mellitus in adults and for other endocrinopathies, including thymomas, in children with recurrent or chronic candidal infections is indicated. As there is an association with bacterial infections in some immune disorders, patients with recurrent bacterial skin infections should be examined for candidosis as well as for evidence of immune deficiency.

#### REFERENCES

Bhaskaram, C., and Reddy, V.: Cell-mediated immunity in iron and vitamin deficient children, Br. Med. J. 3:522, 1975.
**Iron deficiency accompanies impaired cell-mediated immunity.**

Bodey, E. P., and Luna, M.: Skin lesions associated with disseminated candidosis, J.A.M.A. **229**:1466, 1974.
**77 severely ill patients with 10 showing yeast-containing nodules in dermis.**

Cawson, R. A.: Induction of epithelial hyperplasia by *Candida albicans*, Br. J. Dermatol. **89**:497, 1973.
**Is it precancerous?**

Clark, R. A., Root, R. K., and Kimball, H. R.: Defective neutrophil chemotaxis and cellular immunity in a child with recurrent infections, Ann. Intern. Med. **78**:515, 1973.
**Mucocutaneous candidosis since childhood and negative delayed cell-mediated immunity to *Candida*.**

Clayton, Y. M.: Therapy of fungal infections: Comment, Br. J. Dermatol. **89**:423, 1973.
**A good assessment of topical systemic agents available**

deVille, R. L., and Lewis, C. W.: Candidiasis seminar, Cutis **19**:69, 1977.
**Easy to read, comprehensive review.**

Evans, E. E. V., Richardson, D. M., Odds, F. C., et al.: Relevance of antigenicity of *Candida albicans* growth phase to diagnosis of systemic candidiasis, Br. Med. J. **4**:86, 1973.
**The mycelial phase and the yeast cell phase are antigenically different.**

Higgs, J. M., and Wells, R. S.: Chronic mucocutaneous candidiasis: new approaches to treatment, Br. J. Dermatol. **89**:179, 1973.
**Two groups, immune-deficient patients, and mouth, skin, and nail candidosis.**

Kirkpatrick, C. H., Rich, R. R., and Bennett, J. E.: Chronic mucocutaneous candidiasis: model building in cellular immunity, Ann. Intern. Med. **74**:955, 1971.
**Practical omniscience: a guideline for future efforts.**

Mackie, R. M., Cochrane, R., and deSouza, M: The treatment of chronic mucocutaneous candidosis with transfer factor, Scottish Med. J. **20**:278, 1975.
**Successful in patients with impaired cell-mediated immunity.**

Ray, T. L., and Wuepper, D. K.: Activation of the alternate (properdin) pathway of complement by *Candida albicans* and related species, J. Invest. Dermatol. **67**:700, 1976.
**Immunochemical evidence of complement activation.**

Rebora, A., Marples, R. D., and Kligman, A. M.: Experimental infection with *Candida albicans*, Arch. Dermatol. **108**:68, 1973.
**Local occlusion and high humidity.**

Toala, P., Schroeder, S. A., Daly, A. K., et al.: *Candida* at Boston City Hospital: clinical and epidemiological characteristics and susceptibility to eight antimicrobial agents, Arch. Intern. Med. **126**:983, 1970.
**Laboratory evidence and study on 41 patients with presumptive infections.**

## DEEP FUNGAL INFECTIONS

### Actinomycosis

The causative organism is an anaerobic gram-positive filamentous bacterium *Actinomyces israelii*, which exists normally in the throat and tonsillar crypts of normal individuals, in a worldwide distribution. It has not been identified outside the human body and must be considered as producing an endogenous infection, often initiated as a result of dental or oropharyngeal trauma. The structure is pleomorphic, occurring in short rods and in long branched filaments.

Lesions of actinomycosis occur in tissues of face, neck, lungs, pleura, and ileocecal and anorectal areas. Bony, cardiac, and most other tissues can be involved. The cervicofacial area is most frequently affected because of proximity to the tonsillar home of the organism. It spreads to other affected sites by pulmonary or gastrointestinal routes.

Multiple episodes of minor trauma, dental extractions, foreign bodies, and recurrent pyogenic infections of gingivodental tissues allow the bacteria to initiate their own infection. This forms channels beneath the membrane surface and gradually extends, with fibrosis to the outside, so that on the skin surface the lesions are indurated granulomatous swellings that become necrotic, discharging purulent material through sinus tracts to the skin surface. Microscopic examination of the pus reveals "sulfur granules" composed of closely packed, multiple fine filaments that are minute colonies of bacteria distributed in a radial pattern.

#### *Diagnosis*

If care is used, an anaerobic culture of pus or excised tissues will show *A. israelii*, but it will die quickly on exposure to oxygen. If sulfur granules are seen, these offer a higher rate of possible successful culture.

#### *Differential diagnosis*

The infection is to be distinguished from tuberculosis, blastomycosis, osteomyelitis, nocardiosis, and other granulomatous diseases. It is a rare disease.

#### *Treatment*

Penicillin G in adequate doses is the treatment of choice for cervicofacial actinomycosis. It is given intravenously in the range of 50 to 75 mg./kg. daily or as a procaine penicillin intramuscularly 20 mg./kg. daily. Oral penicillin therapy then should be continued for several months after the lesions are healed.

Pulmonary and abdominal forms should be treated with larger doses. Surgical excision of tumor masses may be necessary.

## Coccidioidomycosis

*Coccidioides immitis* is a fungus that lives in the soil of certain areas in the semiarid southwest United States and South America, where this disease is endemic. It is capable of producing infection in man when inhaled. Werner and his colleagues reported 61 of 103 archeology students who contracted the disease from inhalation of dust during an expedition in the Sierra foothills of northern California.

The disease may take several forms. The most common is a short, self-limiting, primary pulmonary infection that then imparts a lifelong immunity. This primary infection is usually asymptomatic, but may be associated with an influenza-like syndrome and the cutaneous lesions of erythema nodosum or erythema multiforme. Erythema nodosum, for unknown reasons, is much more common in females. Arthralgia is also present, and, with pneumonia, these constitute "valley fever." Ninety-five percent of patients recover from this infection, and half or less of the remainder develop residual pulmonary disease.

Dissemination of the disease to other organs may occur in 1 out of 100 adult white males with symptomatic infection. It is more common in other races. It frequently consists of subcutaneous abscesses that rupture to form cutaneous ulcerations, vegetations, and granulomatous lesions. Bone abscesses may be present. The course may be fulminating and fatal or produce a chronic illness.

The coccidioidin skin test becomes positive some weeks after the primary infection and has a similar significance to the tuberculin test. The organisms can be cultured from the sputum or the cutaneous lesions. Less than half of the ill students reported by Werner and his colleagues showed positive skin or serological tests.

Skin eruptions occur in the flexures, palms, and soles of children chiefly prior to development of immunity. Erythema nodosum or multiforme appears shortly after.

### *Diagnosis*

1. Demonstration of organism in pus from abscesses or biopsies
2. Skin tests to coccidioidin supportive only
3. Serologic tests: increasing titer important

### *Treatment*

Cases of severe spreading disseminated coccidioidomycosis are best treated with amphotericin B intravenously, with the amount and duration of therapy being dependent on the form of disease and its response to therapy. Miconazole and amphotericin B methylester are currently being judged in this disease for treatment of disseminated forms. Bed rest and conservative management are best for mild and moderate forms, although experience consultant advice must be sought (Hermans, Hoeprich).

## Sporotrichosis

Sporotrichosis is a disease caused by *Sporothrix schenckii*, an aerobic fungus found in soil or on vegetation. The human lesions are usually initiated by trauma inoculating the organism into subcutaneous tissues and are found chiefly in farmers and plant handlers. Richards reported 12 cases in Ontario in 1971.

The primary lesion begins days or weeks after the initial traumatic episode and consists of a painless, enlarging pustule that forms an ulcerated, indurated lesion. Fingers, hands, feet, or legs are usual sites. Shortly after its appearance, the ulcer is followed by a series of red, firm, painless nodules, appearing in a line along the chain of lymphatics draining the site (Fig. 14-11). These may also form ulcers. However, the cutaneous lesions are frequently atypical, and the diagnosis may be obscure. The localized lesions rarely heal spontaneously, but do not tend to affect the health of the patient. Rarely a disseminated form may occur.

Culture of the lesions is essential and will reveal the specific diagnosis. The organism can be demonstrated in the tissue or seropurulent exudate by PAS staining or fluorescent antibody techniques. It is found in immunodeficient or suppressed patients.

### *Diagnosis*

1. The classic form should be diagnosed by clinical appearance.

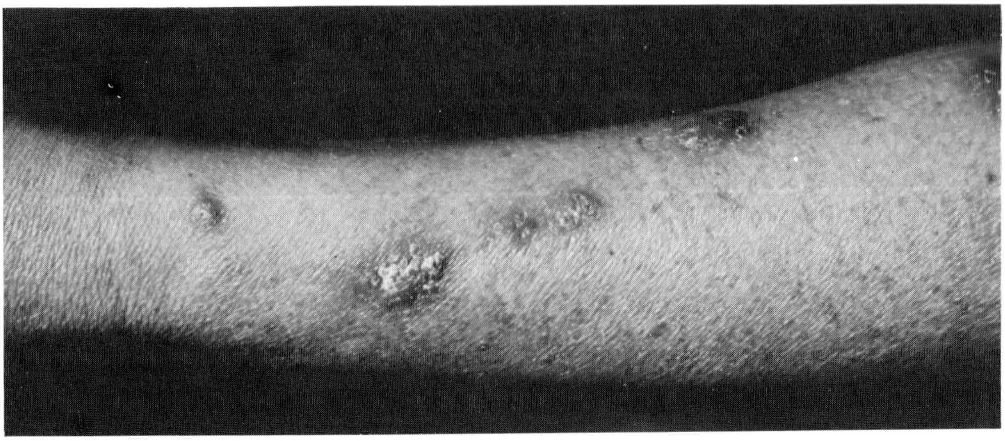

**Fig. 14-11.** Sporotrichosis. Linear distribution of lesions following lymphatic channel (Courtesy Dr. Raymond Lessard, Quebec City, Quebec.)

2. Culture, isolation, and identification of *S. schenckii* from pus or sputum.

### *Differential diagnosis*

Differential diagnosis includes atypical mycobacterial infections, North American blastomycosis, actinomycosis, localized granulomatous diseases, and bacterial skin infections.

### *Treatment*

The lesions ordinarily respond well to a saturated solution of potassium iodide, administered three times daily from an initial smaller dose and increasing to 9 to 12 Gm. daily, and continued for 1 month after the infection is cleared. The medication is added to milk or water and given after meals. Nausea, vomiting, parotid swelling, sneezing, and gastrointestinal reactions are frequent. Amphotericin B and 5-fluorocytosine have been used in disseminated sporotrichosis.

## North American blastomycosis

The causative fungus of the disease, *Blastomyces dermatitidis*, is disseminated by inhalation of spores. The disease occurs in men whose occupations keep them in close exposure to the environment.

The most common form of North American blastomycosis is one of systemic involvement, with cutaneous lesions. It begins as a single nodule that ulcerates and extends peripherally. Subsequently, the lesion becomes verrucous. It slowly heals centrally, with an atrophic scar surrounded by an elevated reddish purple margin. The hands, face, and feet are most commonly involved (Fig. 14-12).

There may be a general dissemination of nodules that ulcerate, discharging blood and pus. Associated joint pains, fever, and anemia are present. Other organs involved include lungs, kidney, prostate gland, central nervous system, and bones.

### *Diagnosis*

The organism may be cultured on Sabouraud's medium or on blood agar. The budding cells are present in the purulent exudate. It is recognized in microscopic sections as a clear spherule, usually within microabscesses.

### *Treatment*

Preferred treatment is slow intravenous drip of amphotericin B in 5% glucose solution. It is started with 0.25 mg./kg. daily and gradually increased to 1 mg./kg. daily over a period of a week, until 2 Gm. are given. Also used intravenously is 2-hydroxystilbamidine.

## Mycetoma (Madura foot)

Mycetoma is a tumor-like indolent bacterial and fungal infection characterized by the ap-

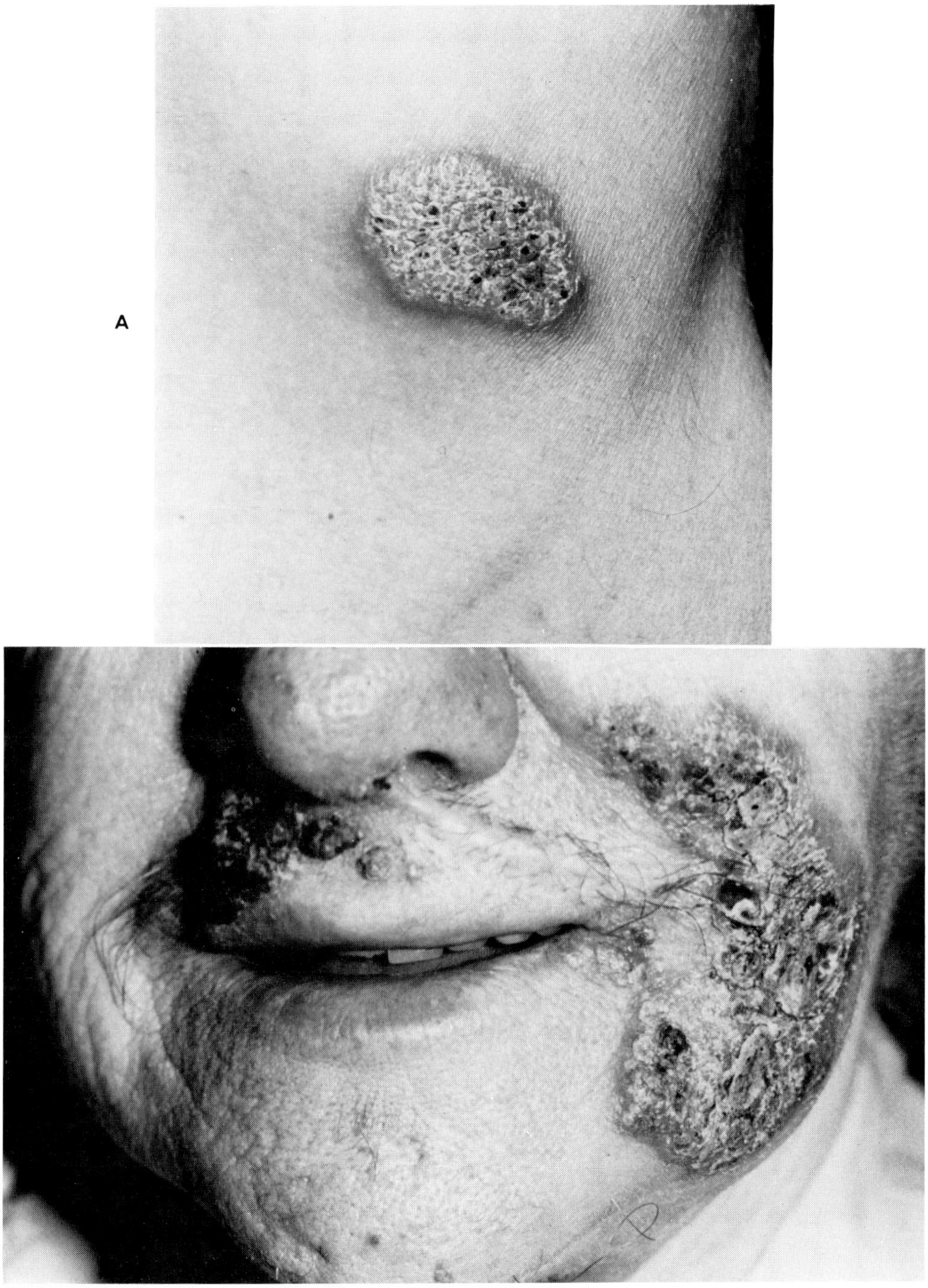


**Fig. 14-12.** North American blastomycosis. **A,** Peripheral and, **B,** facial lesions. (Courtesy Dr. Raymond Lessard, Quebec City, Quebec.)

pearance of "grains" or granules, which can be seen on examination. It is caused by any of several species of soil saprophytes, each of which has its own distinctive colored grain, either white, yellow, red, or black.

It occurs chiefly on the foot or the hand, but may be found elsewhere. Although usually reported from underdeveloped countries, cases have been found in Canada, the United States, and Great Britain.

The lesion is an indolent, painful ulcer, with a raised or verrucous periphery, resulting from the breakdown of a nodule that may be single or multiple. Depending on the causative organism, there may be deformity of the part, with bone destruction, swelling, or little surrounding involvement. Sinus tracts are common sites of infection, and grains or granules of different colors are discharged to the surface in these channels.

Fungi and filamentous bacteria causing this disorder include *Actinomycetes, Nocardia, Actinomadura, Madurella, Phialophora, Allescheria*, and perhaps others.

### *Diagnosis*

Diagnosis is made by microscopic examination of the grains from the lesion and culture of the organisms, although each has its own cultural characteristics. Since some are higher bacteria and others fungi, the diagnosis becomes a microbiologist's challenge.

### *Treatment*

Therapy is dependent on the causative fungus, but amphotericin B, griseofulvin, penicillin, sulfonamides, and tetracycline, combined with surgical excision of the infected area, have been used. Cases must be individualized largely because of the wide range of causative organisms.

### REFERENCES

Bennett, J. E.: Chemotherapy of systemic mycoses, N. Engl. J. Med. **290**:30-32, 320-323, 1974.

Catanzaro, A., Spitler, L., and Moser, K. M.: Immunotherapy of coccidioidomycosis, J. Clin. Invest. **54**:690, 1974.
**Four patients, all became positive reactors after transfer factor collected from donors with cell-mediated immunity to *Candida*.**

Gonçalves, A. P.: Sporotrichosis, coccidioidomycosis and blastomycosis; cosmopolitan fungous infections of tropical interest. In Canizares, O., editor: Clinical tropical dermatology, Oxford, 1975, Blackwell Scientific Publications.
**Brief knowledgeable disease summaries.**

Hermans, P. E.: Antifungal agents used for deep-seated mycotic infections, Mayo Clin. Proc. **52**:687, 1977.
**Amphotericin B, 2-hydrostilbamidine, flucytosine, and newer drugs, as well as various combinations discussed.**

Lynch, P. J., Voorhees, J. J., and Harrell, E. R.: Systemic sporotrichosis, Ann. Intern. Med. **73**:23, 1970.
**Cutaneous inoculation begins most.**

Pappagianis, D.: Coccidioidomycosis. In Hoeprich, P. D., editor: Infectious diseases, Hagerstown, Md., 1977, Harper & Row, Publishers, p. 389.
**All necessary information well presented.**

Richards, R. N.: Sporotrichosis, Can. Med. Assoc. J. **106**:1097, 1972.
**Canadian cases.**

Sarosi, G. A., Hammerman, K. J., Tosh, F. E., et àl.: Clinical features of acute pulmonary blastomycosis, N. Engl. J. Med. **290**:540, 1974.
**The early and subsequent course of the disease.**

Utz, J. P.: Blastomycosis. In Hoeprich, P. D., editor: Infectious diseases, Hagerstown, Md., 1977, Harper & Row, Publishers, p. 399.

Utz, J. P.: Mycetoma. In Hoeprich, P. D., editor: Infectious diseases, Hagerstown, Md., 1977, Harper & Row, Publishers, p. 1142.
**Concise, informative.**

Werner, S. B., Pappagiakis, D., Heindl, I., and Mickel, A.: Epidemic of coccidioidomycosis among archeology students in northern California, N. Engl. J. Med. **268**:507, 1972.

CHAPTER 15

# Viral infections

A virus is an ultramicroscopic organism without an enzyme system that exists as an intracellular parasite. It consists of protein and nucleic acid. The nucleic acid is the core and is either ribonucleic acid (RNA) or deoxyribonucleic acid (DNA). The protein is the shell or capsid. In addition, some viruses have an outer envelope of lipoprotein. Many of the small viruses behave like simple chemicals and can be crystallized. After a virus penetrates a cell, it takes off its capsid and disappears without apparent trace. The invaded cell may appear completely normal in all respects. After entry, the virus, now consisting only of the nucleic acid core, may then stimulate the host cell to form more virus material. The virus is not capable of reproducing by itself. The steps in the replication process include (1) adsorption, in which the envelope is important, (2) penetration into cell and loss of capsid, (3) transcription and accumulation of viral nucleic acids in cell nucleus, (4) synthesis of viral structural protein in cell cytoplasm, (5) aggregation of viral nucleic acid and protein to form virus particles, and (6) ejection from the cell. (Estimates of 20,000 or more finished infectious virus particles produced per cell have been calculated in herpesvirus infections.)

This process may result in the death of the cell, or the cell may show no subsequent sign of disease. The cell, however, has a defense against this invasion. When the virus stimulates the host cell to make more virus particles, the cell may respond by producing interferon. This substance then leaves the cell and enters the neighboring cells, and when virus particles also enter the new host cell, the interferon prevents them from replicating new viruses. The spread of virus particles thus ends. Interferon stimulated by one virus is effective against other viruses.

Various viral diseases have been observed to increase in frequency in individuals whose immune system is impaired for any reason. Zoster, herpes simplex, warts, mollusca, varicella, orf, vaccinia, and cytomegalovirus have been described.

The division of viruses into two general classes—those containing RNA and those containing DNA—is significant in respect to treatment measures, since an agent that successfully attacks one variety may have no effect on the other. This virus protein may be similar antigenically to the host cell, or at least so similar that it cannot be destroyed without destroying host cells. Also, since some chemotherapeutic agents cannot differentiate between virus and cell, they impair both.

A primary viral infection may be asymptomatic or may produce a severe systemic reaction. Since all virus particles contain a number of distinct protein antigens, antibodies are formed by the primary infection in a manner similar to the way they are formed by bacteria.

Recurring viral diseases such as herpes simplex may not necessitate a reinfection to produce symptoms, but only require the appropriate "trigger mechanism" (for example, sunlight) to cause a multiplication of the virus within the cell. The newly formed viruses are clumped together and are visible under a light microscope as an *inclusion body*.

A viral infection of the skin takes place in the epidermal cell, which may react with inflammation and vesiculation (herpes simplex) or by proliferating to form growths consisting of virus-filled cells (molluscum contagiosum). The same virus may present different clinical pictures (Table 5). The varicella-zoster virus may cause either chicken-pox or herpes zoster. The wart virus may produce large acu-

**Table 5.** Virus groups producing cutaneous disease

| Group | Size | Species | Nucleic acid component | Cutaneous disease |
|---|---|---|---|---|
| Herpesvirus | 100 to 200 nm. | Herpes simplex | DNA | Herpes simplex |
| | | Varicella-zoster virus | — | Varicella and zoster |
| | | Epstein-Barr virus | | |
| | | Cytomegalovirus | | |
| Poxvirus | 120 to 300 nm. | Virus of variola | DNA | Smallpox |
| | | Virus of vaccinia | — | Vaccinia |
| | | Virus of cowpox | — | Cowpox |
| | | Virus of molluscum contagiosum | — | Molluscum contagiosum |
| | | Virus of contagious pustular dermatitis | — | Pustular dermatitis (orf) |
| | | Paravaccinia virus | — | Milker's nodules |
| Paramyxovirus | 150 nm. | Rubeola virus | RNA | Measles |
| Papovavirus | 35 to 55 nm. | Wart virus | DNA | Wart |
| Picornavirus | 20 to 30 nm. | Coxsackievirus | RNA | Hand-foot-and-mouth disease |
| | | | | Macular, vesicular, petechial |
| | | Echovirus | — | Macular, vesicular, petechial |
| Togavirus | 40 to 70 nm. | Rubivirus | DNA | Rubella |

minate growths on the prepuce or anal mucosa, or brown flat lesions on the face.

## ANTIVIRAL AGENTS

There is a growing suspicion that Hodgkin's disease and perhaps lymphomas are viral infections. The following seven compounds are potential or available antiviral agents.

***Idoxuridine (IDU, Stoxil, Herplex, Dendrid).*** By preventing certain aspects of DNA synthesis, this agent inhibits propagation of the virus without affecting normal cellular activity. Juel-Jensen indicated that it may be of help topically in treating varicella-zoster, 40% IDU in dimethyl sulfoxide (DMSO). It is used topically in treating skin and eye herpes, most particularly herpes keratitis. Systemic IDU is too toxic for use.

Keratitis recurrences and viral resistance are encountered commonly.

***Amantadine hydrochloride (Symmetrel).*** This amine inhibits the penetration of cells by RNA viruses. It is useful in treating influenza type A and some tumor viruses. The efficacy of amantadine in influenza epidemics allows its use at the time of the epidemic, which is an obvious advantage, since vaccination for influenza must be given 1 to 2 months prior to an epidemic. Its action, however, is chiefly prophylactic.

Its adverse effects are dose related and include insomnia, dizziness, unsteadiness, slurred speach, inability to concentrate, depression, and detachment.

It is given orally and may produce mouth dryness and gastrointestinal discomfort.

***Methisazone (Marboran).*** This agent inhibits bits the replication of the virus by preventing its assembly into a final complete virus. Methisazone is useful in treating some poxvirus infections, particularly for the prevention of smallpox and in the therapy of complications of vaccinia. Interestingly, the drug does not influence the course of primary immunization with vaccinia. It is not given parenterally. Nausea and vomiting seem to be the only important side effects.

***Adenine arabinoside (Vidarabine, ara-A, Vira-A).*** Effective against poxviruses, oncomaviruses, and rhabdoviruses. It is most useful against herpes simplex and varicella-zoster viruses. It appears to be effective topically in herpetic keratitis, but initial trials on cutaneous lesions were not impressive, probably because it does not penetrate the epidermis. A problem arises in its deamination by the host, which lessens its effectiveness. Drugs to prevent this (Co-Vidaribine) will be available shortly. Improved related compounds are being assessed.

It is currently the most effective agent for herpes encephalitis and disseminated vaccinia. It may leave some neurologic sequelae. Nausea, vomiting, weakness, and bone marrow effects are reported.

***Ribavirin (Virazole).*** Many viruses are inhibited by this drug, both RNA and DNA. Uncontrolled studies would seem to indicate that it may have some use topically, but these need confirmation. It is possibly effective in influenza B prophylaxis.

***Interferon.*** Interferons are proteins produced by cells that have harbored viruses. Interferon is active against *all* known viruses. It escapes from the cell of its origin, penetrates other cells in the vicinity, and stimulates production of antiviral protein, which inhibits the virus replication in the new cell. Therapeutic use is limited by their short half life after injection.

Recent developments have enlarged our knowledge of interferon to realize that there are many such compounds. Most cells make these substances and they differ between cells and types of cells. There are several fibroblast interferons, for example. It is now possible to manufacture human interferons in a cell-free system and we look forward to learning a great deal more about them.

***Immune globulin.*** Vaccinia immune globulin (VIG) is prepared from the blood of adults taken 4 to 6 weeks after primary vaccination. This agent is used in treating the complications of smallpox vaccination, specifically, accidental inoculation of a susceptible person, and generalized progressive vaccinia. Pooled gamma globulin modifies infections from measles, hepatitis, rabies, poliomyelitis, and others. It acts by interfering with the entry of the virus particle into the cell.

#### REFERENCES

Becker, Y.: Antiviral drugs. Mode of action and chemotherapy of viral infections of man, Monogr. Virol. **11**:1, 1976.
**A detailed exposé of the villains!**

Hermans, P. E.: Antiviral agents, Mayo Clin. Proc. **52**:683, 1977.
**Amantadine, methisazone, IDU, ara-A, and others.**

Kaufman, H. E.: Antiviral drugs (review), Int. J. Dermatol. **16**:464, 1977.
**Amantadine, Marboran, IDU, ara-A, TFT, PAA, interferon, photoinactivation.**

Notkins, A. L.: Viral infections. Mechanisms of immunological defense and injury, Hosp. Pract. p. 65, Sept. 1974.
**Clearly illustrated superb description of general principles. A must.**

Proceedings of the Third Conference on Anti-viral Agents, Ann. N.Y. Acad. Sci. **284**, 1977.
**An exciting view of work in progress and preview of coming events.**

Vianna, N. J., Greenwald, P., Brady, J., et al.: Hodgkin's disease: cases with the features of a community outbreak, Ann. Intern. Med. **77**:169, 1972.
**A long incubation period, intra–high school personal contacts.**

## HERPES SIMPLEX (FEVER BLISTER, COLD SORE)

Herpes simplex (Plate 30) is an acute vesicular infection of the mucous membranes and skin by either of the two types of herpesvirus.

The primary infection, which occurs chiefly in infants and children but not uncommonly in adults, may be a painful acute gingivostomatitis with lymphadenopathy, malaise, localized mucosal ulcers, and a nonspecific febrile episode. If the primary infection is genital, there is inguinal lymphadenopathy, dysuria, soreness, and spread to adjacent vulvar skin in females. *In the newborn period it may be fatal,* with viremia and involvement of the viscera. Primary infections in children and in adults also occur in the eye, as a follicular conjunctivitis, or on the skin, where it may be extensive, or on a fingertip (herpetic whitlow). Herpes simplex encephalitis is usually a primary infection and has been reported as the most common identified cause of severe or fatal encephalitis of a sporadic nature.

### *Natural course*

The lesion commonly known as a "cold sore" is a recurrent lesion in that a primary lesion has occurred previously. The cold sore consists of grouped vesicles on an erythematous base associated with a moderate degree

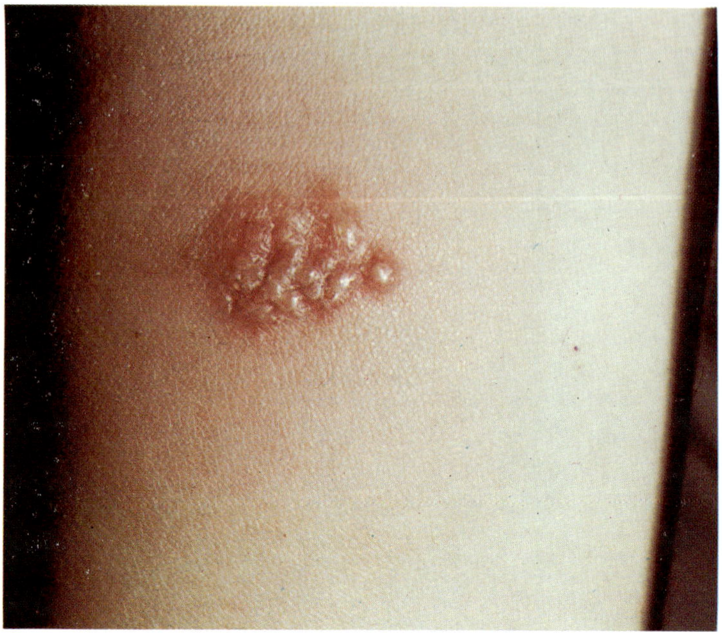

**Plate 30**

Herpes simplex. Multivesicular, compound lesion on the intact skin.

of pruritus. A serous fluid, which crusts and dries over a 7 to 10-day period and may become secondarily infected, exudes from the ruptured vesicles. Regional adenopathy is present early. Frequently, the eruption tends to recur at the same site, with eventual scar formation. The areas most commonly infected are the lips, the cheeks (Fig. 15-1), and the genitalia (Fig. 15-2). Female genital lesions may be labial, urethral, vaginal, or cervical. In the male, lesions may be preputial, urethral, on the glans, and in the coronal sulcus. However, herpes simplex can occur on any part of the skin surface or mucous membrane as a recurrent lesion. The cornea, where the recurrent infection may cause blindness, is one of the frequently involved sites.

A recurrent lesion of herpes simplex may be initiated by one of numerous trigger mechanisms such as trauma, sunlight, fever, or menses. It may be transmitted from one person to another by direct contact during the vesicular phase. Genital herpes can be transmitted by sexual intercourse, and neonatal herpes is almost always acquired from infections of the maternal birth canal. Erythema multiforme is a not uncommon sequel to a recurrent herpes lesion. Successful treatment of the herpetic lesion may avoid appearance of erythema multiforme.

People with atopic dermatitis are especially susceptible to a generalized disseminated vesicular eruption attributable to a primary infection with the herpes simplex virus, type I, which may be fatal (5% to 15%) (Kaposi's varicelliform eruption) (Fig. 15-3), eczema herpeticum (see p. 309).

Individuals with immune-system impairment, or with malignant lymphomas, or who are on immunosuppressive therapy, may develop severe forms of herpes.

*Encephalitis* from herpesvirus infection is not rare and is being recognized with increasing frequency. The diagnosis may be made clinically by a rise in the complement-fixing antibodies, since this is for the most part a

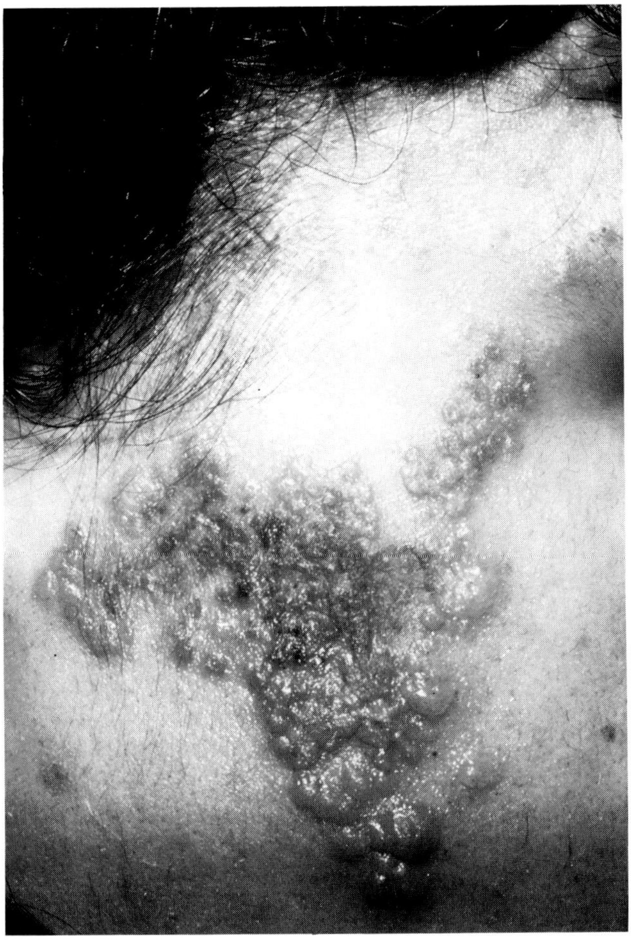

**Fig. 15-1.** Herpes simplex. Extensive involvement on nonmucous membrane surface.

primary infection. There may be a 50% or greater mortality. Cutaneous lesions are not usually a part of this picture.

### *Pertinent information*

Current studies of the virus producing herpes simplex have become among the most exciting and illuminating sources of information concerning virus behaviors. They have greatly expanded our view of the range and extent of virus activity.

The herpesvirus group consists of more than 50 herpesviruses capable of infecting 30 different vertebrates. Seven herpesviruses affecting man are known. These have a distinctive many-sided shape and form characteristic intranuclear inclusions. They have an affinity for ectodermal cells, growing readily in skin and mucous membranes and spreading to the nervous system. The virus travels by neural routes, perhaps using the nerve sheath cells. Some of this family of viruses affect only man, and some are oncogenic, particularly in unnatural hosts.

*Viremia* may occur at the time of cutaneous lesions and at recurrences and may or may not be associated with disseminated lesions. Several generalized herpesvirus infections in debilitated people has resulted in disseminated intravascular coagulation.

After the primary infection and between recurrent infections, the problem arises of determining where the virus hides to avoid detection. Recent studies indicate that the virus

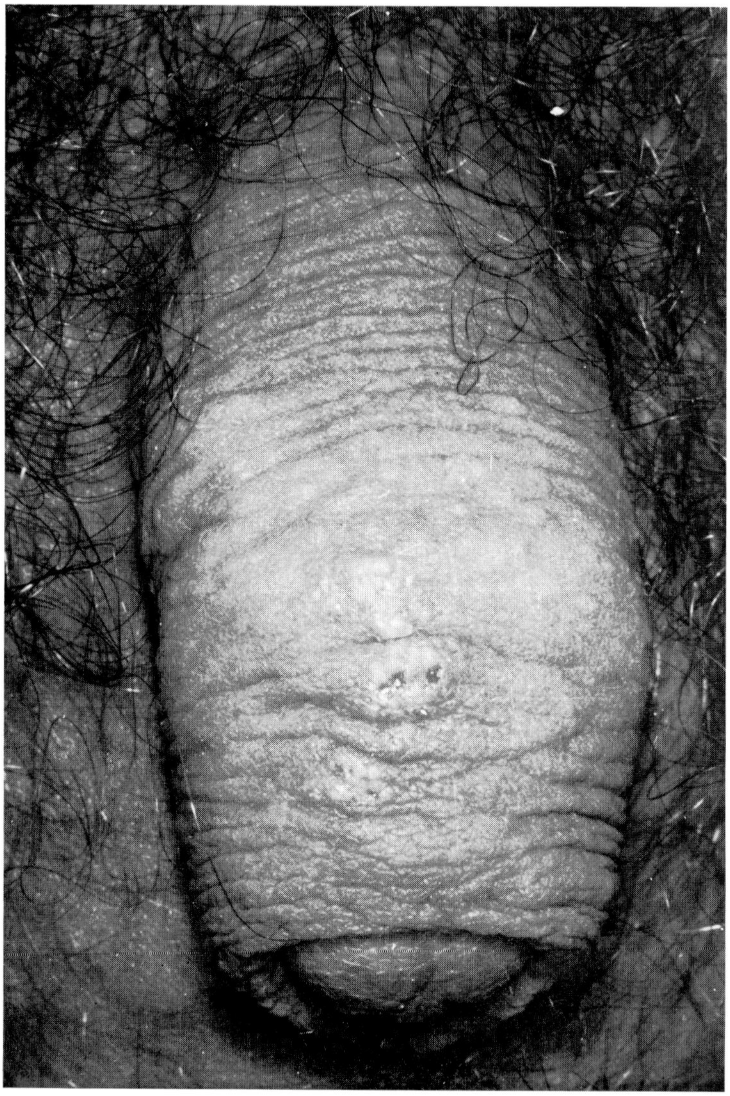

**Fig. 15-2.** Herpes simplex. This is the commonest cause of genital vesiculoulcerative disease. Usually recurrent.

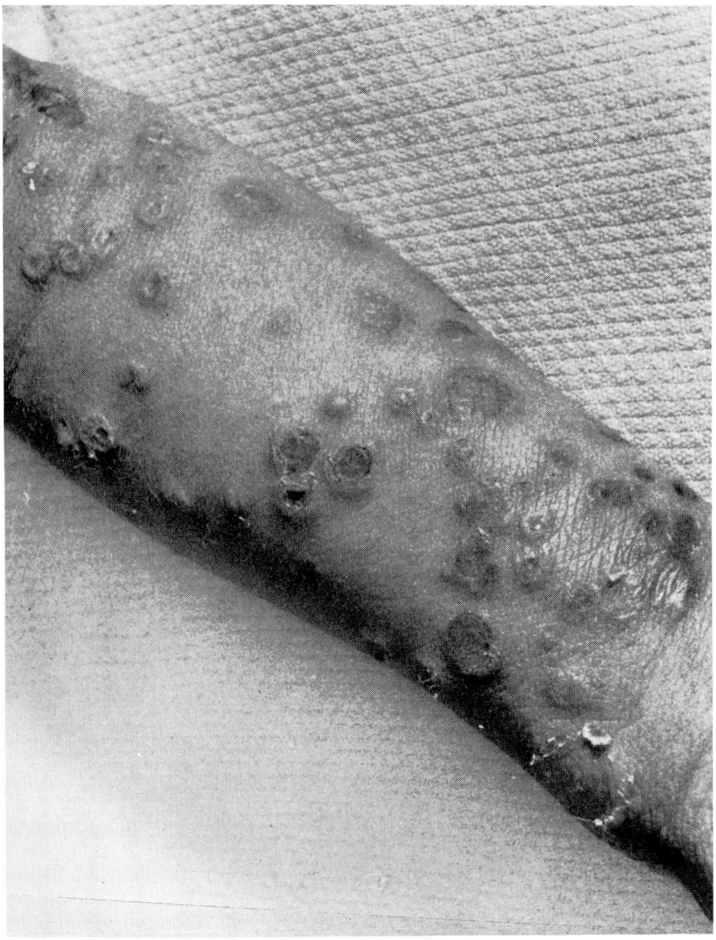

**Fig. 15-3.** Kaposi's varicelliform eruption (eczema herpeticum) caused by herpesvirus in an atopic individual.

may remain in a static or nonreplication state, harbored in ganglia. Barigan and Swoveland recovered herpes simplex virus from trigeminal ganglia of six out of seven cadavers.

A continuing enigma is our inability to produce an effective immunity against this organism. This may be attributable to (1) host dysfunction, (2) neurotropic and secretive nature of the virus, and (3) cell-to-cell viral transfer in the body, thus the virus escapes the defenses. Evidence (Bierman) indicates a possibility of (1) and no evidence of (2); that is, Why does zoster not recur? Probably (3) is the answer.

Some viruses, for example, polio, have the help of host genes that code cells (such as human chromosome 19) for permissive viral entry; so genetic factors are important.

An antibody-dependent cell-mediated cytotoxicity, acting against this and other viruses, without complement has been described. The effector cell does not appear to be either lymphocyte or monocyte. Also, there is some effect of humoral immunity measurably reducing the number of virus particles within ganglion cells and the number of cells infected in animals.

By the use of a variety of serological techniques, *Herpesvirus hominis* (HVH) strains can be differentiated into two distinct antigenic types, designated types 1 and 2. The two types of HVH also demonstrate a number of different biological properties. Of particular clinical and epidemiological significance has been the finding that type 2 HVH occurs chiefly in association with genital infection and is venereally transmitted. On the other hand, type 1 HVH is associated with most nongenital herpetic infections and with eczema herpeticum.

Complement-fixing antibodies to herpes simplex virus are present in the serum of over 80% of adults over 30 years of age, although this percentage varies geographically and in socioeconomic groups.

There has been considerable discussion recently concerning the association of herpesvirus infections and carcinomas. Herpes simplex virus 2 is suspected, but not proved, to have an association with cervical carcinoma, the evidence for which is reviewed well by Poste and colleagues. Other tumors have been brought into the discussion. In man, the Epstein-Barr virus, another herpesvirus, is linked with Burkitt's lymphoma and nasopharyngeal carcinoma. Some viruses have an oncogenic effect in unnatural hosts.

### *Diagnosis*

A diagnosis of herpes simplex infection can be made by examination of scrapings from the base of the vesicles spread on a glass slide and stained with hematoxylin and eosin. Search is then made for giant cells with the diagnostic large eosinophilic intranuclear inclusions.

Immunofluorescent studies can identify the presence of herpes antigen in vesicle fluid or tissue within a very short time and are satisfactory for diagnosis.

Electron microscope examination will rapidly identify the herpesvirus.

### *Microscopic findings*

Multiloculated vesicles are present in the epidermal cells. There are so-called balloon cells present in all of these lesions, which are pathognomonic of a virus infection. These are swollen epidermal cells with a homogeneous eosinophilic cytoplasm that have become separated from each other. Acidophilic intranuclear inclusion bodies are found in the degenerated epidermal cells (Lipschütz bodies).

### *Differential diagnosis*

***Impetigo.*** Impetigo produces multiple crusted facial lesions on normal-appearing skin. It is caused by mixed bacterial infection and may accompany a lesion of herpes simplex.

***Zoster.*** Zoster is a painful lesion with vesicles and bullae that follow a segmental nerve distribution.

***Nummular eczema.*** Circular, pruritic, erythematous vesicular patches occur in nummular eczema, most commonly on the dorsa of the hands and legs.

***Syphilitic chancre.*** A nontender, nonpruritic ulcer, syphilitic chancre is most common on the genitalia but may occur on the lips. *Treponema pallidum* is found on dark-field examination of the serous discharge.

***Squamous cell carcinoma.*** A persistent, indurated, ulcerated papule, often on the lower lip, characterizes squamous cell carcinoma.

### *Treatment*

***Primary infection.*** Mucous membrane lesions are probably best treated with supportive care only. Viscous lidocaine (Xylocaine) hydrochloride may relieve discomfort at mealtime. Juel-Jensen suggests 5% IDU in orabase, or 40% IDU in DMSO (not available in North America), for oral lesions and topical ocular IDU for primary herpes lesions of conjunctivae or corneas. If viremia appears to threaten, ara-A is now the recommended therapy.

Encephalitis is now treated with ara-A under close control, the details of which are not available.

***Recurrent herpes simplex.*** Treatment consists first of detection and elimination of the initiating trigger factor. A detailed history and follow-up and a carefully kept diary of foods, drugs, and activities of the patient are often necessary to elicit the association. Another trigger mechanism, sunlight, can be avoided by the use of an adequate sunscreening agent prior to sun exposure.

If applied frequently, 70% *alcohol* will dry the lesion and prevent secondary infection. Ether has also been used successfully (Sabin).

Very potent glucocorticoids, such as fluocinolone, 0.2% cream, applied topically every half hour, will abort most common cutaneous cold sores. However, effectiveness of the glucocorticoids will only be determined when properly controlled clinical studies have been carried out. At present, there are no such reports available. Weaker concentrations will do little and may allow the infection to spread. Although we have found this therapy to be highly effective, we must point out that systemic glucocorticoid therapy suppresses host defenses and is generally undesirable in viral infections. *Glucocorticoids administered topically must not be used in the eyes for herpetic lesions.* Glucocorticoids should not be used in patients with reduced immune responses.

Certain dyes, when applied to herpes lesions and exposed to ordinary light, will inactivate the virus. An 0.1% solution of neutral red or methylene blue is applied to ruptured vesicles, and 20 minutes later the lesions are exposed to a 30-watt incandescent or fluorescent light for 15 minutes. The light exposure alone is repeated in 4 hours. The recurrence rate of lesions thus treated is said to be lower than control rates. Recent studies cast doubt on the effectiveness of this treatment approach.

IDU can be used topically in the treatment of recurrent herpes simplex. It is probably most satisfactory if used early and frequently in the infection in 0.1% aqueous solution. If dimethyl sulfoxide is available, it can be used as the solvent and is reported to increase the penetration of the drug. Its use in cutaneous localized herpes simplex is of benefit since most infections have been shortened by it and some recurrences prevented. It must be applied very frequently—every half hour.

Other forms of therapy such as smallpox vaccines have failed to demonstrate benefit. Controlled studies with these and ribavirin (Virazole), BCG vaccine, levamisole, or transfer factor are not available.

#### REFERENCES

Aronson, M. D., Phillips, C. F., and Gump, D. W.: Vidarabine therapy for severe herpes virus infections, J.A.M.A. **235**:1339, 1976.

**Effective at 15 mg./kg. daily in six immunosuppressed patients with life-threatening infections.**

Baringer, J. R., and Swoveland, P.: Recovery of herpes simplex virus from human trigeminal ganglions, N. Engl. J. Med. **288**:648, 1973.

**A notable revelation in six of seven cadavers.**

Bierman, S. M.: The mechanism of recurrent infection by herpesvirus hominis, Arch. Dermatol. **112**:1459, 1976.

**Discussion of immunological dysfunction and neurotropic nature. Good.**

Jacobs, E.: Anal infection caused by herpes simplex virus, Dis. Colon Rect. **19**:151, 1976.

**An increasing problem in our society.**

Juel-Jensen, B. E.: Virus disease, Practitioner **213**:508, 1974.

**IDU must be used in 40% concentration and early, as it works only on the replicating virus.**

Lehner, T., Wilton, J. M. A., and Shillitoe, E. J.: Immunological basis for latency, recurrences, and putative oncogenicity of herpes simplex virus, Lancet **2**:60, 1975.

**Herpes 1 and lip carcinoma.**

Nahmias, A. J., Shore, S. L., Kohl, S., et al.: Immunol-

ogy of herpes simplex virus infections, Cancer Res. **36**:836, 1976.
**The most recent evidence of oncogenicity of herpes.**

Niragi, S., Jackson, G. G., and Jonasson, O. M.: Viremia with herpes simplex type I in adults: 4 nonfatal cases, Ann. Intern. Med. **85**:165, 1976.
**Viremia in normal adults is probably more frequent than appreciated.**

Poste, G., Hawkins, F., and Thomlinson, J.: Herpesvirus hominis infection of the female genital tract, Obstet. Gynecol. **49**:871, 1972.
**The spectrum of HVH disease, its treatment, and its ramifications.**

Sabin, A. B.: Misery of recurrent herpes. What to do? Editorial, N. Engl. J. Med. **293**:986, 1975.
**Confirmation of the application of perfume by generations of women.**

Shore, S. L., Black, C. M., and Melwicz, F. M.: Antibody-dependent cell-mediated cytotoxicity to target cells infected with type I and type II herpes simplex virus, J. Immunol. **116**:194, 1976.
**Nonlymphocyte, nonmonocyte cell-mediated immunity.**

Taylor, P. K., and Rodin, P.: Herpes genitalis and circumcision, Br. J. Vener. Dis. **41**:274, 1975.
**Circumcision appears to reduce the likelihood of acquiring genital herpes.**

Walz, A. M., Yamamoto, H., and Notkins, A. L.: Immunologic response limits the number of cells in sensory ganglia infected with herpes simplex virus, Nature **264**:554, 1976.
**By 90%.**

Wheeler, C. E., and Abele, D. C.: Eczema herpeticum, primary and recurrent, Arch. Dermatol. **93**:162, 1966.
**Still as valid as when written.**

## VARICELLA (CHICKEN POX)

Varicella is a common, contagious, vesicular eruption caused by the varicella-zoster virus, occurring in nonimmune individuals, chiefly young children.

### *Natural course*

There is an incubation period of approximately 2 weeks, after which there may be a 24-hour period of mild prodromal symptoms of fever and malaise. The skin eruption appears after this stage and consists of papules that rapidly develop into small vesicles on an erythematous base (dewdrops on a rose petal!) filled with a fluid that is first clear and then becomes turbid (Fig. 15-4). By the fourth day the lesions become crusted. New lesions

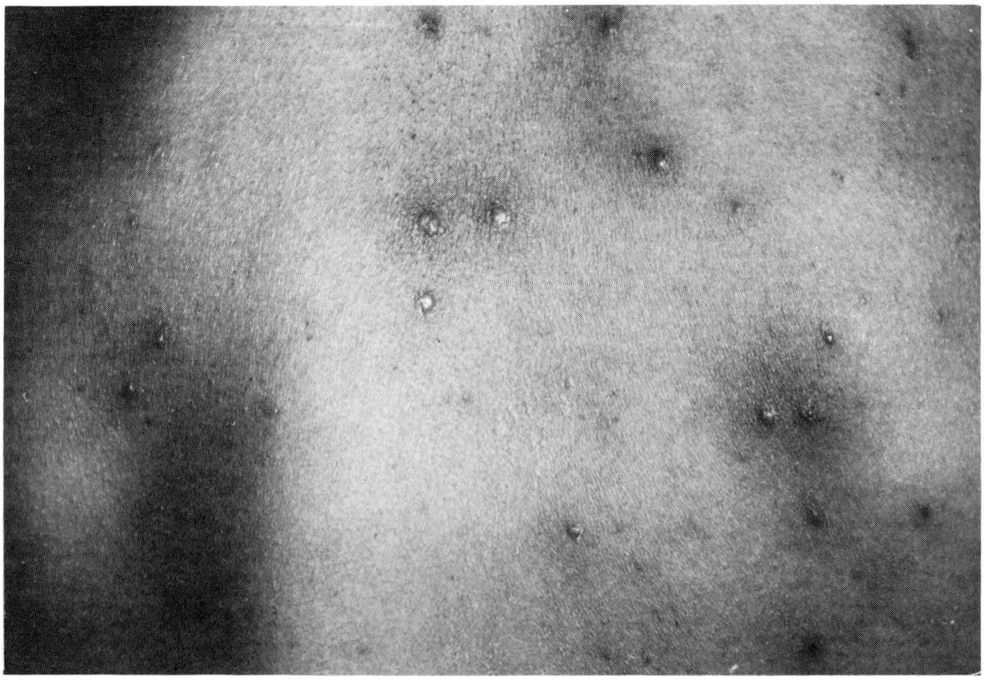

**Fig. 15-4.** Varicella (chicken pox).

continue to appear in crops for the first 3 days; consequently, lesions in various phases of development are seen. The lesions first form on the chest and back and then may extend to the face and extremities. Ulcerations may be present on the buccal mucosa. The vesicles are pruritic and may become secondarily infected as a result of scratching. Chicken pox is infectious from 24 hours before the eruption and for 3 or 4 days. The disease is much more severe in adults than in children.

Complications are uncommon: pneumonia in 1 of 4 adults, pleural effusions in 1 of 10, central nervous system involvement occurs in 1 of 10 of all cases, more seriously in 1 of 100 of these. Renal, cardiac, and platelet abnormalities are rare, although a transient nephritis is not uncommon. If varicella develops in a person taking glucocorticoids, it is more likely to be severe, with dissemination to the central nervous system and viscera. However, the dosage of glucocorticoids should not be stopped immediately upon exposure to this disease, but reduced to low from high levels. Varicella may be serious in the immunocompromised host.

### *Pertinent information*

Varicella and zoster are caused by the same virus. Only man is susceptible, and there appears to be only one antigenic viral type. Varicella occurs in nonimmune individuals and imparts immunity. Zoster is then a manifestation of the infection in an immune individual. The virus replicates in deeper layers of the epidermis where the cells are more active metabolically.

There are other members of the notorious herpesvirus family; such relatives include herpes simplex, Epstein-Barr (EB) virus of infectious mononucleosis, and cytomegalovirus, all of which tend to persist in the host for long periods.

### *Diagnosis*

Scrapings of the base of the vesicle produce characteristic cells with nuclear inclusions. Multinucleated giant cells are present. Electron microscopy of vesicle fluid is rapid and dependable. Only herpes simplex virus cannot be differentiated from varicella-zoster virus.

An indirect fluorescent antibody technique is available if the patient is capable of a normal host response.

### *Differential diagnosis*

***Variola (smallpox).*** Variola consists of deep-seated vesicles, commonly starting on the face and extremities, and is characterized by its toxicity at onset. Electron microscopy of the vesicle fluid or immunofluorescent studies to identify the antigenic viral components present, are diagnostic and rapid.

***Kaposi's varicelliform eruption.*** Kaposi's varicelliform eruption is a generalized vesicular eruption occurring in atopic individuals exposed to herpesvirus or vaccinia virus. History of contact with a vaccinated person or one with active herpes simplex is usually obtained.

***Enterovirus vesicular eruptions.*** The vesicles are noncrusted and smaller. They are chiefly summer eruptions.

### *Treatment*

Since the disease is self-limited, treatment should be symptomatic and should consist of simple measures to relieve itching and prevent secondary infection. Zinc oxide or calamine lotion with lukewarm, brief baths are effective.

For pruritus, trimeprazine (Panectyl, Temaril) tartrate elixir, 2.5 mg. per teaspoonful, or cyproheptadine (Periactin) elixir, 2 mg. per teaspoonful, is given two to three times daily. Antibiotics, as culture and sensitivity studies indicate, should be prescribed readily for any bacterial infection of the lesions.

If chicken pox is diagnosed in an individual or in an immunosuppressed patient, zoster immune globulin should be obtained from the proper public health branch and administered. The immunosuppresive drugs should be discontinued.

## ZOSTER

Zoster is an acute infection with neurocutaneous manifestations, caused by the varicella zoster virus in a partially immune person (one who has had chicken pox).

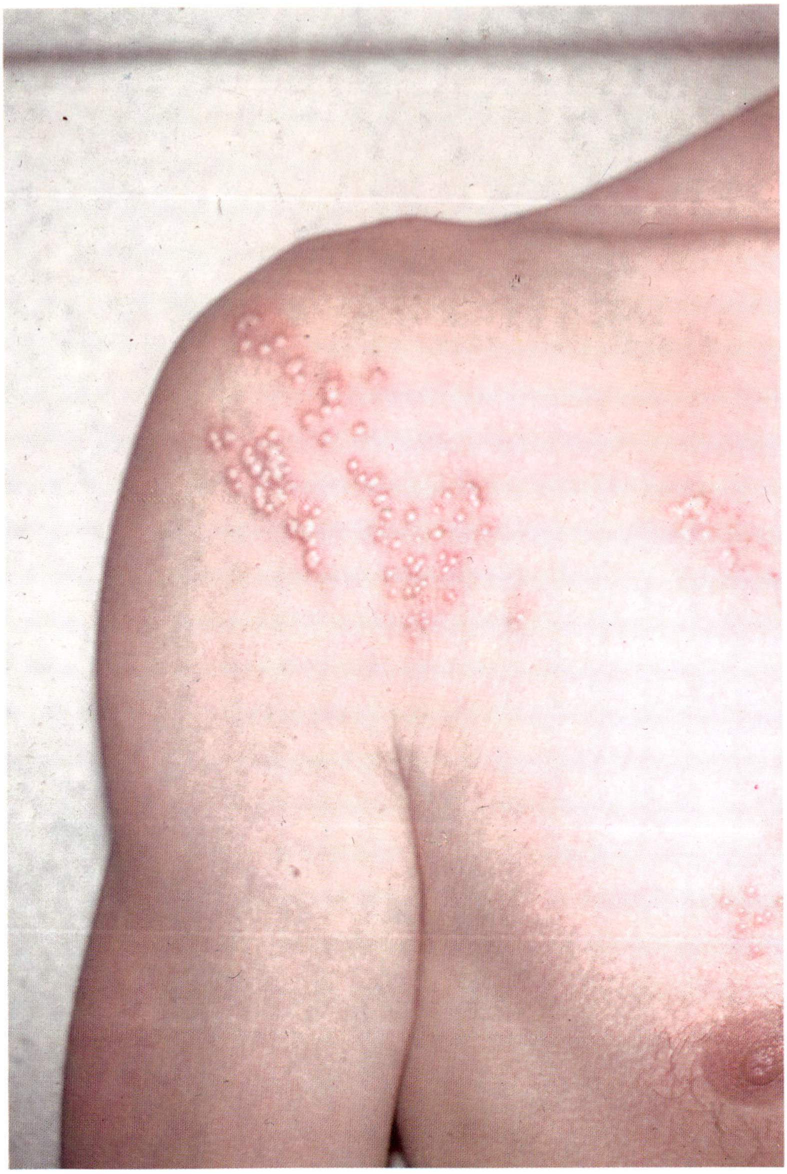

**Plate 31**
Zoster.

*Natural course*

There are prodromal symptoms of pain, burning, or itching prior to the onset of other clinical signs. Subsequently, vesicles develop on a tender, erythematous skin along the segmental distribution of a sensory nerve (Plate 31). The area of involvement is hypersensitive. The vesicles regress and become crusted over a period of 5 to 10 days. The lesions in the affected area may heal with scarring in severe cases. The eruption is unilateral and is associated with regional adenopathy. Stevens and Merigan showed that the extent and duration of the lesions seems to correlate with the lev-

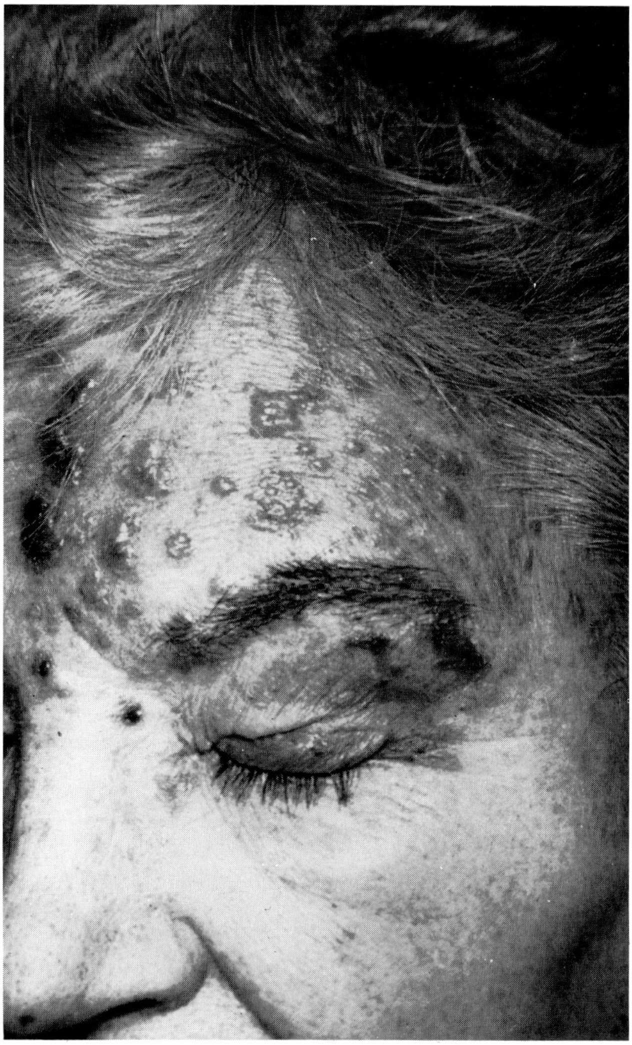

**Fig 15-5.** Ophthalmic zoster. Note eyelid and nose tip lesions, which signify possible corneal involvement.

els of interferon in the vesicles. One episode tends to provide immunity.

Zoster is more common in adults than in children. The site most frequently affected is the thorax. In 20% of cases the trigeminal and cervical regions are involved. Infection of the trigeminal nerve may lead to painful corneal ulceration that may cause loss of sight by involvement of the nasociliary branch. When the eruption involves the side and tip of the nose, there will be corneal involvement as well (Fig. 15-5). Older patients are prone to develop postzoster neuralgia, an agonizing persistent pain remaining in the affected area for weeks to months or longer. It is common in patients over 60 years of age but unusual in younger age groups. They may also develop areas of superficial gangrene along the distribution of the involved nerve. The pain of postzoster neuralgia resolves in 3 to 12 months and may produce depression. It is believed to be central in origin.

The Ramsay-Hunt syndrome results from involvement of the facial and auditory nerves, zoster vesicles affect the ear, and there is facial paralysis with auditory impairment.

It has been clearly shown that there are histological changes in the nerve fibers in the site affected by zoster. An 0.1 ml. intradermal injection of 1:100,000 solution of histamine phosphate produces a flare in normal individuals and mild cases of zoster, but the flare will be reduced or absent in those patients likely to have severe pain and postzoster neuralgia. This may be a helpful test in selected cases.

The zoster virus may involve the lower motor neuron and create paralysis. Goodman and Kendrick have reported that delay in recognizing motor involvement allows complications to develop. It occurs in about 1% of patients, may last several weeks to months, and should be recognized so that muscle stimulation and appropriate treatment can be started. Zoster encephalomyelitis is probably quite common, as are headache and nuchal rigidity in cervical involvement.

Infrequently, a generalized zoster with chicken pox–like vesicles may develop (generalized herpes) when the infection is associated with leukemia, the lymphomas, Hodgkin's disease, or cancer of the lung, gastrointestinal tract, or breast. It has been suggested that inadequate interferon production helps to disseminate zoster.

### Microscopic findings

The infected epidermal cells increase in size and become detached from each other (*ballooning degeneration*). These enlarged cells then degenerate, forming intraepidermal vesicles that are bordered by epidermal cells with nuclear inclusions. The regional ganglion shows inflammation and cellular necrosis, and the associated fibers show degeneration. There may be inflammatory changes in the posterior horn of the spinal cord.

### Pertinent information

The attack rate in individuals exposed to zoster is supposed to be about 15%. Some 4% to 5% of patients with Hodgkin's disease in some series have an episode of zoster. Almost 60% of patients with *disseminated* zoster lesions may have hematological malignancies, whereas 8% of hospitalized patients may show this association with only localized zoster. Zoster is significant as a complication of immunosuppressive therapy, as used for renal transplant procedures.

### Differential diagnosis

***Herpes simplex.*** A patch of small, grouped vesicles most frequently found on the lips and about the mouth is seen in herpes simplex, which frequently is recurrent.

***Dermatitis herpetiformis.*** Grouped pruritic vesicles are present on the scapular areas, buttocks, and arms. Dermatitis herpetiformis is chronic and recurrent and heals with pigmentation.

### Treatment

Zinc oxide, or calamine lotion, and lukewarm brief baths are beneficial. Good nursing care with consideration for the severe discomfort, particularly in an elderly patient in a nursing home, is very important.

Administration of 0.3 Gm. of acetylsalicylic acid, or 15 mg. of codeine sulfate, may be needed for relief of pain.

Epstein injected triamcinolone (2 mg./ml. of saline per treatment) subcutaneously beneath the zoster lesions to provide relief of pain and rapid healing of the disease. His paper should be read before one uses the method.

In the more severe cases, the judicious systemic use of glucocorticoid hormones is of benefit in the reduction of the incidence of postherpetic neuralgia and thus is beneficial in patients over 60 years of age, who have the greatest morbidity from this complication. Prednisone should be used over a 3-week period and *must* be started early in the disease. Marcy suggests 1 mg./kg. daily for a week and then reduced by half weekly for 3 weeks. After the vesicles have begun to develop a crust, it is doubtful whether glucocorticoid hormones are beneficial. Steroids should not be used until it has been determined that there is no underlying disorder affecting the immunity.

Juel-Jensen described his impressive results in patients over 60 years of age by using 40% IDU in DMSO topically. A dressing is soaked with the solution and kept on, but it is resoaked daily throughout the course of the disease. None of 12 elderly patients developed postherpetic neuralgia.

If the trigeminal nerve is involved, ophthalmological consultation should be sought regarding potential corneal ulceration. Secondary bacterial infection can be tragic.

Ophthalmic zoster that threatens to be severe and possibly blinding should be treated as is disseminated severe zoster in a patient with impaired immune responses. The drug of choice at present is adenine arabinoside. Whitley et al. have shown that in 87 patients cutaneous signs, at least, were shorter in the treated group. It should be given in the first 6 days of the disease.

Patients with atypical zoster should be thoroughly examined for possible malignancies or blood dyscrasias, Hodgkin's disease particularly. Serum copper levels fall a very long time prior to zoster in patients with Hodgkin's disease.

#### REFERENCES


Eaglestein, W. H., Katz, R., and Brown, J. A.: The effects of early corticosteroid therapy on the skin eruption and pain of herpes zoster, J.A.M.A. **211**:1681, 1970.

**Pain is reduced; the course is not.**

Epstein, E.: Treatment of herpes zoster and postzoster neuralgia by the intralesional injection of triamcinolone. A computer analysis of 199 cases, Int. J. Dermatol. **15**:762, 1976.

**Uncontrolled but very impressive.**

Goodman, C. E., and Kenrick, M. M.: Herpes zoster with motor paresis, South. Med. J. **67**:1171, 1974.

**Five cases.**

Juel-Jensen, B. E., and MacCallum, F. O.: Herpes simplex, varicella, and zoster: clinical manifestations and treatment, London, 1972, William Heinemann Medical Books, Ltd.

**An excellent little book.**

Luby, J. P.: Varicella-zoster virus, J. Invest. Dermatol. **61**:212, 1973.

**Detailed, full researched review.**

Marcy, S. M., and Kibrick, S.: Varicella and herpes zoster. In Hoeprich, P. D., editor: Infectious diseases, Hagerstown, Md. 1977, Harper & Row, Publishers, p. 744.

Thorling, E. B., and Thorling, K.: Serum copper in Hodgkin's disease before and after herpes zoster, Lancet **2**:1396, 1974.

**Four months before shingles, the serum copper begins to fall.**

Whitley, R. J., Ch'ien, L. T., Dolin, R., et al.: Adenine arabinoside therapy of herpes zoster in the immunosuppressed. NIAID collaborative study, N. Engl. J. Med. **294**:1193, 1976.

**Shortened duration of virus on skin and lesions in compromised patients receiving ara-A.**


## VARIOLA (SMALLPOX)

Variola, caused by a virus of the poxvirus group, as recently as 1967 affected approximately 10 million people throughout the world, at least one fourth of whom died. The authoritative voice of the International Journal of Epidemiology in 1976, reported that for most practical purposes, this disease has been eradicated. The World Health Organization has decreed that two smallpox-free years should elapse before a country can be declared free of the disease. Three countries, Nigeria, Indonesia, and Ethiopia, still report smallpox in remote villages.

### *Natural course*

The incubation period averages slightly less than 2 weeks, but may last up to 3. The severe and sudden onset produces signs of pronounced toxicity, severe muscular pain, and prostration. There are transient characteristic petechial eruptions that involve the inguinal and axillary regions. By the fifth day of illness the eruption begins with erythematous macules; these then rapidly progress to umbilicated vesicles. The lesions will have attained a pustular appearance by the tenth day, and crusts begin by the twelfth day. The distribution of the lesions shows a concentration on the face and extremities and points of pressure. There may be a second febrile peak, when the lesions become pustular, around the end of the first week.

The vesicles are firm and spherical and have a sensation of depth in the dermis.

Hemorrhage and confluent forms of smallpox indicate a poorer prognosis, with mortality up to 100%. In ordinary epidemics, the mortality is approximately 25%.

### *Pertinent information*

The successful eradication of smallpox has been attributable to techniques in preventive medicine.

Currently, speed of travel creates one of the remaining problems. Travelers, after contracting the disease, may arrive in a smallpox-free area within the time of the incubation period. This offers problems in diagnosis for physicians unfamiliar with the manifestations of the disease.

In such instances, all close contacts of the person suspected of having variola should be vaccinated or revaccinated. The virus of smallpox is highly infectious, and because it survives in the skin until late convalescence, it can be spread by many methods, including clothing, bedding, dust, and flies.

### *Investigation*

In the first 2 days after onset, prior to the appearance of the rash, laboratory tests for virus antigen and for the virus can be carried out quickly on blood or, after the appearance of the first lesions on the skin, from skin scrapings. These can be sent to the laboratory on a glass slide. Vaccinia and smallpox viruses cannot be differentiated by serological means.

### *Microscopic findings*

Deep-seated, intraepidermal, multilocular vesicles form and affect the dermis so as to result in scarring. The vesicle is not different from those found in varicella or herpes. The affected cells contain intracytoplasmic inclusions.

### *Diagnosis*

Clinical:

1. Possible exposure to smallpox
2. Febrile prodrome of 2 to 4 days
3. Evidence of past vaccination
4. Rash conforms clinically—centrifugal, single-crop, round, deep, shotty lesions

### *Differential diagnosis*

***Varicella.*** The eruption in varicella is more superficial and proceeds more rapidly. The trunk is chiefly affected. Microscopic examination of varicella virus vesicles shows typical intranuclear inclusions of the herpesviruses. Electron microscopy of vesicle fluid differentiates this rapidly from smallpox.

***Vaccinia.*** A history of recent vaccination and spread of vesicular lesions, either in the pattern of a secondary inoculation from scratching or in an atopic individual (eczema vaccinatum), will indicate a vaccinia diagnosis.

### *Treatment of persons exposed to smallpox*

***Methisazone (Marboran).*** An effective oral antiviral agent, methisazone, has shown great promise in the treatment of persons exposed to smallpox before the fever and skin rash appear. It has been helpful when given up to 6 days after exposure. It produces a 94% reduction in incidence of the disease in these individuals. Two doses of 3 Gm. each are given in a single day, or 1.5 Gm. is given twice daily for 4 days. It may produce nausea, vomiting, and transient alterations in liver function.

***Immune globulin.*** Immune globulin (vaccinia immune globulin, or VIG), when given to susceptible smallpox contacts before fever and skin rash appear, will suppress both of these manifestations. It is used for treatment of susceptible contacts and reduces by 75% the incidence of the disease in these individuals.

Vaccination at, or shortly after, the initial exposure may modify the disease.

### *Prophylaxis*

***Antismallpox vaccination.*** Antismallpox vaccination uses the vaccinia virus, which is antigenically similar to the smallpox virus. The procedure should be performed every third year in those with risk of exposure. Patients with *active* atopic eczema should *not* be vaccinated because of the danger of eczema vaccinatum, another cause of Kaposi's varicelliform eruption.

*Complications resulting from antismallpox vaccination and specific treatment measures are as follows:*

1. Generalized, transient toxic erythemas are the most common complication. Treatment includes aspirin and bed rest.

2. Vaccinia associated with mild, scattered, self-inoculated lesions requires no treatment.

3. For vaccinia that is generalized, severe, and accompanied by fever and prostration, treatment consists of vaccinia immune gamma

globulin (VIG) 0.3 ml. per pound intramuscularly for children and less for adults, and methisazone given orally for 1 to 4 days, which results in arrest of the progression of generalized vaccinia.

4. Postvaccinia encephalitis is seen in older children and adults. There is no treatment for this rare complication.

5. Ulceration at the vaccination site (vaccinia gangrenosa) may occur in patients unable to form antibody. Treatment is with VIG, 0.3 ml. per pound for children and less for adults, and methisazone.

6. Kaposi's varicelliform eruption (Fig. 15-6). An effective agent is available for the control and suppression of reactions to vaccinia virus, if necessary. It is immune gamma globulin (VIG), taken from donors 4 to 8 weeks after a successful vaccination. It is not freely available, but can be obtained through the Canadian Health Protection Branch and through the Blood Program of the American Red Cross.

### *Contraindications to vaccination*

1. *Active* atopic dermatitis in the patient or in a household member
2. An immunodeficiency state as in Hodgkin's disease, lymphoma, or leukemia
3. Patient receiving radiation therapy
4. Patient receiving systemic glucocorticoids
5. Patient receiving immunosuppressive drugs
6. Pregnancy
7. Acute febrile illness

Vaccination as a routine measure in childhood is at present under critical evaluation. However, complications such as encephalitis are much less common in children than in adults.

#### REFERENCES

Blank, H., David, C., and Collins, C.: Electron microscopy for the diagnosis of cutaneous viral infections, Br. J. Dermatol. **83**:69, 1970.

**An outstanding clinically oriented diagnostic approach to viral disease.**

Editorial: Eradication of smallpox, Int. J. Epidemiol. **5**:6, 1976.

**Eradication campaigns have been mounted by international control agencies against malaria and yellow fever, but most striking success has been against smallpox.**

Henderson, D. A.: Surveillance of smallpox, Int. J. Epidemiol. **5**:9, 1976.

Lane, J. M., Ruben, F. L., and Neff, J. M.: Complications of smallpox vaccination, 1968, N. Engl. J. Med. **281**:1201, 1969.

**572 with complications; morbidity and mortality highest in infants.**

## KAPOSI'S VARICELLIFORM ERUPTION (ECZEMA VACCINATUM, ECZEMA HERPETICUM)

Kaposi's varicelliform eruption is a generalized vesicular eruption that occurs in atopic individuals exposed to the vaccinia virus (eczema vaccinatum) (Fig. 15-6) or the herpesvirus (eczema herpeticum) (Fig. 15-3). It is the reason for witholding vaccination from children with active atopic dermatitis and is most common under the age of 5 years.

### *Natural course*

One to 2 weeks after contact with either virus, umbilicated vesicles begin to appear, and in a day or so fever and systemic symptoms develop. Vesicles continue to appear for a very few days and go on to crusting and healing over in approximately 10 days (Fig. 15-6). Vesicles tend to appear first at sites of active skin inflammation, but may become generalized. Viremia and encephalitis may occur. Death follows in a small percentage of cases. There has been a 12% mortality in eczema vaccinatum in children under 5 years of age. Wheeler and Abele have noted that eczema herpeticum may be recurrent, but if so, it is a milder disease with a much less severe prognosis. In eczema vaccinatum, the areas of active dermatitis are first affected.

### *Pertinent information*

Although atopic individuals are most likely to develop this complication while their dermatitis is in an active phase, some with no apparent active lesions may also do so. Spread of the virus from scratching is not the whole cause of the disorder.

Atopic adults or children should be pro-

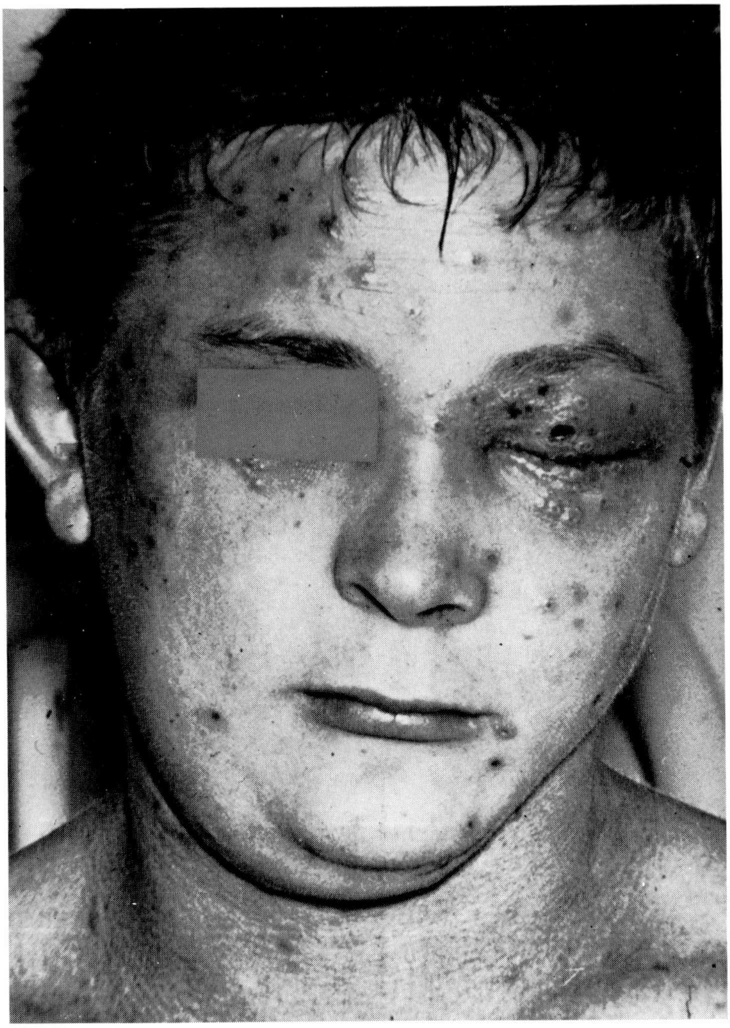

**Fig. 15-6.** Kaposi's varicelliform eruption (eczema vaccinatum) caused by vaccinia virus in atopic individual.

tected from patients demonstrating active herpes simplex lesions or having recent vaccination.

### *Treatment*

These patients should be isolated from other susceptible family members, and supportive care should be given, with rest and comfortable surroundings. Admission to a hospital may be indicated in most cases. Good dermatological nursing care with observation for secondary infection is important.

If severe and accompanied by fever and prostration, this disorder is treated with VIG, 0.1 to 0.3 ml. per pound, and methisazone given orally for 1 to 4 days. In infants with eczema who have had close contact with vaccinated individuals or who themselves have to be vaccinated, VIG should be administered to prevent complications. Dosage is 0.1 to 0.2 ml. per pound. VIG may also be of benefit in atopic infants exposed to herpes infection, if it seems indicated.

#### REFERENCES

Copeman, P. W. M., and Wallace, H. J.: Eczema vaccinatum, Br. Med. J. **2**:906, 1964.
**A 12% mortality from accidental contact!**

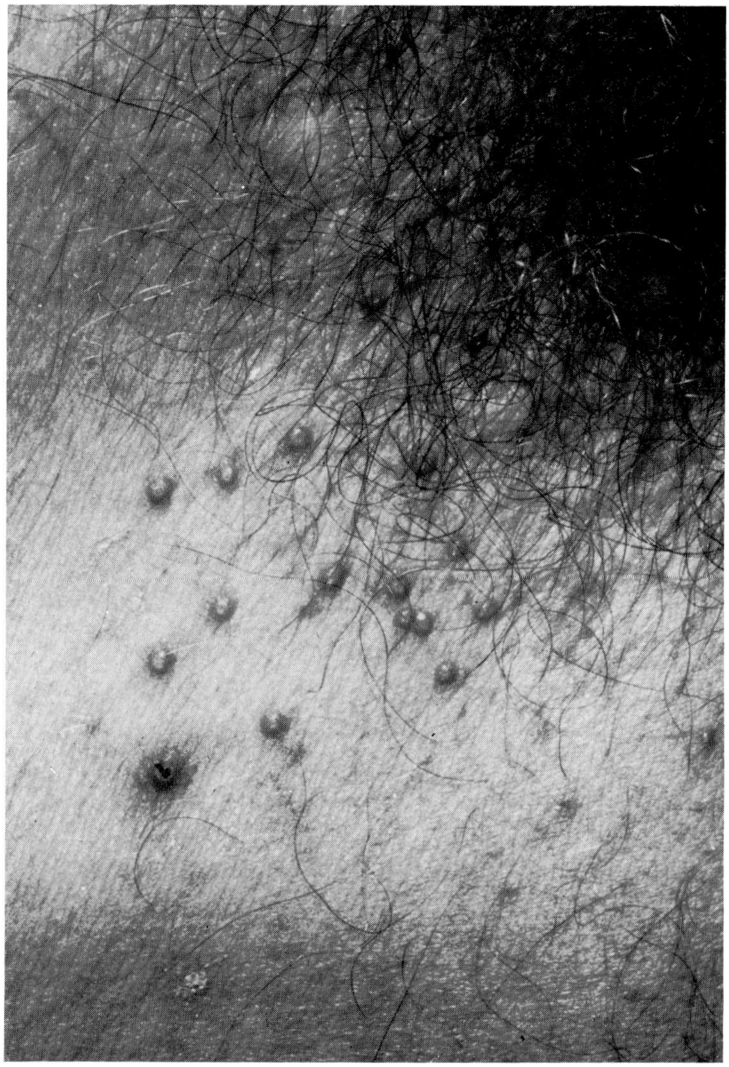

**Fig. 15-7.** Molluscum contagiosum.

London, I. D., and Monsky, D. B.: Eczema vaccinatum, J. Med. Assoc. Alabama **37**:1164, 1968.
**Atopic patients clear of disease contracted eczema vaccinatum. Responded to VIG.**

Wheeler, C. E., Jr., and Abele, D. C.: Eczema herpeticum, primary and recurrent, Arch. Dermatol. **93**:162, 1966.
**Two cases illustrating the disease.**

## MOLLUSCUM CONTAGIOSUM

Molluscum contagiosum (Fig. 15-7) is a contagious viral disease producing discrete, minute, globular cutaneous lesions.

### *Natural course*

The lesion is a characteristic, slightly pink, smooth, round-domed papule, 1 to 3 mm. in size, with a slight apical depression. The mature lesion contains a soft central plug that may easily be expressed. It is found on normal skin, but may have, on occasion, an erythematous base resulting from irritation or secondary infection. The lesion is autoinoculable and contagious, so that a multiplication of lesions on various areas of the skin results. The most commonly involved sites are the abdomen and inner thighs, eyelids, and perianal region.

The lesions may be discrete or grouped, and sometimes only a single lesion is seen. The usual case consists of less than 50 lesions. It is chiefly seen in children, but more often in recent years in young adults, where it often has a genital location in the pubic hair, on the penis, or on the inner thighs.

### *Pertinent information*

The causative agent is one of the largest viruses that affects man. It is an intracytoplasmic invader that stimulates the epidermal cells to undergo a decreased transit time. The incubation period is 2 or more weeks. Recurrent infections are uncommon. Epstein demonstrated antibodies by an immunofluorescent technique in 87% of patients with the disease.

It is associated with atopic disease and with immunodeficient or immunosuppressed patients more often than would be predicted. It is also a sexually transmitted disease.

### *Microscopic findings*

The lesion consists of virus-infected epidermal cells in small tumor masses that are encapsulated by the dermis. These cells contain typical hyalinized intracytoplasmic molluscum bodies. In the mature lesion these bodies form the center of the mass, producing the umbilication seen clinically. Epidermal cell renewal is increased as the infected cells move upward synchronously.

### *Differential diagnosis*

***Intradermal nevus.*** Intradermal nevus is a persistent, skin-colored, firm nodule without a central depression.

***Verruca vulgaris (common wart).*** A skin-colored papular lesion, verruca vulgaris has a rough surface.

***Verruca juvenilis (flat wart).*** Verruca juvenilis is a flat-topped, fawn-colored, smooth papular lesion, chiefly occurring on the face or dorsum of the hand in children.

### *Treatment*

The lesions may clear without treatment, but as a rule some destructive modality must be used. This may be done best by removal of the mature lesion with a sharp dermal curet. (This can be done with a minimum of discomfort. Mature soft lesions come away easily.) Liquid nitrogen has also been used with excellent results.

#### REFERENCES

Ive, F. A.: Treatment of skin infections and infestations, Br. Med. J. **4**:477, 1973.
**A summary of current knowledge.**

Molluscum contagiosum, leading article: Br. Med. J. **1**:459, 1968.
**The infectious nature emphasized.**

## CONTAGIOUS PUSTULAR DERMATITIS (ORF)

Cutaneous pustular dermatitis (Fig. 15-8) is a disease of sheep handlers and persons in contact with infected sheep. The causative agent is a DNA poxvirus that produces epithelial hyperplasia in man, sheep, and goats. Human infections occur on the fingers, hands, or eyelids and begin as a papulovesicular lesion that ulcerates.

Microscopically, there is viral involvement of superficial endothelial and epithelial cells. The lesion may take several weeks to heal. Paronychia is also seen. The lesions are usually painless. In sheep, the disease affects young lambs in areas not covered with wool and on the oral mucosa.

No treatment is necessary since this is a self-limiting disease running a course of 3 to 5 weeks.

Immunity is produced in both sheep and man after the primary infection.

#### REFERENCE

Leavell, U. W., Jr., McNamara, M. J., Muelling, R., et al.: Orf: report of 19 cases with clinical and pathological observations, J.A.M.A. **204**:109, 1968.
**The name basically means 'scab'; the disease occurs in sheep and goats.**

## MILKERS' NODULES

Infected cows have pustular udder lesions that may be transmitted to milkers' hands and fingers as red-brown, painless nodules. They develop after an incubation period of 1 to 4 weeks and may last up to 2 months. There may be associated lymphadenopathy. Recently a viral etiology has been proved. The agent ap-

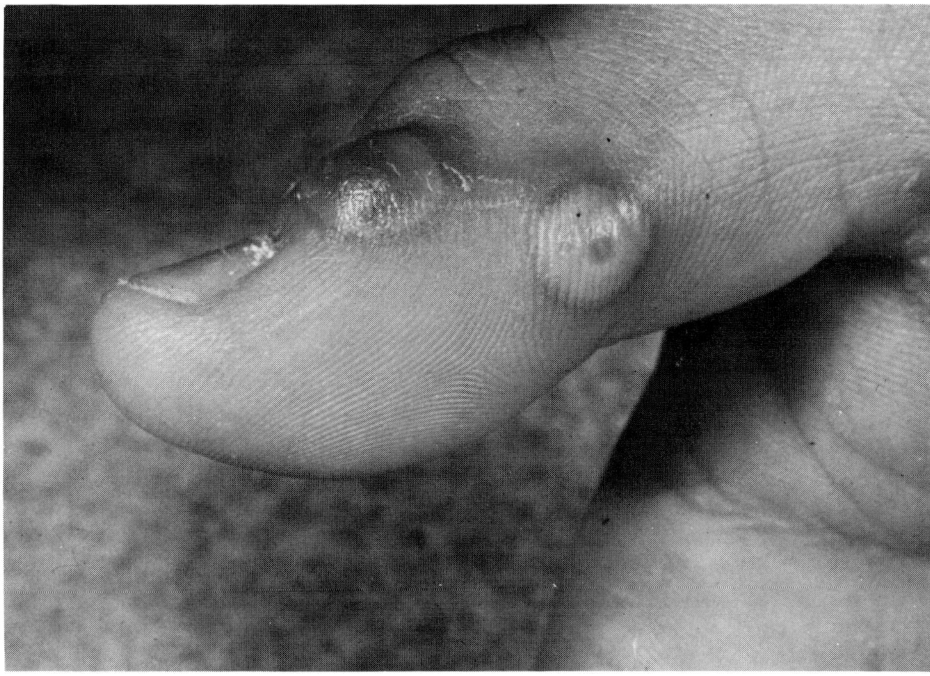

**Fig. 15-8.** Orf.

pears to belong in the poxvirus group and has morphological similarity to orf virus.

No treatment is necessary.

## RUBEOLA (MEASLES, MORBILLI)

Rubeola is a contagious viral childhood infection of worldwide distribution and may have serious complications. If live attenuated measles virus vaccine were administered to all susceptible children, this disease could be eliminated.

### *Natural course*

The incubation period is 10 to 14 days, after which the patient develops fever ranging from 38.5° to 40° C, with a nasal discharge, lacrimation, photophobia, congestion of the mucous membranes of the throat, and a persistent dry cough. The anterior cervical lymph nodes are enlarged and tender. Twenty-four to 36 hours prior to the development of skin lesions, pinhead-sized white spots on an erythematous base are found on the buccal mucosa opposite the molars, and on the mucous membrane inside the lower lip (Koplik's spots) in some 60% of the cases. The skin eruption consists of pruritic red macules that enlarge and coalesce, with a resulting blotchy appearance. It begins on the face and extends to the neck, trunk, and extremities. The rash reaches its peak in 3 to 5 days and then gradually fades, accompanied by a drop in temperature and subsidence of the other symptoms. The disease occurs most frequently in children under 5 years of age and is a greater threat to them than to older children.

The mucosal and cutaneous eruption is a result of direct epithelial cell invasion by the myxovirus. Multinucleated giant cells and characteristic intranuclear virus tubules can be demonstrated in the lesions.

Measles infection alone is rarely fatal, except among socioeconomically deprived children in tropical countries. There mortality may be 10% to 15% and severe complications are common. In most temperate areas, however, it still may lead to the serious bacterial complications of otitis media and pneumonia or to viral pneumonia in 7% to 10% of cases.

Encephalitis occurs in from 0.1% to 0.01% of cases and has a 15% mortality. Central nervous system sequelae frequently occur after encephalitis. The disease is spread by droplet infection. One episode of measles produces a lifelong immunity.

Antibodies from the mother provide infants with a passive immunity to measles that lasts 3 months.

### *Differential diagnosis*

***Roseola infantum.*** An infection of infancy, roseola infantum is characterized by fever lasting 2 to 3 days. When the fever subsides, a diffuse red macular eruption begins.

***Rubella (German measles).*** The symptoms of rubella are milder than those of rubeola, and Koplik's spots are not present. Postauricular and occipital lymph nodes are involved.

***Echovirus exanthem.*** A disease similar in all respects to rubeola may be produced by echovirus. Diagnosis is made by virological studies of material from throat or stool. The incubation period is shorter, being 3 to 5 days.

***Infectious mononucleosis.*** The eruption of infectious mononucleosis may closely resemble rubella and could be confused with rubeola. The heterophil antibody test is most helpful.

***Erythema infectiosum.*** This eruption begins on the cheeks (slapped cheeks) as an erythematous papular eruption that coalesces over a 2- to 4-day period and then fades as a mottled maculopapular eruption extending to the arms and forearms. Course is 5 to 8 days.

### *Prophylaxis*

Gamma globulin may be administered to those who have been exposed to rubeola but have not been immunized. To modify the disease, 0.02 ml. of immune globulin per pound may be given within 6 days or less of exposure to produce a mild episode of the disease. To prevent the disease, 0.1 ml. of immune globulin per pound may be given within 6 days, or less, of the exposure.

For all susceptible children over 12 months of age, measles vaccine (live attenuated virus vaccine) is recommended to avoid measles and its complications. It should also be given to older children and adults who have not had measles. It can be given in combination with rubella and mumps virus (MMR) attenuated vaccine. Its use is contraindicated in debilitated children, glucocorticoid therapy, active tuberculosis, leukemia or malignancy, immunocompromised individuals, pregnancy, and severe illness. These individuals may now be given inactivated vaccine as a preparation for the subsequent use of live vaccine.

### *Treatment*

Treatment consists of bed rest and symptomatic relief.

Because of the incidence of serious subsequent bacterial infections, adequate protective antibiotic therapy should be provided for children under 3 years of age or for debilitated patients.

Aspirin, with dosage regulated for age, should be given for relief of symptoms, as well as antihistaminics for sedative and antipruritic effect. A mixture containing 5 mg. of codeine per dose is beneficial as a cough inhibitor.

Topical antipruritic therapy consists of applying a soothing lotion, such as the following:

| | |
|---|---|
| Menthol | 0.25% |
| Zinc oxide | 15 Gm. |
| Talc | 15 Gm. |
| Glycerin | 10 ml. |
| Alcohol | 30 ml. |
| Water | 50 ml. |

Apply as needed for relief of itching.

#### REFERENCES


Marcy, S. M., and Kilbrick, S.: Measles. In Hoeprich, P. D., editor: Infectious diseases, Hagerstown, Md., 1977, Harper & Row, Publishers, p. 691.
**Viral, clinical, therapeutic, and preventive aspects.**

Suringa, D. W. R., Bank, L. J., and Ackerman, A. B.: Role of measles virus in skin lesions and Koplik's spots, N. Engl. J. Med. **282:**1139, 1970.
**Viral microtubular aggregates in cells in each area.**


## RUBELLA (GERMAN MEASLES)

Rubella is a widespread contagious viral infection that is significant chiefly for its ability to produce congenital defects in children of mothers contracting the disease in the first trimester of pregnancy.

### *Natural course*

The incubation period lasts 14 to 21 days, after which there may be mild prodromal symptoms of headache, malaise, and fever. Many patients develop small erythematous macules on the palate just prior to the appearance of the rash. In about 24 hours there develops on the face a dusky red, blotchy, macular eruption that rapidly extends to the trunk and extremities. The eruption completely involutes in 72 hours. The occipital and postauricular lymph nodes are characteristically enlarged and tender, a significant point in differential diagnosis. The adenopathy may persist for months. Although the eruption is carefully described and considered highly characteristic, a variety of proved rubella infections have demonstrated petechial, acneiform, and other eruptions.

Arthritis frequently affects adults, particularly women, with the disease. Transient thrombocytopenia is seen.

### *Pertinent information*

The virus can be recovered from the pharynx 7 days before to 14 days after the exanthem.

Birth defects occur in 25% of cases in which the mother was infected with rubella in the first trimester. There is no relationship between the severity of the infection in the mother and the type of defect that occurs in the infant. Rubella in pregnant women may cause eye defects, deafness and mutism, cardiac malformations, mental abnormalities, and microcephaly in the infant. It also increases the likelihood of abortions, stillbirths, and infant deaths.

## Congenital rubella

A syndrome including growth retardation, generalized purpura, encephalomyelitis, hepatosplenomegaly, and bony changes has also been demonstrated recently in these infants. Maternal virus can pass to the fetus at certain stages of gestation. The fetus then develops viremia, which results in *persistent viral infection*, *vascular damage*, and *tissue damage*.

Rubella virus can be cultured from the throat and urine of the affected child at birth, 6 months after the disease occurred in the mother. These affected children continue to disseminate the virus to persons, even through brief contact. Neonatal mortality is high, 25% to 30% in the first year of life.

Because of these facts, exposure of preadolescent girls to the disease is desirable, and avoidance of exposure of nonimmune pregnant women to the disease is essential. The disease confers a long-term immunity. However, reinfection of previously immune individuals does occur. Such infections may maintain immunity, rather than only one episode being responsible.

A hemagglutination-inhibition test, which is quite widely available, is now used to identify an individual's immune status within 2 weeks of exposure.

### *Diagnosis*

Clinical diagnosis may still be the best so far. A good dependable diagnostic test awaits further observation and study of immunofluorescent techniques. Hemagglutin-inhibition (HI) antibodies are the earliest to show elevation in the disease.

### *Differential diagnosis*

***Rubeola.*** The symptoms in rubeola are more severe than those of rubella, and Koplik's spots are present on the buccal mucosa. There is not the pronounced lymphadenopathy seen in rubella.

***Drug eruption.*** Drugs (for example, salicylates) may cause a diffuse macular eruption, but there is no enlargement of the occipital lymph nodes, and fever rarely is noted.

***Roseola infantum.*** Roseola exanthem is preceded by a 2- to 3-day fever. It occurs almost exclusively in infants.

***Infectious mononucleosis.*** The eruption of infectious mononucleosis may closely resemble rubella. The heterophil antibody test is most helpful.

***Erythema infectiosum.*** This eruption begins on the cheeks (slapped cheeks) as an erythematous papular eruption that coalesces over a 2- to 4-day period, then fades as a mottled maculopapular eruption extending to the arms and forearms. Course is 5 to 8 days. It may occur in several family members and friends.

### *Prevention*

A new intranasal attenuated live vaccine RA 27/3 and several older live vaccines are available as single-dosage treatments for the prevention of mumps, measles, and rubella. Antibody levels produced were not so high as those found with the naturally occurring disease, but the new vaccine will correct these lower levels. Pregnancy should be averted for 3 months after vaccination.

Immunization is recommended for children from 15 months to puberty and seronegative mature girls and women, if pregnancy can be prevented for 3 subsequent months.

***Rubella in pregnancy.*** Immune serum globulin may be of value in preventing fetal infection after maternal exposure. Vaccine is contraindicated in pregnancy and anticipated pregnancy.

### *Treatment*

Rubella is a self-limited disease for which there is no satisfactory medication that will alter its course once it has begun.

Symptomatic therapy consists of bed rest, if indicated, and administration of aspirin (with dosage regulated for age) for relief of symptoms, as well as antihistaminics for antipruritic and sedative effect.

#### REFERENCES


Hardy, J. B.: Rubella and congenital rubella. In Conn, H. F., editor: Current therapy, Philadelphia, 1975, W. B. Saunders Co., p. 57.
**Succinct, knowledgeable coverage of the subject.**

Heggie, A. D.: Pathogenesis of rubella exanthem: isolation of rubella virus from the skin, N. Engl. J. Med. **285**:664, 1971.
**Erythematous macules demonstrate the virus.**

Marcy, S. M., and Kibrick, S.: Rubella. In Hoeprich, P. D., editor: Infectious diseases, Hagerstown, Md., 1977, Harper & Row, Publishers, p. 701.
**The expanded rubella syndrome.**

Modlin, J. F., and Herrmann, K.: Risk of congenital abnormality after inadvertent rubella vaccination of pregnant women, N. Engl. J. Med. **294**:972, 1976.
**The attenuated virus recovered from fetus.**


## WARTS (VERRUCAE)

Warts are the most common viral infection of the skin and are characterized by localized epithelial hyperplasia, unpredictable course, and eventual spontaneous complete resolution (Fig. 15-9).

### *Natural course*

Warts begin as minute, smooth-surfaced, skin-colored lesions that enlarge for a period of time, but remain stationary after attaining a certain size. Repeated irritation will cause a wart to continue enlarging. The surface takes on a roughened, finely papillomatous texture.

The course is completely unpredictable. A single wart may remain unchanged for months, only to suddenly develop satellite lesions. Warts may continue to appear at a steady rate in some individuals. They occur in 7% to 10% of the population.

This infection is most common in children and young adults, usually occurring on exposed areas such as the fingers, hands, and face, as well as the sole.

### *Pertinent information*

The causative virus is of the papovavirus group, small DNA icosahedral bodies that grow slowly in host cell nuclei. They induce proliferation and produce chronic infections. They have been grown in epithelioid cells. Incubation periods are from 1 to 20 months or more. The majority of persons with warts have IgM antibodies, but with prolonged infection, IgG antibodies appear. Cell-mediated immunity is active during wart regression.

Two thirds of untreated warts disappear within 2 years with no trace of their presence, although it is not unusual to have a wart last many years.

There appear to be several viruses, at least five of which have been immunologically identified, partly because of variations in DNA structure. There is a higher incidence in patients undergoing immunosuppression, those on glucocorticoids (systemic and local),

A

B

C

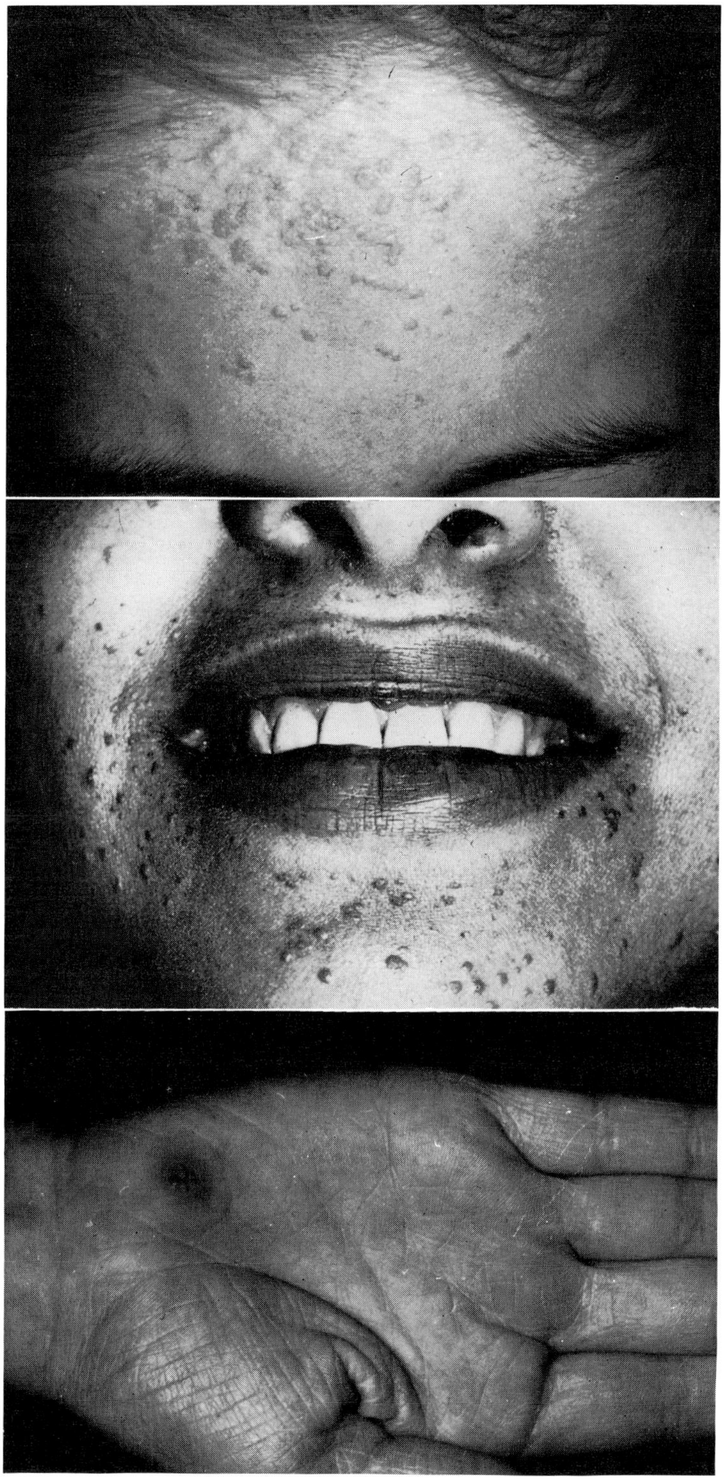

**Fig. 15-9.** Warts. **A,** Juvenile (plain, flat) warts of forehead. **B,** Juvenile warts of chin. **C,** Common wart (verruca vulgaris) of palm.

those with malignancies, particularly Hodgkin's disease, and those who for some reason or another are immunodeficient. Patients with warts may show decreased cell-mediated immunity compared with controls.

Another problem with warts arises because of the oncogenicity of the virus. They do produce cellular proliferation and are related to papilloma-producing viruses in animals. They have prolonged intracellular existence in humans, and genital cancer is preceded by condylomas in 10% of cases investigated. Giant condylomas in the genital area are clearly associated with carcinomas.

### *Regression*

Greenberg and colleagues sensitized four patients with warts to dinitrochlorobenzene (DNCB). After topical challenge by DNCB, the warts disappeared.

***Plane warts.*** Berman has examined flat warts undergoing spontaneous regression and found mononuclear cells in a pattern suggesting cell-mediated immunity. This confirms earlier clinical concepts by Tagami and others. Takigawa has examined spontaneous regression with the electron microscope and described first degeneration and then regeneration from adjacent unaffected tissue.

A

B

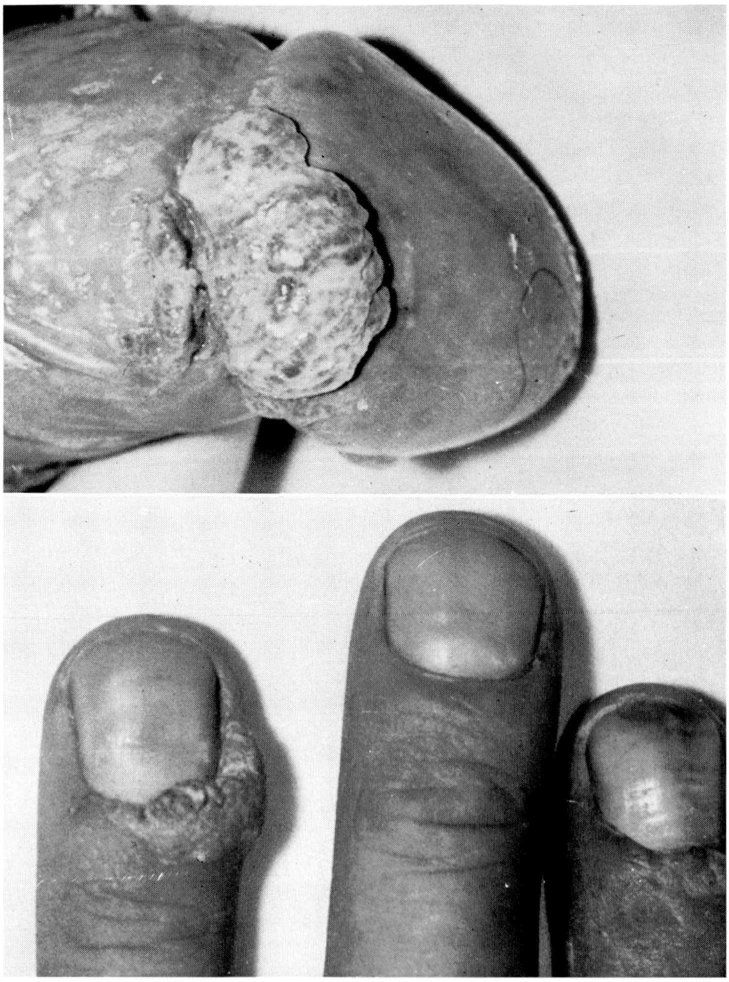

**Fig. 15-10. A,** Verruca acuminata of penis. **B,** Warts at base of nail fold.

Mononuclear cells were limited to the area of regenerating epidermis. Tagami (1977) records that this is distinct from the process of regression described in common warts and is the same process in all despite variations in treatment.

***Common warts.*** Matthews and Pyrhonen both felt humoral immunity was significant in the regression of common warts. There is some evidence that irritating treatment like salicylic acid topically may invoke a stronger immune response.

### *Variations*

The characteristics a wart assumes depend chiefly on its anatomical site.

***Common wart (verruca vulgaris).*** A skin-colored to brown, rough-surfaced epithelial growth, the common wart may be single or multiple and is usually asymptomatic. The sites most frequently involved are the dorsal and palmar surfaces of the hands, the fingers, and the area surrounding and beneath the nails (Fig. 15-10, *B*).

***Plantar wart (verruca plantaris).*** The plantar wart has the appearance of a sharply circumscribed callus that is usually tender. It occurs for the most part on weight-bearing areas on the sole. Close examination reveals multiple tiny black dots that tend to bleed when the surface is removed. These are the blood vessels in the hypertrophied dermal papillae of the wart. Plantar warts are frequently surrounded by a collar of hyperkeratosis. A second category of plantar warts forms predominantly scaling plaques and cover a wide area of the sole. These are known as *mosaic warts.*

***Flat wart, or juvenile wart (verruca plana).*** Flat wart is a skin-colored to brown, slightly raised, smooth, asymptomatic lesion, 1 to 5 mm. in diameter. The lesions are multiple and are commonly found on the face and on the dorsum of the hands in children (Fig. 15-9).

***Digitate wart (verruca digitata).*** Digitate wart is a cornified, hornlike, projecting lesion, 1 to 10 mm. in length and capped with multiple fingerlike projections. Commonly a single lesion is present, usually located on the angles of the mouth, eyelids, neck, bearded area, or scalp.

***Genital wart, or venereal wart (verruca acuminata).*** The verruca acuminata type consists of a group of moist, red, soft papillary projections producing cauliflowerlike growths on the mucous membranes of the penis (Fig. 15-10, *A*), vulva, and perianal region. This form of wart is found in moist areas at the junction of skin and mucous membranes. A remarkable and comprehensive review by Oriel establishes genital warts as a venereal disease unassociated with cutaneous warts elsewhere. He described an infectivity rate of 64% in genital warts from intercourse. Their incubation period appears to be 4 to 6 weeks. He differentiates genital warts (condylomas) from common warts, similar in appearance to those elsewhere on the skin, that appear on the nonmembranous penile shaft and the labia in women. He dismisses the likelihood of spread from hands to genital mucous membranes. They did, however, tend to spread from the genitals to the perianal area and did increase in size in a persistently moist environment.

### *Microscopic findings*

Upward proliferation of the dermal papillae occurs, associated with marked hyperkeratosis, acanthosis, and papillomatosis. Intranuclear and intracytoplasmic basophilic inclusion bodies in the epidermal cells produce a characteristic appearance. The wart is limited to the epidermis.

### *Differential diagnosis*

***Seborrheic keratosis.*** Seborrheic keratosis is characterized by a brown or black warty growth that has the appearance of being "stuck on" the skin. The lesions are usually multiple and are commonly found on the forehead or temples and on the back and chest of elderly people.

***Molluscum contagiosum.*** A small, smooth-surfaced nodule that has a depression in the center distinguishes molluscum contagiosum. The lesions are usually multiple and are found on the trunk, thighs, and arms in children.

***Lichen planus.*** Lesions in lichen planus are

flat-topped, reddish purple papules commonly found on the flexor surface of the wrists. There may be bluish white, lacy patches on the buccal mucosa.

***Callus.*** Callus is a yellow hyperkeratotic lesion on the sole, usually on the weightbearing areas. It is sometimes very difficult to distinguish from plantar warts. It has no black punctate areas, and the dermal ridges, or fingerprints, separate to surround the wart tumor.

***Skin tag.*** A small, skin-colored pedunculated lesion, skin tag usually consists of multiple lesions that are found on the neck in women past 30 years of age.

***Cutaneous horn.*** Cutaneous horn consists of a conical horny growth that is usually single and is found on the face and forehead in elderly individuals.

### Treatment

Warts continue to display one of the great paradoxes in clinical medicine. They are a proved viral infection, contagious, inoculable, and aggravated by irritation. They can, however, disappear within a remarkably short time, leaving no trace behind, even after being present for years. Most interesting of all, they can be "witched" away by suggestion within a few days, again leaving no trace of their existence. All methods of treatment must be attempted with the benign nature of these lesions in mind.

However, warts are more likely to recur if they are treated at the time of continued appearance of new warts, that is, the period of low resistance. The procedure will be more successful if carried out during a period of wart inactivity.

Destructive, scar-producing methods must not be used in such a way that irreversible changes less desirable than the wart are produced. A 10-year-old girl does not realize how she will despair of scars on her hands at 18, from warts removed at her pleading 8 years before.

Any physician treating warts should review Bunney's 1,800-patient, carefully followed trial of 11 therapeutic regimens. Simple new uncomplicated warts a few weeks old will respond favorably to many treatments. Also, most treatments can produce rapid disappearance of the wart, but often will achieve success only after weeks of therapy.

***Common wart.*** Salicylic acid (40%) plaster applied daily or every other day and then removed together with the macerated tissue beneath, will slowly clear most warts.

Salicyclic acid 16.7% with lactic acid 16.7% in flexible collodion (Duofilm) is often the easiest and certainly is satisfactory. It should be applied daily (Bunney).

Electrodesiccation under anesthesia with 2% xylocaine or other local anesthetic will successfully remove most warts. However, a significant recurrence rate must be expected. This procedure should be used with caution on weight-bearing areas on the sole because of scarring.

Solid carbon dioxide or liquid nitrogen applied directly to the lesions for half a minute or less is a commonly employed and successful method of therapy. One treatment, however, does not usually suffice, and second treatments should follow at less than 3 weeks. Three treatments are required on an average.

***Plantar wart.*** Salicyclic acid (40%) plaster is applied to the wart surface under a plastic waterproof occlusive tape and removed by the patient every night, together with the macerated tissue beneath. This then should be examined and friable tissue curetted away at 3-weekly intervals by the doctor.

Formaldehyde, commercial grade, 1 teaspoon in 1 pint of water in a dishpan used as a soak 10 minutes a day, may have to continue for up to 3 months. The dried wart will spontaneously fall off.

The salicyclic-lactic acid in collodion preparation used in common warts is useful in simple plantar warts as well, with an 81% cure in Bunney's trial. In mosaic warts, her successes fell to 40%, and other treatments were also undramatic.

Surgical excision often is unsatisfactory, leaving scars in which the wart reseeds itself.

***Flat wart.*** Benzoyl peroxide (10%) cream is applied twice daily, over a period of at least 2 to 3 weeks. Liquid nitrogen applied gingerly so as to avoid blister formation, but planned so as to repeat the procedure three or four times in 1 to 2 months, is our procedure.

***Digitate wart.*** The most satisfactory treatment consists of electrodesiccation under 2% xylocaine anesthesia, with curettage of the base, or liquid nitrogen therapy.

***Genital wart (verruca acuminata).*** Podophyllin, 20% to 25% in tincture of benzoin compound, is applied carefully to the lesion, but must be washed off by the patient 6 hours later. This is a very satisfactory method of therapy. Liquid nitrogen also is very useful here but will probably be required three or four times.

***Resistant warts.*** After therapy, there are still 10% to 20% warts, particularly plantar warts, still resistant. Hudson has described the careful use of bleomycin, also used in Japan for warts. Bunney describes Monson's use of 20% idoxuridine under occlusion in a cream base. She decries radical vigorous therapy as being no more rewarding. Greenberg describes careful dinitrochlorobenzene sensitization as a mode of therapy for these resistant cases.

### REFERENCES

Berman, A., and Winkelman, R. K.: Flat warts undergoing involution: histopathologic findings, Arch. Dermatol. **113**:1219, 1977.
**Mononuclear cell infiltration and areas of epidermal necrosis.**

Bunney, M. H., Nolan, M. W., and Williams, D. A.: An assessment of methods of treating viral warts by comparative treatment trials based on a standard design, Br. J. Dermatol. **94**:667, 1976.
**1,802 patients in this milestone study were treated with 11 regimens. Salicyclic-lactic acid in collodion came out best. Not much helped mosaic plantar warts.**

Chamberlain, M. J., Reynolds, A. L., and Yeoman, W. B.: Toxic effect of podophyllin application in pregnancy, Br. Med. J. **3**:391, 1972.
**Severe peripheral neuropathy and fetal death.**

Greenberg, J., Smith, T. L., and Katz, R. M.: Verrucae vulgaris rejection, Arch. Dermatol. **107**:580, 1973.
**Dinitrochlorobenzene sensitization may be a problem.**

Hudson, A. L.: Treatment of plantar warts with bleomycin, Arch. Dermatol. **112**:1179, 1976.
**100% over 6 months, at 0.1 to 1 mg. with expanded distance and a jet injector.**

Johansson, E.: Warts are more prevalent in patients with SLE, Br. Med. J. **1**:74, 1977.
**Rheumatoid factor may interfere with host-wart resistance.**

Matthews, R. S., and Shirodaria, P. V.: Study of regressing warts by immunofluorescence, Lancet **1**:689, 1973.
**IgG and perhaps IgA seem to be important in regression.**

Oriel, J. D.: Natural history of genital warts, Br. J. Venereol. Dis. **47**:1, 1971.
**332 patients, 191 men and 141 women, in a careful study.**

Pass, F.: Biology and current therapy, Minn. Med. **57**:844, 1974.
**A sophisticated overview ending in molecular biology.**

Perry, T. L., and Harman, L.: Warts in diseases with immune deficits, Cutis **13**:359, 1974.
**Luxuriant warts suggest immune deficiency.**

Pyrhonen, S., and Johannson, E.: Regression of warts. An immunologic study, Lancet **1**:592, 1975.
**Cure of warts is partly immunologic, with complement-fixing antibodies, but it can also be a nonimmune process.**

Rhatigan, R. H., and Saffos, R. O.: Condyloma acuminatum and squamous cell carcinoma of the vulva, South. Med. J. **70**:591, 1977.
**Three cases of vulvar cancer and condyloma, one with dysplasia.**

Sanders, B. B.: Warts, diagnosis and treatment, J.A.M.A. **235**:2859, 1976.
**A good balanced review of a problem for 1 in 10 individuals.**

Sutton, R., Jr.: Treatment of plantar warts with formaldehyde, Schoch Letter no. 26, October 1976.
**May have to be continued up to 3 months.**

Tagami, H., Takigawa, M., Ogino, A., et al.: Spontaneous regression of plane warts after inflammation. Clinical and histologic studies, Arch. Dermatol. **113**:1209, 1977.
**Similar process in all, despite varied therapeutic agents and spontaneous occurrence.**

Takigawa, M., Tagami, H., Watanabe, S., et al.: Recovery processes during regression of plane warts, Arch. Dermatol. **113**:1214, 1977.
**Two phases are apparent: degeneration and recovery.**

## ENTEROVIRUSES (PICORNAVIRUS)

As a group, the enteroviruses produce human diseases with a wide variety of cutaneous and other manifestations. The classification of these has been a striking advance in clinical medicine. The properties shared by these viruses that lead to grouping them together are their ability to proliferate in the gastrointestinal tract, their similar morphological structure, and their common pathogenic effect on tissue cultures.

They multiply in lymph nodes or lymphatic tissue, enter the bloodstream, and attain entry to one of the following target tissues: meninges, ganglion cells, striated muscle, or skin. They produce pharyngitis, cutaneous signs, myalgias, aseptic meningitis, and myocarditis. They are single-stranded RNA viruses, resistant to acid, bile, and some chlorination.

## Coxsackievirus infections

The discovery in 1947 of the coxsackievirus, named for the town of Coxsackie, New York, led to new techniques in virus propagation and study. These resulted in the definition of two groups of coxsackievirus, designated A and B, each associated with certain types of lesions.

***Diseases caused by group A viruses.*** Herpangina is chiefly a disease of the summer months, occurring in children under 10 years of age. The etiological agent may be one of several types of group A coxsackieviruses. It is associated with a sudden febrile onset, muscular pains, and headache, and there is a vesicular eruption of the palate, fauces, and pharynx. It does not extend onto the lips. The lesions, usually small, are vesicular on an erythematous base; they rupture and leave eroded areas.

Group A, *type 16 coxsackievirus* has been demonstrated to be the causative agent in a form of *hand-foot-and-mouth disease*. In this disease, described first in Toronto, children develop a triad of symptoms: (1) low-grade fever, (2) stomatitis or shallow ulcerations on buccal mucosa or tongue, and (3) vesicular erythematous eruption of the dorsa of the hands or feet, of the palms, soles, periungual area, and heels, or between fingers and toes. In approximately one fourth of those affected, this condition lasts a week or so, clearing without apparent sequelae. Throat swabs, rectal swabs, or vesicle fluid can be used to isolate the virus.

The lesions associated with type *A9* may resemble varicella. At least one epidemic has been described, however, in which there was a malar flush and maculopapular eruption of the thorax.

Other group A coxsackievirus infections have been shown to produce maculopapular eruptions, morbilliform (measles-like eruptions) (Fig. 15-11), and fine petechial cutaneous lesions in association with fever. It appears that the cutaneous lesions are more likely to affect young children, whereas adults may escape them.

***Diseases caused by group B viruses.*** Group B is responsible for minor respiratory illnesses and some accompanying vesicular and papular, erythematous, transient eruptions. The viruses affect muscles (Bornholm disease, or epidemic pleurodynia), central nervous system (aseptic meningitis), myocardium, and pericardium and produce febrile illnesses.

## Echovirus infections

Infections with the echoviruses follow six major disease patterns: (1) aseptic meningitis, (2) paralysis, (3) summer febrile illnesses, (4) diarrhea, (5) rashes, and (6) respiratory illness.

Those infections with a major manifestation of skin eruptions are macular and papular, resemble rubeola, and are often epidemic in form. The lesions tend to appear first on the face, spread to the chest, back, and extremities, involve the palms and soles, and then clear fairly rapidly, disappearing without pruritus or desquamation.

Aseptic meningitis caused by echoviruses is frequently associated with a cutaneous eruption, usually maculopapular or morbilliform.

Infection with *type 16 echovirus* can also cause a sore throat and palatal or tonsillar ulcerations.

Infection with *type 9 echovirus* has been very prevalent in recent years, with a rash seen chiefly in young preschool children. It is associated with aseptic meningitis and affects families. Initial nausea, vomiting, and fever is

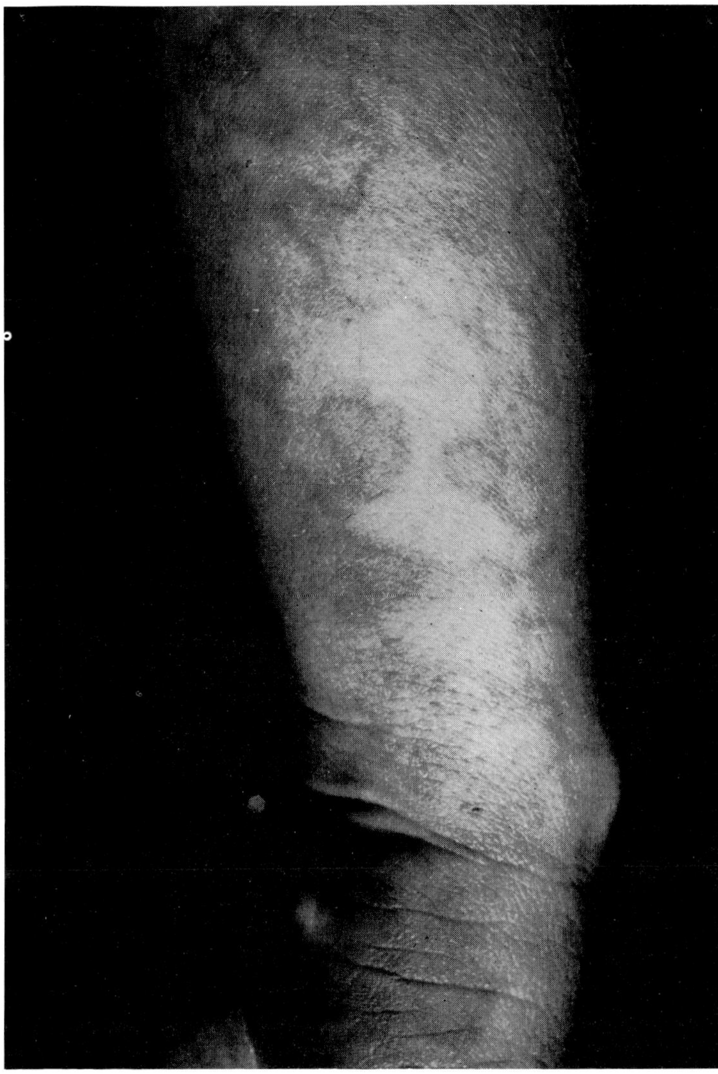

**Fig. 15-11.** Enterovirus dermatosis; morbilliform transient eruption.

followed by a lull, and then cutaneous involvement appears. It is macular or maculopapular, involving face, neck, and chest and then the extremities. Petechiae may be present. The palms and soles may be involved. Approximately one third of patients have buccal mucosal lesions identical to Koplik's spots.

*Boston exanthem* is, like other enterovirus infections, flulike in adults and erythematous to macular in children. It involves the face and thorax and may have buccal mucosal ulcers. Vesicles may occur on the hands and feet.

Echovirus exanthems should be suspected when a cutaneous eruption is maculopapular, occurs in summer, and is associated with similar symptoms and short incubation periods (less than a week) in other family members.

## Foot-and-mouth disease

The virus causing foot-and-mouth disease is of only low infectivity for man, but is found quite commonly in cattle and other domestic as well as wild animals. Very young children or elderly and debilitated individuals are most susceptible to the disease, which is contracted by drinking infected milk or from contact with infected cows.

In man, the cutaneous manifestations appear as large vesicular lesions on the lips and buccal membranes, between the fingers and toes, and on the fingers around the nails. The lesions ulcerate and easily become secondarily infected.

The disease is self-limited.

## Cat-scratch disease

Cat-scratch disease is a relatively common, benign infection, the chief manifestation of which is regional lymphadenopathy.

The etiological agent is presumed to be a virus that enters the skin through an abrasion. This may or may not be a scratch from a kitten, since only 80% of affected patients give this history. The incubation period is up to 2 weeks, which is followed by a local nonspecific inflammation or papule that may ulcerate. The lymph nodes then enlarge, to subside in 4 to 6 weeks. Usually a fever and some poorly defined systemic symptoms are present. A skin test with an antigen specific for the disorder should give positive results in almost 100% of the cases.

There is no specific treatment. Antibiotics are of doubtful help and glucocorticoids do not appear to be justified.

### REFERENCES

Carithers, H. A., Carithers, C. M., and Edwards, R. O., Jr.: Cat-scratch disease: its natural history, J.A.M.A. **207**:312, Jan. 1969.
**152 patients.**

Deseda-Tous, J., Byatt, P. H., and Cherry, J. D.: Vesicular lesions in adults due to echovirus II infections, Arch. Dermatol. **113**:1705, 1977.
**Clinically suspected of being herpes simplex.**

Froeschle, J. E., Nahmias, A. J., Feorino, P. M., et al.: Hand, foot, and mouth disease (coxsackievirus A16) in Atlanta, Am. J. Dis. Child. **114**:278, 1967.
**Clinical virologic-epidemiologic features in 30 patients.**

## CHAPTER 16

# Infestations

Certain parasites puncture the skin for the purpose of sucking blood, injecting venom, or laying their eggs. This process is accomplished by the use of substances foreign to the victim, who may develop an allergic sensitivity to the foreign substance. Thus the presence of certain parasites may be associated with pruritus, urticaria, or systemic reactions, depending on the degree and type of allergic sensitivity. Some insects may produce a toxic reaction. Bagnall and Rook discuss the investigation of the patient suspected of having arthropod mites, the immune response, and its consequences in a valuable approach to this common, but plaguing subject.

The individual bite of a parasite on cutaneous surfaces is ordinarily a matter of little significance to the individual. Cutaneous reactions to parasites do, however, attain importance if (1) they cause symptoms that interfere with the patient's normal activities (for example, the effects of a spider bite), (2) they signify the presence of a contagious skin disease (such as scabies), or (3) if the parasite involved is able to transmit other diseases (for example, ticks transmit Rocky Mountain spotted fever).

Although complications and infections are more prevalent in a nonhygienic environment, they are also frequently seen among scrupulously clean individuals. Patterns of cutaneous involvement by specific parasites may be greatly altered so as to require careful observation in persons who wash frequently. For example, the classical interdigital scabies lesions may not be seen in a compulsive hand washer.

Finally, when the diagnosis of an infestation is made in a clean individual or in the family of a conscientious housewife, the physician must be prepared for an unbelieving or even hostile patient, unless he can present the circumstances diplomatically but without any doubt as to the cause and treatment of the disorder.

## DERMATOSES CAUSED BY MITES AND TICKS (ORDER ACARINA)

### Scabies (Sarcoptes scabiei)

Scabies, an intensely pruritic infestation, has a characteristic history of spread from other family members, bed partners, or intimate contacts, or between schoolchildren. Infestation with mites from cats, dogs and other small animals also occurs. These are ordinarily short lived with loss of animal contact.

#### *Natural course*

The initial infection with *Sarcoptes scabiei* may produce no immediate symptoms. It is only after about a month that the pruritus and discomfort appear to produce the characteristic complaints. On a second attack, however, the symptoms may begin within a day or so of contracting the infestation.

The primary lesion is the mite's burrow, which is a minute, linear, gray-brown threadlike lesion a few millimeters in length. This is usually seen only with difficulty. The more apparent lesions, however, are the punctate discrete excoriations secondary to the pruritus. There are also papules and vesicles present. Urticarial wheals are less common, and infections of the traumatized skin are frequent in the unclean individual (Plate 32).

The infestation and the lesions are most apparent in certain areas. These are the interfinger webs (Fig. 16-1), flexures of the wrist, anterior axillary folds, the penis, and the buttocks. In the adult woman the nipples and areolae are particularly susceptible. Lesions do not ordinarily extend to the face.

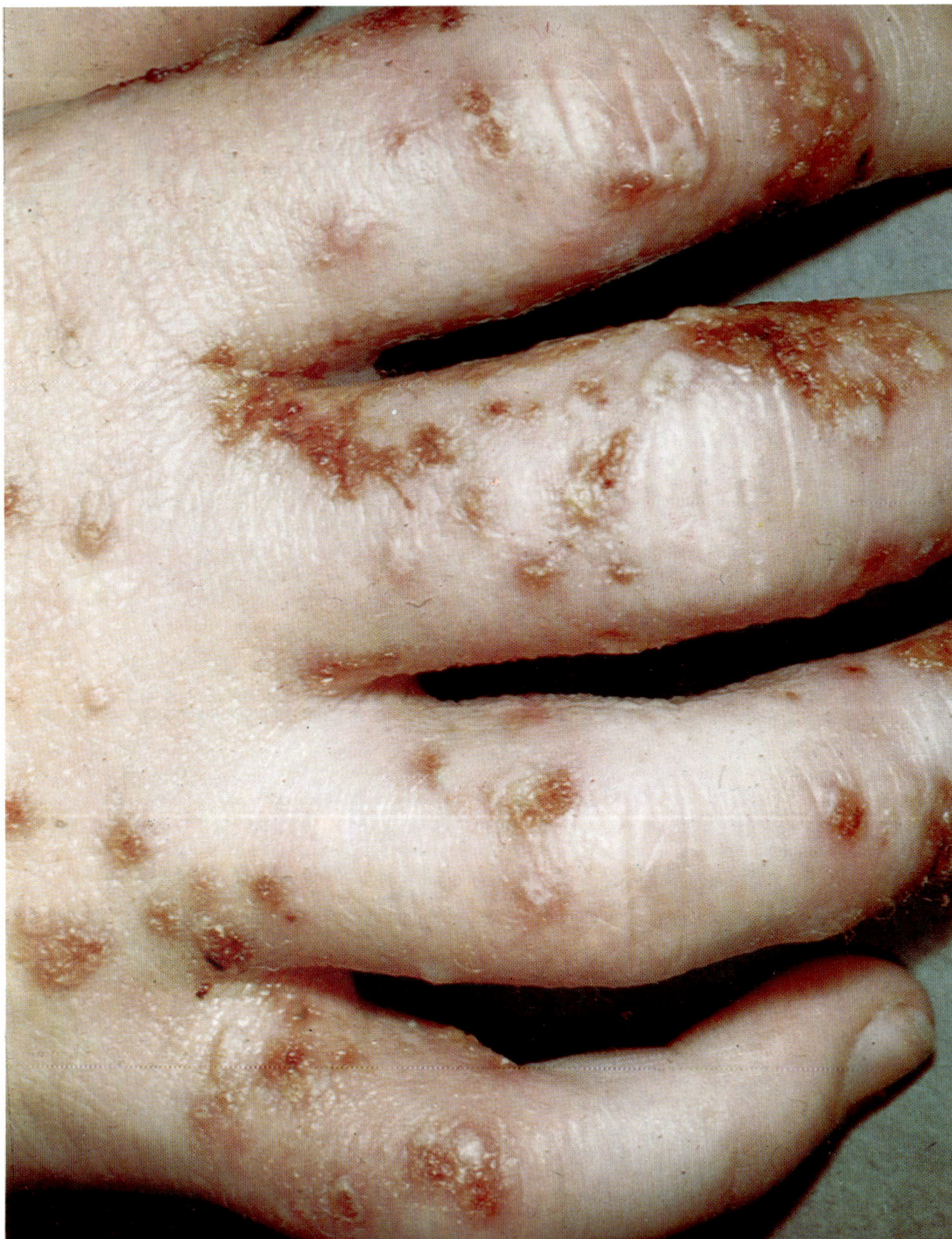

**Plate 32**

Scabies infestation with secondary impetiginization.

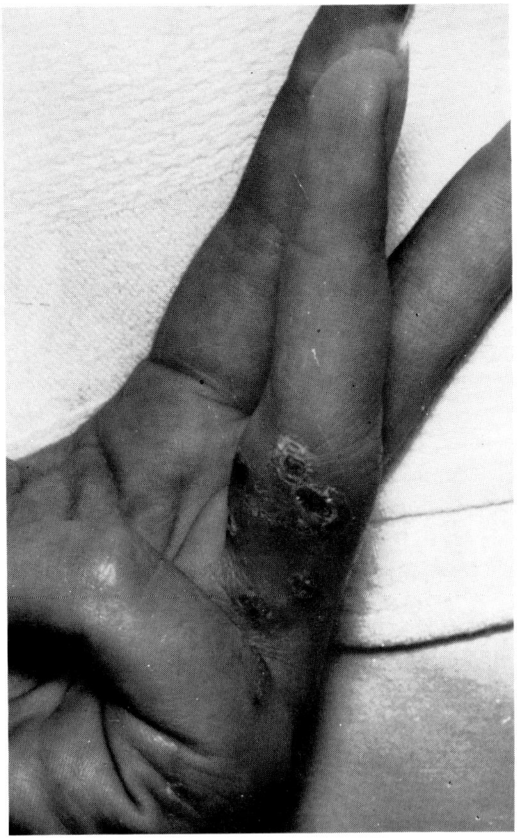

**Fig. 16-1.** Scabies. A characteristic location, often secondarily infected.

The intense pruritus is at first intermittent and then consistent, with peaks at night after retiring. Persistent itching nodules develop in 5% to 10% of cases, children included, even after adequate treatment. Commonest sites in Konstantinov's series were axilla 50%, scrotum, abdomen, chest, groin, and penis. They may take more than 3 months to resolve.

Infestation from animal mites produces a rather different eruption. It may be papular or vesicular and pruritic and is usually localized to waist, arms, and torso. Burrows characteristic of human scabies are not present.

*Norwegian scabies* identifies cases of clinical scabies with immense numbers of mites and often a reduced inflammatory reaction in the host. These individuals serve as significant reservoirs of mites to the surrounding community, as anyone who has looked after them in a hospital is aware. Espy records it in renal transplant patients.

***Pertinent information***

Bagnall and Rook review the rise and fall in scabies infestation incidence in humans over 25 years and the causes. Cases of Norwegian scabies, nonimmune hosts, crowded conditions, some sexual transmission, and physician inexperience are important.

In his interesting tale of the life cycle and activities of the scabies mite (Fig. 16-2), Mellanby follows the female mite, which moves on the skin surface, traveling as far as 1 inch per minute. It takes her approximately 1 hour to burrow into the stratum corneum at the site she selects. She seldom leaves that site. She burrows along the horny outer layer at the rate of 1 mm. or more a day, laying eggs as she goes. The eggs take 3 to 4 days to hatch, and the larvae then leave the burrow. It is probably a minimum of 3 weeks, and usually more, before the second generation of adult mites appears. The adult mites are passed from one person to another by skin contact, not by clothing or sheets. Not all persons are equally susceptible to scabies, and on occasion one individual in a family will remain unaffected, although all about him are scratching furiously.

In doubtful cases one can establish the diagnosis by inserting the point of a needle gently along a burrow to the end. Mellanby describes the burrow as a raised, whitish oval with dark pigmentation at its front. Diagnosis is confirmed if the mite, with gray-white body 0.33 to 0.5 mm. in diameter, is seen at the point of the needle on removal. According to Hoke and Muller, the incidence of positive diagnosis is increased when immersion oil is applied to the unexcoriated papule, or burrow, which is then scraped or sliced with a scalpel and examined in the oil on a slide under a cover slip. In cases of infestation by animal mites, the parasite is demonstrated by scrapings or brushings from the infested animal (Hewitt).

The mean for numbers of parasites in cases of human scabies is very small, between 11 and 12 per case. In nearly 900 patients studied

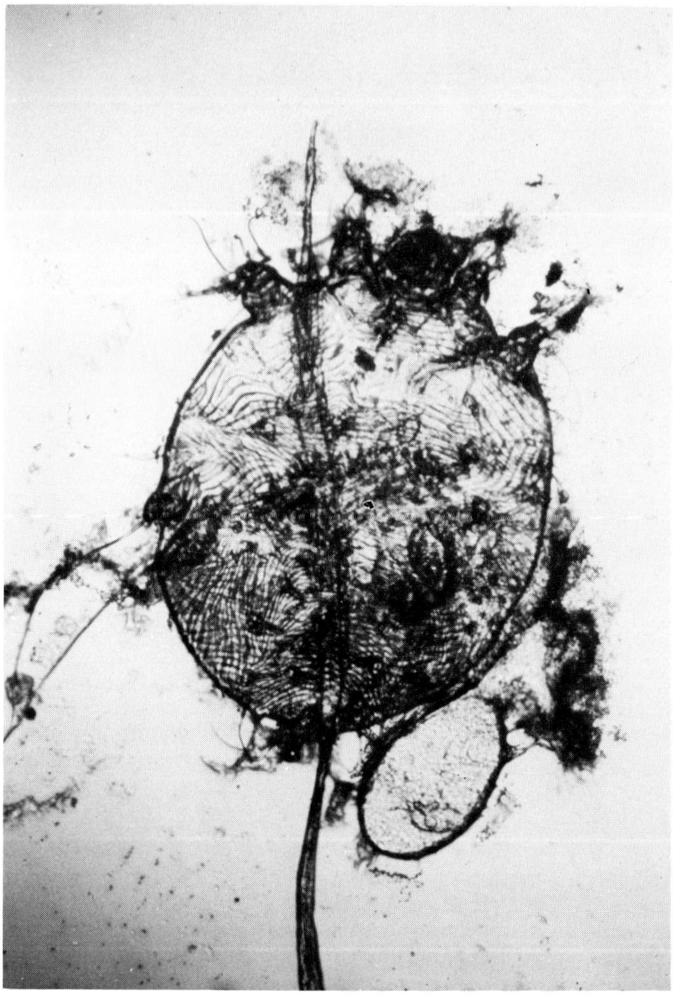

**Fig. 16-2.** Scabies mite, as seen clinically when removed from its burrow.

by Mellanby, 60% of mites were found on the hands and wrists, 11% on extensor aspects of elbows, and 9% on genitals and feet. The mite stays on the skin because of the warmth. If it strays to clothing or blankets, its behavior is such that it will find its way back to the skin.

### *Differential diagnosis*

***Generalized pruritus.*** Multiple excoriations with little in the way of primary lesions can be seen in generalized pruritus, a disorder resembling scabies. The characteristic scabies distribution is not present, and careful inspection reveals no burrows or mites.

***Urticaria.*** Transient migratory wheals without papules or excoriations will reveal the diagnosis.

***Pediculosis, flea bites, and other bites.*** The characteristic bites of insects, with resultant discrete erythematous papules and central puncta, separate these lesions from scabies.

### *Treatment*

The most consistently satisfactory therapy for killing the mite is the use of 20% to 25% benzyl benzoate emulsion, applied, after a bath and subsequent drying of skin, over the entire cutaneous surface from the neck downward. It is left on for 48 hours and then washed off with less time allowed for infants and young children. After 2 days with no treatment, the procedure is repeated. This solution is irritating to the average skin and will not quickly reduce the pruritus. Patients should be made aware that they are likely to be uncomfortable for some weeks. After therapy is completed, application of a bland ointment may give some relief.

All potential cases in the family must be treated simultaneously.

Gamma benzene hexachloride in a vanishing cream base (Kwell, Kwellada) may be applied as just described for benzyl benzoate. However, serious neurotoxicity is reported from this compound in children. Younger children are in general more severely affected. It should not be applied after a hot bath, or for longer than necessary, and not at all in infants or pregnant women. See Solomon.

Crotamiton (Eurax, *N*-ethyl-*o*-crotonotoluide) is a suitable antiscabies preparation in cream form and is less irritating than benzyl benzoate emulsion. Application is as described for the other scabicides.

Sulfur ointment (10% precipitated sulfur in petrolatum or in a vanishing cream base) is an old but reliable remedy. It is applied twice, as with benzyl benzoate.

Ten-percent thiabendazole is used in Mexico and South America. Its toxicity has not been well evaluated. It is rapidly effective.

## Infestations with other mites

***Cheyletiella.*** One species, formerly a rabbit parasite, also occurs transiently in other animals and in man. Some members of this family live on dogs and cats. They produce an eruption of pruritic papules on the arms and trunk that can be confused with dermatitis herpetiformis. The mite has been identified in house dust. The parasite can be classed with scabies or mange mites (Hewitt).

***Chigger (Trombicula) infestation.*** Several species of reddish mites are found throughout the world. They are common in the southern part of the United States, but extend at least to the Canadian border. They are found on grass and bushes, chiefly blackberry bushes. The mite attaches itself to the legs or thighs and punctures the skin to obtain blood. The dermatitis consists of papules with surrounding urticaria, excoriations, and subsequent pustules. There may be pronounced erythema.

***Fowl mite (Dermanyssus) infestation.*** Mites infesting the feathers of birds may attack human beings, particularly children, producing pruritic papules, wheals, and vesicles that most commonly are found in the inguinal area, around the nipples and areolae, and on the face. Birds so infested may be chickens, canaries, pigeons, starlings, and such.

***Grain itch mite (Tyroglyphus) infestation.*** Harvesters, packers, and other person in contact with straw, wheat, oats, and the like may be attacked by the grain itch mite, which lives on the insects that infest grains and vegetation. The dermatitis so produced is often generalized and actively pruritic. It is finely vesicular and urticalial and may be pustular. Fine petechial hemorrhages may accompany the eruption.

### *Treatment*

Prevention of infestation by mites lies in disinfestation of the known sources. For elimination of grain itch mites, 25% benzyl benzoate emulsion, as used in scabies, is satisfactory, although the pruritus will remain for a time, subsiding slowly if further irritation is avoided. Gamma benzene hexachloride 1% (Kwell or Kwellada cream or lotion) can be used with precautions re toxicity. See Solomon.

## Infestation with ticks (Dermacentor, Ornithodoros)

Ticks are parasites that feed on the blood of man, animals, birds, and sometimes reptiles (Fig. 16-3). For man they have significance because they carry pathogenic bacteria, viruses, and rickettsiae; they can cause paralysis by injection of a salivary toxin; and they produce *firm, discrete, intensely pruritic nodules* at the site of their attachment to the skin. They may also cause urticaria or persistent localized erythema. Microscopically, tick bites may show an eosinophilic granuloma appearing at the site.

In North America the hard-bodied wood tick *Dermacentor andersoni* is found in wooded areas on grass and brushes, from which it attaches itself to passing animals and

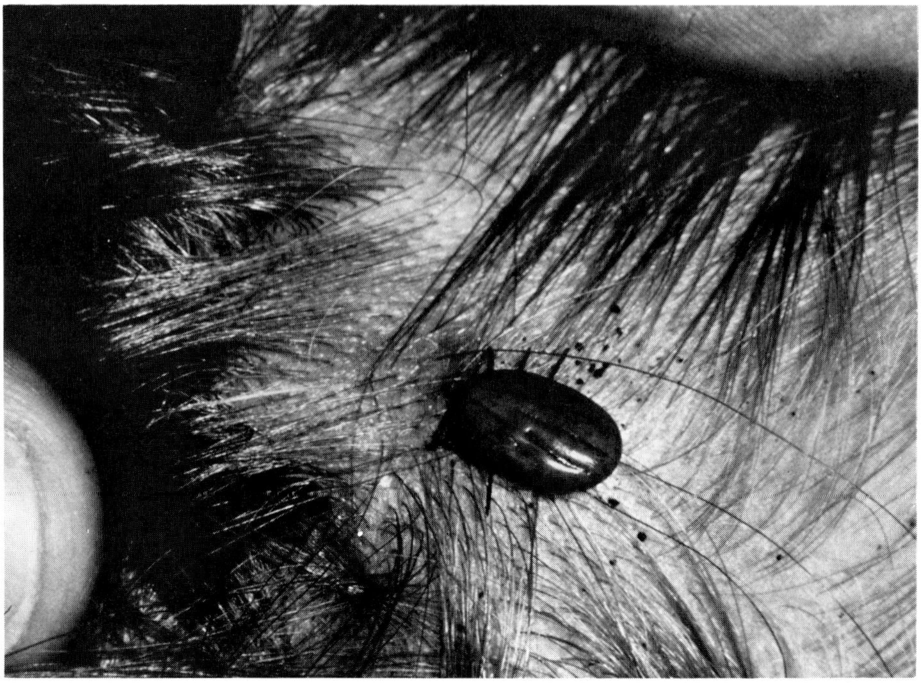

**Fig. 16-3.** Blood-filled tick.

people. It carries *Rocky Mountain spotted fever* and *Q fever* in the western United States and Canada. A soft-bodied tick, *Ornithodoros*, carries the spirochete causing *relapsing fever* in the central and western United States and western Canada. This tick-borne disease is associated with a 24-hour macular eruption over the trunk and proximal parts of the extremities. It has recurrent febrile episodes.

### *Treatment*

Removal of ticks must be carefully accomplished to ensure that the head and mouthparts are removed as well. Heat applied to the body of the tick usually causes it to withdraw its head from embedment in the skin.

Repellants applied to the skin provide little protection from ticks.

#### REFERENCES


Anolik, M. A.: Scabies simulating Darier's disease in an immunosuppressed host, Arch. Dermatol. **112**:73-74, 1976.

**Very atypical: two biopsies and scraping to diagnose.**

Bagnall, B., and Rook, H.: Arthropods and the skin. In Rook, A., editor: Recent advances in dermatology, No. 4, Edinburgh, 1977, Churchill Livingston.

**A thorough overview of the subject including investigation of scabies, demodicidosis, pediculosis, fleas, bees, wasps, ants, moths, thrips, butterflies, and caterpillars.**

Espy, P. D., and Jolly, H. W.: Norwegian scabies occurrence in a patient undergoing immunosuppression, Arch. Dermatol. **112**:193, 1976.

**After kidney transplant.**

Habler, W. R.: Epidemic Norwegian scabies, Arch. Dermatol. **112**:179-181, 1976.

**The clinical picture and its management.**

Hernández-Pérez, E.: Topically applied thiabendazole in the treatment of scabies, Arch. Dermatol. **112**:1400, 1976.

**10% solution in 40 patients; rapidly effective.**

Hewitt, M., Barrow, G. I., Miller, D. C., et al.: Mites in personal environment and their role in skin disorders, Br. J. Dermatol. **89**:401, 1973.

**A rogues' gallery: any of nine mite varieties in 50% of 253 patients investigated.**

Hoke, A. W.: Scabies scraping, Arch. Dermatol. **108**:424, 1973.

**Immersion oil and a slice.**

Konstantinov, D., and Stanoeva, L.: Persistent scabious nodules, Dermatologica **147**:321, 1973.

**One to 15 present on each patient, mostly on axilla or scrotum.**

Mellanby, K.: Scabies, ed. 2, Hampton, Middlesex, Eng., 1972, E. W. Classey, Ltd.
**The mite's innermost habits and secrets.**

Muller, G., Jacobs, P. H., and Moore, N. E.: Scraping for human scabies, Arch. Dermatol. **107**:70, 1973.
**Oil and scraping.**

Orkin, M., and Maibach, H. I.: Scabies and pediculosis, Philadelphia, 1977, J. B. Lippincott Co.
**Pitfalls to successful therapy enumerated.**

Solomon, L. M.: Gamma benzene hexachloride toxicity: a review, Arch. Dermatol. **113**:353, 1977.
**Important: To be used with extreme caution, if at all, on infants, pregnant women, and widely damaged skin.**

## DERMATOSES CAUSED BY SPIDERS (ORDER ARANEIDA)

Virtually all dangerous spider bites on the North American continent are caused by two kinds of spiders, the black widow *(Latrodectus mactans)* and the brown recluse *(Loxosceles reclusa)*. A few other species and genera have been reported to bite man but, although the bites are painful, they are harmless and probably amount to less than 1% of all significant cases of spider bite on this continent. The black widow is found almost universally throughout the United States and in southern Canada.

The female black widow is recognized by a red or orange marking on its underside. It lives in old lumber, unused sheds, and outdoor privies, where most reported bites occur. It may be found inside houses, in attics, closets, rolled up clothing, or drawers. It avoids light and bites only in defense; the bite is not often apparent immediately.

The black widow bite results from injection of venom through a clawlike appendage. The area becomes swollen, painful, and erythematous. Dizziness, weakness, and abdominal pains ensue. A minimal local necrosis may produce a small ulcer at the site of the bite. The venom is neurotropic and causes delirium, paralysis, convulsions, and, particularly if a large amount of a potent venom has been absorbed, death.

The brown recluse is found east of the Rocky Mountains in the United States and is apparently enlarging its territory. This spider is small, fawn to dark brown, and has a light, fiddle-shaped mark on its head. This spider hides in houses, in drawers and closets. It bites people who are dressing in a dark area or while they are sleeping.

After 2 to 8 hours the brown recluse spider bite may cause intense pain, nausea, arthralgia, local tissue necrosis, and bullae that eventually heal with scarring. Grafting may be necessary.

A recent report by Berger describes two cases of brown recluse spider bites that produced mild effects only. This changes our concepts of the range of reactions that may be produced by the bite of this small, unobtrusive spider.

### *Treatment*

Berger has questioned the value of glucocorticoids in treatment of the brown recluse spider bite, inasmuch as rabbits given spider venom showed no benefit from prednisone therapy. This needs to be reviewed and further therapeutic measures must be evaluated as well.

***Black widow.*** Specific treatment consists of antivenom given parenterally for neutralization of the toxin. It should be used for young children and debilitated or elderly individuals. Local treatment appears to be of little value.

Treatment of muscle spasm and hypotension includes the intravenous administration of 10% calcium gluconate. Secondary infection is sometimes present.

***Brown recluse.*** Prompt administration of oral parenteral glucocorticoids in more than average doses should be maintained for 8 to 10 days. The use of heparin, edetate, and epsilon-amniocaproic acid is being investigated.

#### REFERENCES

Berger, R. S.: The unremarkable brown recluse spider bite, J.A.M.A. **225**:1109, 1973.
**Some are unremarkable.**

Berger, R. S.: A critical look at therapy for the brown recluse spider, Arch. Dermatol. **107**:288, 1973.
**Perhaps the severity is less than formerly believed.**

Harves, A. D., and Millikan, L. E.: Current concepts of therapy and pathophysiology of arthropod bites and stings, Int. J. Dermatol. **14**(8):543-562; **14**(9):621-634, 1975.
**The best summary now available on this subject.**

## DERMATOSES CAUSED BY SCORPIONS (ORDER SCORPIONIDA)

Scorpions, which are limited to the southern United States and Mexico on this continent, are nocturnal and photophobic. They sting by means of a hooked caudal stinger that discharges venom. They attack when brushed against or stepped on, and some species are more venomous than others. These are usually found in the southwest United States. Symptoms include local pain, erythema, induration, and a severe burning. Muscle twitching and spasm, vomiting, convulsions, and mental disturbances may also occur. In most cases, symptoms subside in a few hours, but fatal cases have been reported in infants and debilitated adults.

### *Treatment*

Treatment includes delaying absorption of the venom by applying tourniquets for 10 to 15 minutes and submerging the extremity in cold water. Suction of larger wounds will help to extract venom. Ice packs will be of benefit if the foregoing measures cannot be carried out. Specific antivenin, if available, should be given in severe cases.

Supportive therapy to minimize shock and dehydration is indicated.

## INFESTATION WITH FLEAS (ORDER SIPHONAPTERA)

The flea is a wingless insect with a siphon tube and mouthparts adapted to sucking blood. Because of its ability to infest animals and humans, it is able to complete the life cycle of certain organisms, and it serves as a transmitter of bacterial, rickettsial, and parasitic diseases, as well as producing an irritating dermatitis as a result of its bites. Transmission of *plague* and of *rickettsial murine typhus* is probably achieved by rodent fleas, although infected human fleas have been found on persons dying of the plague.

Although human fleas *(Pulex irritans)* are universal in distribution, much of the problem of flea control arises from dog, cat, bird, or other domestic animal fleas. Any of these insects may attack man. The range of flea population found on dogs was 187 to 500 (Kalkofen).

Flea bites are usually innocuous, but in large enough numbers or in a sensitive individual they can produce a clinical problem. The usual reaction to a flea bite is a small wheal with a hemorrhagic punctum. In susceptible persons a flea bite produces larger wheals and urticarial lesions, an intensely pruritic papular lesion, a bulla (Fig. 16-1), or even a small necrotic ulcer. The bites are characteristically grouped in patterns of three.

Certain characteristics of the flea account for the clinical facts of the disease. The eggs ordinarily develop on the ground or floor. The larva goes through three stages and, depending on environmental conditions, may take up to a year to reach the adult stage. Even after reaching this stage, a flea can survive for many months without food, thus explaining the persistence of fleas in areas such as unused basements or attics.

The adult flea is attracted by moving objects and leaps to attain them. This often places it on an ankle or lower leg, rarely higher. It then penetrates the skin, feeds, and crawls to a higher location until stopped by a belt or other area constricted by clothing.

The distribution of flea bites includes a concentration around the ankles, legs, and waist, with scattered lesions elsewhere.

### *Treatment*

Environmental control of fleas in floors or other areas is achieved by use of solutions such as chlordane 1%, dimpylate (Diazinon) 1%, lindane 1%, malathion 3%, methoxychlor 5%, ronnel 1%, or trichlorfon 1% in kerosene fuel oil. Dogs and cats may be dusted with malathion 4% powder, rotenone 1% dust, or methoxychlor 10%. One of the above powders, dusted on infested areas such as dog and cat living quarters, upholstered furniture, room corners, basements, and attics, is usually sufficient to eliminate these insects quickly. The procedure should be repeated after a 2-week interval in order to eliminate newly hatching fleas. The animals should also be regularly dusted, although cats must be prevented from licking or eating the powder.

Deet and Off are effective commercial flea repellants.

An antipruritic lotion, such as calamine, can be applied to the affected areas on the skin for immediate relief of pruritus. The following is more effective:

| | |
|---|---|
| Menthol | 0.5% |
| Phenol | 0.5% |
| Hydrocortisone | 1.0% |
| Unibase | q.s. ad 30 Gm. |

## DERMATITIS CAUSED BY BEETLES (ORDER COLEOPTERA)

Vesicant, or blister, beetles produce irritation and blistering if they are crushed or damaged while on the skin surface. This is achieved by release of a toxic principle in the insect's body fluids, not by biting.

## DERMATITIS CAUSED BY CATERPILLARS (ORDER LEPIDOPTERA)

Caterpillars of more than 50 different species are equipped with spines having on or in them a venom capable of producing a dermatitis on human skin. More or less severe reactions result, both locally and systemically, depending on the species and the amount of venom received by the victims.

These caterpillars are universally distributed, one or another species being present in most areas of the world. In the United States and Canada the most common form of caterpillar dermatitis is produced by the tussock moth and puss caterpillar, flannel moths, or silkworm moths.

The venom is biologically very active, showing histamine-release properties, anticoagulants, fibrinolysis, plasminogen activation.

Contact with the venom occurs from contact with the insect or its nest, or by windblown hairs. The venom produces a stinging sensation, followed by swelling and erythema of the part. Papular lesions or urticaria may develop at the site and elsewhere. If toxin contacts the conjunctiva, very painful persistent nodules are formed.

## REACTIONS TO STINGING INSECTS (ORDER HYMENOPTERA)

The sting of the bee, wasp, hornet, yellow jacket, or ant results from a puncture of the skin by the insect's sharp stinging apparatus and the injection of a chemically complex venom.

The usual sequel of the sting is the familiar one of temporary pain, local inflammation, and fairly rapid subsidence. However, some individuals even after a first sting, may show a systemic reaction. Such people often have a history of drug sensitivity or a familial history of allergy.

The allergic reaction may be of the *immediate* anaphylactic type, varying from mild to severe, or *delayed*, occurring from 1 to 4 days after the sting and consisting of urticaria, purpura, and serum sickness type of allergic manifestations. Most dangerous or fatal reactions are in older adults, from a sting on the face, head, or neck of an atopic individual, and occur within a few minutes of receiving the sting. They consist of tachycardia, hyperpnea, chest tightness, dizziness, pallor, nausea and vomiting, weakness, sweating, and unconsciousness. In the majority of cases the reactions are IgE mediated, and atopic patients are more often affected than nonatopic patients.

Huang reports that fluorescein-tagged antibodies to bee venom have been demonstrated in the internal organs of beesting victims. The venom has been demonstrated to contain a variety of antigens, so that desensitization procedures may not protect against all types of stings.

The honeybee and some wasps leave part of the sting and the poison sacs in the wound, which intermittently discharge more venom and penetrate farther.

### *Treatment*

The stinging apparatus should be carefully removed if it is seen to have been left in the wound.

Urticarial and mild immediate systemic reactions may be treated by antihistaminics orally or parenterally. Allergic patients stung by these insects should be treated as an emergency, since the reaction may be sudden (within minutes) and overwhelming. Severe immediate reactions should be treated as any severe shock. Epinephrine may be indicated to counter the effects of histamine already liberated. It is given hypodermically, but in severe cases may be given slowly intravenously, 0.3 to 0.5 ml. of 1:1,000 solution.

Calcium gluconate, 10 ml. of 10% solution, can be given intravenously for immediate effect. Oral or, if necessary, parenteral glucocorticoids may be used to prevent further histamine release.

Oral antihistaminics should be started at this point and maintained for some 3 days.

A generalized reaction, urticarial or otherwise, is indication for desensitization with polyvalent insect extracts.* Desensitization is a prolonged procedure, to be carried out over a period of 3 years, and results are conflicting.

Multiple bites producing localized rather than systemic allergic reactions should be treated with local glucocorticoid ointments applied every 2 hours. If this does not alleviate the symptoms of pruritus and discomfort, oral corticosteroids in a dosage equivalent to 5 mg. of prednisone three times daily may also be given temporarily.

*Available from Omega Laboratories, Town of Mount Royal, Quebec; Bencard Allergy Unit, Weston, Ontario; and Hollister-Stier Laboratory, Spokane, Washington.

#### REFERENCES

Barnard, J. H.: Studies of 400 Hymenoptera sting deaths in the U.S., J. Allergy Clin. Immunol. **52**:259, 1973.
**70% attributable to massive obstructive edema.**

Hewitt, M., Walton, G. S., and Waterhouse, M.: Pet animal infestations and human skin lesions, Br. J. Dermatol. **85**:215, 1971.
**A most useful article concerning flea bite.**

Huang, I.: Fluorescent antibody studies in three patients dying from honeybee sting, J. Allergy **47**:198, 1971.
**May be valuable procedure.**

Kalkofen, U. P., and Greenberg, J.: Public health implications of *Pulex irritans* infestations of dogs, J. Am. Vet. Med. Assoc. **165**:903, 1974.
**Repayment for man's best friend: 80% of fleas on dogs are the human variety.**

Smith, K. G. V.: Lepidoptera in insects and other arthropods of medical importance, London, 1973, British Museum (Natural History), p. 405.
**An excellent survey of many different caterpillars.**

## LESIONS CAUSED BY MOSQUITOES AND FLIES (ORDER DIPTERA)

### Effects of mosquito bites

Mosquitoes are well known for their role in transmitting the viral diseases *yellow fever*, *dengue fever*, and *encephalitis* and the parasitic diseases *malaria* and *filariasis*. They also frequently produce an irritating dermatitis.

Mosquitoes are attracted by lights, dark clothing, and the presence of warmblooded creatures. They zero in on human targets, as a reaction to olfactory and thermal stimuli. They have been shown to light on a warm, wet sack in preference to a warm, dry sack or a cold, wet sack.* Movement interests them, and an increase in carbon dioxide concentration in their environment excites them. There is a distinct difference in day-flying mosquitoes, which go directly to their target, feed, and leave, and nightflying mosquitoes. The latter, as any victim knows, approach in ever-decreasing circles over the most attractive area to light and feed. Except for a few species, the female is the bloodsucker, requiring blood containing epinephrine or serotonin in order to ovulate.

The ordinary mosquito bite produces local irritation and an erythematous papule of only transient discomfort. Large numbers of bites are more significant, and pruritus in the patient with multiple lesions will be relieved by the topical therapy outlined below.

At times, persons will show a hypersensitive reaction to mosquito bites, with production of urticaria or even symptoms of serum sickness, presumably caused by foreign protein material.

Lesions are produced by the mosquito's penetration of the skin and the droplets of mosquito saliva introduced prior to removal of blood. These lesions are commonly on the exposed areas of hands, arms, face, neck, and legs.

*Personal communication: R. H. Wright, former Head, Olfactory Responses Investigation Unit, British Columbia Research Council.

*Treatment*

Prophylactic therapy with commercially available insect repellents is useful for a short time. When applied to the exposed skin, they are diluted by perspiration after 1 to 2 hours and become less effective and must be reapplied frequently. These compounds include indalone, dimethylphthalate, Rutgers 612, and *N,N-diethyl-meta-toluamide* (Deet, Off) for all-purpose use. The preparation should contain more than 20% of the chemical.

Itching from multiple lesions is relieved by topical glucocorticoid ointments to which 0.5% menthol and phenol have been added. A standard shake lotion is preferred by many dermatologists, as follows:

| | |
|---|---|
| Menthol | 0.5% |
| Phenol | 0.5% |
| Zinc oxide | 15 Gm. |
| Talc | 15 Gm. |
| Glycerine | 10 ml. |
| Alcohol | 40 ml. |
| Water | 40 ml. |

Apply with fingers or a soft brush.

The preparation should be applied every 1 to 2 hours.

Serum sickness or systemic reactions require systemic antihistaminics and oral or parenteral glucocorticoids.

## Lesions caused by biting flies

On the North American continent there are innumerable biting flies (chiefly of three families: the blackflies, *Simuliidae;* the horseflies, deerflies, and gadflies, *Tabanidae;* and the dog fly or stable fly, *Muscidae).* Some of these are bloodsucking insects, but in general not so many are carriers of significant disease as in other parts of the world. Most of them are day or dusk feeders, attacking in swarms on the exposed parts of the face, neck, and arms.

The lesions are ordinarily painful and remain irritating and pruritic for some days. Urticaria may be associated, presumably as a reaction to the protein-containing salivary gland secretion deposited in the wound. The blackfly and horsefly can produce a painful, slow-healing wound.

Diseases transmitted by these flies include *tularemia* in the central and western United States.

*Treatment*

Avoidance of these bites may be achieved to some extent by adequate protection and proper clothing. Insect repellants containing more than 20% *N,N*-diethyl-*meta*-toluamide (Deet, Off) are satisfactory for short intervals. This chemical can be applied to skin and to clothing.

Local wounds can be relieved and secondary bacterial infection reduced by topical drying preparations such as described in the previous section for mosquito bites.

## Diseases caused by nonbiting flies

Nonbiting flies, including the common housefly, have habits of feeding at open wounds, exudates, and chronic ulcers, as well as ingesting human food, feces, and infected and decaying organic material, and thus they transfer common bacteria to open and traumatized areas. They also produce *myiasis,* or invasion of tissue, in their larval stages.

Only a few varieties on this continent will produce larvae that are invasive to human tissues. The screwworm fly, found in central and southern parts of the United States, will hatch larvae on injured skin that produce deep, infected, purulent wounds. Flesh flies will deposit larvae on nasal and conjunctival secretions or the diaper area of infants, with resulting swellings and local reactions when the larvae invade the cutaneous tissues.

*Treatment*

Cleanliness, protection, and prevention are the important aspects of treatment in these parasitic diseases.

### REFERENCES

Bagnall, B., and Rook, A.: Arthropods and the skin. In Rook, A., editor: Recent advances in dermatology, ed. 4, London, 1977, Churchill Livingstone, pp. 59-90.
**A comprehensive review of this subject.**

Maibach, H. I., Khan, A. A., and Akers, W.: Use of insect repellants for maximum efficacy, Arch. Dermatol. **109**:32, 1974.
**A perceptive treatise concerning the many problems surrounding the development of a successful all-purpose insect repellent.**

## INFESTATION WITH BEDBUGS (FAMILY CIMICIDAE)

Only two species of bedbugs are of dermatological importance because they invade human habitations—*Cimex lectularius* and *Cimex hemipterus*. These bloodsucking insects feed preferably on man, although they will also attack other mammals. They are nocturnal in their habits and leave their daytime hiding places in cracks and crevices to obtain blood meals at night. The adults require from 10 to 15 minutes after puncturing the skin to gorge themselves and may not disturb the victim. The bites are arranged in a straight line and consist of erythematous papules with a central punctum. The buttocks, back, and extremities are most often involved. Urticaria may accompany the lesions.

Because the infestation is often in unhygienic individuals, secondary infection and pyoderma are not uncommon.

### *Treatment*

Attention to personal hygiene and prevention of infection are important. Further local therapy is usually not necessary.

To disinfect the habitation, a thorough spraying with a pesticide is necessary in crevices of furniture, walls, and floors, as well as mattresses. DDT, chlordane, or a substitute may be used. These pesticides have fallen into disfavor, and a special permit is required for their use; however, there is nothing so satisfactory to take their place. Malathion, carbamide, and dimpylate (Diazinon) are available in kerosene-based sprays, but must be used carefully to prevent oil spotting.

## DERMATOSES CAUSED BY LICE (ORDER ANOPLURA)

An intensely pruritic reaction results from the bites of pediculi, bloodsucking insects that commonly infest the scalp, body, and pubic region in man.

***Pediculosis capitis.*** Infestation of the scalp by *Pediculus humanus* var. *capitis* begins with an itching of the scalp that may vary from moderate to severe in intensity. The saliva of the louse produces the strong pruritus. Excoriations are produced, and these soon become secondarily infected, with crusting. The posterior aspect of the scalp commonly shows the greatest degree of involvement, and the posterior occipital nodes are enlarged and tender. Children are most frequently affected and usually have an associated impetigo of the face.

Close examination of the hair shaft will show minute white eggs (nits) firmly attached in series. They fluoresce under Wood's light. The adult louse is slender, 2 to 4 mm. long, and found only with difficulty.

***Pediculosis corporis.*** Infestation of the body by *Pediculus humanus* var. *corporis* is characterized by pruritus and by parallel linear excoriations that are frequently secondarily infected. The primary lesion, which is seldom found because of the excoriations, is an urticarial wheal with a central hemorrhagic punctum. In cases of prolonged infestations the skin becomes dry, scaly, and hyperpigmented (vagabond's disease).

The adult louse, which measures 1 to 4 mm. in length, feeds on the skin, but lives on the seams of clothing. It is associated with unhygienic environmental conditions. When long pruritic excoriations on the body are found, the clothes should be carefully examined for lice.

***Pediculosis pubis.*** Infestation by *Phthirus pubis*, or the crab louse, is primarily manifested by itching. The urticarial lesions and secondary infections are seldom found with this type of infestation. In severe or longstanding cases, the lice may infect the chest and axillary hair, as well as the eyelashes. A feature of the condition is the reddish brown "dust" apparent on underclothing, which is formed from the excreta of the insects. On close examination, the 1 to 2 mm. long reddish brown louse may be found with its head buried in the hair follicle. The nits are darker than those found in head and body infestations. Dusky gray-blue macules (*taches bleuâtres*, or maculae caeruleae), 1 to 3 cm. in diameter, often may be observed on the trunk, thighs, and axillae. These are a result of the reaction of the insect's saliva on bilirubin, converting it to biliverdin.

Transmission is by close personal contact, usually by sexual intercourse.

### *Pertinent information*

The two species of lice that infest the head, body, and pubic region differ in size and appearance, but their eggs (nits) are similar. The scalp louse, which may lay as many as 300 eggs, cements each egg to a hair shaft. The body louse differs in attaching its eggs to the seams of clothing. The nit stage lasts for some 9 days, the adult about 30 days. Newly hatched lice must feed within 24 hours in order to survive. Transmission of this infestation is by skin-to-skin contact, wearing of infested clothing, or using infested combs or hats, and the lice move readily from person to person.

Lice are vectors for *relapsing fever* and *typhus*, because the causative organisms may be contained in the gastrointestinal tract of the insect and excreted onto the skin surface.

### *Differential diagnosis*

***Scabies.*** In scabies there are small excoriated lesions in the interdigital webs of the fingers and on the wrists and the penis.

***Flea bites.*** Excoriated papular lesions caused by fleas are usually limited to the lower half of the legs.

***Infestation with bedbugs.*** The papular lesions caused by bedbugs are uniform in size, with central puncta, and arranged in rows on exposed areas.

***Tinea capitis.*** Tinea capitis produces hairless, discrete areas of scalp involvement. Depending on the type of fungus, the lesions may be crusted, swollen, and tender and may appear secondarily infected. The fungus will be found on microscopic examination and culture of the infected hair.

### *Treatment*

The adult lice and their ova are best attacked by use of a preparation containing gammabenzene hexachloride.

***Pediculosis capitis.*** Gamma benzene hexacloride (Kwell, Kwellada) shampoo should be used to cleanse the scalp. It should also be used in cream or lotion form, massaged onto the scalp after shampooing and left on overnight. Shampoo is repeated the next day, and again in 1 week if necessary. Benzyl benzoate 20% emulsion can be used as well in the same way.

***Pediculosis corporis.*** The patient should have a bath. All clothes and bedding should be throughly laundered and clothing seams should be ironed with a hot iron. If this is impossible, the infested bedding and clothing may be dusted with 1% gamma benzene hexachloride in talc, to be repeated after an interval of 2 weeks.

An antipruritic lotion, such as the following is applied:

| | |
|---|---|
| Menthol | 0.5% |
| Phenol | 0.5% |
| Zinc oxide | 15 Gm. |
| Talc | 15 Gm. |
| Glycerin | 10 ml. |
| Alcohol | 40 ml. |
| Water | 40 ml. |

Apply with fingers three times daily.

***Pediculosis pubis.*** Satisfactory treatment consists of application of 25% benzyl benzoate emulsion or gamma benzene hexacloride (Kwell) on 2 successive days. Kwell is available either as a lotion or as a shampoo.

Infested eyelashes may need to be treated by the daily application of yellow oxide of mercury or an ophthalmic ointment containing 0.25% physostigmine.

#### REFERENCES

Fisher, I. *Phthirus pubis* infestation, Br. J. Vener. Dis. **46**:326, 1970.

Maguire, J.: Head infestation in school children: extent of the problem and treatment, Community Med. **128**:374, 1972.

Peck, S. M., Wright, W. H., and Gant, J. Q., Jr.: Cutaneous reactions to the body louse *(Pediculus humanus)*, J.A.M.A. **123**:821, 1943.
**These three articles cover lice infestations involving the head, body, and pubic areas.**

## DERMATITIS CAUSED BY CERCARIAE
## Swimmer's itch (schistosome dermatitis, cutaneous schistosomiasis).

Swimmer's itch is an allergic cutaneous reaction to contact with schistosome cercariae from swimming or wading in infested fresh water.

### *Natural course*

In infested waters the cercariae, which are the free-swimming form of the schistosome, penetrate the skin of bathers, causing a

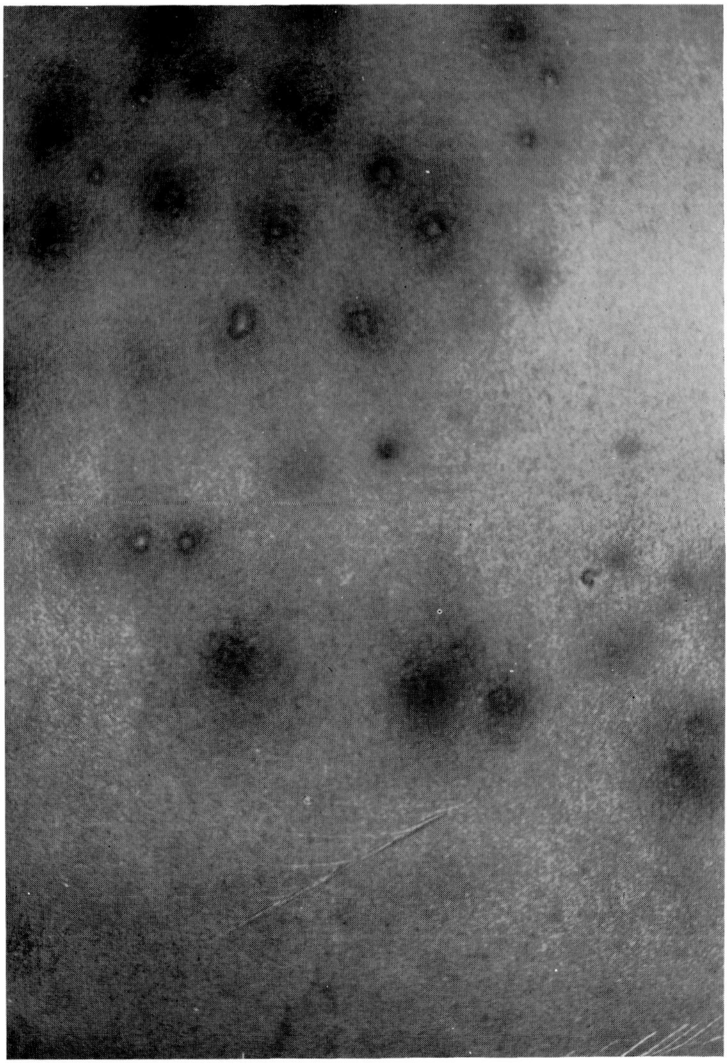

**Fig. 16-4.** Swimmers' itch (schistosome dermatitis). Contracted from freshwater swimming.

prickly pruritus. The organism dies in the skin and its breakdown products produce a cutaneous allergic reaction. The first exposure produces a period of sensitization, and the reaction is delayed for 5 to 13 days. On subsequent exposures, the degree of reaction is intensified, resulting in urticarial wheals occurring immediately. These are followed by papules with an erythematous halo, vesicles, and pustules (Fig. 16-4). The lesions subside within a week.

Birds, especially ducks, and some rodents are the most common definitive hosts of schistosomes. The schistosomes infest snails, and during the warm months cercariae are released from the snails.

### *Differential diagnosis*

***Sea bather's eruption.*** Sea bather's eruption is an acute pruritic dermatitis occurring under the bathing suit area. It is found in the Caribbean area and involves many bathers when it occurs. The lesions are urticarial.

***Seaweed dermatitis.*** An unusual dermatitis

observed in persons swimming in ocean water off Honolulu, seaweed dermatitis is caused by contact with marine algae.

### *Treatment*

Showering and subsequent thorough toweling of the skin immediately after emerging from the water is an excellent prophylactic measure.

Symptomatic treatment includes topical application of an antipruritic lotion, such as the following:

| | |
|---|---|
| Menthol | 0.5% |
| Phenol | 0.5% |
| Hexachlorophene | 1.0% |
| Zinc oxide | 15 Gm. |
| Talc | 15 Gm. |
| Glycerin | 10 ml. |
| Alcohol | 40 ml. |
| Water | 40 ml. |

Oral antihistaminics in adequate dosage may be helpful.

#### REFERENCES

McMullen, D. B.: Studies on schistosome dermatitis: distribution and epidemiology in Michigan, Am. J. Hygiene **47**:259, 1948.

Ramos, S. F.: Late cutaneous bilharziasis, S. Afr. Med. J. **47**:2103, 1973.
**Swimmers' itch, the ubiquitous and transient dermatitis common to swimmers in the lakes of North America, has a more serious counterpart in other geographic areas.**

## INFESTATION WITH PINWORMS

## Enterobiasis (oxyuriasis)

The human pinworm, *Enterobius* (formerly *Oxyuris*) *vermicularis*, has been known since ancient times for its part in the causation of pruritus ani.

### *Natural course*

The intense pruritus produced in the perianal and perineal areas of children commonly begins in the evening or after sleep has begun. It may be associated with a colicky pain in the rectum. The repeated rubbing and scratching may provoke excoriations, lichenification, and infection.

This is a very common family infestation, often affecting first the children and subsequently the parents. Continual reinfection is the rule if the organism is not eliminated.

### *Pertinent information*

The pinworm is found worldwide but is more common in temperate than the tropical climates.

The worms inhabit the small intestine and cecum, ordinarily without symptoms, until the female migrates through the large intestine to the anus in order to lay her eggs. She emerges to crawl on the perianal skin and deposit ova. The eggs, which hatch in a few hours, are transferred by fingers and fingernails to the mouth, where the intestine is thus reinfected. Other individuals become infected from bedclothes, towels, and so forth.

Diagnosis is most effectively made by use of a transparent adhesive-tape swab, rolled over the perianal skin at bedtime and examined microscopically for ova.

Direct examination of the anal orifice at this time may reveal the small white worms just inside the sphincter.

### *Treatment*

Piperazine adipate (Entacyl), 1 to 3 teaspoonsful three times daily, or another form of piperazine (such as Pripsen or Antepar) is given according to the weight of the child.

Pyrvinium pamoate (Povan, Vanquin), 50 mg. or 5 mg./kg. of body weight, is given in a single dose. It will color stools red and may stain clothing or bedding.

## CREEPING ERUPTION (LARVA MIGRANS)

Creeping eruption is an infestation of the epithelial layers of the skin of man by the larval forms of certain roundworms, *Ancylostoma braziliense, Ancylostoma duodenale,* and *Necator americanus*—the cat, dog, and human hookworms, respectively. These are common in the southern United States and in many other parts of the world. Other hookworms are causative agents as well.

The lesions are produced in the unprotected skin and may be single or multiple, sometimes numbering in the hundreds, in the

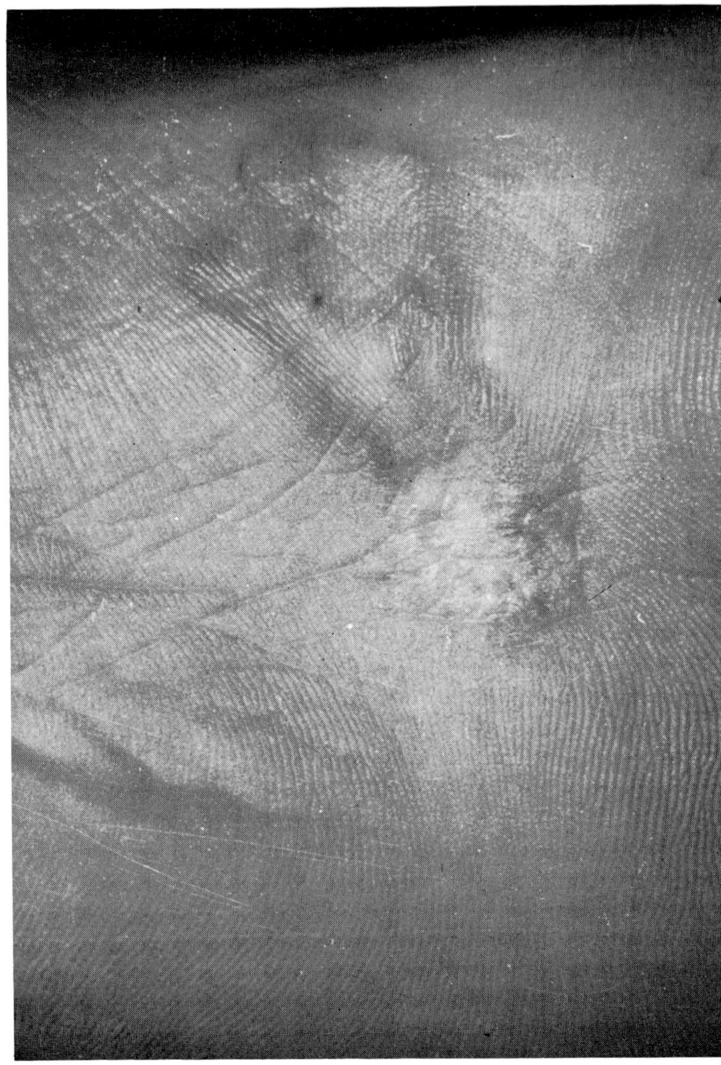

**Fig. 16-5.** Creeping eruption on sole of foot.

form of irregular wandering tunnels, with overlying erythema, vesiculation, and crusting. Although lesions may persist actively for weeks or even months, more than half of the active new lesions may disappear spontaneously in 2 weeks. Thus one must consider the natural cause of the disorder in assessing effectiveness of medications. Lesions are commonly found on the feet, legs, and hands and are intensely pruritic (Fig. 16-5). Systemic involvement occurs in some cases, as a result of the parasite migrating to the lungs and other organs.

Infection is contracted in moist sandy areas or where infected dogs or cats have defecated.

### *Treatment*

Freezing with ethyl chloride spray, solid carbon dioxide, or liquid nitrogen is used for individual lesions when only a few are present. Also, the topical application of oral thiabendazole suspension works satisfactorily in most areas. The use of 2% lindane (Gammexane) cream or 25% piperazine ointment is effective.

Thiabendazole systemically reversed the previously unhappy prognosis of victims of this and some other nematode diseases. It is a medication of high effectiveness, although evidence of hepatotoxicity is reported. It should be used with caution in patients with liver disease or decreased liver function. It can produce dizziness, nausea and vomiting, and headaches. It is given over 2 to 4 days, 25 mg./kg. twice daily. A 15% thiabendazole solution in a water-soluble base topically four times daily produces inactivity of lesions within 72 hours in mild cases.

## REFERENCES

Faust, E. C., Russell, P. F., and Jung, R. C.: Craig and Faust's clinical parasitology, ed. 8, Philadelphia, 1970, Lea & Febiger.
**Medically oriented.**

Harman, R. R. M.: Tropical skin diseases in temperate climates—helminthic diseases (larva migrans). In Rook, A., editor: Recent advances in dermatology, ed. 4, London, 1977, Churchill Livingstone, p. 119.
**The most comprehensive survey on the subject.**

Smith, C. C.: Creeping eruption. In Maddin, S., editor: Current dermatologic management, St. Louis, 1975, The C. V. Mosby Co., p. 102.
**A knowledgeable clinical presentation in terms of treatment.**

## CHAPTER 17

# Keratinization disorders

### KERATINIZATION

This is the process of differentiation by which epidermal cells transform themselves into the firm compact barrier of the outer stratum corneum (Fig. 17-1). This maturation process clearly demonstrates the vertical orientation of the epidermal cell and the "column" of cells from adjacent basal cells at the bottom to "stacked" corneocytes in the outer compact layer. Basal cells synthesize and incorporate new protein, add lipids, and increase in cell mass as they move independently to their destination at the surface (Fig. 17-2). Their initial alpha-keratin filaments, bundled into tonofibrils, become enmeshed in an amorphous glue. The cell membrane thickens and the whole structure flattens, interdigitates with adjacent cell neighbors, and loses its cellular identity to become a part of the firm resilient compact layer. There are two stages in this process, a synthesizing stage and a transitional stage (Matoltsy).

In the earlier synthesizing stage, tonofilaments, membrane-coating granules, and ker-

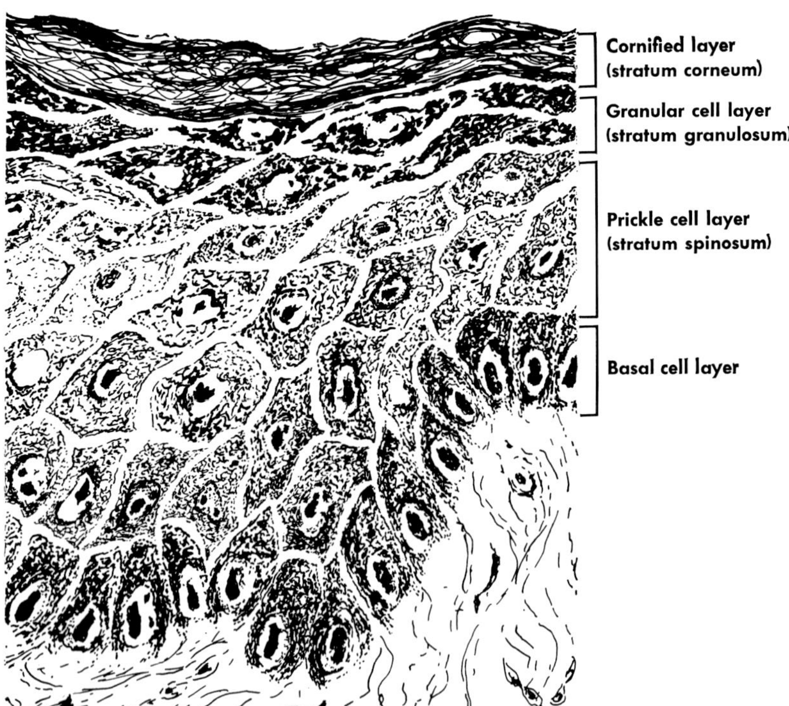


**Fig. 17-1.** Layers of the skin. After mitosis, basal cells migrate upward as components of each layer, finally reaching the surface.

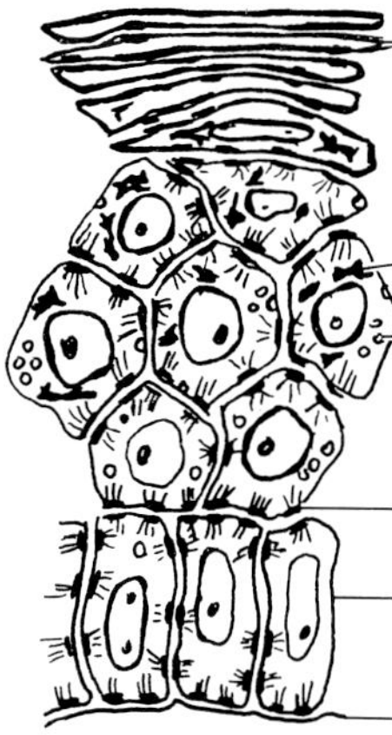


**Fig. 17-2.** Markers of keratinization process.

atohyaline granules are formed from proteins synthesized in ribosomes. By the time the cell moves to the upper spinous layer, small intracytoplasmic membrane-coating granules move to the cell membrane and spread a layered lipid material on the outside of the cell that fills in intercellular nooks and crannies, as one would butter toast. Next the cellular lysosomes discharge their enzymes, which stop cellular synthetic activity, and the cytoplasmic contents consolidate. The nucleus fades. Large irregular dense keratohyaline granules disperse and enmesh the fibrillar material in an amorphous protein glue. The outer cellular membrane thickens, and the intercellular lipid shows pronounced layers. The eventual remarkable strength and resistance of the keratin is related to the disulfide bonds in the amorphous glue, and the insoluble thickened cell membranes. Elasticity and pliability rests with the sulfur-poor fibrils. Aqueous and lipid-soluble substances pass through the laminated intercellular lipid cement. The integrity of the layer is dependent on the tough lipid protein cell membranes.

It has been almost 50 years since essential fatty acid deficiency was observed to cause a scaling dermatosis in experimental animals. Now clinical observations of patients on total parenteral nutrition have confirmed dramatically the importance of these essential fatty acids in the maintenance of skin integrity. A range of findings from severe scaling to exfoliative dermatitis has been observed in infants and adults undergoing supportive alimentary care for gastrointestinal failure, when linoleic and arachidonic acids were omitted (Riella, Prottey). Essential fatty acids are components of cellular structural lipids, cell membranes, and mitochondria. They are found in the reproductive organs, and they give rise to the most potent biologically active substances known, the prostaglandins. Cutaneous manifestations of essential fatty acid deficiency, as noted above, can be completely reversed by topical application of prostaglandins or their precursor, linoleic acid (Prottey), or by their addition to the nutritional supply (Riella). Severe scaling has also resulted in patients placed on hypolipemic drugs, such as triparanol or butyrophenone, which interfere with lipid synthesis (Winkelmann; Simpson and Cranswick).

### REFERENCES

Matoltsy, A. G.: Desmosomes, filaments, and keratohyaline granules: their role in the stabilization and keratinization of the epidermis, J. Invest. Dermatol. **65**:127, 1975.

**Lucid clarification of structure in respect to function.**

Prottey, C., Hartop, P. J., and Press, M.: Correction of cutaneous manifestations of essential fatty acid deficiency in man by application of sunflower seed oil to skin, J. Invest. Dermatol. **64**:228, 1975.

**Three patients with less than 3 feet of small bowel on low fat diets developed scaly eczema. Cleared with topical linoleic acid.**

Riella, M. C., Broviac, J. W., Wells, M., and Scribner, B. H.: Essential fatty acid deficiency in human adults during total parenteral nutrition, Ann. Intern. Med. **83**:786, 1975.

**Fat-free alimentation produced exfoliative dermatitis, ostensibly because of reduced linoleic acid intake.**

Simpson, G. M., and Cranswick, E. H.: Cutaneous effects of a new butyrophenone drug, Clin. Pharmacol. Ther. **5**:310, 1964.

**Ichthyosiform scaling.**

Winkleman, R. K., Perry, H. O., Achor, R. W., et al.: Cutaneous syndromes produced as side effects of triparanol therapy, Arch. Dermatol. **87**:372, 1963.

**Interferes with normal endogenous lipid synthesis.**

Yardley, H. J., and Goldstein, K. J.: Changes in dry

weight and projected area of human epidermal cells undergoing keratinization as determined by scanning interference microscopy, Br. J. Dermatol. **95**:621, 1976.

**Epidermal cells increase in mass probably through lipid and protein synthesis in upper epidermis.**

## ICHTHYOSIS

Ichthyosis is a very common inherited disorder, characterized by varying degrees of dryness, scaling, and exfoliation of the skin.

### *Natural course*

*There are four patterns of inheritance of ichthyosis*, arranged and introduced by Wells and Kerr to form a basis for clinical classification of these disorders, thus producing a more reasonable approach to this disease than a purely morphological one.

To this reasonable basis have been added further sophisticated biological measurements confirming the rationale of the classification. These have been concisely reviewed by Frost (1973).

Thus observations on the functional state of epidermal turnover, cell-transit time from mitosis to outer surface, rates of transepidermal water loss, and microscopy all confirm the correctness of this classification. The categories are listed in Table 6.

***Ichthyosis vulgaris (dominant).*** The dominant form of the disease (dominant ichthyosis vulgaris) is the most common. It is first observed after the first 3 months of life, is not sex linked, and tends to diminish in severity during adult life. It is distinguished by a fine scaling of the skin or only a tendency to dryness. The areas of most severe involvement are the elbows, knees, sides of arms and thighs, palms, soles, and forehead. Follicular hyperkeratotic lesions are present over the extensor surfaces of the extremities. The hair and scalp are dry. The disorder is most apparent during

**Table 6.** Four patterns of inheritance of ichthyosis, forming the basis for clinical classification of the disorder

| | | | Ichthyosiform erythroderma | |
|---|---|---|---|---|
| | **Dominant ichthyosis vulgaris** | **Recessive male sex-linked ichthyosis** | **Nonbullous recessive (lamellar ichthyosis)** | **Bullous dominant (epidermolytic hyperkeratosis)** |
| Incidence | 1:1,000 | 1:6,000 | Rare | Rare |
| Onset | Childhood | Infancy | Birth | Birth |
| Distribution | Extensor aspect of extremities, face; palmar markings accentuated; flexures spared | Anteroposterior thorax and abdomen, total extremities; flexures spared | Generalized | Erythrodermatous palms and soles; flexures affected |
| Scaling | Small, thin, light scale | Flat, larger, dirty brown scale | Large, adherent, thin scale | Thick, course, warty, linear scale |
| Associations | Atopic dermatitis | Posterior capsule opacities on slit-lamp examination of eyes in patients and female carriers | Prematurity, ectropion | Vesicular and bullous lesions |
| Prognosis | Improves | Persists | Persists | Improves partially, then limited to flexures |
| Treatment | 40% propylene glycol in water under occlusion | 40% propylene glycol in water under occlusion | Topical retinoic acid, 40% propylene glycol in water under occlusion | Topical retinoic acid |

the winter months. Those patients with atopic dermatitis who have an associated ichthyosis have this form of the disease. Pruritus may be a feature.

*Microscopically*, hyperkeratosis is present, with diminution of the granular layer. There is follicular plugging. These changes are less pronounced than in other forms of the disease.

***Sex-linked ichthyosis.*** The sex-linked *recessive* form of ichthyosis (recessive ichthyosis vulgaris) affects only males, becomes apparent shortly after birth, and involves the entire cutaneous surface, sparing the palms and soles. The affected areas are dry and scaling, with large dark plate-like scales that shed easily. The scalp, neck, and sides of the face are involved in children, whereas the abdomen and legs are the areas chiefly affected in adults. Sever, Frost, and Weinstein correlated the four types of ichthyosis with eye changes. They observed that individuals with this disorder demonstrate deep corneal opacities on slit-lamp examination, but these do not appear to affect vision (Fig. 17-3, *A*).

*Microscopic studies* reveal changes similar to those of the dominant form, with the addition of branching and elongated rete ridges and more plugging.

***Ichthyosiform erythroderma.*** A third form

A

B

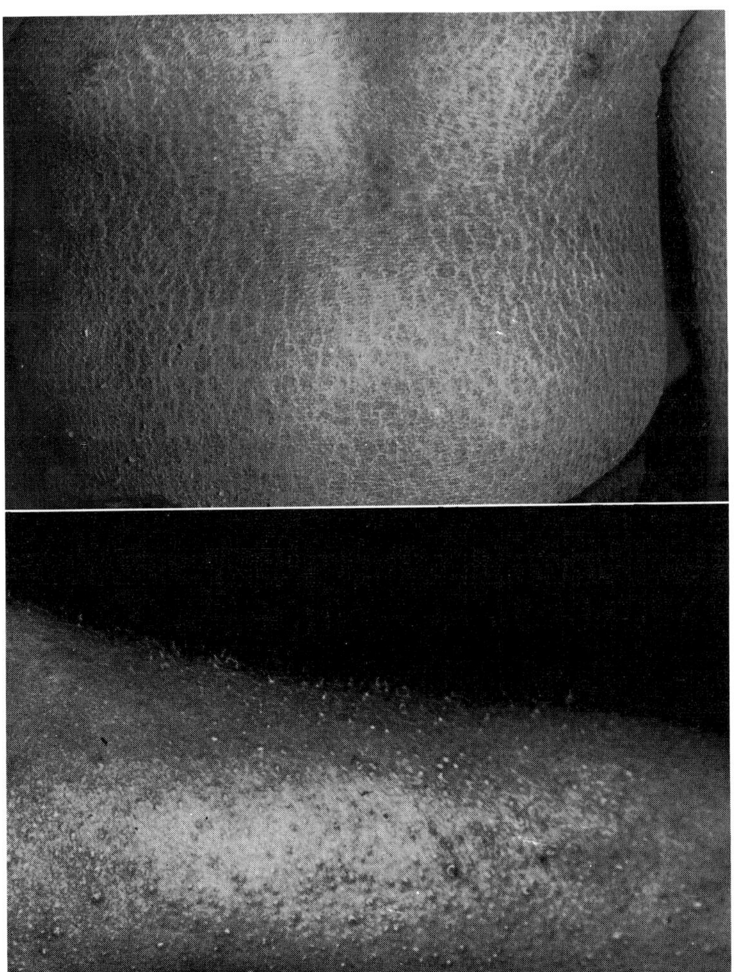

**Fig. 17-3. A,** Ichthyosis, sex-linked recessive form. **B,** Lichen spinulosus.

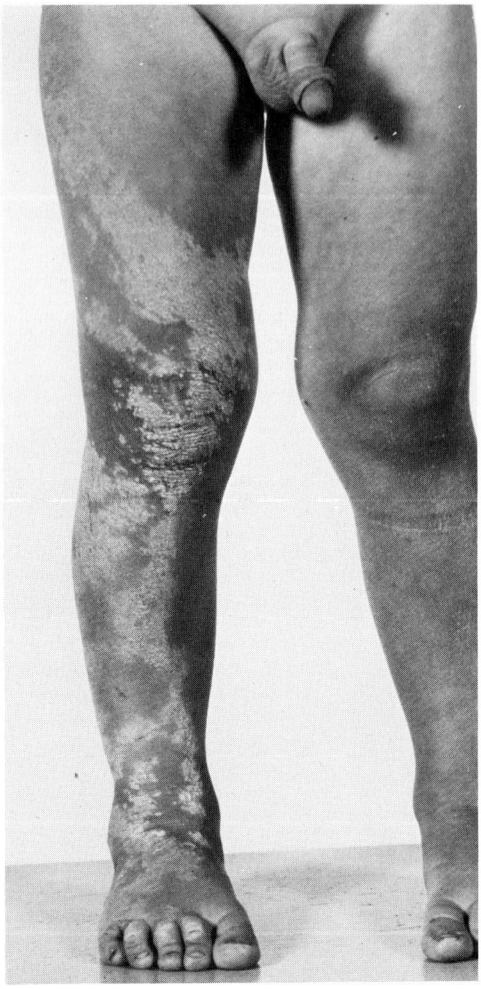

**Fig. 17-4.** Bullous dominant ichthyosiform erythroderma. Localized form, with thick verrucous scales.

of ichthyosis appears at birth. It has in the past been separated from the first two types under the name of *ichthyosiform erythroderma* (ichthyosis congenita). It occurs in a *dominant bullous* and in a *recessive nonbullous* form.

*Bullous ichthyosiform erythroderma (dominant) (epidermolytic hyperkeratosis)* (Fig. 17-4). The bullous form may show early minimal evidence of vesicle and bulla formation, or these blisters may dominate the clinical picture. They are more severe early in life and indeed may result in secondary infection and death during infancy.

If the disease is compatible with life, it will demonstrate varying proportions of erythema and hyperkeratosis, essentially for life. Some children improve to the extent of having a relatively normal skin. Thick, gray-brown, verrucous scales, most prominent in the flexures, are the distinguishing feature. These may slough off in infancy, leaving a moist surface, only to be replaced in childhood. Hair growth may be vigorous or sparse. Thickening of palms and soles is a feature. Ichthyosis congenita may be patchy. These individuals may demonstrate deafness, vascularizing keratitis, physical retardation, and peripheral neuropathy.

Microscopic findings include a diagnostic vacuolation of the epidermal cells in the granular layer and midepidermis. Bullae are formed by rupture of the vacuolated areas. Large keratohyaline granules are present. Extreme hyperkeratosis, papilloma, and acanthosis are seen. There is rapid turnover of epidermal cells.

*Nonbullous ichthyosiform erythroderma (recessive) (lamellar ichthyosis).* The *recessive nonbullous* form is characterized by a dry skin with large scales that are easily shed. The face and flexures are involved, as are the palms and soles. There is less underlying erythroderma. This form is perhaps more widely referred to as lamellar ichthyosis, and we will use this title here.

*Lamellar ichthyosis* is a recessive form of ichthyosis (Fig. 17-5) appearing at birth, with features of ectropion, fixity of the mouth, palm and sole involvement, and envelopment in a shining, dry, thin layer that has been likened to collodion. This layer may be found in other forms of ichthyosis as well. It is not a diagnostic feature of lamellar ichthyosis. Large, coarse, yellow scales with raised corners cover most of the body and are easily shed. The palms, soles, and face have accentuated markings and thickened epidermis. The state persists. Most collodion babies in Larregue's study of 29 infants, developed this pattern.

Microscopic findings include a definite granular layer, hyperkeratosis, acanthosis, and keratin-filled follicular orifices. Some

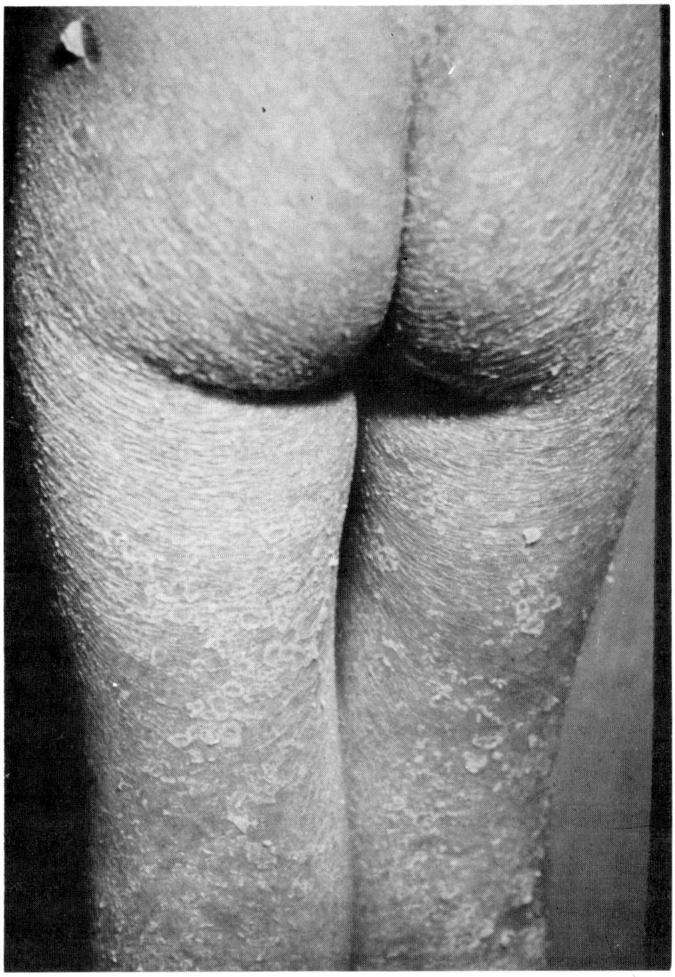

**Fig. 17-5.** Recessive lamellar ichthyosis. Large scales with raised corners.

perivascular infiltrate is seen. No vacuolation of cells is apparent. There is rapid turnover of epidermal cells.

As the child grows older, the chief clinical characteristic is a fine scale with a distinct underlying erythroderma.

Other associated types of ichthyosis that have an autosomal-recessive inheritance include those associated with central nervous system abnormalities, mental retardation, eyelid and corneal changes, and the rarer syndromes that incorporate localized ichthyotic changes in their findings.

The microscopic findings are distinctive and may serve to connect many linear nevi, local hyperkeratoses, and warty isolated lesions, with similar microscopic appearances. These changes occur through a wide range of epithelial lesions.

Goldsmith has begun, with our current knowledge, to relate clinical abnormalities to structural and genetic faults. Only where this is on a sound basis can we try to correct the underlying problem.

### *Differential diagnosis*

***Ichthyosis.*** Forms of ichthyosis may occur associated with Hodgkin's disease, leprosy, and other malignancies.

***Psoriasis.*** Psoriasis may present as a generalized, thickly scaling erythroderma of fairly long standing. The response to sunlight, nail involvement, and family history will differentiate it from ichthyosis.

Some forms of generalized erythroderma in the neonatal period may be generalized psoriasis.

***Exfoliative dermatitis.*** Exfoliative dermatitis is ordinarily of fairly recent onset, worsens rapidly, and is often preceded by a specific cutaneous disease.

***Generalized dermatitis.*** Generalized dermatitis such as develops from a contact dermatitis, autoeczematization of a localized process, atopic dermatitis, or seborrheic dermatitis may present as a generalized, red, scaling eruption. Generally, however, these are of more recent onset than ichthyosis.

### *Treatment*

For the severe bullous form of ichthyosiform erythroderma, systemic glucocorticoids may be lifesaving in infancy. In other forms, they are of no value. Antimetabolites have not been helpful in the management of these disorders.

Prolonged exposure to hot weather is very beneficial in the dominant and the sex-linked recessive forms of ichthyosis, but in ichthyosiform erythroderma heat is uncomfortable.

Baden and Goldsmith have successfully used 40% to 60% propylene glycol in water under occlusion in the treatment of ichthyosis vulgaris, sex-linked ichthyosis, and to some degree in nonbullous ichthyosiform erythroderma. It is used for a week under occlusion, then only every third night for maintenance therapy.

Medication for all forms includes the following ointments:

| | |
|---|---|
| Urea | 10% |
| Unibase | q.s. |

Apply after bathing while skin is moist, or three to seven times weekly.

| | |
|---|---|
| Salicylic acid | 2% |
| Hydrophilic ointment | q.s. |

Apply after bathing while skin is moist, or three to seven times weekly.

Brief but regular baths, using commercially available bath oil preparations, are of distinct benefit for some patients.

Topical retinoic acid, 0.05% to 0.1% in propylene glycol and in a cream base, has been tried and found successful, although its effect may diminish over several weeks. It is useful only in the bullous and nonbullous forms of ichthyosiform erythroderma.

Early clinical trials suggest that oral 13-*cis*-retinoic acid (oral synthetic retinoid) may be of benefit in these patients with keratinizing disorders. Peck and Yoder report that all five patients with lamellar ichthyosis demonstrated excellent improvement. However, this drug is not yet available for general use, and there is also evidence that suggests that untoward side reactions may limit its adoption.

#### REFERENCES

Ackerman, A. B.: Histopathologic concept of epidermolytic hyperkeratosis, Arch. Dermatol. **102**:253, 1970.
**Specific pathologic features that occur in a wide clinical range of disease.**

Briggaman, R. A., and Wheeler, C.: Lamellar ichthyosis. Long-term graft studies on congenitally athymic nude mice, J. Invest. Dermatol. **67**:567, 1976.
**Epidermal proliferation and abnormalities maintained independent of dermal effect.**

Flint, G. L., Flam, M., and Soter, S. N.: Acquired ichthyosis, Arch. Dermatol. **111**:1446, 1975.
**The ichthyosis may be helpful in monitoring the patient's response to therapy of the malignancy.**

Frost, P.: Disorders of cornification. In Moschella, S. L., Pillsbury, D. M., and Hurley, H. J., editors: Dermatology, Philadelphia, 1975, W. B. Saunders Co., p. 1056.
**The best in-depth coverage of the subject that is presently available.**

Frost, P.: Ichthyosiform dermatoses, J. Invest. Dermatol. **60**:541, 1973.
**Classification and treatment. Well illustrated.**

Goldsmith, L. A.: The ichthyoses, Prog. Med. Genet. **1**:185, 1976.
**Genetics emphasized, as well as association with malignancy, dietary deficiency, drugs, and psoriasis.**

Goldsmith, L. A.: Molecular mechanisms of genetic disorders of keratinization, Arch. Dermatol. **112**:375, 1976.
**An attempt to relate structure to function and inheritance.**

Goldsmith, L. A., and Baden, H. P.: Propylene glycol with occlusion for treatment of ichthyosis, J.A.M.A. **220**:479, 1972.
**Safe, effective, excellent, particularly for localized areas, and when complemented by daytime creams in sex-linked ichthyosis and ichthyosis vulgaris.**

Jay, B., Blach, R. K., and Wells, R. S.: Ocular manifestations of ichthyosis, Br. J. Ophthalmol. **52:**217, 1968.
**62 patients studied—all sex-linked ichthyosis cases over 25 had corneal changes.**

Larregue, M., Charlie, J., Daniel, Y., et al.: The collodion baby: development of 29 cases, Ann. Dermatol. Syphiligr. (Paris) **103:**31, 1976.
**The collodion baby most often develops a recessive nonbullous ichthyosiform erythroderma.**

Mirrer, E., and McGuire, J.: Lamellar ichthyosis—responses to retinoic acid (Tretinoin), a case report, Arch. Dermatol. **102:**548, 1970.
**Successful, but may be transient.**

Muller, S. A., Belcher, R. W., and Esterly, N. B.: Keratinizing dermatoses, Arch. Dermatol. **113:**1052, 1977.
**Beneficial effect of topical 0.1% retinoic acid cream compared with 2% salicyclic acid in lamellar ichthyosis and with ichthyosis vulgaris.**

Peck, G. L., and Yoder, F. W.: Treatment of lamellar ichthyosis and other keratinizing dermatoses with an oral synthetic retinoid, Lancet **2:**1172, 1976.
**This interesting report from two workers at the National Institutes of Health is not only of therapeutic interest, but also is provocative. This specific therapy confirms the recent classification of ichthyosis.**

Schorr, W. F., and Papa, C. M.: Epidermolytic hyperkeratosis, Arch. Dermatol. **102:**253, 1970.
**Topical retinoic acid therapy at 0.05% was successful in restoring the skin's appearance to normal.**

Van Scott, E. J., and Yu, R. J.: Control of keratinization with alpha-hydroxy acids and related compounds, Arch. Dermatol. **110:**586, 1974.
**Best results were on lamellar ichthyosis, ichthyosis vulgaris, and sex-linked ichthyosis. Good results remained as long as the topical therapy was maintained.**

Wells, R. S.: Ichthyosis. In Maddin, S., editor: Current dermatologic management, ed. 2, St. Louis, 1975, The C. V. Mosby Co., p. 190.
**A clinically oriented presentation with major emphasis on diagnosis and management.**

Wells, R. S., and Kerr, C. B.: Genetic classification of ichthyosis, Arch. Dermatol. **92:**1, 1965.
**A significant advance.**

Wells, R. S., and Kerr, C. B.: The histology of ichthyosis, J. Invest. Dermatol. **46:**530, 1966.
**Microscopic confirmation of the classification.**

## KERATOSIS PILARIS

Keratosis pilaris is a very common hereditary disorder of keratinization, producing a gooseflesh appearance (Fig. 17-6) on the upper arms and thighs.

### *Natural course*

The lesion is a hyperkeratotic papule at the orifice of the hair follicle. It is symmetrical, multiple, and usually seen as discrete horny papules on the outer aspect of the arms and thighs. When the examiner's fingers are passed over these papules, there is a rough sensation as though passing over a nutmeg grater. There are no subjective complaints, and there are no ill effects to the general health. Keratosis pilaris occurs at all ages and in both sexes and is brought to our attention most often by females during the summer months, because summer clothing makes it easily apparent. It is actually more pronounced in cold weather. It is an autosomal-dominant characteristic. There is a frequent association with ichthyosis.

### *Microscopic findings*

Microscopic findings consist of hyperkeratosis of the follicular orifice, with dilatation and plugging. There may be a coiled or broken-off hair in the center of the papule.

### *Differential diagnosis*

***Lichen spinulosus.*** Lichen spinulosus is a rare, patchy, follicular hyperkeratosis with small horny spines, which occurs in children and involutes spontaneously.

***Pityriasis rubra pilaris.*** Scaling, thickening, and erythema of the face and neck, and horny papules of the dorsa of the fingers are manifestations of pityriasis rubra pilaris, which occurs in adults.

***Keratosis follicularis (Darier's disease).*** In keratosis follicularis, a rare disorder, the areas most often involved by greasy, brown, isolated hyperkeratotic lesions are the back, neck, and scalp.

***Ichthyosis.*** A hereditary, dry, generalized scaling disorder, ichthyosis vulgaris becomes apparent at birth or shortly thereafter. Keratosis pilaris and ichthyosis are frequently associated.

### *Treatment*

Reassurance of the parents and the patient of the benign nature of the condition is important; treatment with drugs is usually not necessary.

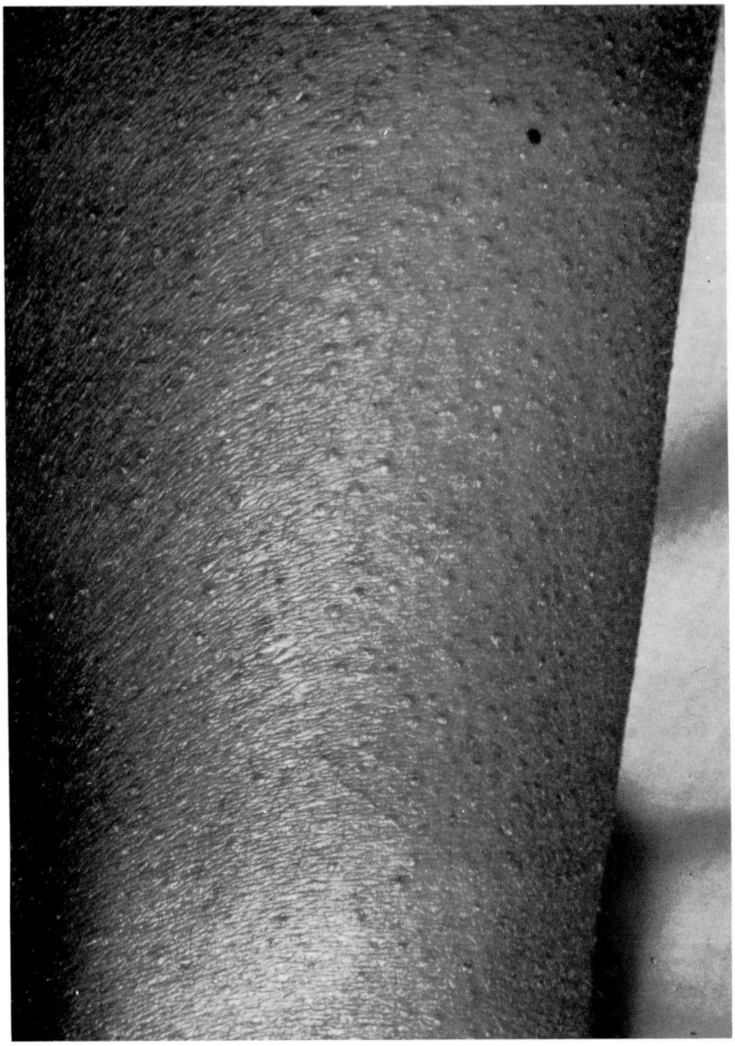

**Fig. 17-6.** Keratosis pilaris. May be seen in the dominant form of ichthyosis vulgaris.

Avoidance of hot baths, soap, wool, and rough clothing prevents aggravation of the condition.

If treatment is indicated, the following preparations are useful:

| | |
|---|---|
| Salicyclic acid | 2% |
| Hydrophilic ointment | q.s. |
| Apply twice daily. | |
| Lactic acid | 4% |
| Dermabase | q.s. |
| Apply twice daily. | |

## LICHEN SPINULOSUS

The primary lesion of this rare follicular eruption is a horny spine extruding from follicular flesh-colored papules (Fig. 17-3, *B*). The asymptomatic papules are in patches, symmetrically distributed over the neck, lateral surfaces of arms, abdomen, and legs. It is found in children. The lesions involute slowly, causing no deleterious effects to the general health.

Microscopically, lichen spinulosus is characterized by a perifollicular hyperkeratosis.

### *Treatment*

We recommend the use of a keratolytic agent such as 2% salicylic acid in hydrophilic ointment or lactic acid 4% in Dermabase, as either is helpful. If this proves unsatisfactory,

1% hydrocortisone in a hydrophilic petrolatum, q.s., may be applied.

## PITYRIASIS RUBRA PILARIS

Pityriasis rubra pilaris is a rare, chronic, exfoliating disease.

### *Natural course*

Pityriasis rubra pilaris may develop in children as a mild, inherited keratinization disorder or in adults at middle age as a disease with a sudden onset and subsequent severe chronic course, generalized involvement, and exfoliation. Its etiology is unknown.

The primary lesion is a reddish, hyperkeratotic, perifollicular papule through which a hair may be found protruding. The lesions are multiple, tending to coalesce gradually into scaling red plaques.

The eruption commonly begins on the scalp and extends to the face, posterior aspect of the neck, trunk, and extremities. It may become generalized. A clinical finding that is of considerable diagnostic assistance is the presence of firm papules with horny follicular plugs over the dorsal surfaces of the fingers. Concomitantly, there is a pronounced thickening and fissuring of the palms and soles. There may be no subjective complaints other than occasional itching and the discomfort of a generalized branny exfoliation. There is no systemic involvement.

### *Microscopic findings*

Microscopically, there is a follicular hyperkeratosis with a degeneration of the basal cell layer. There is perivascular inflammation.

Radioactive labeling has demonstrated decreased transit times through the skin.

### *Treatment*

Treatment has not been of noticeable benefit in many cases of this disease.

High oral doses of vitamin A in the range of 200,000 to 400,000 units daily may produce a remission in adult cases. If no effect is produced in 6 to 8 weeks, then it should be discontinued. Toxicity will occur on longer therapy. Children should receive much lower doses, and the drug must be discontinued at intervals because of toxicity.

Early results indicate also that oral 13-*cis*-retinoic acid may produce remission in pityriasis rubra pilaris. This drug is not available commercially as yet.

Oral methotrexate has been used here, as in extensive psoriasis, with good results. Its toxicity must be balanced against possible beneficial effects.

Oral glucocorticoids in short courses may reduce the active erythrodermic aspect.

Hunter advocates the use of azathioprine in extensive cases, an initial dose of 150 to 200 mg. daily, reduced to 100 mg. or even 50 mg. daily as warranted. The usual precautions must be observed when one uses this potent agent.

#### REFERENCES

Brown, J., and Perry, H. O.: Pityriasis rubra pilaris, Arch. Dermatol. **94**:636, 1966.
**Methotrexate has proved successful.**

Hunter, G. A., and Forbes, I. J.: Pityriasis rubra pilaris. In Maddin, S., editor: Current dermatologic management, St. Louis, 1975, The C. V. Mosby Co., p. 248.
**Recommends azathioprine in severe unrelenting cases.**

Peck, G. L., and Yoder, F. W.: Treatment of lamellar ichthyosis and other keratinizing dermatoses with an oral synthetic retinoid, Lancet **2**:1172, 1976.
**One patient with pityriasis rubra pilaris responded, beginning within 2 weeks.**

## KERATOSIS FOLLICULARIS (DARIER'S DISEASE)

A rare hereditary dominant epidermal defect, keratosis follicularis usually begins in childhood and tends to become progressively more severe.

The primary lesion is a papule that develops around and between hair follicles. It becomes a greasy dark brown papule that increases in size and may form warty masses with a rancid odor. These multiply to form confluent, greasy, crusted masses of lesions. The sites of predilection are the seborrheic and sun-exposed areas, the postauricular area, face, neck, chest, upper back, axillae, and inguinal area. Frequently the disease becomes worse in summer with sun exposure and tends to improve with the onset of cold weather. Oral and genital mucous membranes may be involved. Patchy nonpigmented forms with minimal involvement are seen but may clear spontaneously.

### *Microscopic findings*

There is abnormal keratinization and follicular hyperkeratosis associated with clefts (lacunae) in the epidermis and the projection of papillae into these spaces. There are small, dyskeratotic, eosinophilic-staining grain-like cells (grains), and round clear cells that have lost their prickles (corps ronds).

### *Treatment*

Therapeutic response is poor. The most consistent results are obtained with Grenz radiation. Avoidance of sunlight, however, is advisable.

Topically applied 1% vitamin A acid in equal parts alcohol and propylene glycol, under plastic occlusion for 48 hours, has provided encouraging results. This treatment may be repeated when necessary.

Bathing with a hexachlorophene-containing soap tends to decrease the odor.

## PALMAR AND PLANTAR HYPERKERATOSIS

Keratosis palmaris et plantaris is a hereditary disorder resulting in thickening of the palms and soles (Fig. 17-7). There are many forms of this disease, with different heredity and manifestations. Striate lesions, punctate lesions, associated blisters, and so forth, occur in unexplained patterns of heredity and may

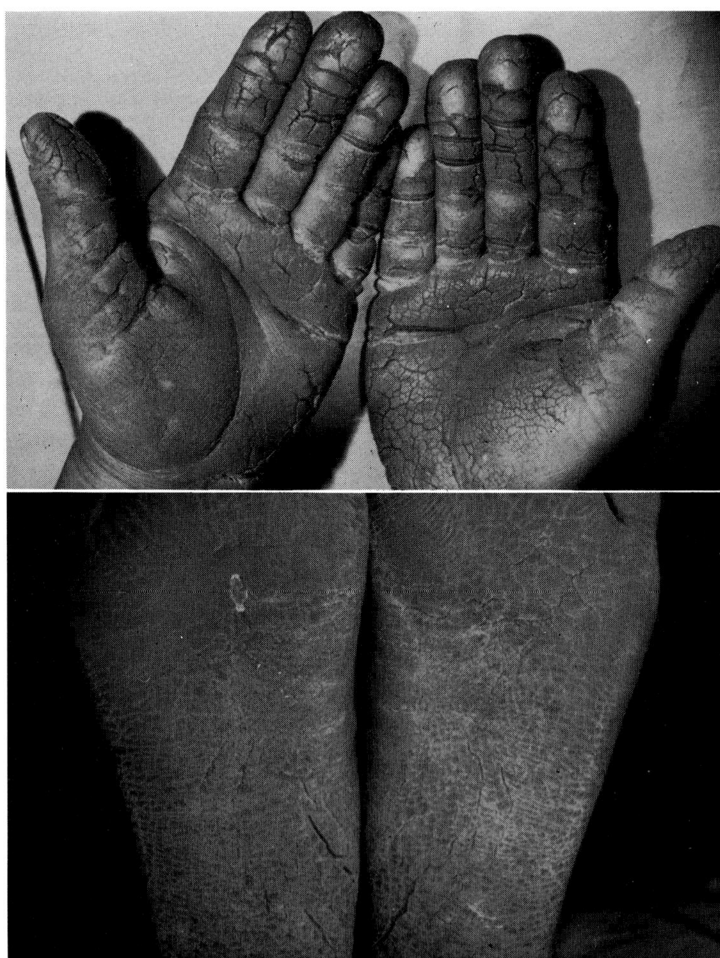

**Fig. 17-7.** Keratosis palmaris et plantaris of palms and soles.

be associated with significant lesions elsewhere. A comprehensive and thoroughly understandable review of the types and their differential diagnosis has been presented by Ebling and Rook.

### *Natural course*

In childhood there is a symmetrical initial redness of the palms and soles, which progresses slowly to a thickening of these tissues by puberty. The epidermis becomes yellow or brown and dry, with fissures developing in the creases. The normal skin ridges are distinctly seen. There is an abrupt transition to normal skin at the sides of the fingers and the sides of the fingers and the sides of the hands. Normal or even increased sweating is present. The disease demonstrates all degrees of involvement, from a mild dryness and scaling to a great thickening and reduced flexibility of the hands. There are punctate forms in which isolated small lesions distributed over the palms and soles are present in an otherwise normal skin. The disease has a dominant inheritance pattern. It is aggravated by manual labor.

The chief clinical features of the fully developed syndrome are the painful fissures and reduction of flexibility of the hands and fingers. It has been postulated that the abnormal keratinization originates from the intraepidermal portion of the sweat glands.

The association of palmar-plantar hyperkeratosis and esophageal carcinoma is well known. However, there are now reports linking this condition with other neoplastic diseases (Gould).

### *Microscopic findings*

Microscopically, one sees an unremarkable acanthosis and hyperkeratosis.

### *Differential diagnosis*

***Psoriasis.*** Psoriasis can produce a dull, red, thickly scaling, patchy involvement of the palms and soles. Psoriasis is seen elsewhere, particularly on the knees, elbows, and scalp.

***Arsenical punctate keratosis.*** Long after arsenic ingestion or exposure, punctate areas of brownish hyperkeratosis and dyskeratosis may appear, some of which progress to malignancy. A cutaneous hyperpigmentation is often also present.

***Contact dermatitis.*** Chronic contact dermatitis may eventuate into a fixed, thickened, scaling, erythematous dermatitis of the palms or soles, with fissuring of the creases. The history here is helpful.

***Epidermophytosis.*** Long-standing fungal infection of palms or soles can result in a chronic dermatitis with thickening and fissuring. Scrapings will reveal the causative fungus.

***Ichthyosis.*** The palms and soles are involved with thickening and fissuring, in association with the generalized skin changes.

### *Treatment*

The disorder is intensified by manual labor and by excessive walking. The less trauma to the areas, the better.

Gunther, an advocate of topically applied retinoic acid in other disorders, has reported successful therapy of this stubborn disorder with 0.1% retinoic acid in petroleum jelly, applied to palms and soles on alternate days for 2 to 4 months. Maintenance applications once or twice weekly are then used.

Bland ointments, preferably those with a slightly greasy base, are most helpful in keeping the area pliable. These can be applied under plastic during the night if comfort permits. Often of distinct help are 5% to 10% salicylic acid ointments in bland, slightly greasy vehicles. To suppress bacterial growth and thus reduce odor, 1% hexachlorophene is helpful.

Heiss and Gross reported successful therapy in one patient, with 0.3% vitamin A acid in petrolatum.

Punctate forms can be treated with the localized application of 40% salicylic acid plasters applied intermittently.

#### REFERENCES

Ebling, F. J. G., and Rook, A.: Disorders of keratinization. In Rook, A., Wilkinson, D. S., and Ebling, F. J. G., editors: Textbook of dermatology, Oxford, 1972, Blackwell Scientific Publications, p. 1178.

**A worthwhile and practical presentation on this subject.**

Gould, D. J.: Hyperkeratosis of the palms and soles asso-

ciated with internal malignancy and elevated levels of immunoreactive human growth hormone, Clin. Exp. Dermatol. 1:363, 1976.
**This report further emphasizes the need for one to be clinically aware when presented with hyperkeratosis of the palms and soles of recent onset in older patients.**

Heiss, H. B., and Gross, P. R.: Keratosis palmaris et plantaris treatment with topically applied vitamin A acid, Arch. Dermatol. **101**:100, 1970.
**0.3% vitamin A acid produced significant relief within 2 weeks.**

## CALLUS

A callus is an acquired area of dense hyperkeratosis formed at a site of repeated pressure or friction. The lesion is elevated, often poorly defined, and yellow, with a normal pattern of skin ridges running over its surface. It is found most frequently on the palms and serves as a guide to the occupation of the individual, with the calluses reflecting sites of most frequent pressure and friction. Loosely fitting shoes and going barefoot predispose to callus formation on the feet.

### *Differential diagnosis*

***Plantar wart.*** Plantar wart is a circumscribed round lesion with a roughened, finely papillary surface, in which, on removal of the outer layers, punctate black dots (the dermal vessels) are seen. There is a hyperkeratosis around most plantar warts.

### *Treatment*

Treatment consists of the application of 40% salicylic acid plaster or ointment, with slight extension beyond the edge of the lesion. This is removed daily, together with the macerated tissue beneath it, and the medication is then reapplied. Bars, pads, or other supportive devices placed in shoes may be helpful. X-ray therapy should not be used.

## CORN (CLAVUS)

A corn is a flat to slightly elevated circumscribed lesion with a smooth hard surface, producing pain on pressure. It appears over bony prominences such as the interphalangeal joints of the toes, at the site of pressure from footwear. Soft corns occur between the toes, characteristically the fourth and fifth, at the site of pressure from a bony spur of the phalanx.

### *Microscopic findings*

Microscopically, the hyperkeratosis is localized and dense, forming a hyalinized cone with the apex extending down and pressing on dermal structures.

### *Treatment*

Application of 40% salicylic acid plaster to the lesion, or salicyclic acid in ether and collodion, is the most effective treatment. A corn can often be shelled out by dissection. Wide, well-fitting shoes and soft foam-rubber pads, worn consistently, will prevent most corns from recurring.

It must be emphasized to the patient that tight, poorly fitting shoes are the almost invariable cause.

CHAPTER **18**

# Lichen planus

Lichen planus is a chronic, pruritic, inflammatory, papular eruption of the skin and mucous membranes that presents a distinctive clinical and histopathological pattern but shows wide variations in its clinical course. Its etiology is unknown.

### *Natural course*

The onset of lichen planus is ordinarily insidious, since the disease begins with the individual appearance of very pruritic, discrete, shiny, reddish violet, flat-topped polygonal papules, 0.5 to 5 mm. in diameter (Fig. 18-1). Close examination reveals pathognomonic gray lines on the flat surface of each papule (Wickham's striae). The papules may become confluent as they appear in larger and larger numbers (Fig. 18-2). The lesions of lichen planus commonly have a symmetrical distribution. The sites of predilection are the flexor surfaces of the wrists and forearms, ankles, abdomen, and sacrum. Only rarely are papules seen on palms and soles. At the site of skin damage, such as a scratch, a linear eruption of lichen planus papules may develop (Koebner's phenomenon).

Variations from these characteristic papules include annular, linear, and hypertrophic lesions. The *hypertrophic* lesions may take the form of pruritic plaques, usually limited to the anterior aspect of the leg, along the bony crest. Occasionally, *bullous* lesions are also seen. Rarely, *atrophic* lesions occur in the course of lichen planus, and these may be associated with cicatrizing scalp lesions that produce permanent patchy hair loss. These variations in the forms of papules, however, are associated with the characteristic flat-topped lesions elsewhere, and these must be sought by the examiner.

There is occasionally an acute onset of a *generalized* eruption of lichen planus.

The average duration of the disease is 15 to 24 months, but it may persist for many years. Localized lesions tend to persist longer than generalized ones, particularly the pruritic hypertrophic lesions of the shins. Healing is followed by residual pigmentation that fades slowly.

Gray, lacy-looking patches are present on the buccal mucosa, tongue, and lips in approximately 60% of cases with skin involvement. When persistent, these patches may thicken and become indistinguishable from leukoplakia. On occasion, the lesions of either the lips or oral cavity are tender, painful, and exceedingly uncomfortable. They may persist for months. Occasional malignant degeneration may occur in about 1 out of 100 cases. Gray lacy lesions or flat red papules occur on the mucosa of the glans penis. Occasionally these mucous membrane lesions produce erosions. Mucous membrane lesions have been recorded in the urinary bladder and throughout the gastrointestinal tract mucosa in association with cutaneous lesions.

*Lichen planus actinicus*, or *subtropicus*, occurs in exposed areas and exhibits a degree of hyperpigmentation. It often presents as circular elevated discrete plaques on the forehead (Fig. 18-3).

The nails may be involved, with a progressive thinning and an increase in longitudinal ridging. They are affected in some 10% of cases, and this involvement may be the only manifestation of the disease. Rarely, nails may be completely shed.

This dermatosis is found much more frequently in adults than in children. Eighty-five percent of cases occur in persons between 30

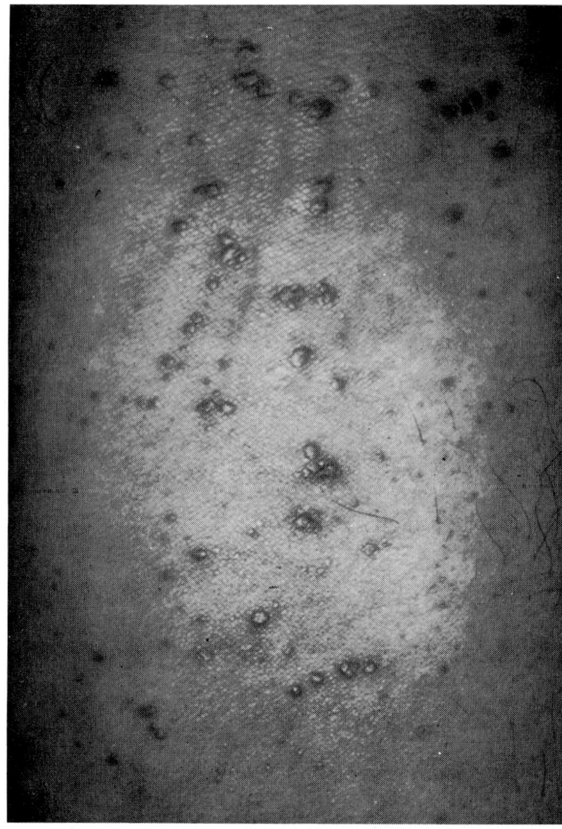

**Fig. 18-1.** Lichen planus. Note polyangular flat-topped papules.

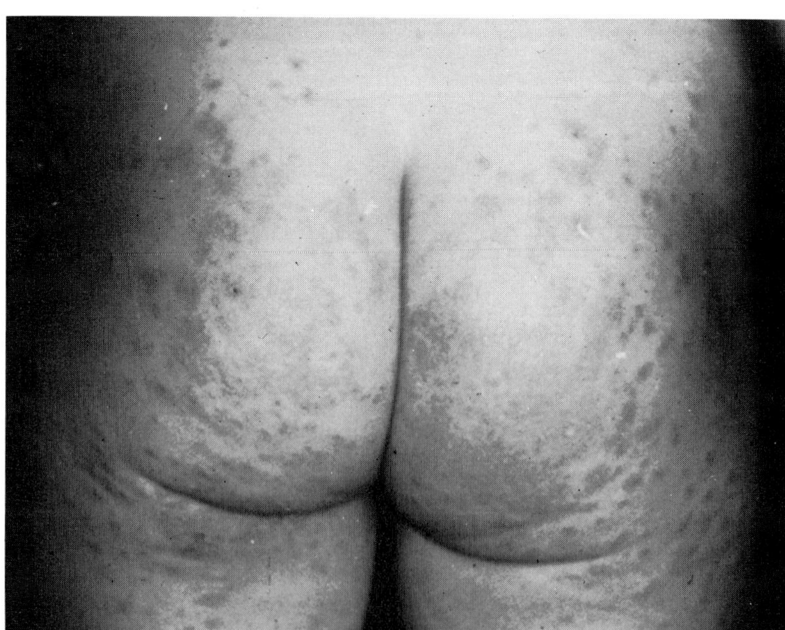

**Fig. 18-2.** Lichen planus involving the buttocks. Large, confluent lesions are apparent.

and 70 years of age. Lesions may be found on the mucous membranes in more than 25% of patients.

A number of interesting variants of lichen planus can sometimes complicate the clinical picture—hypertrophic lesions on the shins; a retiform pattern on the buccal mucosa; bullae and vesicles that may mimic bullous pemphigoid; lichen planus–like drug eruptions; scarring scalp alopecia; and hyperpigmentation of the forehead. There are also well-substantiated cases of lichen planus that cannot be differentiated from lupus erythematosus and increasing numbers of cases of graft-versus-host reaction associated with a lichen planus–like eruption are being reported.

No hereditary influence is apparent in this disease, although instances of multiple cases in families are reported.

### *Microscopic findings*

The histological findings are characteristic, with hyperkeratosis and prominence of the granular layer, together with a jagged, irregular, downward projection of the epidermal rete pegs. There is a sharply demarcated inflammatory infiltrate, consisting mainly of lymphocytes in a band beneath the epidermis. There is degeneration of the basal cell layer.

Electron microscopy reveals a decrease in the number of tonofibrils and desmosomes. Abnormal intranuclear structures, which are nonspecific for lichen planus, are described and may represent a disturbance in cell metabolism, although the presence of a bacterial or viral inclusion has been considered.

### *Pertinent information*

Lichen planus has been studied with varying etiological concepts in mind. Globular deposits of immunoglobulin have been described in the papillary dermis by most observers, in both involved and uninvolved skin. Fibrin is deposited in the active process. Ultrastructurally, the damage is seen to occur in the basal cell layer, first in the nuclei of epidermal cells and melanocytes and then in dermal cells. The cellular infiltrate, probably consisting of lymphoblasts, demonstrates a

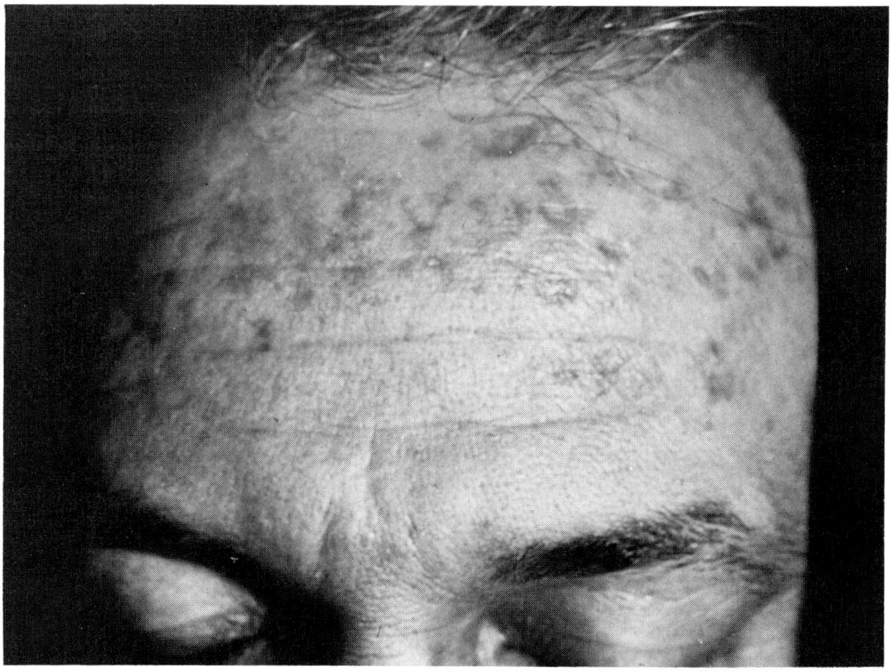

**Fig. 18-3.** Actinic or subtropic lichen planus. Pigmented lesions of forehead.

high labeling index of the order of that seen in allergic contact dermatitis, and one that is three to four times higher than the index seen in psoriasis. These findings could be evidence of an immunological response.

Evidence to suggest a glucose-6-phosphate dehydrogenase deficiency in skin has been reported. Black and Wilson-Jones, who also reported histochemical evidence of reduction in G6PDH activity, believe that microscopic studies indicate a continual pattern of epidermal cell death and replacement on the minute battlefield of a lichen planus lesion. Clusters of repopulating cells crowd in from unaffected areas to fill a deficit in the ranks.

There is IgM and fibrin in the papillary dermis adjacent to the dermoepidermal junction in cases of lichen planus. The ultrastructural presence of viruslike particles in lupus erythematosus has not been demonstrated in lichen planus.

### Diagnosis

Immunofluorescent studies reveal IgG in globules in the papillary dermis, which is an aid to diagnosis. Biopsy of the lesion usually reveals a typical pathologic picture.

### Differential diagnosis

***Drug eruption.*** Identical clinical and microscopic findings can be produced by atabrine, chloroquine, quinidine, mercury, gold, or arsenic. Tetracycline, streptomycin, iodides, para-aminosalicylic acid (PAS), and thiazides may produce a lichen planus–like eruption. Contact with a chemical used in developing color photographs (a substituted paraphenylendiamine derivative) also produces a dermatitis resembling lichen planus in susceptible individuals.

***Psoriasis.*** Psoriasis of the acute guttate type is differentiated by its silvery white scale. It is uncommon for psoriasis to be itchy. Biopsy will establish the diagnosis.

***Early syphilis.*** The lesions of early syphilis are not pruritic and are usually present on the palms and soles. The serological test for syphilis is positive at this stage of the infection.

***Lichen simplex chronicus.*** Lichen simplex chronicus is a single, pruritic, thickened plaque that is usually unilateral and can be differentiated from hypertrophic lichen planus by biopsy.

***Leukoplakia.*** Leukoplakia presents a white thickened plaque on the mucous membrane; it does not have the gray lacy appearance of lichen planus. Later lesions of lichen planus may clinically and microscopically resemble leukoplakia.

### Treatment

First, because of the possibility of drug eruptions, the patient should be taken off all medications presently being used, and substitutions should be made for those that are essential.

Localized lichen planus often responds to topical application of glucocorticoid cream, ointment, or gel in concentrations at least equal to 1% hydrocortisone in effectiveness, under an occlusive dressing. This therapy must be maintained for a period longer than that required to only flatten and fade the lesions. There should be no sign of the lesion by the time the procedure is discontinued.

Intralesional injection of a fluorinated glucocorticoid, such as triamcinolone 5 mg./ml. in lidocaine hydrochloride, is beneficial for localized hypertrophic lesions. (See discussion on intralesional therapy.)

In cases of hypertrophic lichen planus of the legs, a firm occlusive dressing of an Unna boot type (of which there are several easily available commercial preparations), changed weekly, relieves the pruritus and produces flattening of the lesions over a period of weeks.

In patients with generalized lichen planus, systemic administration of glucocorticoids is effective in suppressing the disease. It is of great value in an acute or spreading disease. This should be given with the knowledge that when the medication is stopped, a recurrence may appear. If this happens, the glucocorticoid should be maintained at the lowest possible dose that keeps the dermatitis from recurring but produces a minimum side effect, and attempts should be made to taper off and discontinue the drug at the earliest possible moment.

For widespread lesions, the following lotion may be used in association with systemic therapy:

| | |
|---|---|
| Menthol | 0.5% |
| Phenol | 0.5% |
| Zinc oxide | 15 Gm. |
| Talc | 15 Gm. |
| Glycerin | 10 ml. |
| Alcohol | 40 ml. |
| Water | 40 ml. |

Oral lichen planus may persist for long periods. It may ulcerate. All causes of chronic irritation, for example, roughness of teeth, must be eliminated because secondary malignancy can develop with chronic irritation in the milieu.

If symptoms are present in involvement of mucous membranes, triamcinolone acetonide (Kenalog in Orabase) may be used, applied every 3 to 4 hours.

Griseofulvin, 500 mg. twice daily, has an antipruritic effect and appears to be helpful in this puzzling disease.

We find that painful oral lesions can be benefited by the use of an oral preparation as follows:

| | |
|---|---|
| Soluble betamethasone tablets | 28 |
| Zephiran hydrochloride (21.3%) | 1 drop |
| Peppermint oil | 1 drop |
| Lidocaine hydrochloride | 3% |
| Tragacanth | 4.8 Gm. |
| Distilled water to make | 120 ml. |

¼ tsp. to be swirled around mouth q.3h. (gives 0.1 mg. betamethasone per dose).

## REFERENCES

Abell, E., Presbury, D. C. G., Marks, R., et al.: Diagnostic significance of immunoglobulin and fibrin deposition in lichen planus, Br. J. Dermatol. **93**:117–124, 1975.
**This extensive review of biopsy material on 53 cases of lichen planus emphasizes cytoid body and fibrin deposits in the papillae.**

Altman, J.: Lichen planus and lichen nitidus. In Maddin, S., editor: Current dermatologic management, St. Louis, 1975, The C. V. Mosby Co., p. 200.
**A practical approach to management of this disease and some of its variants.**

Altman, J., and Perry, H. O.: The variation and course of lichen planus, Arch. Dermatol. **84**:179, 1961.
**The study and follow-up of 307 patients. One malignancy in 188 cases of oral lichen planus.**

Black, M.: The pathogenesis of lichen planus, Br. J. Dermatol. **86**:302, 1972.
**A worthwhile presentation on a not uncommon disease of unknown etiology.**

Cawson, R. A.: Oral lichen planus. In Maddin, S., editor: Current dermatologic management, St. Louis, 1975, The C. V. Mosby Co., p. 202.
**Oral betamethasone tablets, 0.1 mg., three times daily, sucked.**

Cotton, D. W. K., Van den Hurk, J. J. M. A., and Van der Staak, W. B. J. M.: Lichen planus, an inborn error of metabolism, Br. J. Dermatol. **87**:341, 1972.
**Glucose-6-phosphate dehydrogenase deficiency.**

Dilaimy, M.: Lichen planus subtropicus. Arch. Dermatol. **112**:1251, 1976.
**Annular pigmented lesions on exposed areas.**

Marks, R., Black, M., and Wilson-Jones, E.: Epidermal cell kinetics in lichen planus, Br. J. Dermatol. **88**:37, 1973.
**Epidermal cell death dominates the picture.**

Medenica, M., and Lorincz, A.: Lichen planus, "an ultrastructural study," Acta Derm. Venereol. **57**:55, 1977.
**Nuclei of epidermal basal cells and melanocytes show the initial damage.**

Romero, R. W., Nesbitt, L. T., Jr., and Reed, R. J.: Unusual variant of lupus erythematosus or lichen planus, Arch. Dermatol. **113**:741, 1977.
**Studies on 11 patients with follow-up indicate that disease cannot be definitely diagnosed and in some patients both diseases may coexist.**

Sehgal, V. N., Abraham, G. J. S., and Malik, G. B.: Griseofulvin therapy in lichen planus, Br. J. Dermatol. **87**:883, 1972.
**Double-blind well-done study that showed a positive benefit of griseofulvin.**

## CHAPTER 19

# Dermatoses produced by light

### EFFECT OF SUNLIGHT ON NORMAL SKIN

Sunlight reaching the earth's surface is composed of wavelengths above 290 nm. The shorter wavelengths are absorbed by the atmosphere. The wavelengths that produce sunburn are those from 290 to 320 nm., whereas those that produce increased tanning are above 320 nm.

Normally, the skin develops sunburn after adequate exposure to sunlight or to an artificial ultraviolet light. This consists of an *erythema* and, if severe, an acute biphasic reaction of pronounced erythema, edema, pain, and tenderness.

The initial erythema appears to be produced by histamine release, but the persistent erythema and perhaps some of the accompanying symptoms appear to be caused, in part at least, by prostaglandins, which are present in excessive amounts in sunburned areas just prior to the appearance of erythema at 48 hours, which coincides with experimental erythema produced by prostaglandin injection. Prostaglandin inhibitors, aspirin and indomethacin locally, will dramatically inhibit erythema formation. The epidermal cell is directly damaged by radiation in the sunburn spectrum, and there is evidence to suggest that the sunburn response results chiefly from epidermal cell damage. The lysosomes, which contain hydrolytic enzymes, appear to release these destructive compounds. Vesicles and then bulla formation may occur, and subsequent exfoliation appears after the acute signs subside.

Within 72 hours after exposure to sun, an increased mitotic rate in epidermal cells begins to produce a thickening of all layers of the epidermis. The increased mitosis stops within 7 to 10 days, and the thickened epidermis returns to normal in 2 months if no further sun exposure occurs.

Tanning, which develops 3 to 4 days after sun exposure, is a result of synthesis of new melanin by the intraepidermal melanocytes. This pigment is passed on to the epidermal cells, which, because of their proliferation, carry it away more rapidly than normal, with the result that the epidermal compartment contains considerably more protective pigment than normal.

Long-continued exposure to the sun will invariably result in permanent changes in the exposed areas of skin (Fig. 19-1). Persons with fair complexions and blond or red hair are especially prone to these irreversible changes, since they have less pigment-producing capacity and thus less protection than darker skinned individuals. Also, people in outdoor occupations and sunny climates characteristically develop these cutaneous effects of sun. Heat appears to accelerate this degeneration; thus hot climates may play a significant part in the production of actinic changes. Wind aggravates and speeds the changes caused by ultraviolet light.

***Actinic skin.*** The cutaneous changes caused by ultraviolet radiation are those usually associated with aging of the skin. It becomes dry, thin, inelastic, and atrophic, with premature wrinkling, telangiectasia, and areas of hyperpigmentation and depigmentation. After this, localized roughened sites of actinic keratosis make their appearance, and these premalignant lesions may then slowly progress to squamous cell carcinoma. These gross clinical changes are accompanied by histopathological findings, which include alteration of the elastic tissue and staining abnormalities of the

A

B

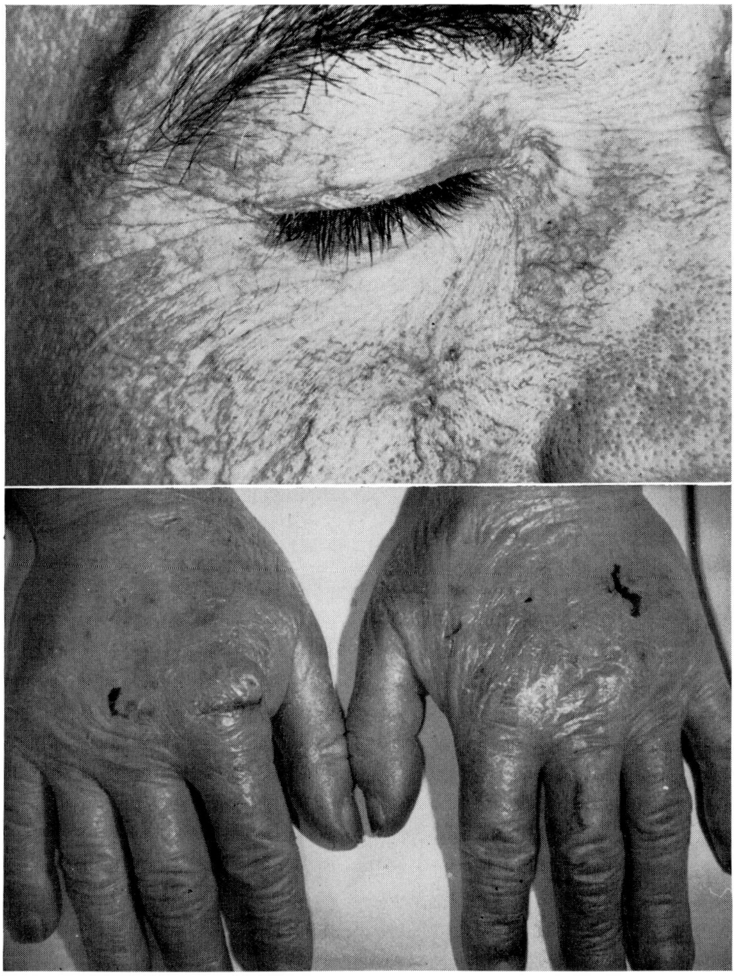

**Fig. 19-1. A,** Telangiectasia from lifelong actinic exposure. **B,** Severe actinic dermatitis. Note thinness and fragility of skin.

dermal collagen. The blood vessels may show some sclerosis and some dilatation. Epidermal cells develop evidence of disorder and depolarization, atypical features, dyskeratosis, and eventual changes. Basal cell carcinoma, squamous cell carcinoma, and also malignant melanoma all may develop in sundamaged skin. Recent work indicates that chronic actinic dermatitis is at least partly reversible.

*Protection* from ultraviolet light is afforded by a combination of factors. The stratum corneum acts as a filter to deflect the harmful rays, which in abraded areas rapidly cause cell death. The melanin situated to protect previous nuclear material absorbs light energy. Repair of damaged DNA begins. The damaged segments are neatly excised and replaced in a progressive process. Melanin production and epidermal thickening are stimulated by multiple light exposures.

## ACTINIC CHEILITIS

Certain individuals develop an acute inflammation with edema and pruritus on the lips with exposure to excessive sunlight. These persons are also more susceptible than the average individual to the chronic effects of sunlight on the lips. Excessive exposure to sunlight gradually results in an atrophic, pale,

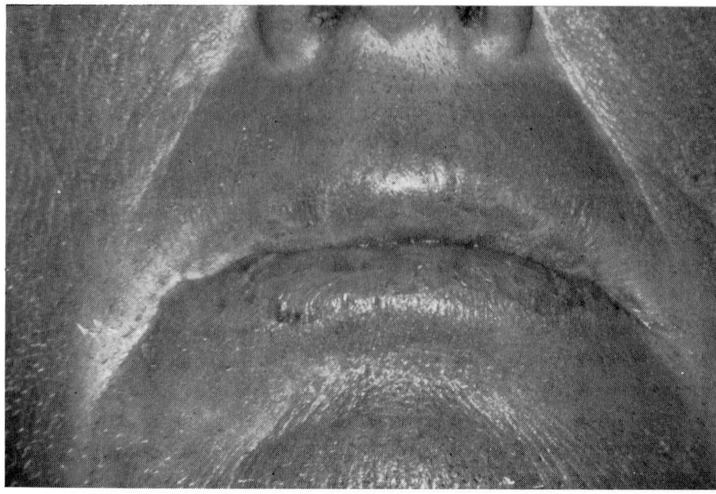

**Fig. 19-2.** Actinic cheilitis.

dry appearance of the lower lip. The membrane is scaling, fissured, fragile, and easily traumatized (Fig. 19-2).

Histologically, the epidermis is very thin and atrophic, and there are degenerative changes in the collagen and elastic tissue. These areas are predisposed to the development of carcinoma.

### *Treatment*

Protection includes remaining indoors and wearing of protective hats and opaque clothing (a surprising amount of sun penetrates the ordinary cotton shirt). Ordinary window glass stops sunrays below 320 nm.

Sunscreens (p. 262) are available in a wide variety of compounds and vehicles. Some are partially successful in filtering out burning rays and allowing a tan to occur, others are not. Para-aminobenzoic acid 5% in ethanol (Presun, Pabanol) and the benzophenones are among the most successful blocking agents.

Women subject to actinic cheilitis should wear a protective coat of opaque lipstick regularly. If the condition is far advanced, surgery to remove the affected areas of dermis and epidermis is necessary to forestall malignant degenerative changes.

## WAYS IN WHICH LIGHT CAN CAUSE CUTANEOUS DISEASE

Light is more damaging to fair whites and albinos than to the more pigmented races and people. Patients with xeroderma pigmentosum have a deficient protective mechanism. Excessive sun exposure varies for each race and individual. In whites and susceptible individuals of other races, it ultimately leads to carcinogenesis and cutaneous malignancy.

Certain chemicals, drugs, foods, plant products, and other substances taken internally or applied topically may produce damage in the skin by themselves being reactive to light. The type of reaction depends on the location of the substance in the skin and its photoreactive peculiarities. *Phototoxic* chemicals may be responsible for damaging lysosome membranes and seem to be taken up by the lysosomes. Release of hydrolytic enzymes from lysosomes to surrounding tissues would be damaging. Prostaglandins also may be involved.

Light may be responsible for the formation of compounds in the tissue that then act as *antigens*, mobilizing an immune response. This is described as a *photoallergic* phenomenon and may result from light alone, in which case it is usually limited to a specific causative wavelength, or it may involve an exogenous intermediate light reactive chemical. The causative chemical may be applied topically and absorbed, or taken internally.

### Photosensitivity

The capacity of certain chemicals to induce a cutaneous reaction to light when ingested or applied topically results from their chemical structure, which allows absorption of light. Energy is produced that is harmful to the biological tissue. The compounds responsible frequently contain three or more connected aromatic rings as a common structural configuration. They often also are fluorescent.

Photosensitizers applied topically ordinarily produce no cutaneous inflammation until light exposure to the area occurs. At a varying time after light exposure, a reaction develops, which may be erythematous, vesicular, pigmented, urticarial, or moist and weeping, coincident with the area of contact with the photosensitizer.

Some cosmetics, perfumes, or lipsticks produce a photosensitizing effect and thus an inflammatory response in association with sun exposure. The surface becomes dry, scaling, thickened and fissured, or simply pigmented.

### Persistent light reactors

Persistent reactions to light occur in some photosensitive patients, who become exceedingly sensitive to even minute exposures to light. Reversion of the skin to normal takes longer after each succeeding episode, until perpetual erythema, thickened, lichenified skin, and chronic pruritus are firmly established. As little as 20 seconds of sun exposure are sufficient to produce a reaction in sensitized patients (Willis).

#### *Topical photosensitizers*

| Substance | Use |
|---|---|
| Bithionol (Actamer) | Antiseptics |
| Tetrachlorosalicylanilide | Antiseptics |
| Dibromosalicylanilide | Antiseptics |
| Tribromosalicylanilide | Antiseptics |
| Hexachlorophene, dichlorophene | Antiseptics |
| Carbanilides | Antiseptics |
| Coal tar derivatives | Dyes, petrochemicals, pitch |
| Furocoumarins, psoralens | Essential oils, perfumes |
| Limes, other citrus fruits, figs | Food handlers |
| Parsnips, celery, parsley | Food handlers |
| Sulfonamides | Antibiotics (not used topically clinically) |

#### *Ingested photosensitizers*

| | |
|---|---|
| Chlorpromazine, chlorprothiazene | Quinine, quinidine |
| Demethylchlortetracycline | Psoralen |
| Griseofulvin | Chlordiazepoxide |
| Sulfanilamide | Cyclamates |
| Thiazide diuretics | Antihistamines |
| Sulfonylureas | |

*When a patient has a dermatitis, acute or chronic, that first affected and is still limited to exposed areas, worsens in summer or with outdoor exposure, and is intensely pruritic, the possibility of photosensitivity must be strongly considered* (Fig. 19-4, A).

## SOLAR URTICARIA

Solar urticaria consists of urticarial lesions that develop within minutes after sun exposure on exposed areas and subside within a few hours. It is analogous to the urticaria produced by drugs. Antihistaminics will reduce the reaction in some patients. In others it may be helpful to prescribe methoxypsoralen tablets, 30 to 40 mg. taken 2 hours prior to sun exposure. These persons must then go into the sun very gingerly for the first few days.

Ramsay has recommended repeated carefully calculated, multiple small daily exposures of small and then progressively larger areas of skin to fluorescent light or natural sunlight, and in so doing, tolerance can be created, inhibiting further urticaria while daily exposures are continued. Patients must be highly motivated to persist. Two of nine were completely successful, and six partly so.

Investigation should include tests for porphyrins especially red cell protoporphyrins.

There are clinical reports that suggest the use of reserpine 0.6 mg. daily, with daily increasing exposures to sunlight, is beneficial for persistent cases of solar urticaria.

## POLYMORPHOUS LIGHT ERUPTION

Polymorphous light eruption identifies a specific dermatological reaction that occurs in a distinctive pattern in certain persons, after exposure to sunlight. It is common—the commonest of the photodermatoses—and has no predilection for age or sex. Its pathogenesis is obscure, as it is not related, to our present knowledge, to any of the known mechanisms

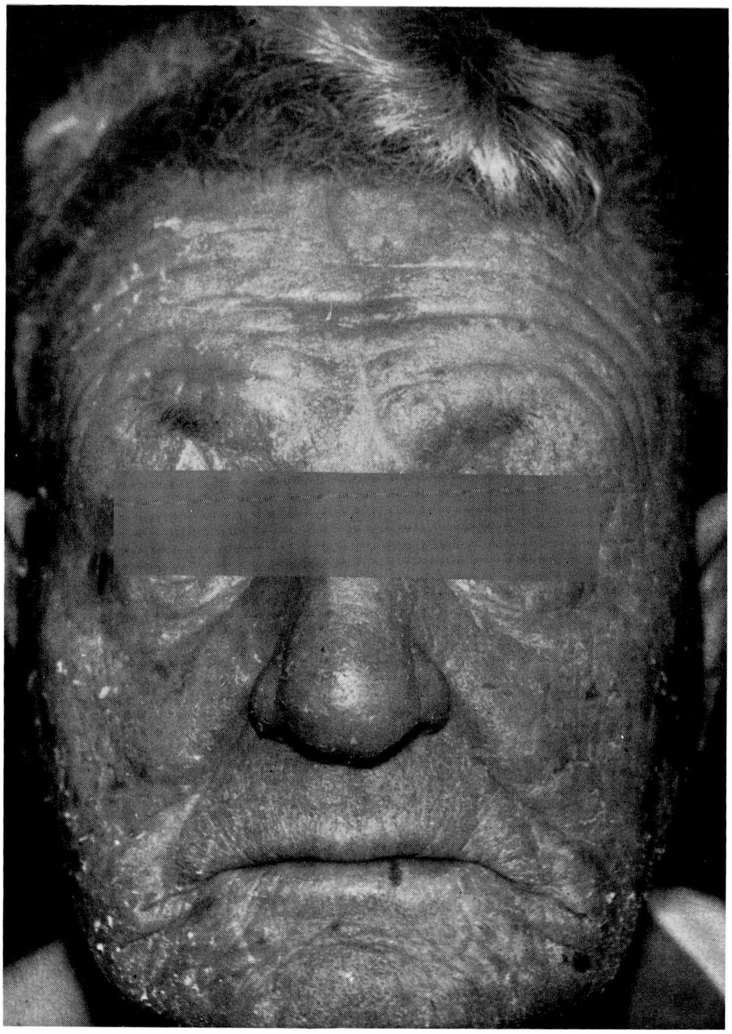

**Fig. 19-3.** Polymorphous light eruption. Vesicular lesions predominated in this man.

of light sensitivity. It is produced by light in the sunburn range and involves a superficial vascular reaction to light. It is a recurrent dermatitis that involves only exposed areas, and it is most often papular or plaquelike, although other forms occur. Vesicular and eczematous forms (Fig. 19-3) also are seen, although less frequently. The reaction appears from within 24 hours to 3 or 4 days of adequate exposure to the sun and then persists for a variable time. There is thus a time lag between exposure to the sun and the appearance of the lesions, which suggests a delayed allergic response. Without any further sun exposure, the lesions involute within 2 weeks.

The usual history emphasizes the first appearance of the dermatitis during the spring and early summer. With repeated exposures, the condition may become progressively more severe.

The lesions are small papules, large papules, vesicles, or elevated discrete erythematous lesions that appear on normal skin. They are characteristically found over the malar areas, the forehead, face, (Fig. 19-4, *B*), forearms, and dorsa of the hands. The individual lesions do not tend to change position, but recur at the same site on repeated exposures. Specific lesions will tend to reappear with sun exposure of other parts of the skin surface.

A

B

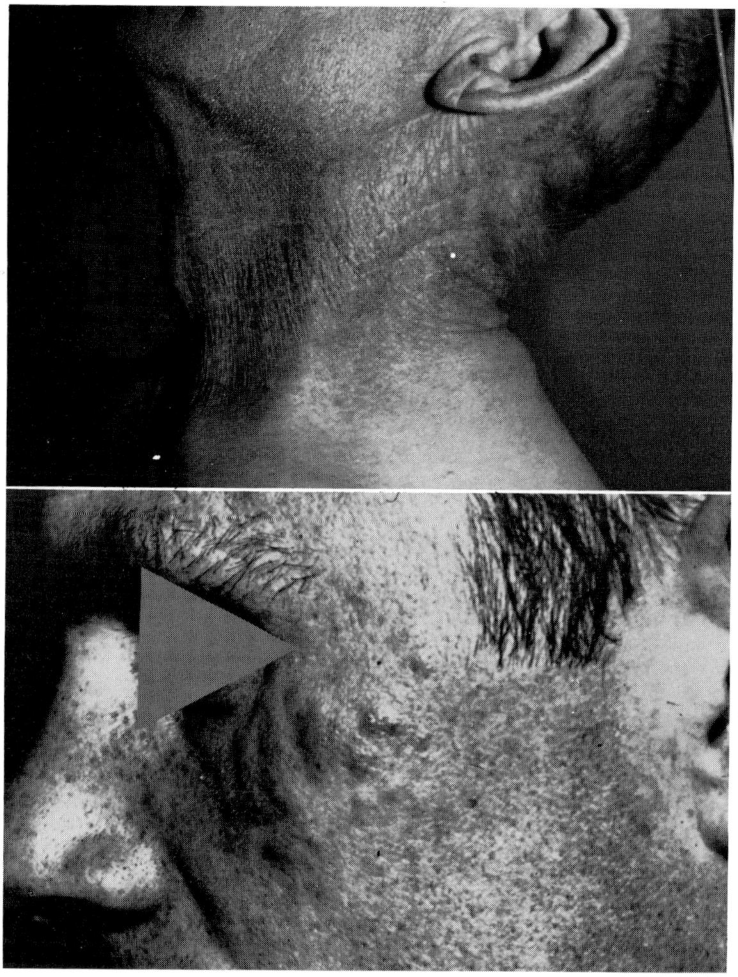

**Fig. 19-4. A,** Photosensitization. Note normal skin below collar in nonexposed area. **B,** Polymorphous light eruption. Plaques and papules predominated in this patient.

The more acute, less severe type of eruption improves as the summer progresses and once the patient is tanned. This has led to the treatment of susceptible persons by artificial tanning in small doses through the winter months in preparation for sun exposure in the spring.

Arthur Birt has described an increasing number of North American Indians subject to a polymorphous light eruption that has all of the criteria of a genetic disorder (Fig. 19-5). It affects the Indians in the central portion of the continent, extending to Central and South America (Plate 33).

There are neither associated abnormal laboratory findings nor association with photosensitizing drugs or topical medications.

The lesions can be reproduced on uninvolved skin by exposure to ultraviolet light under controlled conditions.

### *Differential diagnosis*

These lesions may resemble lupus erythematosus, lymphocytic infiltration of the skin, sarcoidosis, or contact dermatitis.

### *Treatment*

The patient should be instructed to wear suitable protective clothing, such as a broad-brimmed hat, long sleeves, high neckline,

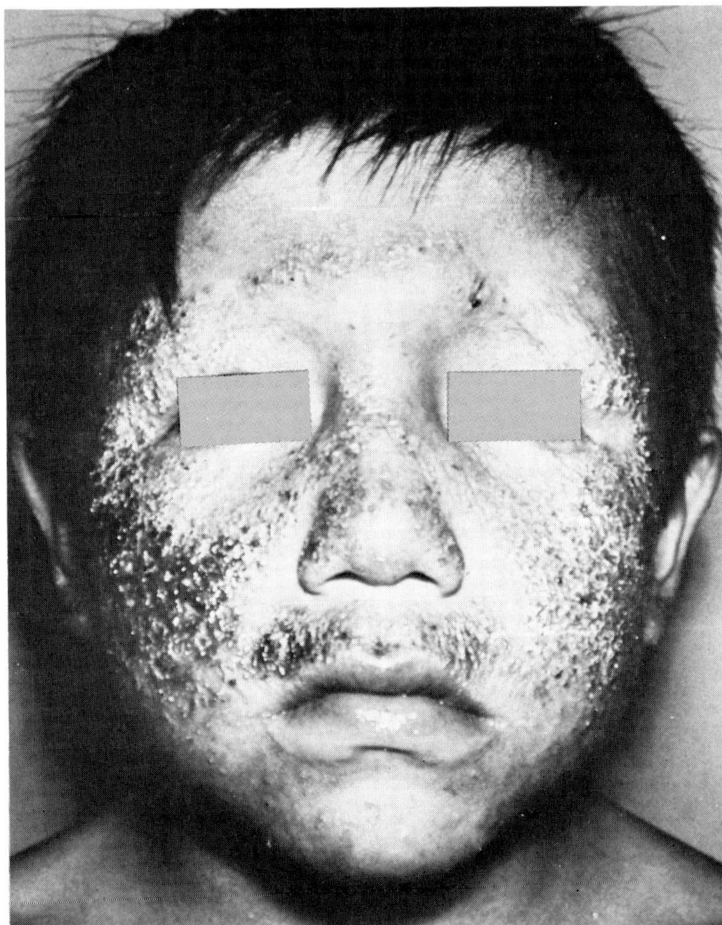

**Fig. 19-5.** Hereditary polymorphous light eruption. (Courtesy Dr. Arthur R. Birt, Winnipeg, Manitoba.)

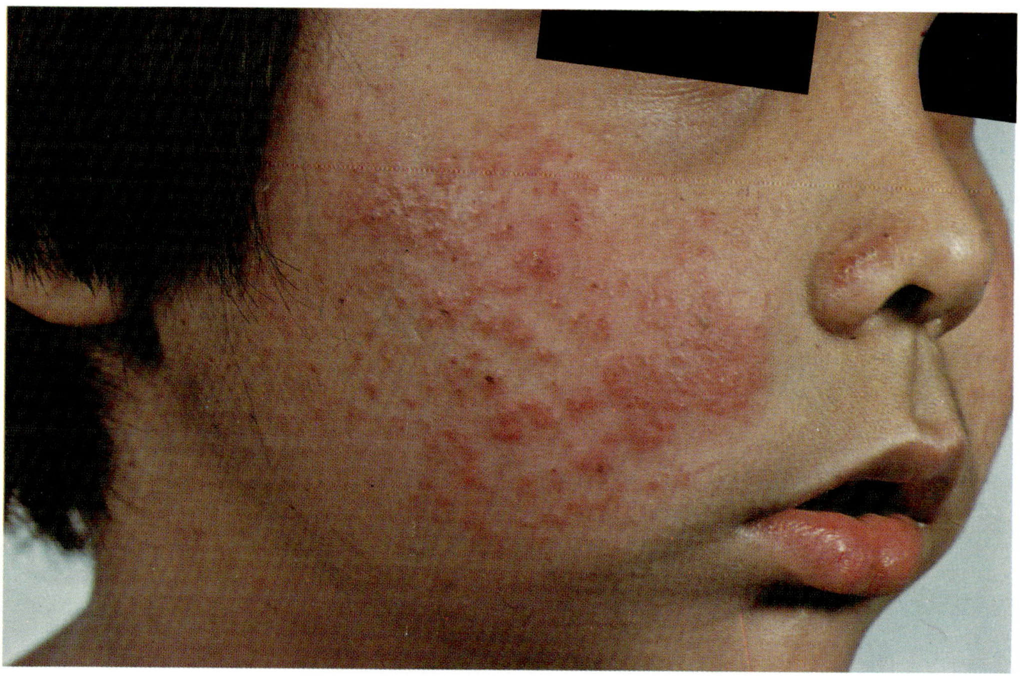

**Plate 33**

Polymorphous light eruption, papular variety. North American Indian from Central Plains.

and gloves when possible. The use of effective sunscreening preparations may be of value in protecting the face, ears, nose, and hands. Of the various protective creams, those containing opaque pigments such as titanium dioxide or zinc oxide are the most effective, although the least desirable cosmetically. Topical creams containing para-aminobenzoic acid (PABA), cinnamates, and benzophenones block the sunburning rays effectively if they are applied frequently. A good preparation is 5% PABA in ethanol. There have been reports of allergic contact dermatitis after the use of aminobenzoic acid esters and to a benzophenone sunscreen (Thompson), but the incidence of such adverse effects is very rare.

Beta-carotene in doses of 90 to 180 mg. daily has proved effective in protecting patients with erythropoietic protoporphyria from the untoward effects of the sun. The use of this drug in other photodermatoses has less benefit. It produces yellow skin discoloration and enough protection so that patients can better tolerate brief exposures. There are no side effects reported from its use.

Mathews-Roth found only one third of her patients got relief, but Swanbeck's patients did better. Thune found also that a third of his patients improved on beta-carotene.

Perhaps the most promising therapy yet reported for polymorphous light eruption is combined treatment with sulisozone, or 5% PABA in alcohol, topically and beta-carotene orally. Patients should be advised to avoid exposure between 10 AM and 4 PM, since ultraviolet radiation is at its maximum between these hours. Although not widely used, partly because of staining, dihydroxyacetone-naphthoquinone topically is also effective in some cases. (See Sunscreens, p. 62.)

The antimalarial agents such as chloroquine, hydroxychloroquine, and related drugs exert a beneficial effect on the polymorphous group of light eruptions. Their ability to stabilize lysosomes in the epidermis against damage may play a significant part in their protection against sun. They are given in dosages of 250 and 400 mg. respectively, once or twice daily. Because of their serious effect on the retina and cornea in some patients, the use of these compounds is restricted to short courses. Ophthalmological examinations should be carried out initially and at regular intervals to discover retinal effects in all patients receiving these drugs. Toxic effects do not ordinarily appear until after several weeks or months of therapy, although attempts are being made to uncover them earlier. These drugs are excreted extremely slowly.

The glucocorticoid drugs in adequate dosage are of benefit in the management of acute and severe or widespread cases of light sensitivity.

## ADVERSE EFFECTS OF SUNLIGHT ON SKIN DISEASES

***Albinism, vitiligo, phenylketonuria.*** Patients with albinism and vitiligo cannot produce pigment (melanin), and burn severely in affected areas when exposed to sunlight.

***Hartnup's syndrome.*** A rare genodermatosis, Hartnup's syndrome has cutaneous changes resembling pellagra. An inflammation on exposed surfaces is present because of the effect of sunlight.

***Herpes simplex.*** Sun exposure, like a febrile episode, can trigger an outbreak of herpes simplex.

***Lupus erythematosus (systemic and discoid).*** Some patients with lupus erythematosis report that the disease process was initiated by severe sun exposure or that exposure caused spread of the existing disease. Worsening of the disease process by sun exposure is well documented.

***Pellagra.*** In pellagra, sun-exposed areas of the body develop erythema, vesiculation, and subsequent hyperpigmentation.

***Porphyria.*** Uroporphyrin or protoporphyrin must be present in the skin before clinical signs develop, with cutaneous fragility, erythema, bullae, and vesicle formation, as well as hyperpigmentation after exposure to sunlight.

***Psoriasis.*** Although benefited by moderate sun exposure, psoriasis is made worse by actual sunburning.

***Xeroderma pigmentosum.*** Xeroderma pigmentosum is an inherited disorder in which the skin is not capable of complete repair of ultraviolet damage to intracellular DNA. It begins in childhood and is produced by exposure to sun. Early, pronounced, actinic changes, epitheliomas, skin carcinomas, and malignant melanomas result, with shortened life span.

## INVESTIGATION OF DERMATOSES PRODUCED BY LIGHT

History is probably the most significant aid to diagnosis of light sensitivity problems. Points to be elicited include age of patient at onset of the condition (porphyria, metabolic, congenital disorders), time of year the problem occurs (summer for polymorphous light eruptions, porphyria), occupation (arc welding causes photosensitivity), use of drugs, cosmetics, soaps, antiseptics (photosensitizing chemicals), and delay after sun exposure (immediate in solar urticaria, delayed in polymorphous light eruption).

Examination at the time of peak of eruption is important. A patient's description is seldom adequate. Absence of erythema in shaded areas is important to determine.

Tests that can be performed to yield pertinent information, but without sophisticated light-testing equipment, include testing with a sunlamp and photopatch testing.

### Testing with sunlamp exposure

Testing to the sunburn range of visible light is possible by use of a standard hot quartz therapeutic sunlamp. The erythema response to a test dose must be known for the lamp used, as well as the composition of the wavelengths produced, so that one can determine if there is an abnormal response to a standard dose. This is indicated in minimal erythema dose (MED). To prove a polymorphous light eruption, the dermatitis should be reproduced by the test dose. All areas not to be tested must be carefully shielded.

### Photopatch testing

To test for photosensitivity, materials suspected of causing contact photosensitivity are applied to the skin in two areas. One is covered, the other is exposed to a suberythemal dose of ultraviolet light beyond the sunburn range. A reaction under the light-exposed patch demonstrates photosensitivity if the covered patch is negative.

#### REFERENCES


Birt, A. R., and Davis, R. A.: Hereditary polymorphic light eruption of American Indians, Int. J. Dermatol. **14**:105, 1975.
**Now up to 128 patients with similar disability.**

Eaglestein, W. H., and Weinstein, G. D.: Prostaglandin and DNA synthesis in human skin: possible relationship to ultraviolet light effects, J. Invest. Dermatol. **64**:386, 1975.
**Prostaglandin $E_2$ and histamine probable mediators of the ultraviolet light–induced inflammation 48 hours after exposure.**

Epstein, J. H. Adverse cutaneous reactions to the sun. In Malkinson, F. D., and Pearson, R. W. editors: Year book of dermatology Chicago, 1971, Year Book Medical Publishers, Inc., p. 5.
**A good source of information.**

Epstein, J. H.: Ultraviolet carcinogenesis. In Giese, A. C., editor: Photophysiology, vol. 5, New York, 1970, Academic Press, Inc., p. 235.

Goldyne, M. E.: Prostaglandins and cutaneous inflammation, J. Invest. Dermatol. **64**:377, 1975.
**Since 1960, revelations of prostaglandin activity from effects of chemicals, ultraviolet light, immunogens, and trauma. Activity is transient and has vascular and cellular effects.**

Harber, L. L.: Reflections and perspectives concerning cutaneous photobiology, Arch. Dermatol. **112**:1668, 1976.
**An informative and challenging précis of the field of photobiology.**

Horio, T., and Minami, K.: Solar urticaria. Photoallergen in a patient's serum, Arch. Dermatol. **113**:157, 1977.
**A review of the immunological aspect of this uncommon form of photoallergy.**

Jung, E. E.: Sun and skin, Dermatologica **151**:257, 1975.
**A brief exposition in perspective.**

Kobza, A., Ramsay, C. A., and Magnus, I. A.: Oral β-carotene therapy in actinic reticuloid and solar urticaria: failure to demonstrate photoprotective effect against long wave ultraviolet and visible radiation, Br. J. Dermatol. **88**:157, 1973.
**Failure of beta-carotene to give photoprotection to five patients tested, despite high carotene levels.**

Mathews-Roth, M. M., Pathak, M. A., Fitzpatrick, T. B., et al.: Beta-carotene therapy for erythropoietic protoporphyria, and other photosensitivity diseases, Arch. Dermatol. **113**:1229, 1977.
**Oral beta-carotene is effective in protecting patients with erythropoietic protoporphyria, less so with other light disorders.**

Swanbeck, G., and Wennersten, G.: Treatment of polymorphous light eruptions with beta-carotene, Acta Derm. Venereol. **52**:462, 1972.
**Good response of eight patients.**

Thompson, G., Maibach, H. I., and Epstein, J.: Allergic contact dermatitis from sunscreen preparations complicating photodermatitis Arch. Dermatol. **113**:1252, 1977.
**Aminobenzoic acid ester and a benzophenone caused the dermatitis.**

Thune, P.: Chronic polymorphic light eruption—particular wavebands and the effect of carotene therapy, Acta Derm. Venereol. **56**:127, 1976.
**Some patients benefited from combined beta-carotene and topical PABA therapy.**

## CHAPTER 20

# Metabolic disorders

## PORPHYRIA

Porphyria is an inherited metabolic disease in which the cutaneous forms are accompanied by an increased sensitivity to sunlight. It has been proposed that the unfortunate patients with congenital porphyria were the origin of the tales of werewolves.

### *Pertinent information*

One of the most fascinating epidemiological tales in medicine is the tracing of 200 genetic pedigrees involving porphyria to a single pair of Dutch immigrants by Dean.

The metabolic disorder in the various forms of porphyria results in sizable increases in the excretion of porphyrins. One of the characteristics of these precursors of hemoglobin is that they combine readily with metals. The chief sites of their metabolism are in the part of bone marrow concerned with erythropoiesis and in the liver, and they are for the most part normally excreted in the bile. If they are produced in excess and cannot be handled, they overflow into the blood, subcutaneous tissues, and urine, where tests can be performed to identify them. Cutaneous lesions in those patients with porphyria who are exposed to sunlight are caused by the presence of *uroporphyrin* or *protoporphyrins* within the skin. Asymptomatic cases occur.

The porphyrin precursors, porphyrinogens (see chart, p. 372) are not photosensitizers. Only after their oxidation to porphyrins in each step are they able to absorb light and dissipate this energy in fluorescence, heat, motion, and chemical changes with peroxide release and inflammation produced: this is the photosensitivity reaction we see in the skin in porphyria, where the light-absorbing compound, uroporphyrin, is present in the dermis.

Certain acquired diseases, such as hematological disorders, hepatic cirrhosis, hepatic tumors, diabetes, and hepatic disease, are capable of giving rise to increased porphyrin excretion.

Alcohol has a deleterious effect in all hepatic porphyrias, and estrogens, tolbutamide, and chloroquine have an adverse effect in porphyria cutanea tarda. Of the common drugs, estrogens, diphenylhydantoin, griseofulvin, meprobamate, barbiturates, and sulfonamides are offenders as precipitating factors of acute intermittent and variegate porphyria.

Laboratory studies of blood, urine, and feces for porphyrins delineate the pattern by which each of the types of clinical disease is identified, in conjunction with the history and physical examination of the patient.

In addition to the abnormal porphyrins, the serum iron level, iron-binding capacity, and saturation percentage are altered as a result of the disorganized manufacture of hemoglobin, particularly in porphyria cutanea tarda. Heme apparently acts as a feedback inhibitor to the formation of δ-aminolevulinic acid (ALA), an early component in the manufacture of heme.

### *Microscopic findings*

Exposed skin, even if grossly normal, possesses dermal amorphous periodic acid—Schiff (PAS) positive deposits. Hyaline material of similar nature is present in superficial pericapillary distribution and thickened dermoepidermal-basement membranes. The microscopic anatomy is significantly similar in all the porphyric states (Epstein).

*Chain of formation of porphyrins to heme manufacture*

**Glycine** ↘ ↙ **Succinyl coenzyme A**

**Glycine succinate**

\+

δ-aminolevulinic acid synthetase

↓

**δ-aminolevulinic acid**

\+

δ-aminolevulinic acid dehydratase

↓

**Porphobilinogen**

\+

Uroporphyrinogen III synthetase and cosynthetase

↓

**Uroporphyrin III** ← **Uroporphyrinogen III**

\+

Uroporphyrinogen III decarboxylase

↓

**Coproporphyrinogen III**

\+

Coproporphyrinogen III oxidase

↓

**Protoporphyrin**

\+

Ferrochelatase

\+

**Iron**

↓

**HEME**

**Porphobilinogen**

\+

Uroporphyrinogen I synthetase

↓

**Uroporphyrinogen I** → **Uroporphyrin I**

\+

Uroporphyrinogen I decarboxylase

↓

**Coproporphyrinogen I**

↓

**Coproporphyrin I**

### *Classification*

Each of the clinical types of porphyria arises because of a biochemical block or enzyme abnormality in the normal chemical chain of formation of heme prior to its combination with globin to form hemoglobin. Most of these blocks are identified or predicted, but final elucidation of all the abnormalities has not quite been accomplished.

The porphyrias can be most readily classified as follows:

1. Erythropoietic protoporphyria—hereditary, dominant
2. Congenital erythropoietic porphyria—hereditary, recessive
3. Hepatic porphyria
   a. Acute intermittent porphyria—hereditary, dominant
   b. Porphyria cutanea tarda (symptomatic)—hereditary, dominant
   c. Porphyria cutanea tarda (latent)—hereditary, dominant
   d. Variegate porphyria (mixed porphyria)—hereditary
4. Others
   a. Turkish porphyria from ingested fungicide—acquired
   b. Bantu porphyria possibly from ingested wines—acquired

***Erythropoietic protoporphyria.*** The disease occurs as soon as 2 years after birth and is inherited as an autosomal dominant trait. The urine is normal, but there is a greater elevation in protoporphyrin levels in the stools and in the red blood cells. Thus the diagnostic tests include examination of the *stools* and *red blood cells* for protoporphyrins. Photosensitivity is the important feature, since sunlight exposure produces a burning pain or pruritus *within 30 minutes*. The exposed areas then develop urticarial wheals, plaques, small crusted vesicles, and eventually the signs of a chronic lichenified dermatitis.

The areas characteristically affected are nose, vermilion border of lips, dorsa of hands, outer ears. Long-standing cases show scarring and waxy thickening of skin in prominent areas. The liver has recently been implicated as a contributor to the excess protoporphyrins and indeed as the cause of death in this disease.

Children with this disease learn early the discomfort associated with sun exposure and, by their own choice, play outside only in the shade and in the evening.

This disorder may be confused with polymorphic light eruptions, atopic dermatitis, photosensitivity dermatitis from other causes, and milder forms of epidermolysis bullosa. Fourteen or more deaths have now been attributed to the deposition of protoporphyrin and subsequent fibrosis.

***Congenital erythropoietic porphyria.*** A very rare disorder, congenital erythropoietic porphyria appears in early infancy. Patients do not survive to middle age. Photosensitivity is striking, and the cutaneous changes are severe. Both teeth and bones demonstrate a red fluorescence. Many circulating erythrocytes show fluorescence. Splenomegaly is pronounced. Urinary and plasma uroporphyrin and fecal coproporphyrin levels are elevated. The urine turns red on standing.

***Acute intermittent porphyria.*** Drugs are by far the most important provocative agents in this form of porphyria, which has an autosomal dominant inheritance. Studies of relatives of patients demonstrate abnormal porphyrin excretion.

The defect here is related to deficient uroporphyrinogen synthetase activity, thus with uroporphyrin, coproporphyrin, δ-aminolevulinic acid, and porphobilinogen in the urine.

Acute intermittent porphyria occurs most frequently in persons from 25 to 30 years of age. The dermatological signs are neither striking nor important. The major clinical features include severe abdominal pain, gastrointestinal tract symptoms, muscle weakness, and central nervous system disturbances. All symptoms of the disease may result from the central and peripheral spinal and autonomic neuropathological changes recorded. Demyelinization is present.

Certain drugs, such as barbiturates, sulfonamides, griseofulvin, meprobamate, diphenylhydantoin, and estrogens, are capable of precipitating an attack. These drugs are contraindicated in this disease.

*The diagnosis is established by the presence*

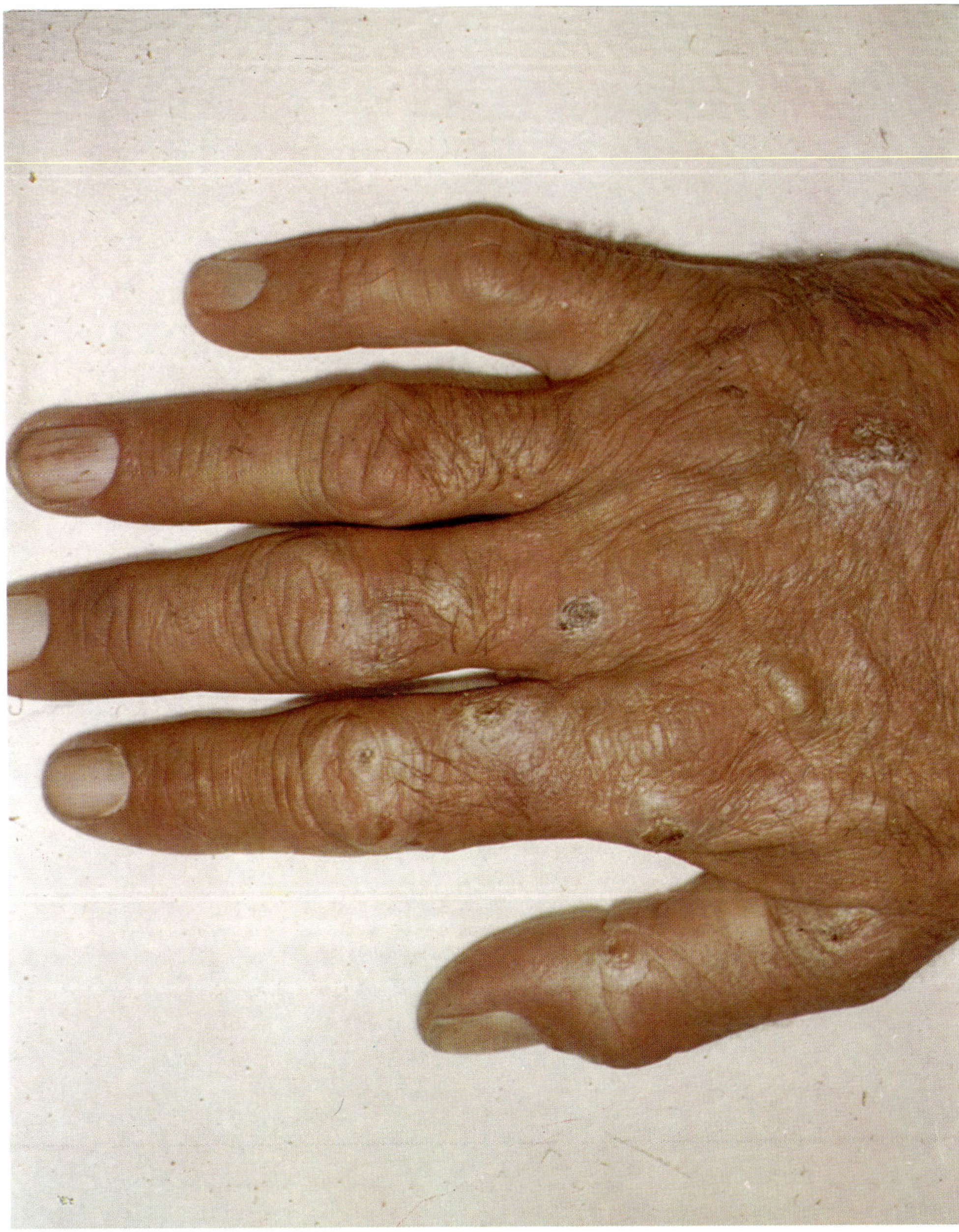

**Plate 34**

Porphyria cutanea tarda. Vesicles, blisters, crusts, and scars occur from light exposure.

*of urinary porphobilinogen in increased amounts.* If the urine is allowed to stand, it frequently becomes a port-wine color or nearly black and may stain clothing. It fluoresces red under ultraviolet light. Porphobilinogen and δ-aminolevulinic acid levels are elevated in the plasma and urine.

***Porphyria cutanea tarda (symptomatic).*** The symptomatic type of porphyria cutanea tarda (Plate 34) is of major dermatological interest in North America. Its most striking clinical manifestation is photosensitivity. Hepatic dysfunction and alcoholism are associated with this form of the disease. It occurs in both

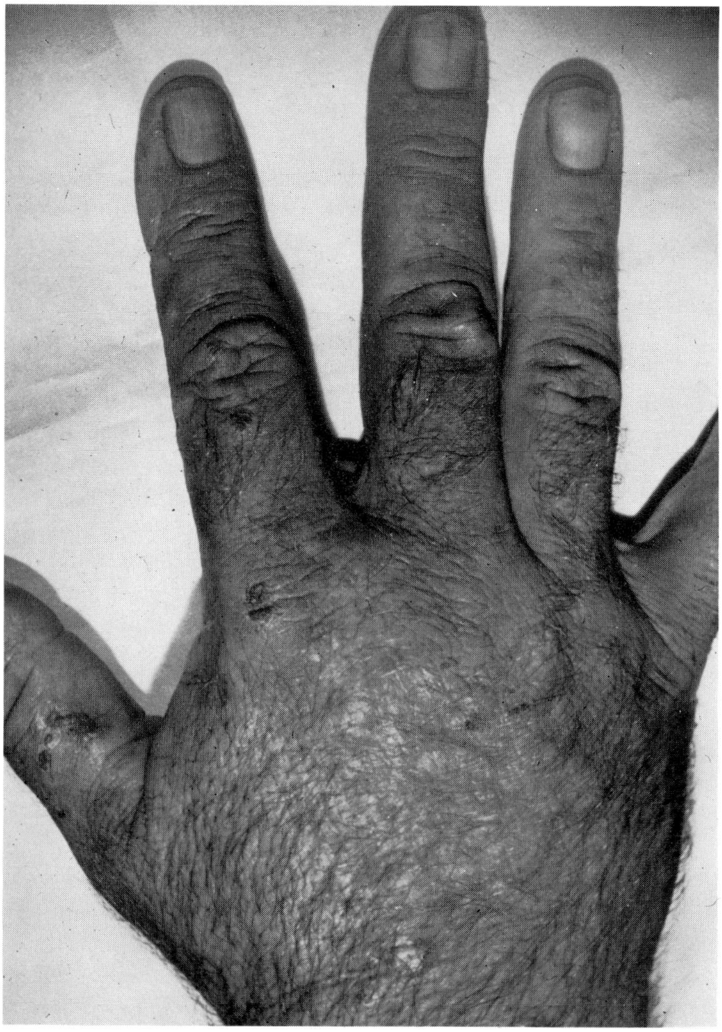

**Fig. 20-1.** Porphyria cutanea tarda, with fragility of skin, hyperpigmentation, and bulla formation.

sexes almost equally, in the 30- to 50-year age group. Porphyria cutanea tarda is reported to be attributable to the combination of an inherited defect in uroporphyrinogen decarboxylase and uroporphyrinogen cosynthetase and an acquired factor, usually siderosis associated with alcoholic liver disease. The disease is latent until there is an excessive accumulation of hepatic iron stores, which explains some clinical features. Kushner and colleagues recently were able to demonstrate that uroporphyrinogen decarboxylase was deficient in six patients with porphyria cutanea tarda, and in unaffected members of the families of three patients with the disease as well. This indicates more than one factor is responsible for revealing the latent disease. One may consider high alcohol ingestion, estrogenic hormones, chloroquin, griseofulvin, and iron as possibilities.

After sun exposure or minor trauma, the affected areas become red, vesicles appear, and not infrequently bullae are produced in the fragile skin. Affected areas are the face, neck, and backs of the hands (Fig. 20-1). Hyperpigmentation, along with a tendency to easy abrasion, is present. Areas of atrophy, along with pigmented scars, usually become apparent over the exposed surfaces. Excessive facial hair growth is another feature. *There is a sharp increase in urinary uroporphyrin and some increase in coproporphyrin.* There is also a derangement of iron metabolism with iron overloading, high serum iron and iron saturation, and polycythemia. Abnormal liver function tests have been reported in most cases, and certainly everything points to deranged hepatic function as the important site of the altered metabolism that results in excessive porphyrins. Necrosis, fibrosis, siderosis, fatty infiltration, and porphyrin deposition have been reported. Diabetes mellitus is present in almost one fourth of these patients.

Infrequently, porphyria cutanea tarda may be found in association with internal malignancies.

Certain chemicals and drugs besides alcohol have been reported to trigger this disease. Hexachlorobenzene, chloroquine, griseofulvin, estrogens, iron, chlorinated insecticides, and phenylhydrazine have been shown to precipitate acute attacks.

It has been proposed that cellular lysosomes in the skin are deranged by the action of irradiated porphyrin compounds, resulting in vesicular and bullous lesions.

MICROSCOPIC FINDINGS. Vascular damage and the deposit of amorphous PAS-positive material in vessel walls close to the effect of ultraviolet light, that is, the superficial dermis, are the result of excessive circulating porphyrins. Epstein believes that these are diagnostic features to experienced eyes and are common to four forms of porphyria reported (1973).

DIFFERENTIAL DIAGNOSIS. The vesicular, bullous, and easily traumatized skin of the patient with prophyria cutanea tarda is limited to exposed areas of the dorsa of hands and wrists, face, and neck. It is often hyperpigmented and has excessive hair growth.

It may be confused with contact dermatitis from airborne allergens, photosensitivity reactions from other causes, epidermolysis bullosa, plant dermatitis, and pellagra.

***Porphyria cutanea tarda (latent).*** Kushner's demonstration of the unrevealed disorder in family members of patients with hepatic porphyria would indicate a latent asymptomatic form of the disease. What such a case would require to produce symptoms is not clear.

***Variegate porphyria (mixed porphyria).*** Mixed porphyria is relatively common in South Africa, occurring as a dominant hereditary disease. The clinical features of both *acute intermittent porphyria* and *porphyria cutanea tarda* occur. In the United States there are somewhat different features to the disease. Patients with mixed porphyria do not appear so far to have a genetic background and may show symptoms of either the acute intermittent or cutaneous disease. There are episodes of abdominal pain, dark urine, and neuropsychiatric changes, while the cutaneous changes worsen on sun exposure, even in remissions. These patients must be carefully differentiated from individuals with acute abdominal problems requiring surgery. Urinalysis shows *elevation of both porphobilinogen and uroporphyrin levels during acute attacks. Fecal protoporphyrin is increased even in remissions, a diagnostic sign.*

### *Diagnosis of cutaneous porphyrias*

Harber describes three rapid tests for red cell porphyrins in erythropoietic protoporphyria, two rapid urinary tests for uroporphyrins, and a rapid test for urinary porphobilinogen.

The following is a correlation of laboratory tests with types of porphyria:

1. *Urine examination for uroporphyrins* (porphyria cutanea tarda and congenital porphyria) and *porphobilinogen* (variegate porphyria)
2. *Stool examination for protoporphyrins* in suspected variegate porphyria, if urine examination is negative (increase of porphyrins in feces in all cutaneous porphyrias)
3. *Examination of erythrocytes for fluorescence,* which is transient, with the fluorescence becoming exhausted after 10 to 15 seconds and with 5% to 30% fluorescing (congenital porphyria and erythropoietic porphyria)

4. *Examination of blood for porphyrins* (erythropoietic porphyria and congenital porphyria)
5. *Liver function tests,* (erythropoietic protoporphyria in late stages, porphyria cutanea tarda, and variegate porphyria)
6. *Serum iron and total iron binding capacity* (porphyria cutanea tarda and variegate porphyria)

### Treatment

***Erythropoietic protoporphyria.*** Beta-carotene (Solatene), orally in doses of 60 to 180 mg. daily, to produce a serum level of 500 to 600 mg./100 ml. and an orange discoloration of the skin, which protects from the causative wavelengths enough to allow most patients with erythropoietic protoporphyria at least three times more sun exposure than that before the drug.

It is not recommended to try to attain these levels of carotenemia by the ingestion of yellow vegetables. Leukopenia and methemoglobinemia have resulted.

***Porphyria cutanea tarda.*** Alcohol and drugs producing exacerbations must be strictly avoided. Complete abstinence from alcohol has led to loss of symptoms and signs of skin fragility. Phlebotomy provides the most satisfactory method of management in patients demonstrating porphyria cutanea tarda or variegate porphyria. At approximately 2-week intervals, 500 ml. of blood is removed until the hemoglobin levels approach 12 Gm./100 ml. Maximum therapeutic benefit was not observed until 6 to 12 months after phlebotomy in Ramsay's trials. Signs of skin fragility and photosensitivity disappear, and the remission appears to be prolonged. Some patients will require retreatment. Hypertrichosis is more resistant.

Chloroquine in relatively low doses has been shown to produce an excretion of uroporphyrin from the liver, with rather extreme speed if the dose is too high. Worrisome signs or worsening of the disease may occur. This should only be used by one with a thorough knowledge of the pathophysiology and pharmacology involved.

Alkalinization of urine to a pH range of 7 to 8 by sodium bicarbonate, 2 tablets, 0.65 Gm., taken orally for more than 3 months, causes increased excretion of the photoactive chemical and relief of cutaneous symptoms. Metabolic alkalinization produced no benefit in two cases of erythropoietic porphyria (Günther's disease) as reported by Stretcher.

### REFERENCES


Bopp, C., Peres, M., Kosminski, B., et al.: Sclerodermaform porphyria cutanea tarda combined with cataracts. Med. Cutan. Iber. Lat. Am. **3**:149, 1975.

**Sclerodermoid changes in exposed areas of scalp, ears, and face, with bilateral nuclear cataracts.**

Brodie, M. J., et al.: Enzyme abnormalities in the porphyrias, Lancet **2**:699, 1977.

**Six authors state that each of the porphyrias represent a different inborn error in metabolism involving hematologic biosynthesis.**

Christensen, K. N., and With, T. K.: Latent cutaneous porphyria, type PCT, in a Caucasian woman, Am. J. Med. **53**:517, 1972.

**Now seen as proof of a genetic origin.**

Dean, G.: The porphyrias. A story of inheritance and environment, London, 1973, Pitman Medical Publishing Co.

**As compelling as any adventure story.**

Eales, L., and Dowdle, E. B.: Clinical aspects of the porphyrias, Br. J. Clin. Pract. **22**:505, 1968.

**A thorough clinical description of these diseases.**

Epstein, J. H., Tuffanelli, D. L., and Epstein, W. L.: Cutaneous changes in the porphyrias: microscopic study, Arch. Dermatol. **107**:689, 1973.

**An excellent compendium of histopathologic material from 40 patients concerning the manifestations of porphyria that are similar and diagnostic in four forms of porphyria.**

Harber, L. C., and Bickers, D. R.: The porphyrias: basic science aspects, clinical diagnosis and management. In Malkinson, F. D., and Pearson, R. W., editors: Yearbook of dermatology, Chicago, 1975, Year Book Medical Publishers, Inc., p. 9.

Kushner, J. P., Barbuto, A. J., and Lee, G. R.: An inherited enzymatic defect in porphyria cutanea tarda: decreased uroporphyrinogen decarboxylase activity, J. Clin. Invest. **58**:1089, 1976.

**Assayed in liver and red blood cells, the enzyme defect was present in families as well as patients with PCT. Subclinical porphyria was revealed in two families.**

MacDonald, D. M., and Nicholson, D. C.: Erythropoietic protoporphyria. Hepatic implications, Br. J. Dermatol. **95**:157, 1976.

**Liver damage corresponds to crystalline protoporphyrin deposits and develops insidiously with minor labo-**

**ratory alteration. Death has occurred in 14 patients.**

Piomelli, S., Lamola, A. A., Poh-Fitzpatrick, M. B., et al.: Erythropoietic protoporphyria and lead intoxication. Molecular basis for difference in cutaneous photosensitivity. Parts I and II, J. Clin. Invest. **56**:1519, 1528, 1975.

**Rewarding cellular biology studies that show mechanisms of protoporphyrin pileup in lead poisoning, iron deficiency, and EPP.**

Ramsay, C. A., Magnus, I. A., Turnbull, A., et al.: Treatment of porphyria cutanea tarda by venesection, Q. J. Med. **43**:1, 1974.

**A technique suggested by Ippen and first reported in 1961 for the management of PCT has been brought up to date and clinically quantitated. Photosensitivity correlated with uroporphyrin levels.**

Scholnick, P. L., Epstein, J., and Marver, H. S.: Molecular basis for the action of chloroquin in porphyria cutanea tarda, J. Invest. Dermatol. **61**:226, 1973.

**Porphyrins form a unique molecular intracellular complex with chloroquine and produce a massive porphyrinuria.**

Stretcher, G. S.: Erythropoietic porphyria, Arch. Dermatol. **113**:1553, 1977.

**Negative therapeutic report on two cases in which metabolic alkalinization has been used.**

The etiology of werewolves, editorial, Can. Med. Assoc. J. **90**:648, 1964.

**A tragic vignette of our attitudes.**

Ying, C., Parrish, J. A., and Pathak, M. A.: Additive erythemogenic effects of middle (280-320 nm.) and long (320-400 nm.) wave UVL, J. Invest Dermatol. **63**:273, 1974.

**Time, course, and intensity of erythema differs in ultraviolet light from different wavelengths. These effects can be shown to be additive, a finding that might explain some light-induced phenomena.**

## XANTHOMATOSES

There is a group of disorders of lipid metabolism that result in the deposition of small amounts of fat in cutaneous lesions *(xanthomas)*. The fat is intracellular, within histiocytes, and forms a variety of lesions.

It is now known that familial derangements of serum lipids are best classified on the basis of paper electrophoresis and analytical ultracentrifugation, rather than as elevations of serum cholesterol, triglycerides, or phospholipids. Although the latter grouping satisfies a chemical subdivision of the serum lipids, the newer Fredrickson classification by lipoprotein groups is a functional and genetic one. Different lipoprotein groups contain varying amounts of triglycerides and cholesterol. Fredrickson has classified familial hyperlipidemias into five types designated I to V.

Cutaneous xanthomas, the clinical manifestations of the dyslipidoses, can be related to elevations of the three lipid components: cholesterol, triglycerides, and phospholipids. This relation is useful in the diagnosis of secondary xanthomas arising as a result of pancreatitis, myxedema, diabetes, liver disease, and so forth.

Clinical descriptions of the xanthomas are as follows:

1. *Xanthelasma.* Yellow, flat, asymptomatic plaques are found on the eyelids. Fifty percent demonstrate normal lipids, 50% elevated serum lipids.
2. *Xanthoma tuberosum and tendinosum.* The predominant lesions are nodules and tumors, yellow to brown or reddish, on the extensor surfaces of the body. They occur on points of pressure, tendon sheaths, dorsa of hands and feet, and some internal organs (Fig. 20-2). Elevated serum cholesterol level or triglycerides, or both.
3. *Tuberoeruptive xanthomas.* The predominant lesion is papular, flatter and less prominent than nodules of xanthoma tuberosum, reddish to yellow in color, small, and grouped or isolated. It is usually found on the neck (Plate 35), axillae, inguinal folds, and trunk. Mucosal surfaces can be involved as well. Elevated triglyceride level.
4. *Eruptive xanthomas.* Raised erythematous to pale papular lesions, usually with an erythematous halo, appearing suddenly in large numbers. They may appear on buttocks, legs, arms, and trunk (Fig. 20-3). Elevated triglyceride level.
5. *Palmar xanthomas.* Yellow nodules and irregular plaques on palms and fingers. Familial hyperlipoproteinemia types II and III.
6. *Palmar crease xanthomas.* Yellow, flat streaks on the creases of fingers, toes, palms, and soles. Elevated serum cholesterol or triglyceride level.
7. *Plane xanthomas.* Yellow plaques and

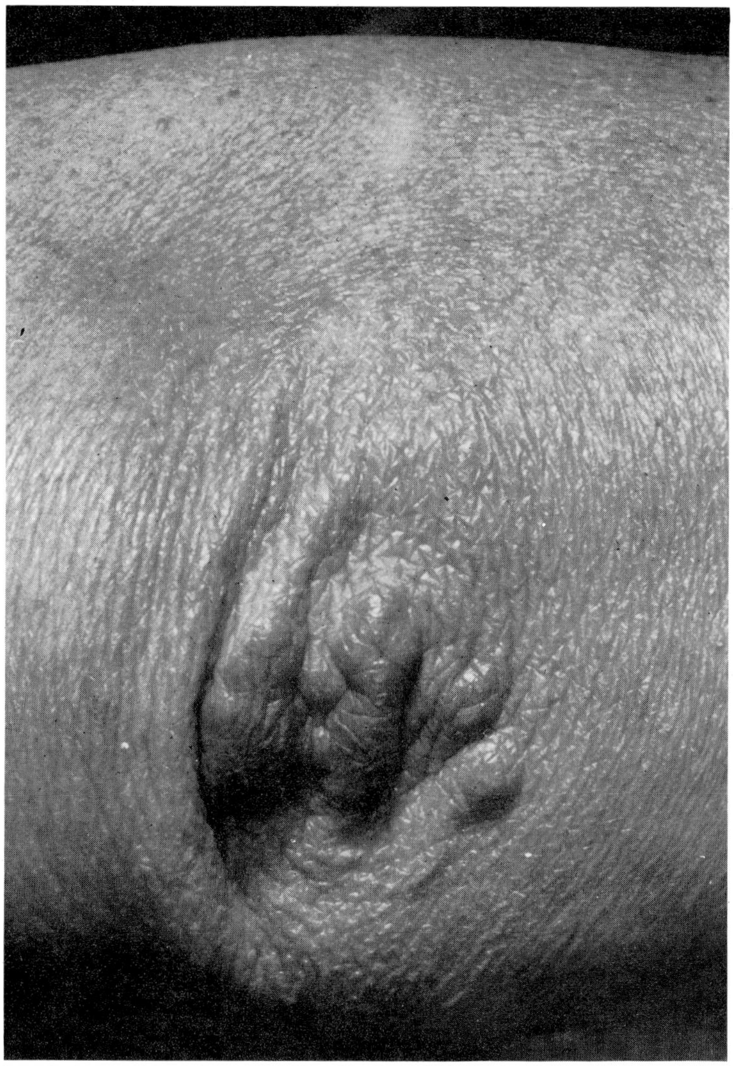

**Fig. 20-2.** Xanthoma tuberosum, with nodules of elbow.

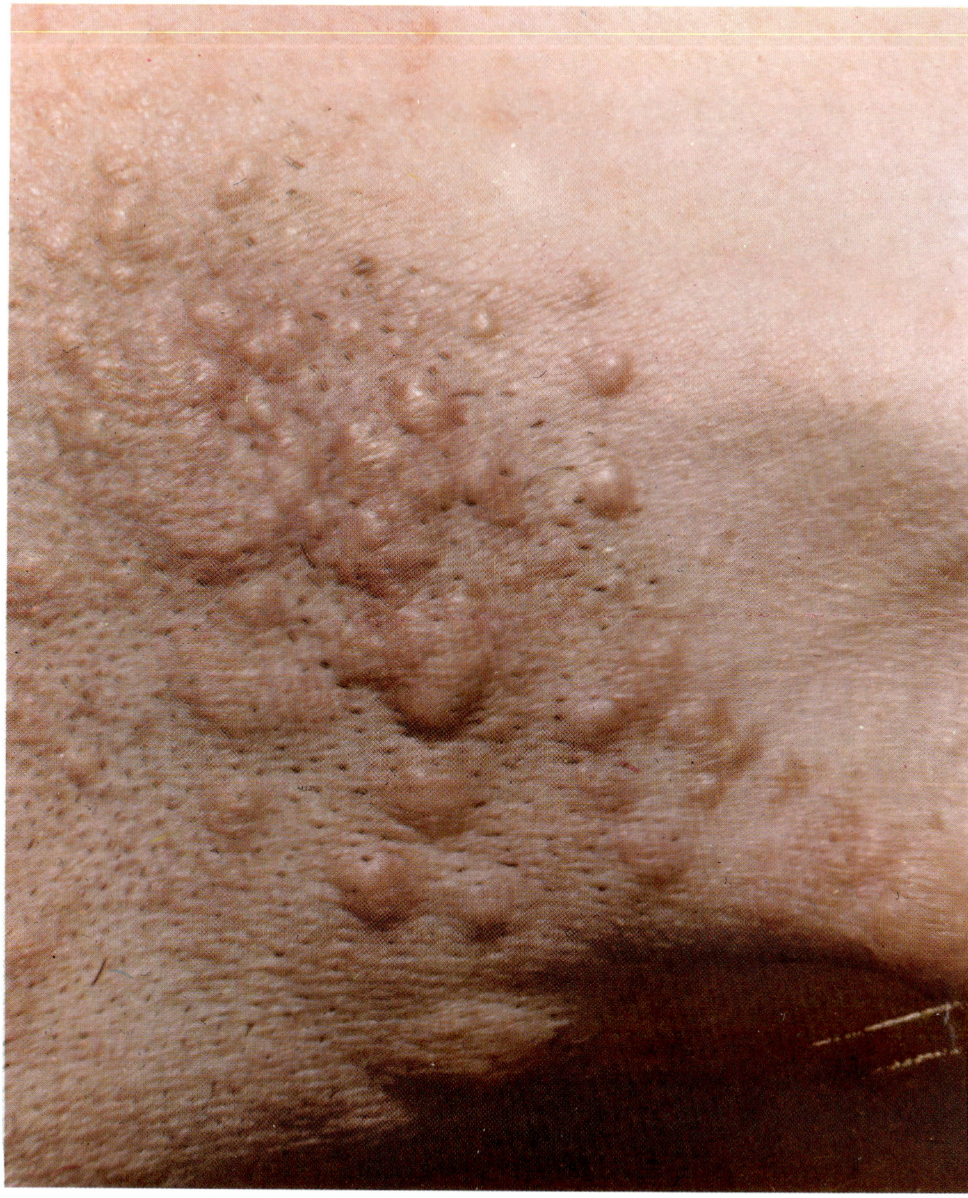

**Plate 35**

Papular xanthomas.

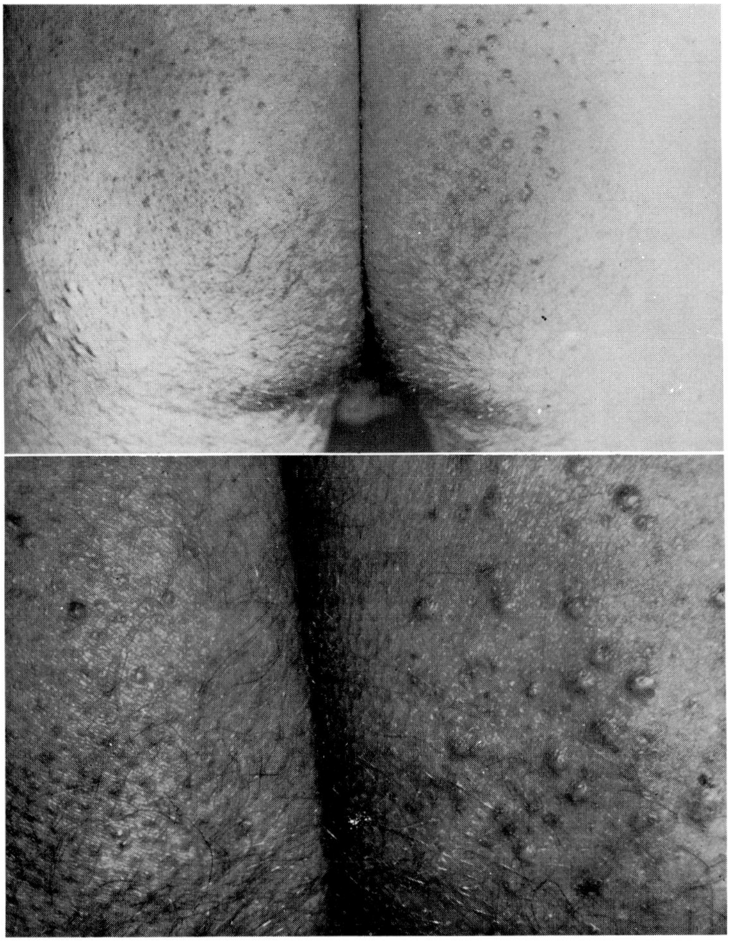

**Fig. 20-3.** Papular xanthomas involving buttocks.

patches, slightly indurated, on the neck, chest, palms, and trunk. Serum may be normal or may have elevated lipid level. Liver disease, myeloma, and leukemia.

The diseases that produce these xanthomas are most easily considered in two categories: those in which an elevated serum lipid fraction is present and those in which serum lipids are normal.

*Investigation*

The following procedures are involved in the investigation of all disorders of lipid metabolism:

1. Causes of secondary hyperlipidemias ruled out
2. Skin biopsy of xanthoma
3. Examination of serum for turbidity
4. Serum cholesterol
5. Serum triglycerides
6. Phospholipids
7. Lipoprotein electrophoresis
8. Glucose tolerance test

## Xanthomas with increased serum lipids

### Essential familial hypercholesterolemia (type II hyperlipoproteinemia of Fredrickson and colleagues)

Essential familial hypercholesterolemia is a hereditary disorder of cholesterol metabolism that may or may not be associated with cutaneous lesions. It is an autosomal dominant trait with a highly penetrant inheritance.

The xanthomas that may appear are *xanthelasma* and tendon xanthomas; papules, nodules, and plaques of *xanthoma tuberosum* (Fig. 20-2). They may also appear in the palmar creases. Corneal arcs are present. The lesions may commence at any age, and they appear to have no sexual predilection.

The course of the disease leads to widespread vascular involvement and cardiovascular renal disease. Coronary occlusion is common.

Serum cholesterol levels are elevated, as are the beta-lipoproteins. Plasma triglycerides are normal. Plasma is not milky.

### Microscopic findings

Microscopically, there is xanthoma or foam cells in the lesions. These are histiocytes filled with lipid droplets. The cells are in large aggregates, often together with some inflammatory cells.

This pattern may also be seen with liver disease, nephrotic syndrome, myeloma, hypothyroidism, and macroglobulinemia.

### Treatment

Individual nodules or plaques may be removed by surgery or electrodesiccation if they are large, tender ulcerating, or unsightly. Lesions may tend to recur in the scar, however.

Maintenance of an ideal weight and a diet low in cholesterol and in vegetable fats are desirable. Clofibrate (Atromid-S) may be of benefit. Other drugs in use are cholestyramine, D-thyroxine, and nicotinic acid.

## Essential familial hyperlipemia (type I hyperlipoproteinemia of Fredrickson and colleagues)

Essential familial hyperlipemia is a very rare hereditary disorder of lipid metabolism that results in a delayed clearing of chylomicrons from the serum. It is frequently recognized in those less than 20 years of age and may be seen in infants.

Xanthelasma is common in this disorder. A lipemia of the retina is apparent on ophthalmological examination, and there is a corneal arcus of fatty substance, as in arcus senilis. Eruptive *xanthomas* may be associated. Other important features include abdominal pain (possibly caused by pancreatitis), hepatosplenomegaly, and cardiovascular involvement. The serum is milky on examination. Plasma triglycerides are elevated and serum cholesterol is essentially normal. There is delayed removal of absorbed chylomicrons from the serum.

### Microscopic findings

Microscopic findings are similar to those in other xanthomas.

### Treatment

Treatment consists of reduction of the serum fat levels with a low-fat diet and avoidance of excessive carbohydrate intake.

## Carbohydrate-induced hyperlipoproteinemias (types III, IV, and V of Fredrickson and colleagues)

Carbohydrate-induced hyperlipoproteinemias are forms of abnormal lipid transport that are combined because there are common features. The disorders are all accentuated by carbohydrate ingestion. Tendinous and tuberous xanthomas, xanthelasma, and corneal arcus are present. In type III of Fredrickson and colleagues, small elevated palmar-crease xanthomas occur as a distinctive feature. Tuberoeruptive and eruptive xanthomas may be seen. Abdominal pain may be a feature of the disease.

Plasma cholesterol is elevated, as well as the triglycerides. The pre–beta-lipoprotein level is elevated. The serum is turbid. The glucose tolerance test is abnormal.

### Treatment

Ideal weight should be maintained, and a low-carbohydrate, low-cholesterol diet with addition of unsaturated fat may be indicated. The xanthomas will disappear on the proper regimen.

Clofibrate may be indicated, depending on the response to diet therapy. Nicotinic acid and D-thyroxine are also used.

## Xanthelasma

Xanthelasma (Plate 36) is the most common type of xanthoma and usually is an isolated

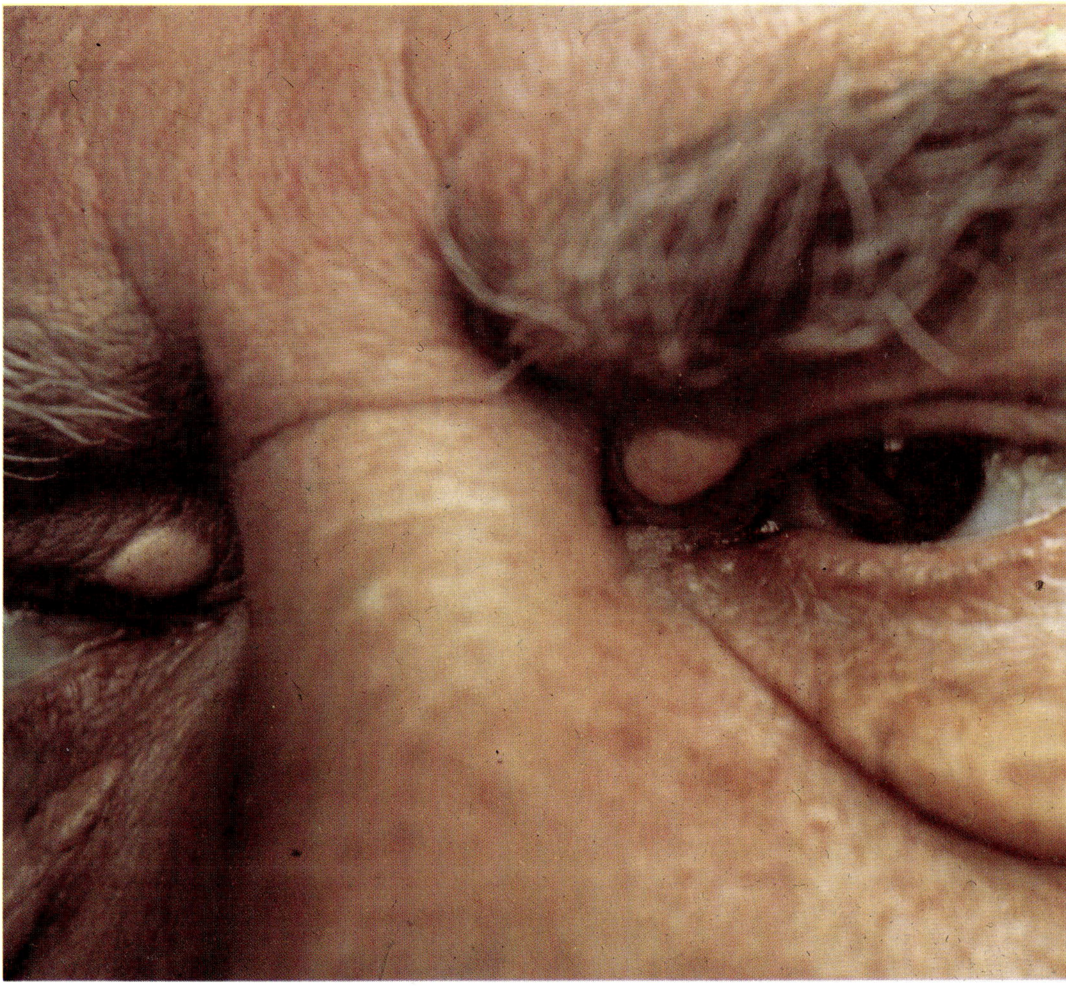

**Plate 36**
Xanthelasma.

lesion. The flat yellow plaques are on upper and lower eyelids and do not extend beyond the orbital area. The lesion may be small, or it may be large enough to cover more than half the eyelid. Xanthelasma is essentially asymptomatic and nonulcerating. At least half the individuals possessing xanthelasma have an abnormal elevation of some fraction of the serum lipids. At least one third of the patients have a family history of clinically apparent cardiovascular disease.

Women are affected more often than men, although they are less likely to demonstrate hyperlipidemia.

***Treatment***

It must be determined whether a recognizable underlying abnormality of serum lipids is present. If so, suitable treatment is initiated.

Surgical excision is not difficult in patients with small plaques and with loose eyelid tissue. There may be recurrences.

Trichloracetic acid application is frequently used, although it must be done *with great care*. The acid must be applied with a wooden orange stick only moistened, not overloaded, with the acid, and it must be applied just to the borders of the lesion, not on normal skin.

There may be no recurrence for several years, if at all.

### Biliary cirrhosis (and obstructive extrahepatic jaundice)

*Plane xanthomas, palmar crease and palmar xanthomas* may appear, relative to elevation of the serum cholesterol. Spider angiomas appear in longstanding cases. Jaundice is present, in association with other clinical findings of obstructive liver disease. Cholestyramine may be effective therapy in reducing the xanthomas, but it is primarily for relieving the associated pruritus.

***Hypothyroidism.*** Papular xanthomas are seen rarely in the hypercholesterolemia associated with myxedema.

### Diabetes mellitus

Eruptive xanthomas may occur in uncontrolled diabetes. There is moderate to pronounced elevation of serum triglycerides, and the serum is milky. Cholesterol is elevated. With control of the diabetes, the cutaneous lesions disappear quite promptly.

### Pancreatitis and lipid nephrosis

Rarely, pancreatitis and lipid nephrosis may be associated with xanthomas. One or more fractions of the serum lipids are elevated.

### Glycogen-storage disease (type I)

Type I glycogen-storage (von Gierke's) disease is a hereditary disorder of childhood, typically manifested by a fat face and an obese abdomen. There may be elevation of cholesterol, triglycerides, and phospholipids. The serum is milky. There may be eruptive xanthomas. The underlying difficulty is in faulty carbohydrate metabolism and increased fat mobilization.

## Xanthomas with normal serum lipids

### Reticuloendothelioses

Papular xanthomatous lesions occur with certain disorders of the reticuloendothelial system. These diseases include Letterer-Siwe disease, Hand-Schüler-Christian disease and eosinophilic granuloma, which are considered to be parts of the more inclusive entity of histocytosis X. Xanthoma dissemination and juvenile xanthogranulomas are sometimes also considered in the reticuloendothelioses.

### Histiocytosis X

Histiocytosis X is a hyperplasia of the reticuloendothelial system, usually involving the skin, bones, lungs, nervous system, and possibly other organs.

The disease usually begins in childhood. The severe forms affect infants and may rapidly progress to death. In the benign forms, adults are first affected, and lesions may be single, asymptomatic, and nonprogressive. Because of the nature of the reticuloendothelial system and its presence in virtually every organ and tissue, any such tissue may be involved.

Cutaneous lesions consist of seborrheic dermatitis–like, greasy, crusted, erythematous macules and papules, which may ulcerate. These affect the scalp, abdomen, chest, back, inguinal area, and axillae. There are purpuric lesions and xanthomas that are usually small, multiple, and papular (Plate 37).

Systemic lesions consist of hepatosplenomegaly, lymphadenopathy, pulmonary infiltrates, bone cysts, and exophthalmos.

Space-occupying pituitary fossa lesions and cranial involvement may lead to diabetes insipidus. This is present in severe forms of the disease.

Laboratory findings include anemia, thrombocytopenia, and normal serum lipids.

Skin biopsy of characteristic lesions will establish the diagnosis.

It is not clear whether this is a form of malignant proliferation or a benign hyperplastic reaction of the reticuloendothelial system to an unknown stimulus. The relationship to fat metabolism and xanthomas is also obscure.

#### *Microscopic findings*

Microscopic examination reveals infiltration of affected areas by large, pale, reticuloendothelial cells and giant cells in very large numbers, associated with an inflammatory

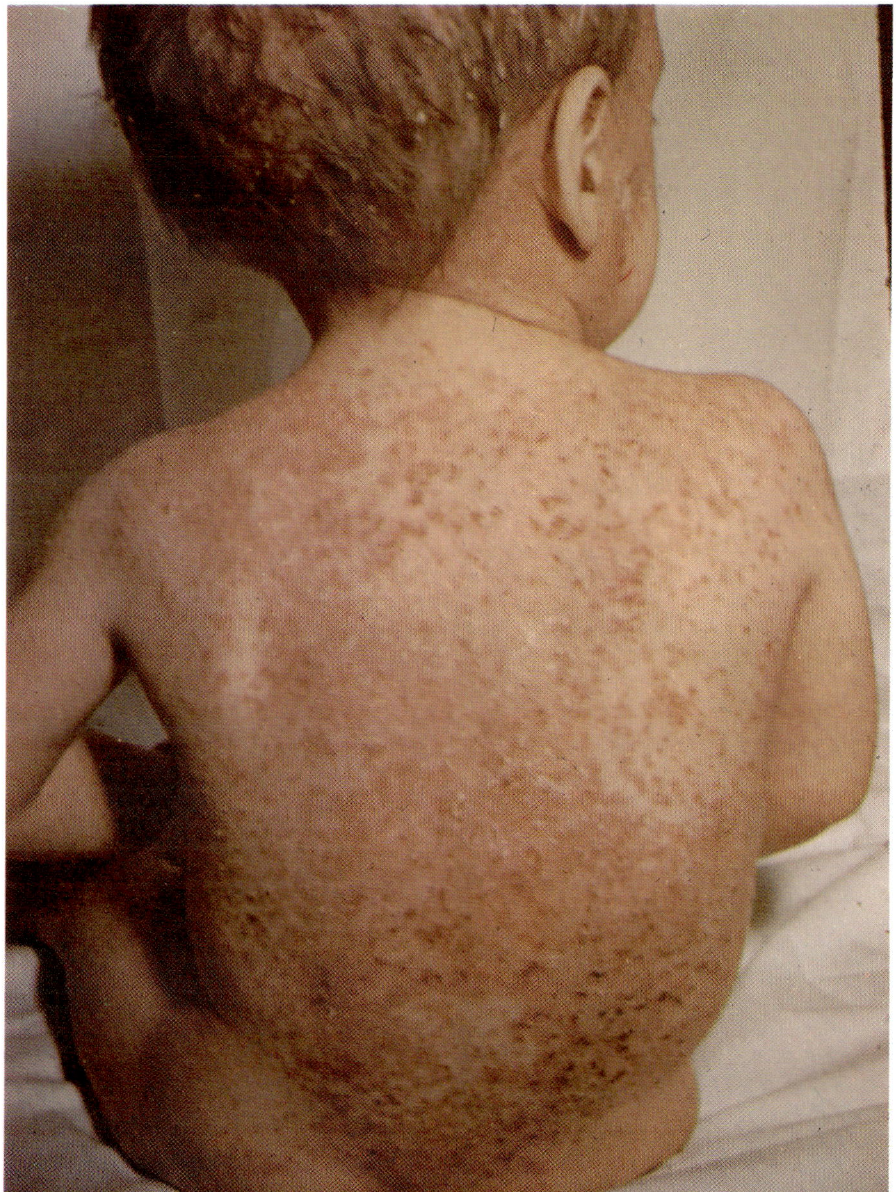

**Plate 37**

Histiocytosis X.

reaction of eosinophils, plasma cells, and neutrophils.

### *Treatment*

Treatment includes antibiotics, topical and systemic adrenocorticosteroids, cytotoxic medications, vasopressin (Pitressin), judicious x-ray therapy, and supportive care, individualized to the specific case.

## Xanthoma disseminatum

A rare, nonhereditary disease that appears to be essentially a proliferative disorder of the monocyte-macrophage system, with secondary lipid accumulation in the skin and elsewhere.

There is a predilection for papular and plane xanthomas to affect the flexural surfaces of neck, axillae, inguinal folds, eyelids, and thorax. There may be mucosal lesions infiltrated plaques. This is a long-standing chronic disorder.

There is said to be no effective treatment, although Mishkel and his colleagues believed that clofibrate was helpful in their patient.

## Juvenile xanthogranuloma

Xanthomas in the form of papular yellow to yellow-orange lesions occur on the face, neck, trunk, and extremities in the first 6 months of life. There may rarely be ocular complications. The disease usually resolves spontaneously without therapy.

### REFERENCES

Bhattacharyya, A. K., Connor, W. E., Mansoff, F. A., et al.: Turnover of xanthoma cholesterol in hyperlipoproteinemia patients, J. Lab. Clin. Med. **87**:503, 1976.
**Xanthomas exchange lipids with plasma. Esterification may occur in xanthoma cells with return to plasma.**

Fleischmajor, R., and Schragger, A. H.: The clinical significance of cutaneous xanthomas, Postgrad. Med. J. **46**:671, 1970.
**An excellent account of normolipemic and hyperlipoproteinemic cutaneous xanthomas.**

Frederickson, D. S., Levy, R. I., and Lees, R. S.: Fat transport in lipoproteins—an integrated approach in mechanisms and disorders, N. Engl. J. Med. **276**:32, 94, 148, 215, 273, 1976.
**The classic in which the various xanthomatoses are classified on the basis of genetic as well as lipoprotein group.**

Mishkel, M. A.: Xanthoma and xanthomatosis. In Maddin, S., editor: Current dermatologic management, ed. 2, St. Louis, 1975. The C. V. Mosby Co. p. 314.
**A most practical and clinically oriented presentation.**

Mishkel, M. A., Cockshott, W. P., Nazir, D. J., et al.: Xanthoma disseminatum. Clinical, metabolic, pathologic, and radiologic aspects, Arch. Dermatol. **113**:1094, 1977.
**Thirteen-year follow-up of a basically histiocytic proliferative disease with secondary lipid accumulation.**

Sims, D. G.: Histiocytosis X, Arch. Dis. Child. **52**:433, 1977.
**Follow-up studies on 12 of 29 survivors of 43 cases of histocytosis presenting in children under 12 years.**

## CHAPTER 21

# Mucous membrane diseases

## EXAMINATION OF MOUTH

An examination of the mouth is seldom done either systemically or consistently. A successful eight-step routine to develop as a habit for this examination follows: (1) Check the lips and vermilion borders, together with the angles and internal commissures. (2) Examine the labial mucosa by holding and everting each lip with a gauze pad; at this point, the tongue is protruded to the right. (3) Grasp the tip with gauze and gently pull further to the right while examining, with the aid of a tongue blade, the left side of the base of the tongue and the floor of the mouth (an important area). (4) Do the same for the right side; the patient then touches the palate with the tip of the tongue, as far posteriorly as possible. (5) This further exposes the vital mouth floor for red or white discolorations; the central gingiva can be seen thus with great clarity. (6 and 7) Again use a tongue blade for each buccal mucosa and lateral vestibule, and (8) tonsillar pillars and posterior pharyngeal wall. A gloved finger should be used whenever suspicious or curious lesions are revealed.

## APHTHOUS STOMATITIS

The lesions that compose aphthous stomatitis are discrete, often recurrent, small superficial ulcerations of the oral mucous membranes. They occur singly or in small groups, last for a few days, and heal without scarring. They are painful, but ordinarily do not become infected, bleed, or produce other complications.

The typical lesion is 2 to 5 mm. in size and is surrounded by a ring of erythema. It is often on the inner surface of the lip, in the vestibule, or on the tongue or buccal mucosa. It may be beneath the tongue or, less often, on the palate. It begins as a reddened, small macule that develops a gray-white center, which ulcerates (Fig. 21-1). The ulcer is exceedingly painful. The course of individual lesions is from 1 to 2 weeks. There is no lymphadenopathy. The microscopic appearance is nonspecific, although the earliest lesions demonstrate lymphocytic infiltration, and a subsequent vasculitis may be present.

The disorder may appear at regular intervals indefinately, one lesion after the other. There may be recurrences associated with the menstrual cycle. Ulcers may also occur on the genitalia, rectal or perianal areas, eyes, or larynx. Behçet's disease may be difficult to differentiate.

### *Pertinent information*

The cause of recurrent aphthous ulcers is unknown. Herpesvirus has been isolated from intraoral herpetiform mucous membrane lesions that, however, are clustered, 1 to 2 mm. in diameter, and round and have a shorter duration. Intranuclear inclusions are not recorded. Many authorities now consider the most likely cause to be a delayed hypersensitivity reaction, possibly autoimmune. Some recent investigations of lymphocyte transformation and lymphocytoxicity of patients' cells toward oral mucosal cells would strengthen this concept. Immunosuppressive agents and immunopotentiating drugs have both been beneficial in treatment.

The cause is possibly multifactorial, because cases have been reported from contact allergens (proved by patch testing), bacteria (streptococci), and immunogens. There appears to be a familial susceptibility to some observers (Ship), and HL-A B12 antigen frequency may be significantly increased.

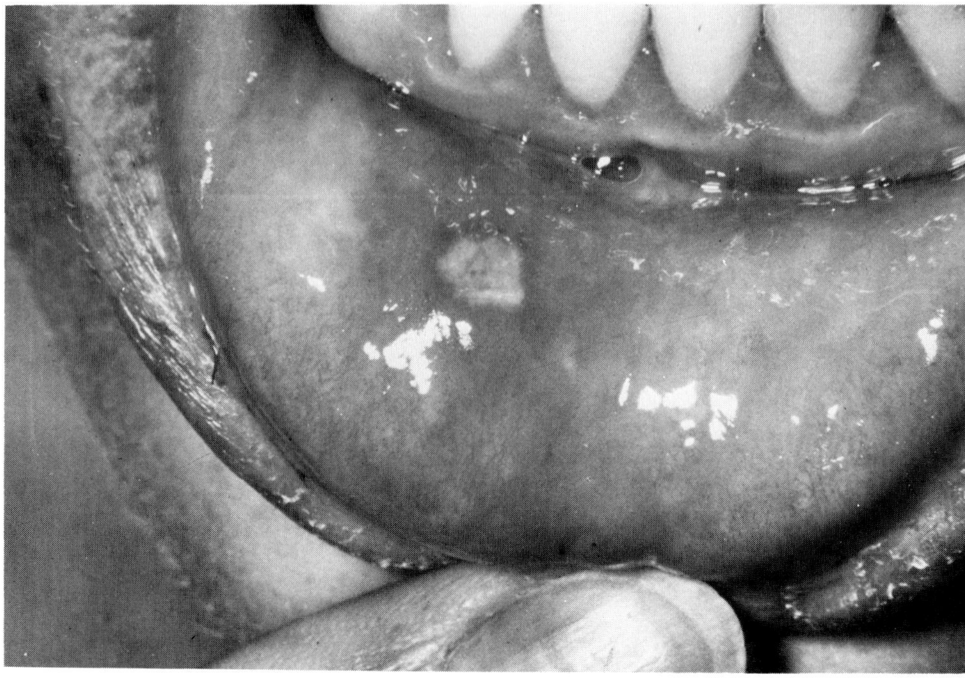

**Fig. 21-1.** Aphthous stomatitis. Gray-white center with erythematous halo.

*Differential diagnosis*

***Behçet's disease.*** This disease has many similar features, but there are systemic overtones, including eye, skin, vascular, joint, neurological, and gastrointestinal lesions which form a quite different prognosis. The lesions on the oral mucous membrane may be identical to aphthous ulcers. There are genital mucosal lesions, iritis, uveitis, and noduloulcerative, cutaneous lesions as well. Minor skin damage may produce inflammation and ulceration. HL-A antigens are different in Behcet's disease and in aphthous ulceration. There is a 75% association with HL-A B5 in Behçet's disease but not in aphthous ulcers.

***Necrotizing gingivitis.*** Raw ulcerated areas covered by a gray pseudomembrane are present on the gum margins and oral mucous membrane. There is a fetid odor to the breath. Transmissable. Probably of bacterial origin.

***Stevens-Johnson syndrome.*** In children and young adults, the Stevens-Johnson form of erythema multiforme produces acute erosions and vesicles on lips, tongue, and oral mucosa, as well as on genital and ocular mucous membranes. The patient may be severely ill (Plate 38). (See p. 212).

***Pemphigus.*** In pemphigus, bullae appear on the skin after the first appearance of erosions on the oral mucosa (p. 133).

***Herpes gingivostomatitis.*** Primary infection is usually seen in children, associated with fever, malaise, and local lymphadenopathy. Gingivitis and multiple small lesions in oral mucosa are present. The gingiva is fiery red, swollen, and may be covered with a serofibrous exudate. Lasts 10 days to 2 weeks. There is good evidence that herpetiform ulcers are recurrent intraoral forms of herpes simplex with clusters of minute vesicles (Weathers).

***Reiter's disease.*** In about 10% of cases of Reiter's disease, after episodes of gonorrheal or nonspecific urethritis there may develop rusted erythematous lesions of the glans penis and erosive lesions of the oral mucosa. The palms and soles may have pustular involvement, followed by brown, crusted lesions. Arthritis is a feature as well.

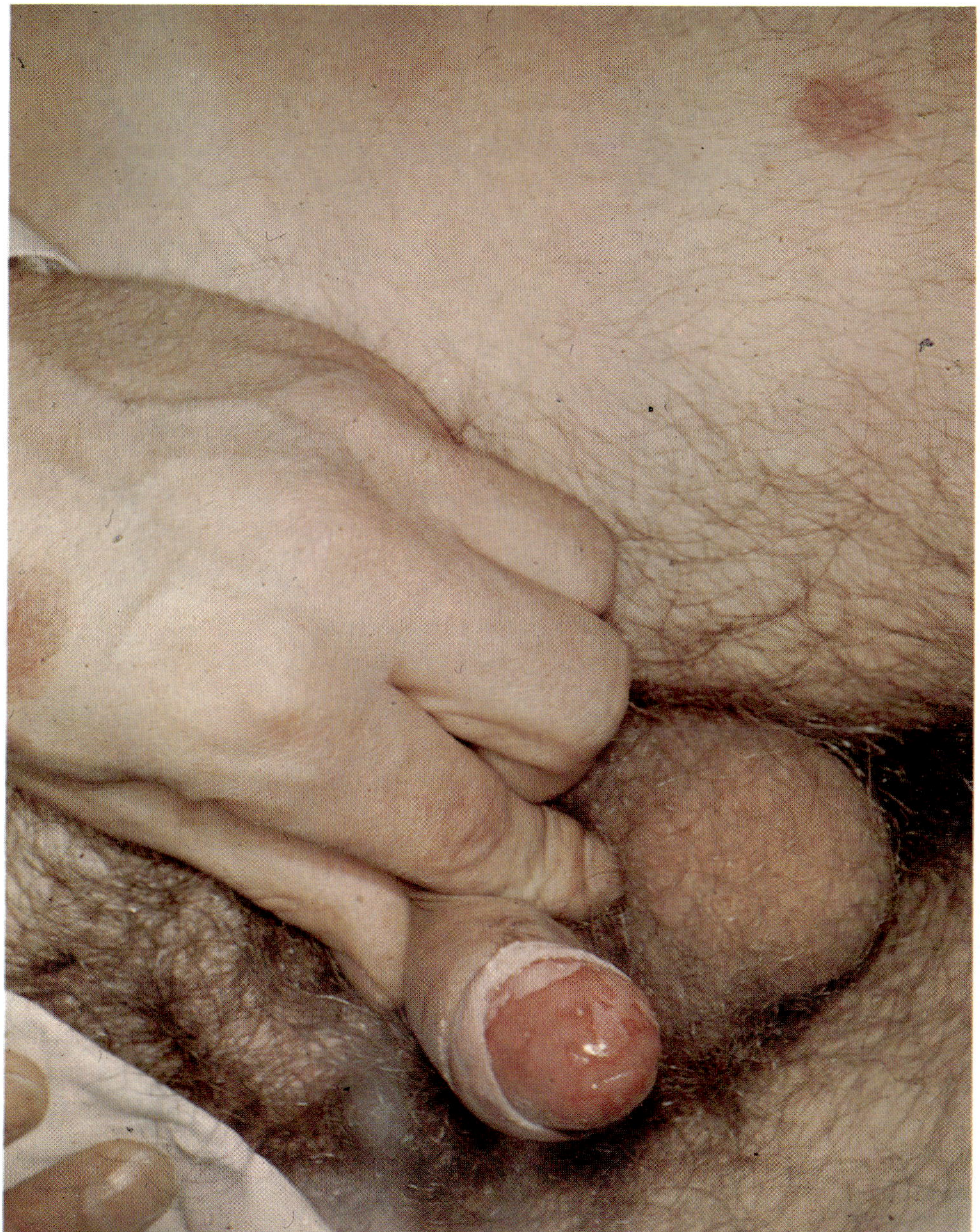

**Plate 38**

Mucous membrane lesion; erythema multiforme. Note hand and thigh lesions as well.

### *Treatment*

The patient should be studied for anemia, ulcerative colitis, or irritative dental factors.

Some episodes of aphthous stomatitis are the result of drug or food sensitivity, which can be ascertained by elimination and then subsequent retesting of the suspected item. Chocolate, cheese, and flavorings are among the more frequent causes. Local trauma from any cause, but particularly from tooth brushing, must be avoided.

Levamisole has been shown by ongoing clinical trials to improve the course of this disorder, but not dramatically so. Its effect is temporary.

Local anesthetics such as viscous lidocaine (Xylocaine) applied to the ulcers prior to eating, give the patient great relief.

Glucocorticoids applied locally in lozenge form may shorten an episode, but do not prevent recurrences. Triamcinolone incorporated into a moisture-resistant vehicle that adheres to the ulcer is very helpful if applied frequently enough (Kenalog in Orabase).

Some authors (Shelley) suggest that tetracycline, given either systemically or in a suspension, may be effective. A suspension of a capsule's contents in water is applied with a pad to the ulcer for 20 minutes, four to six times daily. Tetracycline and demeclocycline have been recommended.

We find that the following formula is very helpful:

| | |
|---|---|
| Soluble betamethasone tablets (0.5 mg.) | 28 |
| Zephiran hydrochloride, 21.3% | 1 drop |
| Peppermint oil | 1 drop |
| Lidocaine hydrochloride | 3% |
| Tragacanth | 4.8 Gm. |
| Distilled water | to make 4 oz. |

¼ tsp. to be swirled around mouth q.3h. (gives 0.1 mg. of betamethasone per dose)

Liquid nitrogen touched for short intervals to new lesions is claimed to hasten recovery without residual scarring.

Merchant found that if zinc levels were down, ulcers would respond well to 220 to 660 mg. of zinc sulfate daily.

## NECROTIZING GINGIVITIS (VINCENT'S STOMATITIS)

Although uncommon, necrotizing gingivitis is the most frequently seen bacterial infection of the oral mucosa.

The clinical appearance is that of an acute inflammatory process involving the dental edges of the gingivae, particularly the interdental papillae. Necrosis and ulceration of the edges occur, with the formation of a pseudomembrane. Bleeding is frequent from the uninvolved areas. There is a characteristic fetid odor. The course may be prolonged.

The disease may be associated with systemic debilitating disorders.

The normal bacterial flora are responsible, since they become pathogenic under conditions of reduced resistance. Bacterial cultures show a variety of organisms, including spirochetes, fusiform bacilli, and streptococci.

Systemic hematological disease such as leukemia or agranulocytosis must be ruled out.

### *Treatment*

Penicillin is the antibiotic of choice. Oral penicillin V may be used in a dosage of 400,000 units four to six times daily for 5 days.

General cleansing measures, periodontal care, and removal of necrotic areas may be carried out by the patient's dentist. It is transmissable to a susceptible host. Some studies have indicated a genetic susceptibility.

Good oral hygiene should be instituted and maintained.

## DENTURE STOMATITIS

Dentures may cause significant problems aside from the annoyance and irritation of a poorly fitting prosthesis. Middle-aged to elderly individuals who have worn false teeth for years without difficulty may develop an angular cheilitis, hyperplasia, alveolar ridge soreness, or persistent, intolerable, hard palate inflammation and tenderness.

***Angular cheilitis.*** Fissuring at the mouth corners where overlap occurs and moisture accumulates, with resulting inflammation, crusting, and fissuring, is characteristic of angular cheilitis. *Candida* is a secondary invader.

Treatment consists of dental procedures to enlarge the vertical height of the dentures and eliminate the overlap. Topical nystatin applied to the area three times daily after drying is effective.

***Denture irritation hyperplasia.*** Poorly fitting or unevenly pressing dentures may traumatize the membrane surface of the maxilla or mandible. A hyperplastic change in the surface follows. Often associated with erythema. Most are on the alveolar ridge. They may be asymptomatic and will subside with correction of the denture.

***Irritation of alveolar ridge and palate.*** A noticeably reddened, diffusely affected area covered by dentures contrasts sharply with the adjacent normal membrane, usually over the vault of the palate. Loose dentures, with local reaction from food particles or minor trauma seems to provide a site favorable to *Candida* invasion. Iron-deficiency anemia seems to enhance *Candida* invasion. Culturing can demonstrate *Candida*.

Treatment consists of nystatin topically, orally, or both, together with correction of the iron-deficiency anemia.

## CICATRICIAL PEMPHIGOID (BENIGN MUCOUS MEMBRANE PEMPHIGOID)

Cicatricial pemphigoid is a chronic bullous and erosive disease of the mucosal surfaces and skin that results in permanent scars.

The disorder occurs chiefly in persons over 65 years of age, although cases in the second decade have been reported.

It begins on mucous membranes or the adjacent skin, particularly the conjunctival and oral mucosa, but may involve vulval, vaginal, or perianal areas, as well as the larynx or even the esophagus. The lesions begin as small vesicles and spread to form large erosions that are slow to heal and leave scars on the mouth. These scars are gray and lacy, whereas in other areas adhesions and strictures may form. Conjunctival lesions may lead to blindness from epithelization of the cornea (Fig. 21-2).

Skin lesions, consisting of bullae, occur in one third of the cases. These, too, may lead to scarring and atrophy.

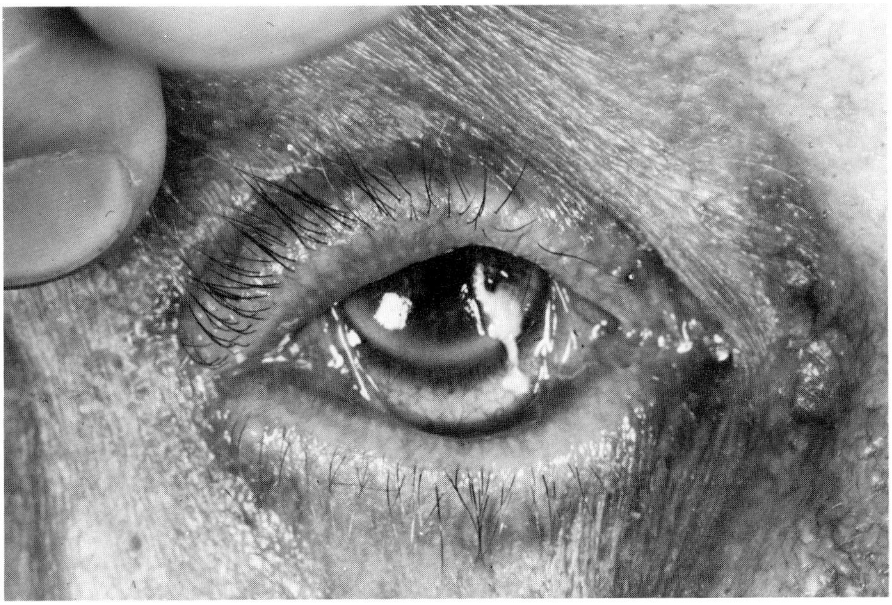

**Fig. 21-2.** Cicatricial pemphigoid.

The course extends over many years and does not carry the fatal prognosis of pemphigus.

Biopsy is indicated for diagnosis. The site chosen for hematoxylin and eosin staining is a very new pustule. For immunofluorescence the site adjacent to a fresh bulla or erosion is most likely to yield best results. Direct immunofluorescent studies reveal positive basement membrane fluorescence with deposition of IgG and complement. Circulating indirect-staining antibodies have been demonstrated as in pemphigus.

### *Differential diagnosis*

***Pemphigus vulgaris.*** In pemphigus vulgaris, lesions develop rapidly, with most of the mouth involved. There are associated large numbers of skin lesions. Acantholytic cells may be demonstrated by scrapings from a bulla. Direct and indirect immunofluorescence studies are positive and diagnostic.

***Bullous pemphigoid.*** In bullous pemphigoid, bullous lesions occur on the groin, limbs, and abdomen, usually sparing the mucosal surfaces. Biopsy reveals basement-membrane fluorescence under the direct immunofluorescence technique. Electron microscopy of the subtle changes may be necessary for confirmed diagnosis. These two disorders may be each a part of the spectrum of a single bullous pemphigoid-cicatricial pemphigoid disorder.

***Erythema multiforme bullosum.*** In erythema multiforme bullosum, skin lesions are associated with mucous membrane lesions and often have a classic iris appearance. There is no diagnostic immunofluorescence.

### *Treatment*

Because of the benign nature of the disease and the relative lack of discomfort, treatment may not always be necessary.

Oral administration of local anesthetics such as viscous lidocaine (Xylocaine) 15 minutes prior to eating will be helpful.

Triamcinolone in an adhesive base such as Kenalog in Orabase may be applied several times daily, or the following formula may be used:

| | |
|---|---|
| Soluble betamethasone tablets (0.5 mg.) | 28 |
| Zephiran hydrochloride 21.3% | 1 drop |
| Peppermint oil | 1 drop |
| Lidocaine hydrochloride | 3% |
| Tragacanth | 4.8 Gm. |
| Distilled water | to make 4 oz. |

¼ tsp. to be swirled around mouth q.3h.

Intralesional injections of glucocorticoids to affected areas of the conjunctiva may prevent adhesions and strictures.

Systemic glucocorticoids are beneficial but high doses are required to produce an effect, and side effects may be unjustifiably severe in this age group.

## BALANITIS

*Acute balanitis* consists of an inflammation of the glans penis, characterized by erythema, edema, and, in more severe instances, weeping, moisture, and vesiculation. Pain, tenderness, and discomfort are present. Rarely, there may be bulla formation.

The inflammation is usually caused by hot water, soap, and excess cleansing and results from primary irritation. Allergic eczematous contact dermatitis is secondary to an allergic process and is caused by medications, rubber, clothing, contraceptive creams, and so forth. *Candida* is a frequent cause of a transient form of balanitis and is transmitted by sexual intercourse. About 10% of the male sexual partners of women with vaginal candidosis were found to have candidal balanoposthitis. *Candida* does not ordinarily survive on the glans penis, particularly in circumcised males, so that untreated balanitis is self-limited to a 2- or 3-day course. Gonococcal infection produces a painful, burning inflammation of the urethral orifice and periorificial glans, with mucopurulent discharge from the meatus. Frequency and dysuria are usually present. Symptoms develop in 1 week to 10 days after exposure to the infection. Diagnosis is made by culture of the distal 2 cm. of urethra and the culture is specially managed (see gonorrhea, p. 251).

*Chronic circumscribed balanitis* has been described as a separate entity, with the inflammation of the glans appearing as a sharply bordered, velvety red patch on the mucous

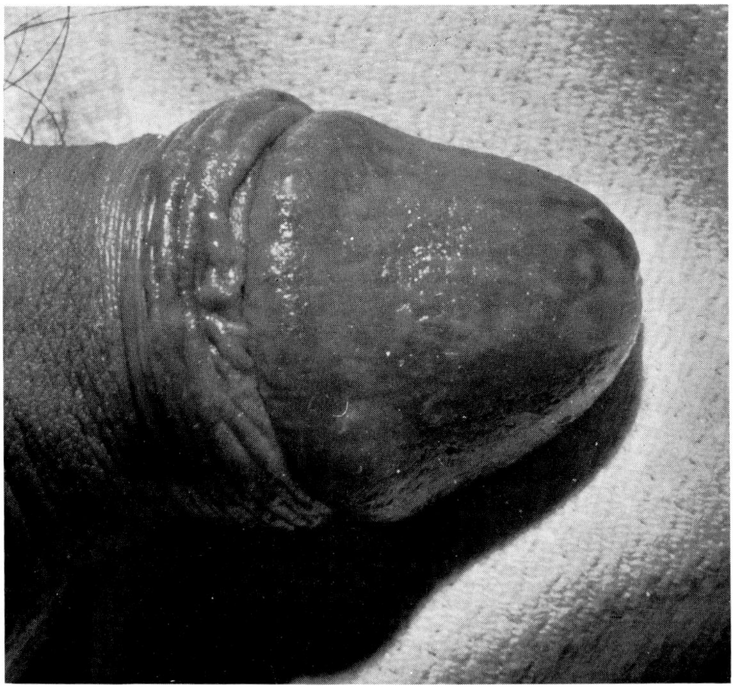

**Fig. 21-3.** Chronic circumscribed balanitis. Note sharp demarcation of normal mucosa distally.

membrane. The adjacent unaffected mucous membrane is normal in appearance. The disorder is persistent and produces continuing discomfort over weeks to months (Fig. 21-3). Bowen's disease or erythroplasia of Queyrat must be ruled out by biopsy.

Microscopically, this lesion is characterized by the large plasma cell component of the inflammatory cellular infiltrate.

### *Differential diagnosis*

***Steroid balanitis.*** Long-term use, and in susceptible individuals not so long-term use, of potentn topical glucocorticoids will produce erythema and a sense of irritation and moisture. There will be a worsening after cessation of the steroid and a slow subsidence over a period of weeks, apart from the initial reason for steroid use.

***Psoriasis.*** Psoriasis presents a red patch on the glans. Often there is an overlying fine scale. Psoriasis is usually present elsewhere.

***Lichen planus.*** Lichen planus may involve the glans penis, causing discrete papules or an erythematous patch. There are characteristic angular papules elsewhere.

***Herpes progenitalis.*** A moist erosion of the mucous membrane, herpes progenitalis begins with a vesicular lesion and lasts for several days.

***Syphilis (chancre).*** Chancre is a localized, firm, painless, inflammatory induration that becomes eroded, usually on the glans or corona. There is noticeable local lymphadenopathy.

***Erythroplasia of Queyrat.*** This is a carcinoma in situ in the epidermis that presents on the glans penis as a sharply bordered, red, velvety patch, which, however, can affect the entire glans.

### *Treatment*

*Acute balanitis* is treated most satisfactorily by avoidance of irritants and possible sensitizing contacts. Friction of rough clothing and trauma should be eliminated.

Burow's solution, in the form of prepared

tablets or packets of aluminum acetate, 1 tablet or packet to a pint of cool water, is used for compresses, which are applied for 15-minute periods three times daily.

Systemic and topical antibiotic lotion or cream, such as clotrimazole (Canestin, Lotrimin) or miconazole (Micatin), should be used after the compresses if there is evidence of infection.

Some individuals experience recurrent episodes of acute and persistent balanitis that can only be cured by circumcision. The sex partner should be examined and treated. An underlying systemic disease such as an undiagnosed diabetes should be kept in mind in recalcitrant cases.

*Chronic circumscribed balanitis* is very unresponsive to topical therapy. Hydrocortisone 1% to 2% in cream is best used, along with a good deal of patience and common sense.

## LEUKOPLAKIA

See also erythroplasia, p. 396.

An area of abnormal keratin on the mucous membranes appears as a white patch. Areas of benign hyperkeratosis may arise from the membrane over vesicles or bullae or a patch of underlying dermatitis. None of these, however, contain atypical cells on microscopic examination.

Although the process of leukoplakia is not well defined, it does indicate microscopic atypia of epithelial cells and a distinct premalignant potential. Dermatologists, pathologists, dentists, and gynecologists have various ways of classifying this disorder. There are progressive steps being taken to unify our thoughts on these matters. We will divide leukoplakia here into *dysplastic*, demonstrating cellular dysplasia, a potentially malignant lesion, and *nondysplastic*, which is an innocent process.

In a study of 3,256 specimens of oral leukoplakia in the United States, a nondysplastic process was observed in 80%, mild dysplasia was present in 12%, and severe dysplastic change amounting to carcinoma in situ was found in 4.5%. Infiltrating squamous cell carcinoma was already present in 3%. Oral cancer comprises 2% to 3% of all cancers. Chronic bullous disease, and oral lichen planus can act as precursors to oral cancer, especially if erosive or chronically inflamed lesions are also chronically irritated by a sharp tooth edge or other similar factor.

The patches of leukoplakia are discrete, sharply defined, and slightly elevated. They may be either single or multiple. They may be small or large and are irregular in outline. The buccal mucosa and alveolar ridges are most commonly involved, followed by the floor of the mouth, the tongue, vestibule, and hard palate. The thickness, size, fissuring, and other features bear no relationship to the malignancy potential, nor do they predict the microscopic atypicality of the abnormal cells, although some clinical and histological correlation is possible. Leukoplakia from the floor of the mouth has a 43% chance of being dysplastic, the tongue 25%, the lip 24%, and palate 18%, according to Waldron's study. Also, we must state that Pinborg believes that speckled leukoplakia and leukoplakia that has a *Candida* infection superimposed stand a chance of demonstrating atypia or malignant changes in 60% or more. *Histological examination is essential in all these lesions.* Leukoplakia is also found on the lips, penile mucosa, and vulva (Plate 39).

### *Microscopic findings*

Microscopically, one finds hyperkeratosis, some evidence of a granular layer, and atypical cells. These are hyperchromatic, irregular in size, shape, and polarity, and characterized by increased numbers of mitotic figures. There is often an intense inflammatory response immediately beneath the epidermis.

### *Differential diagnosis*

***Lichen planus.*** One may have some difficulty in differentiating leukoplakia from lichen planus. Lesions in lichen planus, although usually gray with fine lines and no induration, may present as white plaques. The atypical cells in leukoplakia are the important feature. Other areas are involved in lichen planus.

***Lupus erythematosus.*** Lupus erythematosus produces lip lesions with slightly raised,

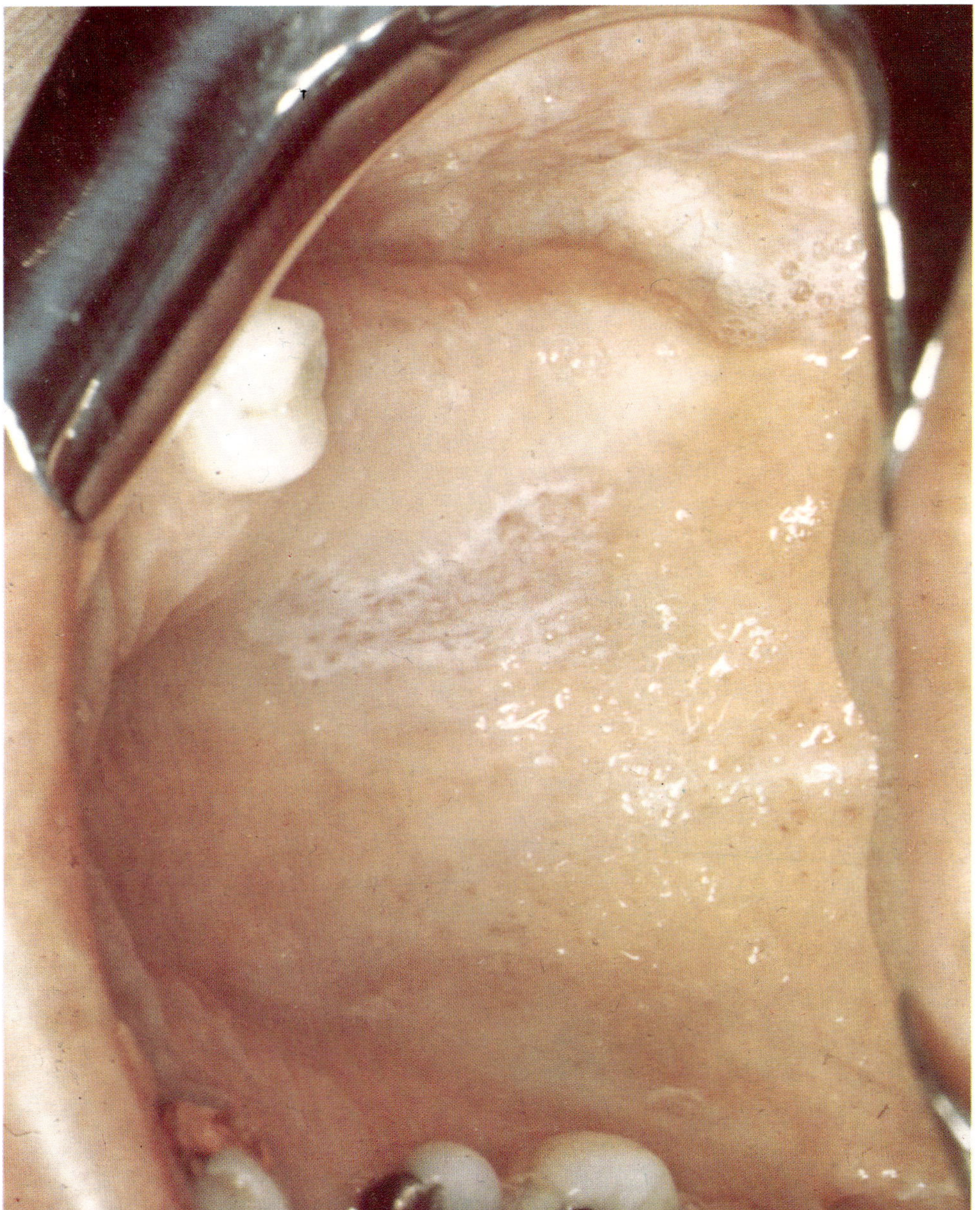

**Plate 39**

Dysplastic leukoplakia, involving hard palate, on left side of vault.

reddened areas covered by a whitish scale. There are ordinarily other more characteristic facial lesions found on the malar area.

***Carcinoma.*** Early squamous cell carcinoma of the lip or mucous membrane may also present a plaque of white hyperkeratosis, which shortly fissures or ulcerates. Biopsy differentiates carcinoma from leukoplakia.

***White sponge nevus.*** A hereditary disorder, white sponge nevus is characterized by a thickened, patchy, white oral mucous membrane with a pebbled surface. It is soft and spongy and can be differentiated from other keratotic oral lesions. It is present from childhood and is benign. No treatment is necessary.

### Treatment

All chronic erosive oral disease should be followed carefully and by multiple biopsies. Irritating contacts and sources of chronic friction must be searched for and eliminated. Treatment consists of attention to teeth, particularly by noting of possible irritation from rough areas on dentures or from smoking, and correction of oral hygiene. A biopsy *must* be done to determine the degree and extent of atypia of the cells. The lesion can then be removed by electrodesiccation, radiotherapy, or surgical excision, depending on the site and size. We cannot emphasize enough that the only way of assessing these lesions satisfactorily is by adequate biopsy and careful microscopic review of the section. More than one biopsy may be necessary.

## ORAL ERYTHROPLASIA

Mashberg believes strongly that we are following the wrong path looking for early carcinoma by investigating leukoplakia. He states unequivocally that erythroplasia, that is, a velvety patch, is the most common sign of early asymptomatic oral carcinoma, 97% of which are found on the floor of the mouth. These lesions are chiefly found in high-risk patients (smokers and heavy drinking males, 40 to 70 years of age). Half of these lesions are 1 cm. or less, and local excision, if complete, results in less than 5% recurrence, excellent statistics for so treacherous a cancer.

## GIANT CELL GRANULOMA

This is a tumor that may be *peripheral,* outside the alveolar or mandibular ridges, or central, inside the ridges. The peripheral tumor is related to trauma or low-grade irritation and results from proliferation of connective tissue elements. It is a pale, firm, benign, slow-growing tumor and is easily traumatized. The central granuloma is also a benign tumor, is red to purple in color and very soft, bleeds easily, and recurs rapidly if incompletely removed.

Microscopically, one sees a loose connective tissue structure, with fibroblastic giant cells and a very vascular matrix. It involves the periodontal membrane, and there may be destruction of the underlying bone.

### Differential diagnosis

***Peripheral fibroma.*** This fibrous, firm, pink, rapidly growing lesion may grow enough to separate teeth. It occurs most commonly on the anterior outer aspect of the alveolar or mandibular ridge.

***Pyogenic granuloma.*** This fleshy, red, soft, friable tumor of the external fixed gingiva results from trauma. It bleeds copiously when damaged.

Common, benign tumors that arise in the mouth and from the gingiva and which can be compressed, include mucous cysts, swelling from apical abscess, pregnancy granulomas, warts, and hemangiomas. Squamous cell carcinoma may originate from the gingiva.

### Treatment

Removal of these tumors must be complete, or they will recur. This is more difficult with the giant cell epulis, which requires more extensive removal of surrounding tissues.

## MUCOUS CYST

A retention cyst of mucous gland origin may be formed as a result of trauma. The trauma, which may be minor and unnoticed, as from biting or chewing, causes ductal obstruction, so that mucus collects within the gland. The lesion is soft and fluctuant and has the color of normal mucous membranes with a bluish tinge; it is commonly seen on the lower lip. A mucous cyst on the floor of the mouth under the tongue is called a *ranula* and is larger than most mucoceles. The lesion is benign. Microscopic examination reveals a mucinous mass contained within a capsule of connective tissue.

### *Treatment*

Treatment consists of electrodesiccation with the patient under local anesthesia, with removal of the fibrous capsule in a procedure analogous to that for sebaceous cysts.

Removal of a ranula is a specialistic surgical procedure.

## ORAL PIGMENTATION

Pigmentation occurs normally in Negroes, but also in other races. It develops by the third decade and is greater in amount with increased skin pigmentation. Nonpigmented gingivae are seen more often in fair-skinned persons. Pigmentation may appear as purplish blue, brown, or light brown macules, or patches, on the gingivae or hard palate and less often on the buccal mucosa (Fig. 21-4).

*Peutz-Jeghers syndrome* may demonstrate macules on buccal mucosa as well as lips and perioral region.

*Addison's disease* is associated with an accentuation of physiological pigmentation of the buccal mucosa.

*Pigmented nevi* are present in the mucous membrane of the oral cavity but are not common. As on the skin, they may appear at adolescence or be present at birth.

*Junctional, intradermal, compound,* and *blue nevi* are recognized. *Malignant melanomas* can develop from these lesions, but less than 2% of melanomas originate here.

*Heavy metals,* silver, lead, and bismuth, produce gingival pigmentation. Silver produces more diffuse pigmentation than do the others.

*Chloroquine, atabrine, and related drugs* produce patchy mucosal melanization.

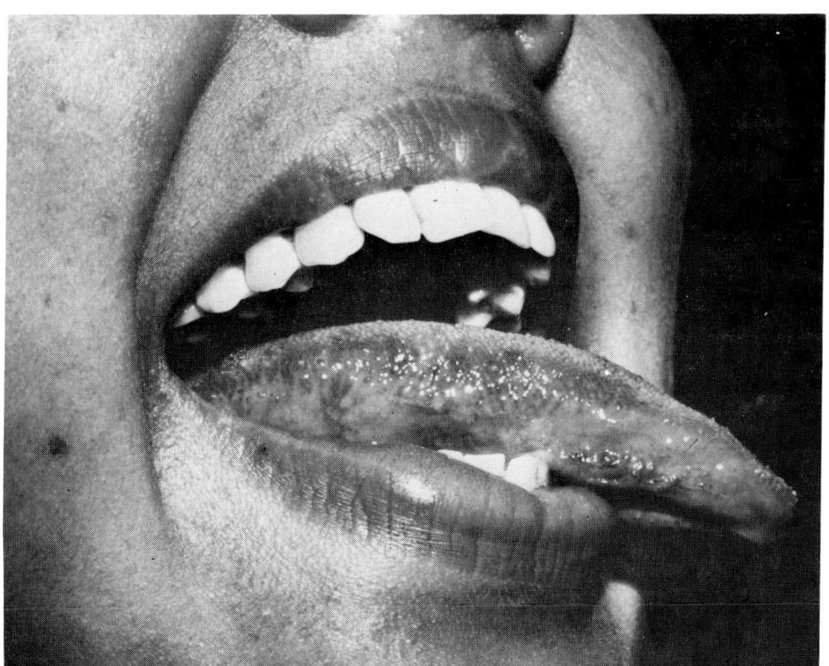

**Fig. 21-4.** Physiologic pigmentation. Brown-black pigmentation of sides of tongue.

**REFERENCES**

Caterall, R. D.: The sexually transmitted diseases. In Rook, A., editor: Recent advances in dermatology, vol. 4, London, 1977, Churchill Livingstone, p. 42.
**The specific findings of Diddle on candidosis and balanitis.**

Challacombe, S. J., Batchelor, J. R., and Kennedy, L. A.: HLA antigens in recurrent oral ulceration, Arch. Dermatol. **113**:1717, 1977.
**HL-A B12 frequency in patients with herpetic ulcerations was increased, perhaps significantly.**

deMeyer, J., Degraeve, M., and Clarysse, J.: Levamisole in aphthous stomatitis. Evaluation of three regimens, Br. Med. J. **1**:671, 1977.
**124 patients demonstrated gradual but significant improvement compared to placebo.**

Griffin, J. W.: Recurrent intraoral herpes simplex virus infection, Oral Surg. **19**:209, 1965.
**Rare, but confirmed of viral origin.**

Lehner, T.: Immunologic aspects of recurrent oral ulcers, Oral Surg. **33**:80, 1972.
**The immunologic aspect is positively endorsed as being causative in recurrent aphthae.**

Lehner, T., Wilton, J. M. A., and Ivanyi, L.: Double blind crossover trial of levamisole in recurrent aphthous ulceration, Lancet **2**:926, 1976.
**64% of patients responded with a decrease in ulcers after 2 months of intermittent levamisole.**

Mashberg, A.: Erythroplasia vs. leukoplakia in the diagnosis of early asymptomatic oral squamous cell carcinoma, N. Engl. J. Med. **297**:109, 1977.
**Erythroplasia is significantly more likely to be, or to become, malignant than leukoplakia.**

McCarthy, P. L., and Shklar, G.: Diseases of the oral mucosa, New York, 1964, McGraw-Hill Book Co

Merchant, H. W., Gangarosa, L. P., and Glassman, A. B.: Zinc sulfate supplementation for treatment of recurring oral ulcers, South. Med. J. **70**:559, 1977.
**Of 32 patients, nine had abnormally low serum-zinc levels, and all showed improvement on zinc therapy—50% to 100% reduction in frequency.**

O'Duffy, J. D., Carney, J. A., and Deodhar, S. H.: Behçet's disease. Report of 10 cases, 3 with new manifestations, Ann. Intern. Med. **75**:561, 1971.
**Vasculitis in mucocutaneous lesions. New associations were pancreatitis, peripheral neuropathy, subungual lesions, and lymphomas.**

Ohno, S, Nakayama, E., Suguiro, S., et al.: Specific histocompatibility antigens associated with Behçet's disease, Am. J. Opthalmol. **50**:636, 1975.
**HL-A B5 found in 75% of patients.**

Olson, J. A., Nelms, C., Silverman, S., et al.: Levamisole. A new treatment for recurrent aphthous stomatitis, Oral Med. **41**:588, 1976.
**50 patients: 6% had long-term benefit; 56% found attacks were reduced in number and severity; 38% showed no response.**

Pearson, R. W.: Advances in the diagnosis and treatment of blistering diseases. In Malkinson, F. D., and Pearson, R. W., editors: Yearbook of dermatology, Chicago, 1977, Year Book Medical Publishers, Inc., p. 15.
**A balanced, readable selective review of benign mucous membrane pemphigoid and bullous pemphigoid.**

Pinborg, J. J.: Atlas of diseases of the oral mucosa, New York, 1973, W. B. Saunders Co.
**Over 450 excellent color photographs and accompanying text.**

Recurrent oral ulceration. Editorial; Br. Med. J. **3**:757, 1974.
**A succinct review and comment on management.**

Rickles, N. H.: Allergy in surface lesions of the oral mucosa, Oral Surg. **33**:744, 1972.
**Cinnamon oil causing aphthous ulcers, positive patch tests, confirmed.**

Rogers, R. S., Sains, W. M., and Shorter, R. G.: Lymphotoxicity in recurrent aphthous stomatitis: lymphocytotoxicity for oral epithelial cells in recurrent aphthous stomatitis and Behçet's syndrome, Arch. Dermatol. **109**:361, 1974.
**Lymphocyte suspensions, cytotoxic in 18 hours for oral epithelial cells, correlated with disease activity.**

Shelley, W. B.: Consultations in dermatology, 2. Chapter on Aphthous stomatitis, Philadelphia, 1974, W. B. Saunders Co. p. 190.
**Strongly favors oral tetracycline compresses and an immune basis for most cases.**

Ship, I. I.: Inheritance of aphthous ulcerations of the mouth, J. Dent. Res. **44**:837, 1965.
**Frequent familial occurrence.**

Silverman, S., Jr.: Lesions affecting oral mucosa. In Maddin, S., editor: Current dermatologic management, ed. 2, St. Louis, 1975, The C. V. Mosby Co. p. 230.
**A practical approach to the management of an often difficult disease.**

Sobel, J. D., Haim, S., Shafrir, A., et al.: Cutaneous hyperreactivity in Behçet's disease, Dermatologica **146**:350, 1973.
**An investigation of the enhanced reaction to cutaneous injury in Behçet's disease.**

Turrell, A. J. W.: Angular cheilosis and dentures, Br. J. Dermatol. **79**:331, 1967.
**A well-documented and practical presentation on an important clinical entity.**

Waldron, C. A., and Shafer, W. G.: Leukoplakia revisited. A clinicopathologic study of 3,256 oral leukoplakias, Cancer **36**:1386, 1975.
**The floor of the mouth is the most dangerous area.**

Weathers, D. R., and Griffin, J. W.: Intraoral ulcerations of recurrent herpes simplex and recurrent aphthae. Two distinct clinical entities, J. Am. Dent. Assoc. **81**:81, 1970.
**Criteria are proposed and defended for the occurrence of these two diseases.**

## CHAPTER 22

# Diseases of the nails

## NAILS

### Embryology

Primate nails are chemically and structurally different from reptilian and avian claws. Nails are constructed from alpha-keratin protein, the filaments of which are oriented perpendicular to the growth axis and related to the degree of lateral curvature of the nail plate (Baden).

The first recognizable nail structure is a smooth rectangular area, present by 10 weeks of intrauterine life, and delineated by depressions or grooves. *Keratinization* begins at 11 weeks on the distal ridge, a site that eventually becomes the subungual portion under the free edge of the adult nail. The *matrix* is mature by the twentieth week and contributes the ventral portion of the nail fold. *Nail formation*, however, is first recognizable by the fourteenth week from the earliest nail matrix.

The keratinizing process that *produces* the hard alpha-keratin of the nails involves keratohyaline granules, accumulation of tonofibrils, and mucopolysaccharides. The fibrous protein filaments are aligned perpendicularly to the growth axis. The resulting nail is a layered structure, partly contributed by the dorsal matrix, partly by the ventral matrix, and partly by the nail bed.

The nail is formed in such a way that it slides distally on the nail bed along the dermoepidermal ridges, which are arranged in parallel longitudinal rows.

### Anatomy (Fig. 22-1)

Externally, the *matrix* is identified by the *lunula* visible chiefly on the thumbs, but often apparent on all nails. The free edge of the nail fold is continuous with the *cuticle*, an extension of the stratum corneum of the dorsum of the finger, and immediately below this is the *eponychium*, which is continuous with the roof of the nail fold. These structures become important in paronychial infections of the area, in which they are separated from the nail by inflammation (Fig. 14-10).

The nail bed lies distal to the lunula and, contrary to previous belief, does appear to participate in nail formation. The most distal aspect, the original distal ridge, is the site of production of a crumbly keratin in some cutaneous disorders.

There is a rich local arteriolar blood supply to the area, with circulation entirely dependent on the two digital arteries

These vessels first traverse the pulp space so that damage to the ball of the finger may threaten the blood supply to the growing nail. An accessory supply arises proximal to the nail fold and can supply the nail bed.

### Growth

Fingernails are replaced, on an average, in 5½ months, whereas toenails take 1 to 1½ years. There is great individual variation in nail growth, which may be temporarily halted by many systemic disorders. Daily rates of recorded growth vary from 0.1 to 1 mm. and from finger to finger and so are perhaps too variable for accuracy. Some disorders result in the formation of transverse grooves, or *Beau's lines*, which may be deep enough to cause separation and loss of the nail.

#### REFERENCES


Baden, H. P.: The physical properties of nails, J. Invest. Dermatol. **55**:115, 1970.

**X-ray diffraction, fiber orientation, elasticity, and water-binding capacity.**

Norton, L. A.: Incorporation of thymidine-methyl-$H^3$ and glycine-2-$H^3$ in the nail matrix and bed of humans, J. Invest. Dermatol. **56**:61, 1971.

**The nail bed does indeed contribute to the layered nail plate.**

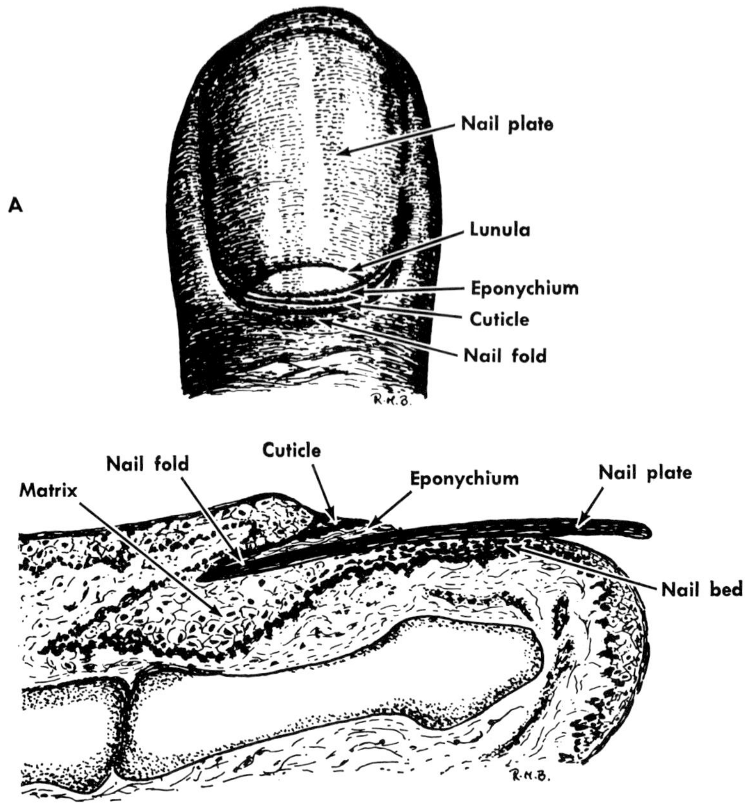


**Fig. 22-1. A,** Nail, dorsal view. **B,** Finger, sagittal section demonstrating nail fold, nail bed, and nail matrix.

## PSORIASIS

Psoriasis is the most important single cause of deformities of the fingernails. Psoriatic nail changes may occur in the absence of typical psoriasis on other areas of the body. Fine pitting is the most common clinical feature observed. The pits are usually small and may be linear or irregularly scattered over the nail plate (Fig. 22-2). They are caused by minute foci of psoriasis affecting the nail matrix and by the formation of scale, which then falls off, leaving its impression on the hardening nail plate.

Psoriasis may cause only color changes in the nail. The normal luster is lost, areas become opaque, and patchy discoloration may occur.

There is a collection of hyperkeratotic material beneath the free edge (subungual hyperkeratosis).

Onycholysis (Fig. 22-7) also occurs in patients with psoriasis. The distal edge of the nail plate is involved. Separation of the nail is often accompanied by a yellow color change appearing in the affected area. The development of gross thickening of the nail plate or psoriasis of the distal nail bed may account for loosening of the nail. *Candida* may be a secondary invader.

### *Treatment*

Treatment of psoriasis of the nails is not satisfactory. Frequently the nails improve when the psoriasis elsewhere clears. Irradiation of the affected nails, although of some therapeutic benefit, is not justified because of the benign and recurrent nature of the disease. Intracutaneous injection of triamcinolone into the nail fold area of affected nails results in improvement over a period of sev-

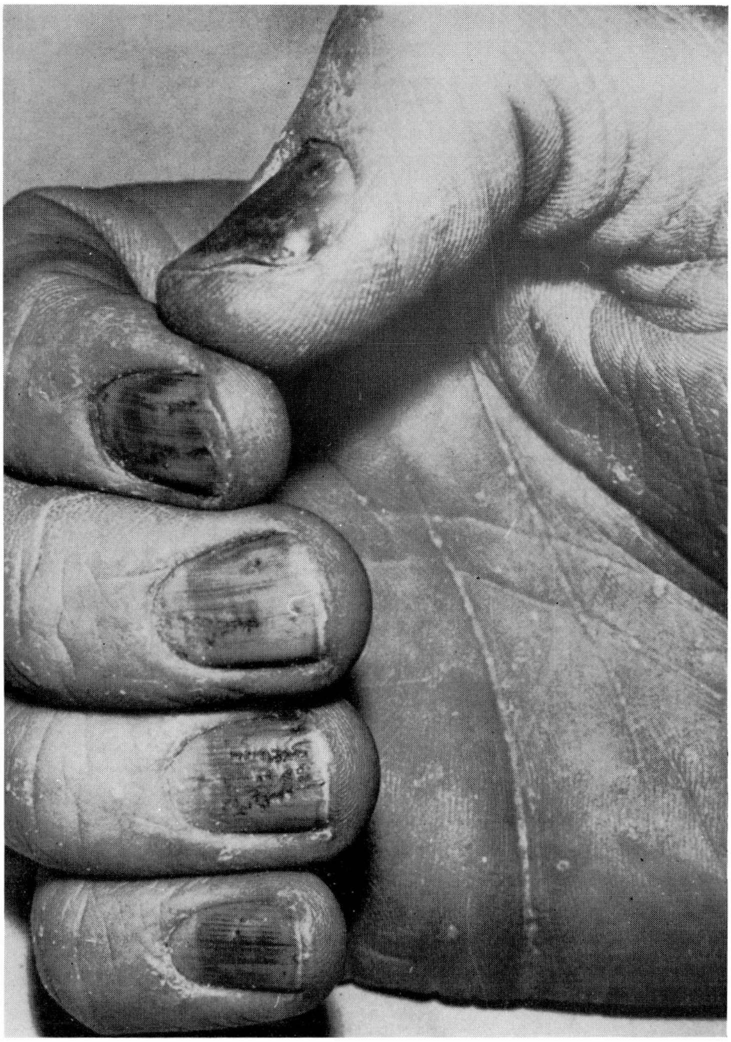

**Fig. 22-2.** Psoriasis of nails. Minimal early involvement in rows of discrete pits.

eral weeks or months. The injection may have to be repeated. Triamcinolone suspension, 5 to 10 mg./ml., is used.

Patient, persistent exposure of the nails to intense ultraviolet light, with close approximation of the light source while the adjacent skin is shielded, has been successful in some of our stubborn cases.

## FUNGAL INFECTION

Fungal infection of the otherwise undamaged nail (Fig. 22-3) is most often caused by *Trichophyton rubrum.* Other fungi causing infection of the nails are *Trichophyton mentagrophytes, T. violaceum, T. schoenleini,* and *Epidermophyton floccosum. Candida albicans* may also produce nail plate changes but probably only after an initial trauma.

Nails infected with fungal elements serve as a reservoir for ringworm of adjacent skin. Recently published work suggests that defective T-cell reactivity may be responsible for inadequate host defense against fungal infection. It is too early to suggest that this possibility

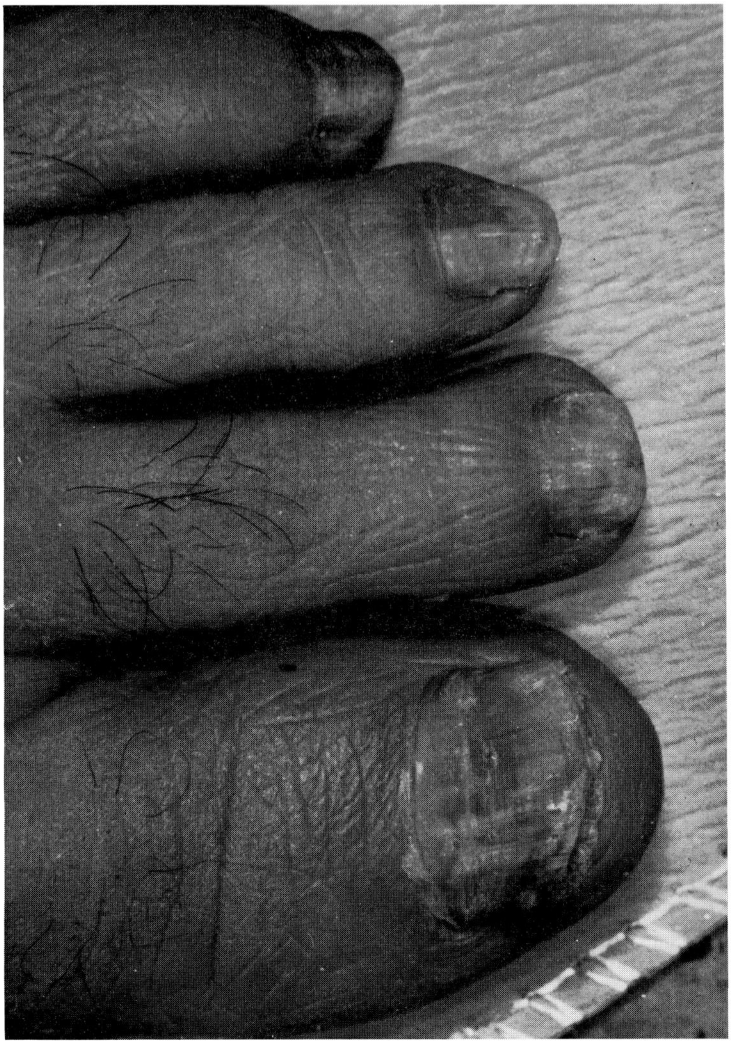

**Fig. 22-3.** Fungal infection of toenails. Note patchy discoloration, distortion, fraying, and opacity.

would explain the relapses and persistence of fungal infection of the nails in some patients.

Some of the earliest changes to appear are brownish discoloration of the edge of the nail plate and thickening and crumbling or breaking away of the nail edge. Usually only one or two nails are involved.

Clinical impression should be substantiated by microscopic examinations and culture of the nail clippings. Direct examination with potassium hydroxide for fungal elements is far more productive of positive results than is a culture.

***Treatment***

The effectiveness of treatment of fungal infections of the nails has been remarkably improved by the introduction of griseofulvin. It must be given in a dose of 1 gm. daily in the micronized form for full therapeutic benefit. It is not unusual for the treatment period to extend over several months, because of the slow growth of the nail. It must be continued until the diseased nail grows out completely (for fingernails, 6 to 8 months; for toenails, 18 to 20 months). Involvement of the toenails is less effectively treated with griseofulvin therapy than infection of the fingernails, and recurrences are common. Topical medications have not as yet proved to be effective.

## DERMATITIS OF THE FINGERS

The nails are very frequently affected by the occurrence of a dermatitis involving the nail fold and the paronychial areas. Long-standing primary irritation dermatitis and atopic dermatitis are the diseases most often responsible.

The appearance of transverse ridging and pitting of the nails commonly accompanies hand dermatitis. Exfoliative dermatitis, if severe and generalized, may lead to all or several of the nails being shed. Onycholysis, or loosening of the nail plate, may also occur in association with a dermatitis of the hands.

A special entity should be mentioned here. This is contact dermatitis of the paronychial and subungual area caused by *nail hardener*. Most of these hardeners contain formalin, a potent sensitizer, which sooner or later, with continued use, will produce an acute dermatitis that causes pain, edema, and onycholysis.

### *Treatment*

The use of the offending agent should be discontinued. Treatment with topical steroids should be instituted, and observation should be maintained until the nail regrows.

## DISTURBED VASCULAR SUPPLY

Not infrequently, a disturbance in the vascular supply alters the nail. Well-established Raynaud's phenomenon, scleroderma, and chronic venous or lymphatic stasis are the disease processes most often responsible.

The nail plate may demonstrate thinning, brittleness, and longitudinal ridging in association with Raynaud's phenomenon. Partial or complete nail loss, an associated chronic paronychia, and nail color changes may appear in patients with scleroderma, Milroy's edema, and arterial impairment, as in diabetes. Nail hypertrophy is not uncommon in cases of long-standing chronic venous insufficiency.

### *Treatment*

Successful therapy is entirely dependent on correcting the underlying disease.

## YELLOW NAIL SYNDROME

As a result of impaired lymph drainage, the nails become slow growing, lusterless, yellow or pale green, and develop a convexity and loss of cuticle. Yellow nail syndrome has been reported in primary lymphedema affecting the fingers, extremities, or face, chronic bronchitis or bronchiectasis, and in association with *pleural effusion* (Plate 40). The pleural effusion may not appear for some time after the development of yellow nails. Hiller reported that three of four patients with yellow nail syndrome at autopsy had developed malignancies.

### *Investigation*

Causes of the primary lymphedema and the presence of pleural effusion should be investigated.

## PARONYCHIA (Fig. 14-10)

Paronychia is a frequent cause of nail distortion. The organisms responsible are mixed. *Candida albicans*, staphylococci, and streptococci predominate. Patients engaged in wet work are most often affected.

Erythema, with induration and swelling of the nail fold, is the most striking clinical feature. One or several fingers may be involved. Pain and tenderness accompany this infection. Purulent discharge may exude from beneath the nail fold. The nail will show some discoloration, pitting, and ridging.

### *Treatment*

Treatment consists of keeping the nail *scrupulously* dry and dropping on a solution of 2% resorcinol in alcohol or 4% thymol in chloroform three times a day. This is usually effective if the wet work can be discontinued or greatly reduced. Much can be achieved if the hands are kept free of water. The oral administration of a suitable antibiotic may also be

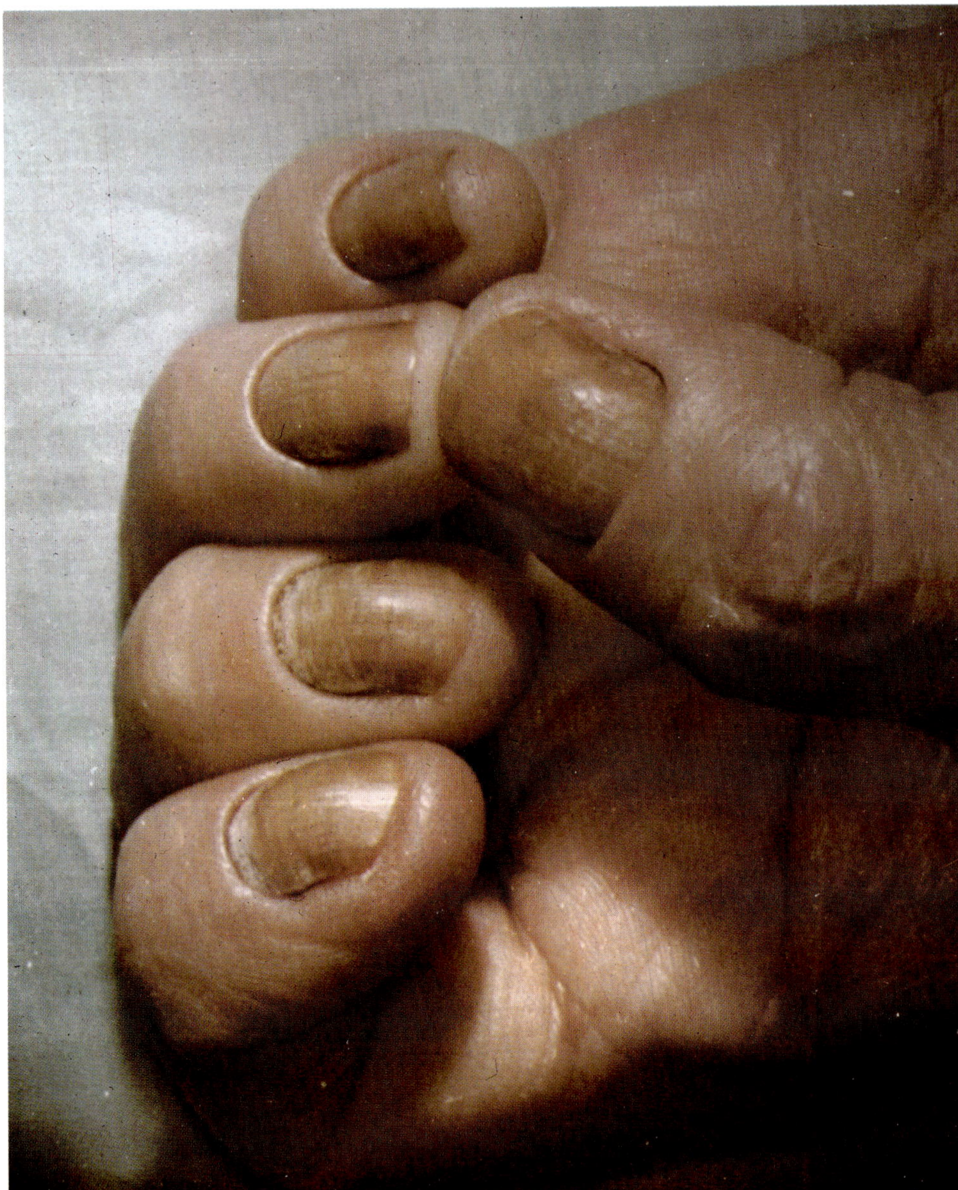

**Plate 40**

Yellow nail syndrome. Intrathoracic systemic associations must be sought.

required if culture reveals susceptible organisms. Seventy percent dimethyl sulfoxide has been recommended as effective treatment applied similarly.

## TRAUMA

Trauma may be responsible for the formation of a hematoma beneath the nail, which may be followed by loss of the nail plate.

### *Treatment*

A *hematoma* beneath the nail plate may cause considerable pain from pressure. This is immediately relieved by a 2 mm. punch biopsy through the nail plate.

## INGROWN TOENAIL

Tight footwear is one of the major causes of ingrown toenail *(unguis incarnatus)* of the large toe.

### *Treatment*

An ingrown toenail is relieved by careful removal of the lateral 3 to 5 mm. of the nail from free edge to matrix under local anesthetic. A temporary tourniquet around the toe will result in a bloodless field, but one must be very careful to remove it before bandaging.

A slightly different technique is to desiccate and curette the inflamed, edematous, soft tissue obstructing the nail growth, lateral to the edge of the nail so that it grows back unimpeded. This produces little or no scarring, and is quite effective.

## NAIL DISORDERS THAT MIRROR UNDERLYING SYSTEMIC DISEASES

***Nail fold telangiectasia.*** Although not strictly a nail disorder, nail fold telangiectasia seems best suited for discussion here. Telangiectasia may be noted on close examination of the nail folds of patients with systemic lupus erythematosus and dermatomyositis.

***Koilonychia.*** Thinning and softening of the nail plate may result in a spoon-shaped nail, which may be associated with hypochromic anemia and Raynaud's phenomenon.

***Beau's lines.*** The appearance of a transverse depression of the nail plate on *all* fingers often reflects a previous *febrile disorder* or systemic disease such as measles. One or several fingers may be involved in cases of severe cold *(frostbite)* and *Raynaud's phenomenon.*

***Onycholysis.*** Distal separation of the nail plate from the nail bed may sometimes be associated with *thyroid dysfunction.*

***Red lunules.*** Red halfmoons have been described in association with congestive heart failure (Terry).

***Finger clubbing.*** Bulbous thickening and broadening of the terminal phalanx, without joint or bone involvement, may occur with diseases of the heart or lungs, biliary cirrhosis, and chronic ulcerative colitis. It may be inherited.

***White nails.*** There may be a diffuse milky ground-glass appearance in the fingernails of patients with hepatic cirrhosis, which can obliterate the lunula. There may be a distal pink band covering no more than 25% of the nail.

***Median nail dystrophy*** (Fig. 22-4). Median nail dystrophy is an uncommon disorder that develops proximally under the nail fold and extends distally, distorting the nail to produce a "fir-tree" deformity. It is usually just off the midline. After months, the nails return to normal although a ridge may remain. Sometimes a history of trauma is available. Recurrences are seen.

***Transverse ridging*** (Fig. 22-5). In addition to Beau's lines, a series of parallel transverse ridges may appear as a result of recurrent local inflammatory cutaneous disease of the nail fold, such as atopic dermatitis or contact dermatitis. Perhaps more often, the same ridges are attributable to a nervous habit of rubbing the sharp edge of the index finger across the soft lunula of the thumb, where it usually occurs.

***Splinter hemorrhages.*** Small, linear, longitudinal hemorrhages may appear beneath the nail intermittently in subacute bacterial endocarditis, as well as numerous other disorders, and occasionally also in normal individuals.

***Paired white bands (Muehrcke's bands).*** Double parallel subungual white bands occur in chronic hypoalbuminemia and ede-

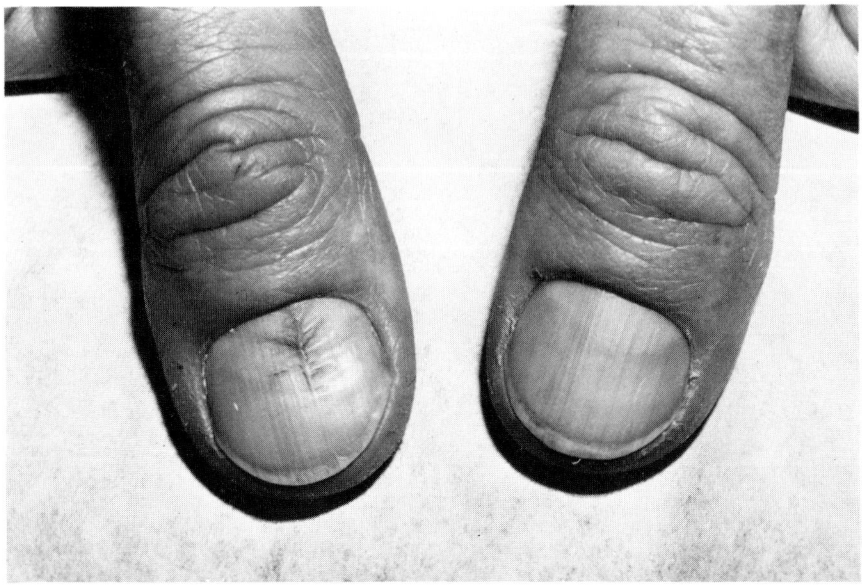

**Fig. 22-4.** Median nail dystrophy. Inverted "fir tree" deformity.

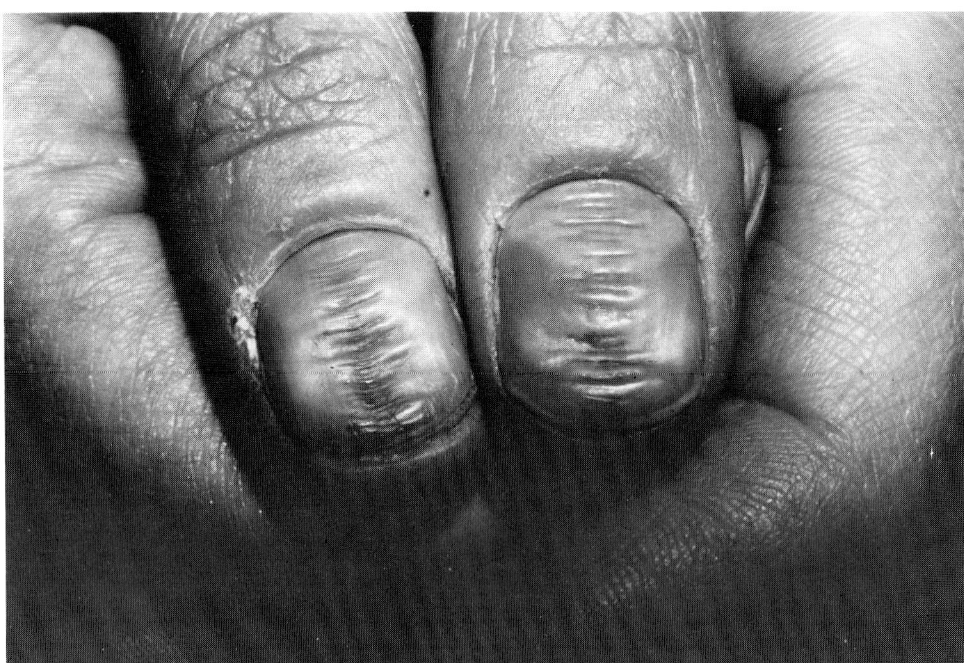

**Fig. 22-5.** Central nail striae, produced by a nervous habit of rubbing the sharp edge of one nail across the soft lunula of the other.

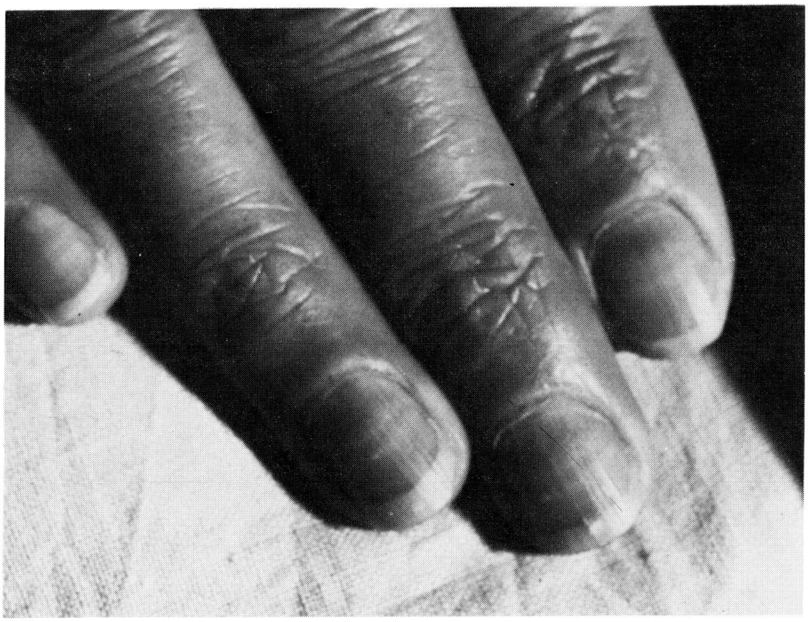

**Fig. 22-6.** Muehrcke's double parallel white bands affecting the nail bed, not the nail plate. Seen in chronic hypoalbuminemia.

ma, as well as in the nephrotic syndrome (Fig. 22-6). They do not grow out with the nail plate.

***Half-and-half nail.*** In azotemia from renal disease, patients may demonstrate nails with distal red, pink, or brown discoloration, whereas the proximal half is white. It may be present on both fingers and toes but is more distinct in the fingers. One study demonstrated brown areas in the distal part of the nails in 35% of patients with established renal disease.

## SUMMARY OF MOST PROBABLE CAUSES OF NAIL PLATE CHANGES

***Pitting of the nail.*** Psoriasis, dermatitis of the hand, paronychia, and alopecia areata are responsible for causing pitting of the nail.

***Onycholysis.*** Psoriasis, trauma, contact dermatitis from nail hardeners, fungal infection, *Pseudomonas* infection, drug eruption (for example, photosensitivity), disturbed vascular supply, and thyroid dysfunction with hyperhidrosis are possible causative factors in separation of the nail plate from its bed (Fig. 22-7). It is often idiopathic.

***Nail discoloration.*** Nail discoloration may be caused by the presence of white spots (leukonychia), brown or black spots from melanin in the nail (pigmentary disorders, nevi, or malignant melanoma), lighter brown patches (caused by psoriasis, fungal infection, and *Candida* infection), or stains (from hair dyes, local medications, nail polish, or cigarette smoking). Green-black discolorations may be produced by *Pseudomonas* or *Candida*.

***Nail thinning.*** Loss of nail substance, thinning, fragility, and longitudinal ridging may be seen with impaired circulation in Raynaud's syndrome, arteriosclerosis, ischemia of other causes, anemia, simple aging, and trauma. It occurs in lichen planus, sometimes with pterygium formation or loss of matrix.

***Hypertrophy.*** Thickening of the nail plate occurs with advancing age (that is, altered vascular supply), psoriasis, fungal infections, trauma from improper footwear, and pachyonychia congenita (inherited abnormality).

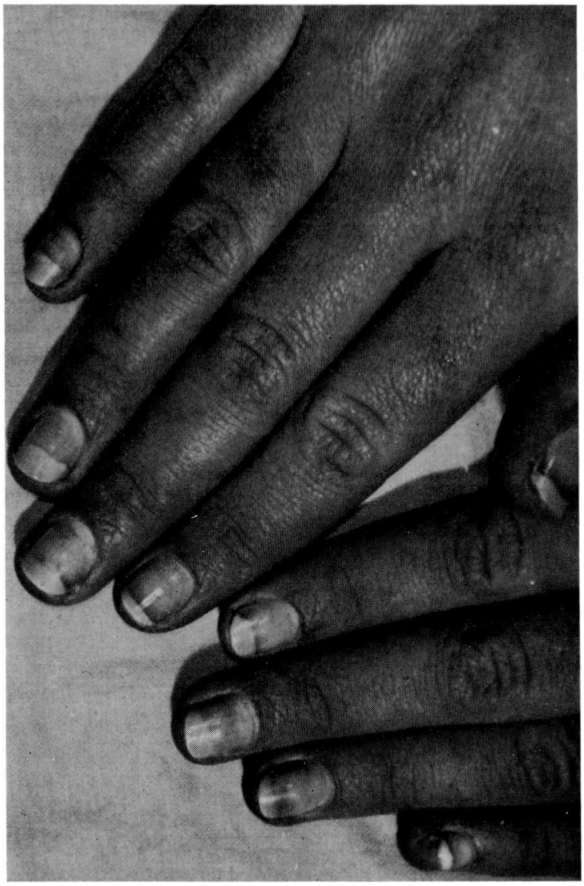

**Fig. 22-7.** Onycholysis. White areas overlie separation of nail plate from nail bed.


## REFERENCES

Abel, E., and Samman, P. D.: Intradermal triamcinolone treatment of nail dystrophies, Br. J. Dermatol. **89**:191, 1973.
**Enthusiastic. Detailed instruction for carrying out this therapeutic procedure, although total dosage not mentioned.**

Dwek, J. H., and Greenberg, G. M.: Yellow nails, lymphedema and pleural effusions, N.Y. J. Med. **73**:1093, 1973.
**A useful review of this subject.**

Hiller, E., Rosenow, E. C., III, and Olsen, M. A.: Pulmonary manifestations of the yellow nail syndrome, Chest **61**:452, 1972.
**Twelve patients described with hypoplastic lymphatic channels. Eight of 12 patients with pulmonary effusion.**

Lindsay, P. G.: The half and half nail, Arch. Intern. Med. **119**:583, 1967.
**Twenty-five patients with a new nail syndrome and renal disease.**

Muehrcke, R. C.: The finger-nails in chronic hypoalbuminaemia, Br. Med. J. **1**:1327, 1956.
**Paired narrow white bands seen that do not move with nail growth. Disappear with abolition of low albumen.**

Samman, P. D.: Nail disorders. In Maddin, S., editor: Current dermatologic management, ed. 2, St. Louis, 1975, The C. V. Mosby Co., p. 221.
**Concise presentation of pertinent diagnostic and therapeutics of nail diseases.**

Samman, P. D.: The yellow nail syndrome, Trans. St. John's Hosp. Dermatol. Soc. **59**:37, 1973.
**Color related to slow rate of growth and edema.**

Samman, P. D., and White, W. F.: The yellow nail syndrome, Br. J. Dermatol. **76**:153, 1964.
**The original description.**

Stewart, W. K., and Raffle, E. J.: Brown nail bed arcs and chronic renal disease, Br. Med. J. **1**:784, 1972.
**A significant dissertation for the diagnosis of renal disease.**

Stobo, J. D., Paul, S., Van Scoy, R. E., et al.: Suppressor thymus–derived lymphocytes in fungal infection, J. Clin. Invest. **57**:319, 1976.
**It is suggested that the T-cell defect hindered clearing of organisms.**

Terry, R.: Red half-moons in cardiac failure, Lancet **2**:842, 1954.
**A significant relationship to congestive heart failure.**

Terry, R.: White nails in hepatic cirrhosis, Lancet **1**:757, 1954.
**Normal pink zone distally. All nails may not be affected.**

CHAPTER 23

# Perioral dermatitis

Over the past decade, perioral dermatitis has been observed as a relatively common disorder, chiefly affecting young adult women (Plate 41).

It consists of a localized grouping of red papules or vesicopapules along the nasolabial folds and upper lip and bilaterally as discrete patches on either side of the chin beneath the outer corners of the mouth. There may be extension of the lesions to the paranasal area and the upper eyelids. The involvement of the eyelids is almost unique, occurring only occasionally in some severe cases of rosacea. It is a frequent occurrence in perioral dermatitis.

The lesions may burn, are rarely pruritic, and may be asymptomatic. Exacerbations and remissions are frequent, without apparent cause. Premenstrual flares are frequent. We have seen this dermatosis worsen with pregnancy and clear slowly with therapy only after delivery. Other dermatoses do not seem to be associated. Heat and perspiration seem to be aggravating factors, but sunlight exposure is neither beneficial nor harmful.

In our experience, perioral dermatitis is frequently a self-limited disorder, disappearing spontaneously 3 to 6 months after onset. Some cases are more aggressive and more prolonged. With the following therapeutic regimen, we find that it can be successfully cleared and the medication discontinued in 2 to 4 months. If the patient has been using potent topical glucocorticoids, there will be a noticeable and disconcerting worsening of the process when they are discontinued.

### *Pertinent information*

As we have become more familiar with the behavior of this disorder, we find that potent topical glucocorticoids behave badly. They will successfully suppress the inflammation and clear the skin, only to have it flare when they are discontinued. With long-continued use, the potent topical glucocorticoids will produce their known adverse effects (p. 204) on the face, and in addition the perioral dermatitis will break through the suppressive effect of the medication, some times with extensive involvement. Hydrocortisone 1% is safe to use and is essential when the major cause of the whole problem has been application of potent topical glucocorticoids, often for a forgotten reason!

Some dermatologists hold to the belief that topical cosmetics cause this disorder.

### *Differential diagnosis*

***Acne vulgaris.*** The presence of comedones and pustules differentiates acne vulgaris.

***Seborrheic dermatitis.*** Although it involves the same areas, seborrheic dermatitis ordinarily consists of patches of erythema and scaling.

***Rosacea.*** In rosacea, pustules and malar and nasal erythema are present.

### *Treatment*

The entity is resistant to therapy and somewhat erratic in its course, so that actual therapeutic benefit is difficult to assess. The following are beneficial in treating perioral dermatitis.

1. Tetracycline, 250 mg., two to three times daily for 1 month and then for 2 weeks out of each month for a further 2 or 3 months.
2. When the cause of the dermatitis is unequivocally the use of potent fluorinated glucocorticoid compounds to the face, as it frequently is, then mild nonfluorinated hydrocortisone compounds should be used to reduce the severity of the "withdrawal" syndrome. We use:

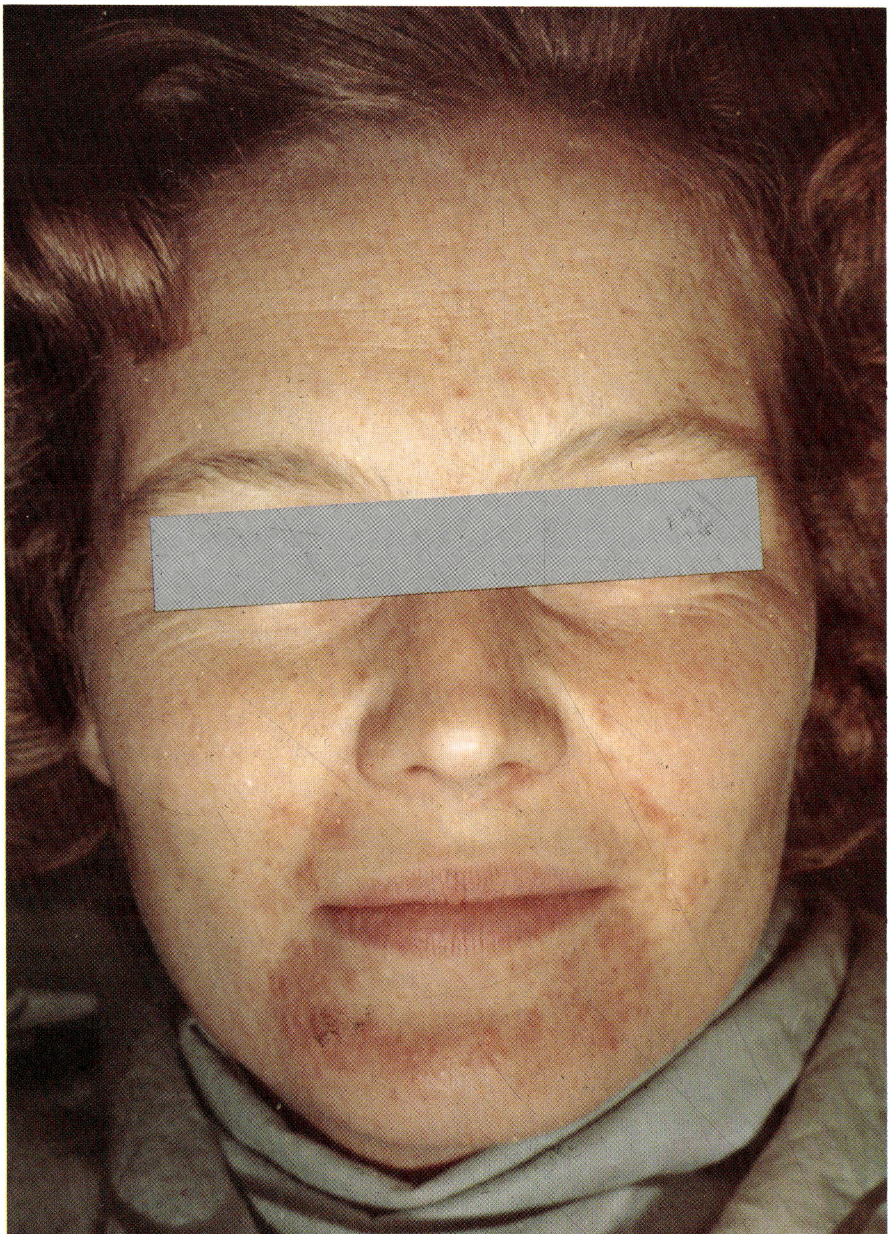

**Plate 41**
Perioral dermatitis.

| | |
|---|---|
| Hydrocortisone | 1% |
| Water | 25% |
| Dermabase | to 60 Gm. |

Apply sparingly three times daily.

3. All cosmetics are discontinued, except for lipstick and mascara.
4. Soap is used for cleansing twice daily.

## REFERENCES

Abele, D. C.: Moisturizers and perioral dermatitis, Arch. Dermatol. **113:**110, 1977.

**A clinical observation by many.**

MacDonald, A., and Fiewel, M.: Perioral dermatitis: etiology and treatment with tetracycline, Br. J. Dermatol. **87:**315, 1972.

**Tetracycline remains a good treatment in this puzzling disorder.**

Weber, G.: Rosacea-like dermatitis: contraindications or intolerance reaction to strong steroids, Br. J. Dermatol. **86:**253, 1972.

**This early warning of untoward side effects of the potent topical steroids still stands!**

CHAPTER 24

# Pigmentation disorders

## PROCESS OF NORMAL PIGMENTATION

The single cell responsible for human skin pigmentation and all its social ramifications is a highly differentiated (specialized) cell in the basal layer of the epidermis, the *melanocyte*. This cell produces a complex polymer that is linked to protein to produce the brown-black color associated with normal skin and hair color, skin tanning, and localized deposits of blue, black, or shades of brown in the moles (congenital spots) in the skin. This cell traveled a long and arduous journey from the neural crest in the tenth to fourteenth week of intrauterine life to find its predestined cutaneous location. The difficulty of that long journey may be guessed by the rather large numbers of melanocytes that did not succeed in arriving but formed congenital pigmented birthmarks or moles in the dermis along the way to their planned location. The cells that do gain the epidermis are fairly uniformly distributed, in numbers surprisingly similar for all races. In its mature form, this highly social octopus-like cell, surrounded by its group of keratinocytes, has no known junction beyond pigment (melanin) production and transference. Some of the melanocytes are dendritic and pass on the pigment packages through hollow tubes of *dendrites* to surrounding epidermal cells. (Fig. 24-1). The *epidermal melanin unit* comprises the pigment cell and 36 or so adjacent keratinocytes that accept the pigment granules by nipping off the proffered dendrite with its pigmented center. Melanocytes present in hair-root papillae also enjoy the active participation of cortical and medullary keratinocytes in transference of pigment to the hair shaft. The melanocytes that remain in the central nervous system are found in the leptomeninges, uvea, or retina, are not dendritic, and retain the melanin they produce. Fitzpatrick and his colleagues have successfully investigated and lucidly described the process of human melanization in normal and in disordered states.

The amino acid tyrosine is the substrate from which tyrosinase begins the process of melanin production. Tyrosinase, an aerobic oxidase containing copper found only in melanocytes, converts tyrosine to dihydroxyphenylalanine (levodopa). This compound is further oxidized by tyrosinase through a complex series of steps to dopa-quinone and finally melanin, a polymer of quinone units. This virtually insoluble pigment is manufactured within the cell after accumulation of the components in the rough, and then the smooth, endoplasmic reticulum. Tyrosinase and the melanin precursors are assembled into well-defined packages, *melanosomes*, where the formation of melanin obscures the filamentous internal structure to a uniformly black electron-dense oval capsule. The size of the melanosome and the degree of melanization varies with race, genetic influence, and ultraviolet light exposure. The darker the overall skin color, the more completely melanized are the capsules found within melanocytes. Blacks also have slightly larger melanosomes than do whites. In addition, the smaller melanosomes are aggregated into clumps bound by a membrane. Light-skinned individuals experience more rapid degradation of melanosomes than do blacks.

As noted above, the melanocytes transfer pigment in melanosomes through their dendrites, which extend between and around epidermal cells to make contact with the 20 to 36 keratinocytes within the functional epidermal

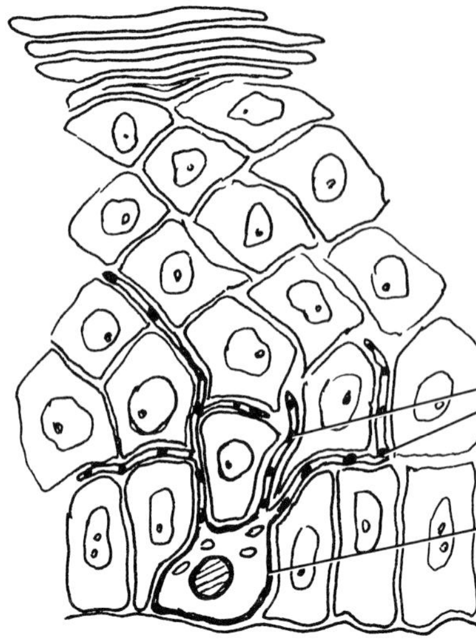


**Fig. 24-1.** Intraepidermal melanocyte responsible for skin pigmentation.

melanin unit. The epidermal cells phagocytose the ends of the dendrites containing melanosomes and retain the melanin capsules, which then move to form a supranuclear cap between the ultraviolet-light source and the cell nucleus where it remains as the epidermal cell differentiates and migrates to the granular layer. Keratinocyte activity increases with acceptance of melanosomes. In hair, the melanocytes present in the hair bulb pass on melanosomes to cortical and medullary structural cells, only during active hair growth (anagen). In the quiescent phase, melanocytes disappear, only to return when growth recommences. Resting "club" hairs, which have a shrunken white top, demonstrate this cessation of melanization at the time of cessation of growth. Pheomelanin, a yellow-red type of melanin that contains sulfur and demonstrates ultrastructural differences, is present in blond hair. Chalones, as described by Bullough, have been considered to control epidermal cellular replication, including that of sebaceous cells, keratinocytes, and melanocytes. By such chemical regulators, the rather fixed ratios of varied cells in the epidermis might be maintained. Voorhees envisages other regulators, such as cyclic AMP and polyamines, as well.

Tanning is produced by immediate darkening of the melanosomes already formed in cells, producing a visible darkening of light skin (immediate pigmentation, IP) and, further, by the formation of new melanin within 2 to 3 days. Ultraviolet light stimulates melanocytes to new melanin production. There is also increased spread upward of melanin with more rapidly proliferating epidermal cells. Melanin absorbs radiation throughout the entire range of visible and ultraviolet light.

Melanin has been described, and some of its known mechanisms of action have been indicated by Menon and Haberman. It is a remarkable compound, able to protect susceptible tissues from enormous doses of ultraviolet radiation, not, apparently, entirely by absorption but also by some as yet unclear active reactions with the ultraviolet light. Melanin may act as a photosensitizer, and indeed at higher doses of radiation, melanin may become cytotoxic. At shorter wavelengths, it has some hemolytic action. Perhaps this in some way relates to the unexplained deaths of those individuals in whom high prolonged doses of phenothiazines were found to mobilize melanin to the bloodstream and deposit it in the monocyte macrophage system where it was seen at autopsy (Satanove).

Pigmentation is thus under genetic control,

which regulates the origin, differentiation, and activity of melanocytes, production of melanosomes and their degree of melanization, and the amount of pigment transfer to epidermis and hair. Forms of albinism reflect defects in various stages of pigment production and transfer.

Ultraviolet-light exposure stimulates tyrosinase activity, pigment production, more melanocytes, more melanosomes per cell, more melanization of melanosomes, and greater transfer of melanin to the epidermis.

Hormonal factors also influence our skin color. The intermediate lobe of the pituitary forms melanocyte-stimulating hormone (MSH), which in combination with sex hormones is responsible for skin darkening in pregnancy. MSH and ACTH cause the hyperpigmentation of adrenal insufficiency.

Disorders of pigmentation obviously may be categorized as hyperpigmentation and hypopigmentation, but they must be examined in the light of our present knowledge of the process of melanin synthesis and transfer. The following are processes that may be responsible:

1. Increased or decreased numbers of melanocytes
2. Increased or decreased normal melanosome formation
3. Increased or decreased melanosome melanization
4. Increased or decreased melanin transfer
5. Increased or decreased melanosome degradation

Increased pigmentation in local areas may be the result of heat, pressure, friction, scratching or rubbing, as well as previous inflammation from a variety of causes. Dark-complexioned individuals pigment more easily than do fair ones, and some persons develop dark areas with any inflammatory cutaneous disorder. This may persist for months but will eventually fade.

#### REFERENCES

Bullough, W. S.: The actions of the chalones, Agents Actions **2**:1, 1971.
**Mitotic activity of the melanocytes is regulated by tissue-specific inhibitory chalones.**

Dewey, D. L.: The melanocyte chalone. In Forscher, B. K., and Houck, J. C., editors: Chalones: concepts and current researchers, Natl. Cancer Inst. Monogr. **38**:213, 1973.

Fitzpatrick, T. B., and Quevedo, W. C., Jr.: Biological processes underlying melanin pigmentation and pigmentary disorders, Mod. Trends Dermatol. **4**:122, 1971.
**Melanocyte and keratinocyte interactions, melanogenesis, melanosome transfer, and melanosome dispersal.**

Menon, I. A., and Haberman, H. F.: Mechanisms of action of melanins, Br. J. Dermatol. **97**:109, 1977.
**Further insight into the paradoxical attributes of these compounds. Excellent references.**

Satanove, A.: Pigmentation due to phenothiazines in high and prolonged dosage, J.A.M.A. **191**:263, 1965.
**Melanin transported by blood vessels to a generalized distribution.**

Sober, A. J., and Fitzpatrick, T. B.: Mechanisms of pigmentation in man. In Moschella, S. L., Pillsbury, D. M., and Hurley, H. J., editors: Dermatology, vol. 2, Philadelphia, 1975, W. B. Saunders Co., p. 1085.
**A careful, fully documented condensation of the physiology of cutaneous pigmentation.**

Voorhees, J. J., and Duell, E. H.: Psoriasis as a possible defect of the adenylcyclase–cyclic AMP cascade, Arch. Dermatol. **104**:352, 1971.
**Mitotic activity in the epidermis is controlled by levels of cyclic AMP.**

## DISCRETE PIGMENTATIONS
## Lesions with accumulation of pigment in the basal cell layer

### Freckle (ephelis)

A freckle is a flat, tan to dark brown, harmless, small superficial lesion accentuated by sun exposure and ordinarily limited to exposed skin surfaces. It first becomes apparent in children 6 to 9 years of age. Freckling is an inherited tendency, most frequently found in persons with red hair. Histologically, there are no more melanocytes in the basal cell layer, but they are larger and have more melanin.

#### *Treatment*

Individuals whose skin becomes freckled should be advised to avoid sunlight or to apply protective sunscreening ointments, since these are the persons who may develop chronic actinic changes. (See sunscreens, p. 62.)

Application of a bleaching cream may be beneficial over a prolonged period.

| | |
|---|---|
| Bleaching cream: | |
| Ammoniated mercury | 10% |
| Unibase | 30 Gm. |

Apply twice daily to small localized areas only.

There is, however, general reluctance to use mercury nowadays because of absorption. Kligman's compound can be used twice daily over a period of 3 to 7 weeks. It contains the following:

| | |
|---|---|
| Retinoic acid | 0.1% |
| Hydroquinone | 5% |
| Dexamethasone (or other steroid) | 0.1% |
| in hydrophilic ointment, or | |
| in propylene glycol, or | |
| in alcohol–propylene glycol | |

### Café-au-lait patch

Café-au-lait patch is a quite uniformly pale, tan, flat, irregularly shaped lesion, usually 2 to 10 cm. in diameter, occurring on any part of the skin surface. It is frequently present as a solitary lesion in otherwise normal individuals, but occurs as multiple lesions in persons with neurofibromatosis (von Recklinghausen's disease). Like freckles, it has no malignant potential.

No treatment is indicated for this lesion.

### Juvenile lentigo

The pigmented lesion of juvenile lentigo is multiple, small, flat, asymptomatic, *not* accentuated by sunlight, and dispersed over covered and exposed areas at random. The pigment is intraepidermal, and there is an increase in the number of clear cells, or melanocytes, in the basal cell layer. They first appear before freckles in children around 2 to 5 years of age. Occasionally, these tan to darker lesions may be found in very large numbers. Persistent numbers of lentigines, particularly in a brunette, must introduce the possibility of *xeroderma pigmentosum*.

Microscopically, there are large numbers of melanocytes in the basal cell layer and an elongation and clubbing of the rete pegs.

No treatment is indicated.

### Senile lentigo

Senile lentigo begins to appear on exposed areas after middle age. It is characterized by multiple, small to dime-sized, gray-brown lesions, often with a roughened surface, that may be associated with actinic or senile skin changes in the dermis. It is most frequently observed on the wrists, dorsa of hands, forearms, and faces of persons after middle age, particularly those with fair complexions. It is ordinarily a benign lesion. Clinical differentiation from junction nevus and from small seborrheic keratoses may be impossible. It is unlikely that it will ever become malignant. The histological appearance is similar to that of juvenile lentigo, except for the changes resulting from actinic damage in the dermis.

#### *Treatment*

Electrodesiccation and curettage may be performed for cosmetic reasons but will leave a small pale scar. Very superficial shave after a local anesthetic is infiltrated will permit full microscopic examination.

### Malignant lentigo

See discussion of superficial malignant melanoma and Hutchinson's freckle on p. 503.

## Lesions with accumulation of pigment in the dermis

### Mongolian spot, blue nevus, and pigmented nevus

For a discussion of mongolian spot, blue nevus, and pigmented nevus (Fig. 24-2), see p. 528.

### Tattoo

Tattoos result from the introduction beneath the epidermis into the dermis of various insoluble substances (for example, carbon or mercury). These are removed slowly or not at all by phagocytosis. These substances vary from the materials of the tattoo artist to dirt and to other foreign matter accidentally introduced by trauma.

#### *Treatment*

The various modalities include plastic surgery, which with selected progressive partial

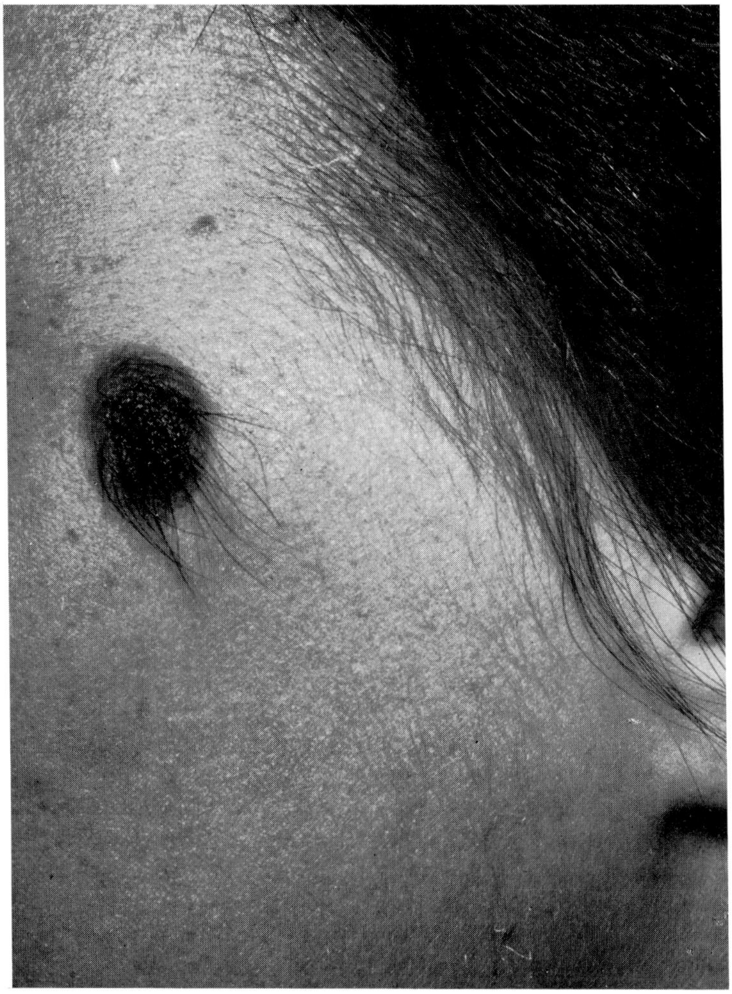

**Fig. 24-2.** Pigmented hairy nevus.

excisions, will remove even larger tattoos that cannot be excised in one procedure. Dermabrasion has been used successfully but tends to produce scarring when carried down into the dermis. Also, it may scatter the pigment particles in the deeper layer, a hazard in the case of allergic reaction to the chemicals used. Salabrasion (Crittenden) can be painful and may produce keloid formation in our experience. Antibiotics orally for a week after the procedure help to prevent secondary infection. Grice has used the Castroviejo keratotome, which is also used to obtain epidermal slices for experimental work, and is pleased with her results. Superficial removal of the tattoo can be followed by compresses, which keep the wound from epithelizing and promote discharge of remaining pigment particles into the overlying moist exudate. Scutt describes in detail a further method, using retattooing with glycerin and tannic acid and then rubbing with silver nitrate. He reports highly successful results.

## DIFFUSE PIGMENTATIONS

### Chloasma

Chloasma (Fig. 24-3) is a mottled brown pigmentation that involves the face of women during and after the childbearing age. The pigmentation is characteristically blotchy, but

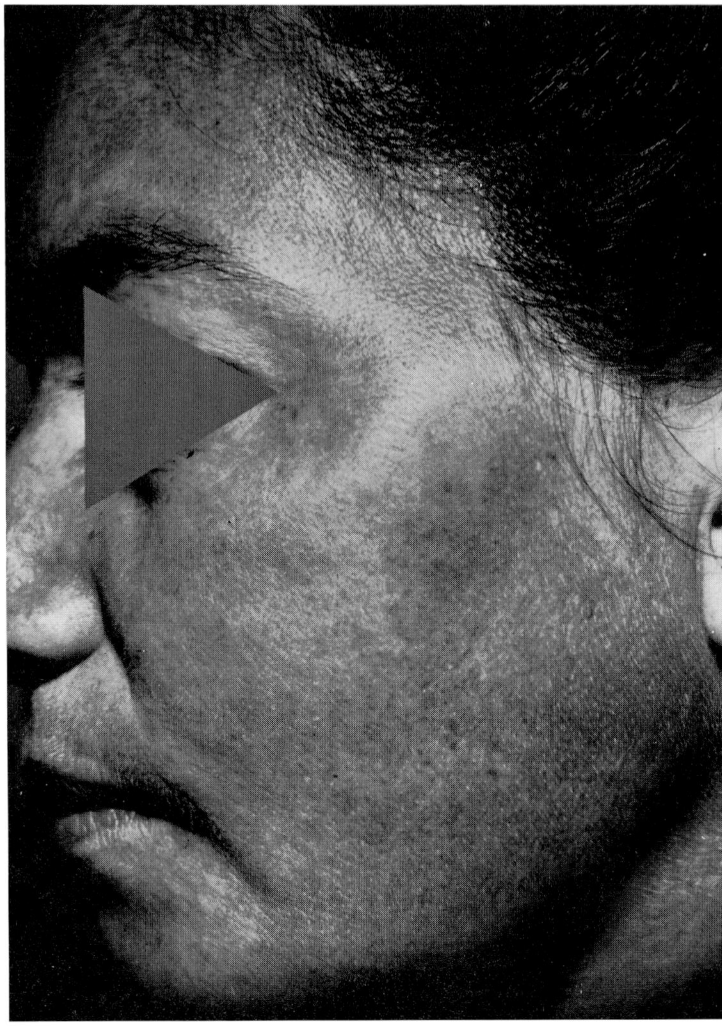

**Fig. 24-3.** Chloasma. Pigmentation affects forehead, preauricular, and supramalar areas.

usually symmetrical, and involves the forehead, malar eminences, and preauricular areas. It less often extends to the upper lip, the chin, and the sides of the neck. Pregnant women, as well as those taking progestogen medication in a rhythmic monthly cycle to control ovulation and the menses, can develop this pigmentation. A similar hyperpigmentation may occur in Cushing's or Addison's disease, some forms of chronic illness, and malnutrition and occasionally in normal individuals. It is exaggerated by sun exposure and therefore is more noticeable in the summer. Melanin is increased in the epidermis, chiefly in the basal cells.

### *Differential diagnosis*

***Tar melanosis.*** There are patchy hyperpigmented areas on sun-exposed regions of the face caused by photocontact dermatitis. The causative agents are tar products or cosmetics or perfume containing tar products.

### *Treatment*

Oral contraceptives must be discontinued to produce fading of the lesions. Protection from direct and reflected sunlight is essential, or the condition will persist. Covermark, sunscreens, makeup, and wide hats all help.

Topical depigmenting medications include hydroquinone, 2% to 4% cream, applied sparingly twice daily. Kligman and Willis have suggested the following formulation of retinoic acid 0.1%, hydroquinone 5%, and dexamethasone 0.1% in hydrophilic ointment or an alcohol–propylene glycol base. They achieved remarkable clinical improvement in the treatment of freckles and melasma. Postinflammatory pigmentation also responded, but not so satisfactorily. The problem, however, is that some return of pigment may appear after therapy along with normal repigmentation.

Bleehen has evaluated a new depigmenting compound (4-isopropylcatechol), which, however, does have sensitizing potential.

The sunscreen that we use is para-aminobenzoic acid 5% and ethyl alcohol 95%, applied twice daily and after swimming or bathing. (See sunscreens, p. 62.)

### Poikiloderma of Civatte

Poikiloderma of Civatte is a very common dermatitis, beginning with patches of erythema of the sides of the face and lateral aspect of the neck, and occurs chiefly in women. There is subsequent dryness and scaling, followed by a reticulated telangiectasia and melanin pigmentation surrounding the hair follicles and extending over the sides of the neck and face. In long-standing cases, linear telangiectasia develops. The cause is unknown, but there may be an element of photosensitivity. The inframandibular region is spared.

### Berloque dermatitis

Application of perfumes and scented cosmetics containing oil of Bergamot, prior to actinic exposure, produces in some individuals a patchy tan pigmentation over the area of contact, usually below the ears, on the sides of the neck, but it may affect any sun-exposed area. Repeated applications and sun exposure produce a deepening of the pigmentation.

### Residual pigmentation after inflammation

Trauma and many dermatoses (from insect bites to dermatitis herpetiformis) may produce subsequent hyperpigmentation of the skin at the affected sites. This occurs relative to the color of the individual's normal skin and the degree of inflammation or injury. Dark-complexioned individuals and Orientals tend to develop hyperpigmentation under these circumstances much more readily than fair-complexioned persons.

### Postirradiation pigmentation

X rays, grenz rays, alpha particles, and all forms of ionizing radiation have the ability to produce cutaneous hyperpigmentation. Up to a certain extent, the softer or less penetrating the radiation, the greater its acute pigment-producing effect. Pigmentation results from increased numbers of melanocytes, as well as increased melanin production of the melanocytes. The duration is 6 months or more, depending on its severity. Chronic radiation changes resulting in atrophy and degeneration of the dermis produce a patchy hyperpigmentation and depigmentation.

### Addison's disease

A characteristic kind of pigmentation develops in which there is a tan to darker brown discoloration of the exposed areas, skin folds, areolae, mucous membranes, and sites of pressure or recent trauma. The buccal mucosa or gums may show streaky areas of hyperpigmentation. The color is attributable to melanin deposition. These patients have none of the normal inhibition of pituitary activity by adrenal steroids, and there is increased secretion of melanocyte-stimulating hormone (MSH), as well as ACTH, from the pituitary gland.

### Pigmentation associated with pregnancy

Pregnant women and women on prolonged estrogen therapy will develop a darkening of the nipple areolae, linea alba, axillae, perineum, and genitalia, and the changes sometimes result in a blotchy pigmentation of the forehead and face (see p. 417). Estrogens, and androgens as well, have a general stimulating effect upon melanin formation.

### Pigmentation in pellagra

Deficiencies of vitamins A and C, as well as of niacin, have all been reported to produce increased melanin formation. In pellagra, the pigmentation appears at the sites of inflammation and with exposure to sunlight, so that clinically the brown areas are preceded by erythema. They involve the hands, face, and neck predominantly.

### Hemochromatosis

A disorder of hyperpigmentation occurring in middle-aged individuals, hemochromatosis is associated with abnormal iron absorption from the gastrointestinal tract. There is an enlarged liver, diabetes mellitus, and elevated serum iron. The diffuse, generalized, dusky gray-brown pigmentation observed in hemochromatosis has usually been considered a result of iron pigment deposition. Recently, however, clinical studies have revealed that both iron and melanin deep in the basal layer are responsible for the color in this condition. The characteristic color is attributable to the depth of the pigment and the overlying epidermis.

### Hypostatic dermatitis

In hypostatic dermatitis the hemosiderin, present as a result of red blood cell extravasation and subsequent destruction, is very su-

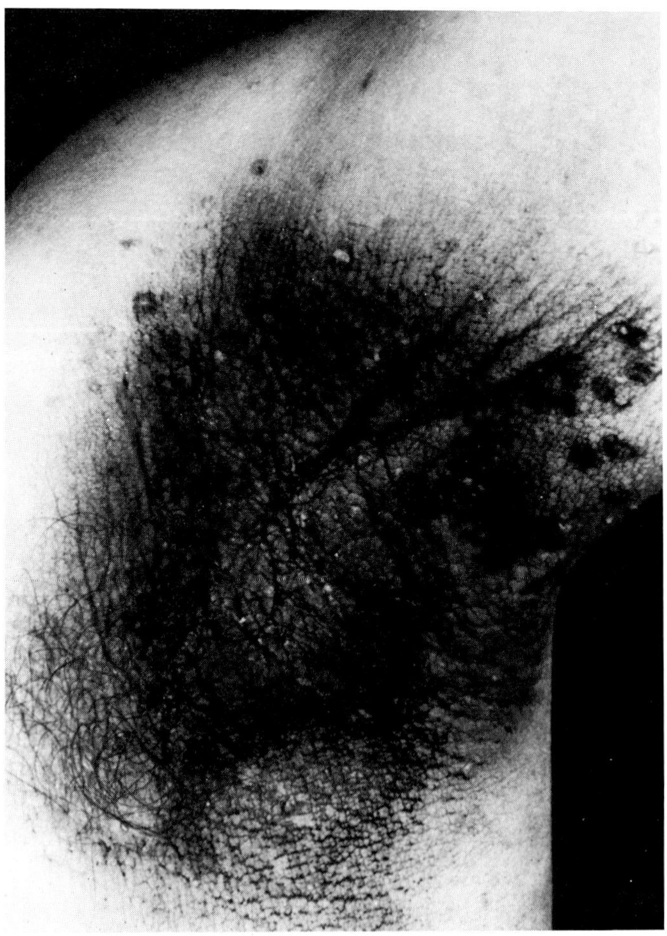

**Fig. 24-4.** Acanthosis nigricans.

perficial and thus clearly seen. It produces a tan-brown color, initially along the course of the veins and subsequently spreading to cover the entire area of the ankle and leg involved by the dermatitis. A part of the pigmentation is caused by melanin.

### Acanthosis nigricans (Fig. 24-4)

Acanthosis nigricans is classified into four types: benign (hereditary juvenile), malignant (associated with internal cancer), pseudoacanthosis (associated with obesity), and acanthosis associated with various endocrinological disorders, of which Cushing's disease is the commonest.

The disorder is characterized by a gray-black, rough, or even papillomatous pigmentation of the axillae, neck, inguinal area, perianal area, and other skin folds. The arms and the mucous membranes of lips and genitalia may be roughened and pigmented. It is microscopically a hyperkeratosis, acanthosis, and hyperpigmentation, with increased melanin in the epidermal basal cells.

The *benign* hereditary form may be present at birth. The highly significant *adult* form associated with internal malignancy may precede the apparent development of the cancer. The cutaneous changes have been shown to recede with treatment of the malignancy. *Pseudoacanthosis* may occur in children or in adults and is associated with obesity. In some cases, endocrine disorders and, more rarely, certain drugs are associated with the characteristic changes of acanthosis nigricans.

### Hyperpigmentation caused by drugs

Arsenic, hydantoin, chloroquin, and chlorpromazine can produce hyperpigmentation. Fixed drug eruptions notoriously leave residual hyperpigmented areas.

#### REFERENCES


Arndt, K. A., and Fitzpatrick, T. B.: Topical use of hydroquinone as a depigmenting agent, J.A.M.A. **94**:965, 1965.
**Satisfactory and effective.**

Bleehen, S. S.: The treatment of hypermelanosis with 4-isopropylcatechol, Br. J. Dermatol. **94**:687, 1976.
**Four of 68 patients developed allergic contact dermatitis. This compound is a potent depigmenting agent.**

Brown, J., and Winkelmann, R. K.: Acanthosis nigricans: a study of 90 cases, Medicine **47**:33, 1968.
**Acanthosis nigricans may be associated with malignancy, 17 of 90 patients, genetic abnormalities, 6 of 90, endocrine disease, 20 of 90, drugs 3 of 90, or idiopathic 43 of 90.**

Crittenden, F. M., Jr.: Salabrasion—removal of tattoos by superficial abrasion with table salt, Cutis **7**:295, 1971.
**Simple, safe, but not entirely satisfactory except for the most superficial marks.**

Grice, K.: Tattoos. In Maddin, S., editor: Current dermatologic management, ed. 2, St. Louis, 1975, The C. V. Mosby Co., p. 54.
**She likes the Castroviejo keratotome for shaving off small superficial marks.**

Kligman, A. M., and Willis, I.: A new formula for depigmenting human skin, Arch. Dermatol. **111**:40, 1975.
**An empiric formulation that is an effective depigmenting combination but can produce considerable inflammation, particularly in East Indians.**

Mehregan, A. H.: Lentigo senilis and its evolutions, J. Invest. Dermatol. **65**:429, 1975.
**A comprehensive clinical and histopathological review.**

Menon, I. A., and Haberman, H. F.: Mechanisms of action of melanin, Br. J. Dermatol. **97**:109, 1977.
**A remarkable presentation of melanin and its mechanism of action with excellent references.**

Scutt, R. W. B.: Chemical removal of tattoo, Br. J. Plast. Surg. **25**:189, 1972.
**The technique produces a slough that contains much of the pigment.**


## DEPIGMENTATIONS

### Albinism

Albinism is a hereditary trait, with lack of pigmentation that may be complete or partial. In *partial albinism* or *piebaldism*, the same area may be affected in more than one member of a family. Hair in the involved areas is nonpigmented, or white forelock may be present. The affected areas are usually linear and unilateral, in a distinctive pattern, unchanging throughout life. It is a dominant characteristic.

In complete, or *universal albinism*, which is a recessive or irregularly dominant trait, there is lack of eye pigment, nystagmus, red or pink nonpigmented iris, and lack of skin and hair pigment. There may be some pig-

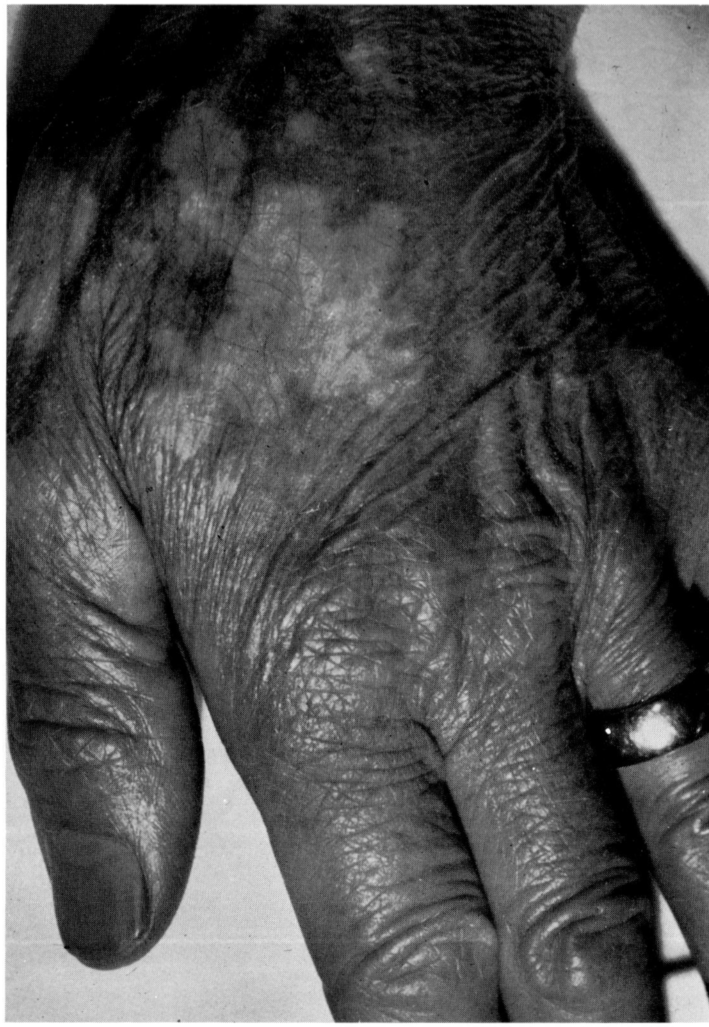

**Fig. 24-5.** Vitiligo. Ordinarily bilateral and tends to appear in flexures.

mentation with increasing age. In climates with much sun, exposure to the outdoors results in premature actinic keratosis and cutaneous malignancy, because of the inability to tan.

In complete albinism, electron microscopy has shown that there are nonpigmented melanosomes within normal melanocytes, so that there is a block in the synthesis of pigment, and melanin is not formed from its precursors.

Partial albinism, however, differs in that no melanocytes are present in the nonpigmented areas.

#### *Treatment*

There is no treatment other than protection from actinic damage.

### Vitiligo

Vitiligo (Fig. 24-5) may be inherited as an autosomal dominant trait, without any sex predominance. The number of new cases of vitiligo increase steadily with advancing age, most often between the ages of 40 and 60 years. It may remain stationary for years, affecting only small areas, or may progress steadily to involve more extensive areas or even the entire skin surface, as well as the hair

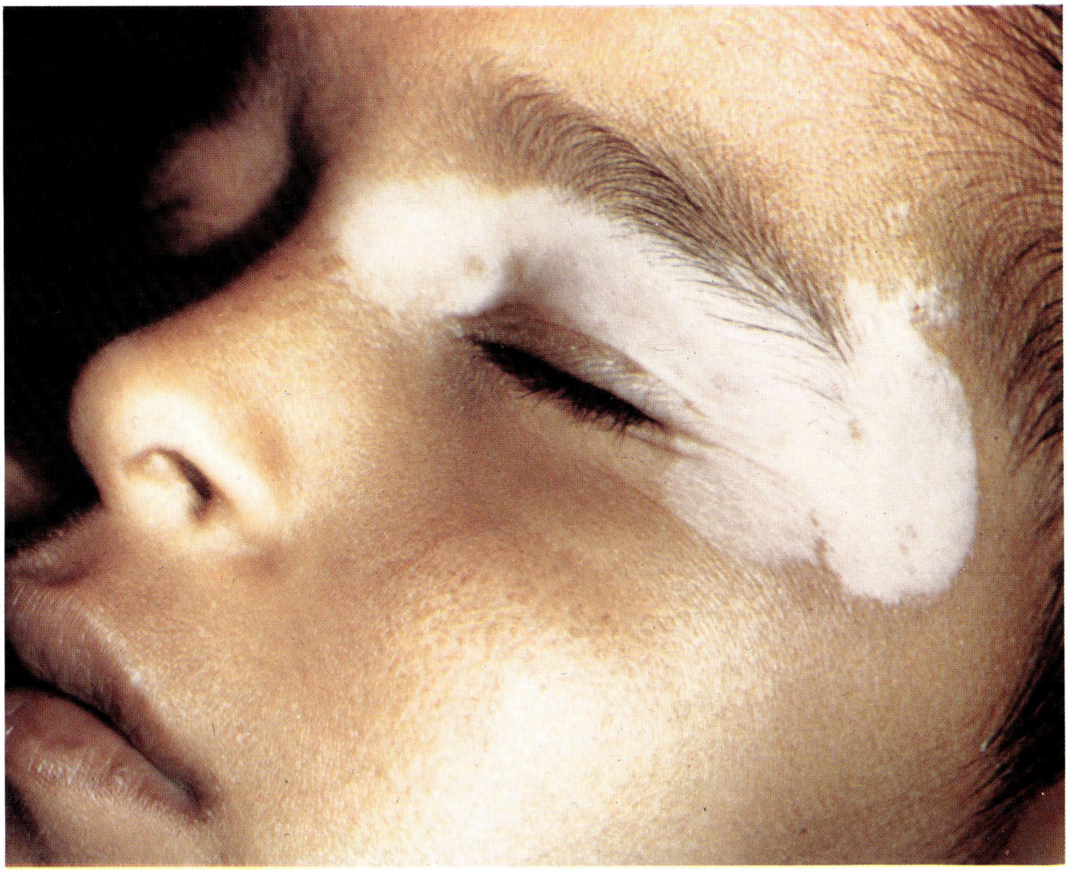

**Plate 42**

Vitiligo. A disease with strong social implications in many parts of the world, among the more deeply pigmented races.

(universal vitiligo). The eyes, however, do not lose their pigment. The lesions are startlingly white, with no pigment (Plate 42), and may have hyperpigmented borders. They are irregular and vary greatly in size.

Certain anatomical areas show a predilection for this disorder, for example, periorbital areas, hands, axillae, perineum, and neck. Vitiligo usually develops symmetrically and may on occasion follow pressure or trauma to an area. Emotional stress is often blamed. The skin is normal except for loss of pigment. Repigmentation occurs not uncommonly, beginning around the hair follicles.

Many theories have been advanced concerning the pathogenesis of vitiligo, but recent work indicates an association with autoimmune disease. There appears to be a significant relationship between vitiligo and thyroid disease, adrenocortical insufficiency, scleroderma, alopecia areata, and pernicious anemia, and a possible relationship with diabetes mellitus. Even in the absence of these autoimmune diseases, a substantially increased frequency of parietal cell, thyroid, and adrenal antibodies has been reported in patients with vitiligo. There is a family history of vitiligo, halo nevi, posttraumatic depigmentation of the skin, or premature graying of the hair in 50% of patients with vitiligo. Melanoma and vitiligo have been observed to occur together, and halo nevi and vitiligo as well. In the light of the recent discoveries of circulating and cell-mediated immune defenses against abnormal melanocytes in melanoma and in halo nevi, one is optimistic that a rationale for the development and course of vitiligo will be demonstrated. *In malignant melanoma, areas of vitiligo or complete depigmentation are looked upon as successful sorties in the battle of host against disease.* Lerner reviews three hypotheses for the etiology of vitiligo, one of which is based on an immune mechanism. Macaroon recently reported five more cases associating insulin-dependent diabetes and vitiligo, and perhaps a hereditary component as well.

Koga has just recently proposed a theory of etiology that divides the disease into two categories: dermatomally distributed and nondermatomally distributed. He believes that the dermatomal category is of neurocutaneous origin, and the other is an immune disorder. His therapeutic responses tend to confirm this belief.

Hertz demonstrated a circulating IgG antibody from the serum of two patients with vitiligo that activated complement and bound to melanocytes, nevus cells, and melanoma cells.

### Microscopic findings

Melanocytes are abnormal and in various stages of cell death at the periphery of the lesions. They are absent in the depigmented areas. Morohashi has demonstrated nerve cell axones in close relationship to these cells, extending into the epidermis—a most unusual behavior for axones, unless some cellular damage has attracted them there. This may relate to the etiology of the disease. Lerner has for years proposed neurocutaneous causation.

### Differential diagnosis

***Partial albinism (piebaldism).*** See discussion earlier in this chapter.

***Acquired leukoderma.*** Depigmentation occurs from contact with a monobenzyl ether of hydroquinone used in the manufacture of rubber products. It is seen in areas of contact with gloves, condoms, and so forth.

***Tinea versicolor.*** Round or oval finely scaling white but not completely depigmented patches are seen on the upper thorax. Wood's light reveals a beige or coral fluorescence, and scrapings possess fungal elements.

### Treatment

Both topical and oral forms of 8-methoxypsoralen have been used in association with carefully graded sun exposure. Severe blistering can occur after the topical use of even minute amounts of this chemical, and it must be used with care. Oral dosage is 40 mg. taken within 2 hours before sun exposure. Initial sun exposure should be limited to 20 minutes or less. If no redness results in 24 hours, one can increase the dosage to 50 mg. 2 hours prior to sun exposure. The normal tendency to begin repigmentation in the summer in vitiligo is used and enhanced by this procedure. Even with good results the return of pigmentation is slow, occurring over many months or years. However, it does repigment. Children demonstrate a quicker response than do adults.

With the advent of PUVA therapy (using psoralens and long-wave ultraviolet light) (see p. 474) cases of hitherto resistant vitiligo do respond. As in psoriasis, maintenance therapy may be required. Repigmentation may take months to years.

The glucocorticoids have been used topically, orally, and intralesionally with varying degrees of success. It would appear that the more potent topical glucocorticoid compounds, applied under occlusion, may bring about repigmentation. However, the usual warnings must be observed, since long continued or widespread usage can create epidermal atrophic change or adrenal suppression. In an immune mechanism of disease, the committed lymphocytes are very resistant to glucocorticoid influence; thus high tissue concentration and potent forms are necessary. If Koga is right, the form of vitiligo may dictate whether ultraviolet light or glucocorticoids should be used.

Covering with waterproof cosmetic agents (Covermark) may be desirable.

#### REFERENCES

Aetiology of vitiligo: Editorial, Lancet **2**:1298, 1971.
**A review of currently plausible etiologies, one of which is inheritance.**

Hertz, K. C., Gazze, L. A., Kirkpatrick, C. H., and Katz, S. I.: Autoimmune vitiligo. Detection of antibodies to melanin-producing cells, N. Engl. J. Med. **297:**12, 634, 1977.

**Both patients demonstrated extensive immune disorder and endocrine faults.**

Howitz, J., Brodthagen, H., Schuartz, M., et al.: Prevalence of vitiligo. Epidemiologic survey on the Isle of Bernholm, Denmark, Arch. Dermatol. **113:**47, 1977.

**A remarkable epidemiologic study revealing vitiligo in 179 of 47,033 patients examined. The prevalence was 0.38% against 1% usually quoted.**

Lerner, A. B.: Vitiligo, Prog. Dermatol. **6:**1, 1972.

**Three theories of causation: autoimmunity neurochemical factors, melanocyte self-destruction.**

Koga, M.: Vitiligo: a new classification and therapy, Br. J. Dermatol. **94:**255, 1977.

**Dermatomally and nondermatomally distributed vitiligo, one neurocutaneous and one autoimmune.**

MacCuish, A. C., and Irvine, W. J.: Autoimmunological aspects of diabetes mellitus, Clin. Endocrin. Metabol. **4:**435, 1975.

**A review of the autoimmune factors associated with diabetes and with vitiligo.**

Macaroon, C., Winter, R., and Traisman, H.: Vitiligo and juvenile diabetes mellitus, Arch. Dermatol. **113:**1515, 1977.

**Five children with both, three had HL-A B8 and four had thyroid adrenal or gastric antibodies.**

Morohashi, M., Hashimoto, K., and Goodman, T. F., Jr., et al.: Ultrastructural studies of vitiligo, Vogt-Koyonagi syndrome, and incontinentia pigmenti achromians, Arch. Dermatol. **113:**755, 1977.

**Dying melanocytes and nerve axons in association with some of them. What does it mean?**

Theodoridis, A., Tsambaos, D., Sivenas, C., et al.: Oral trimethylpsoralen in the treatment of vitiligo, Acta Derm. Venereol. **56:**253, 1976.

**Oral trimethylpsoralen and ultraviolet light over sufficient periods of time will repigment vitiligo. Natural sunlight appeared more effective in children than the artificial light source.**

## SUMMARY OF MELANIN PIGMENTATIONS

### Pigmentation of exposed areas

On exposed areas of the body, pigmentation can result from normal tanning response to sun, photosensitivity to drugs, porphyria, Addison's disease (in addition to hyperpigmentation of creases, folds, and buccal mucosa), acromegaly, argyria and hemochromatosis (in which pigmentation is generalized, but more noticeable on exposed areas), malignant melanoma, ulcerative colitis, pellagra, and xeroderma pigmentosum.

### Generalized pigmentation

Generalized pigmentation may be caused by Hodgkin's disease, Addison's disease, uremia, hemochromatosis, acromegaly, and pituitary tumor.

### Localized pigmentation

Localized pigmentation on the head or face is associated with sprue, pregnancy, female hormones, drugs, pellagra, and nevus of Ota.

On the body, such pigmentation may be caused by radiation therapy, heat, mechanical irritation, dermatitis herpetiformis, urticaria pigmentosa, localized scleroderma, acanthosis nigricans, neurofibromatosis, and mongolian spot.

On the lower extremities, pigmentation may be associated with hypostatic dermatitis, diabetes, heat, mechanical irritation, insect bites, trauma, and lichen planus.

CHAPTER 25

# Pityriasis rosea

Pityriasis rosea is a self-limited disease of unknown etiology that has peaks of occurrence during the spring and fall.

### *Natural course*

Characteristically, a single oval lesion develops first, called a *herald patch*. From several days up to 2 or 3 weeks later, the remainder of the eruption develops on the trunk and extremities. The new smaller lesions are usually similar in configuration to the initial herald patch and are lined up with their long axes parallel and in the direction of the lines of cleavage of the skin (Fig. 25-1). The thorax is the site of greatest frequency of occurrence, but unusual cases limited to the extremities or confined to one area are observed. Lesions on exposed areas are rarely seen.

Individual lesions are pale, erythematous, and macular and have a fine superficial scale. Vesiculation may occasionally be apparent. Papular forms occur, however, and the lesions then may be quite prominent (Fig. 25-2).

The total duration is from 4 to 8 weeks. It is a one-episode disease as a rule, although some recurrences are reported. It is not infectious or contagious. Rarely are two concurrent cases in a family reported.

Pityriasis rosea is less likely to occur on tanned surfaces, and sun exposure appears to hasten the course of the disorder.

Takaki and Miyazaki have reported cytolytic changes in the keratinocyte immediately adjacent to a Langerhans cell in the epidermis of the herald plaque in each of five patients with pityriasis rosea. They have also demonstrated circulating IgM anticytoplasmic antibody, which may be associated with the same cytolytic process. The function of the Langerhans cell is now believed to represent an intraepidermal phagocyte concerned with antigen processing.

### *Microscopic findings*

Findings include a nonspecific inflammation, with a cellular infiltrate in the dermis; some early vesiculation may be seen in the epidermis.

### *Differential diagnosis*

***Seborrheic dermatitis.*** Seborrheic dermatitis consists usually of a diffuse distribution of irregularly shaped, scaling red patches, chiefly on the scalp, face, and midsternum.

***Psoriasis.*** The scale is heavier and the lesions not so uniform in psoriasis, except in the rapidly appearing *guttate* variety. There is no herald patch, and there is usually a previous personal or family history of psoriasis.

***Syphilis.*** Cutaneous lesions of syphilis may closely resemble pityriasis rosea, but again there is no typical herald patch. The patient does not feel well during the cutaneous outbreak. Palms and soles are involved. Serological tests for syphilis are positive.

***Tinea corporis.*** The single herald patch of pityriasis rosea may mimic tinea corporis. The causative fungus is found on microscopic examination and culture of scrapings from the lesion.

### *Treatment*

Treatment is ordinarily unnecessary. Pityriasis rosea is a self-limited disease that is tolerated by most patients when they realize the lesions will disappear in a few weeks.

If pruritus is severe, the following medications may be prescribed:

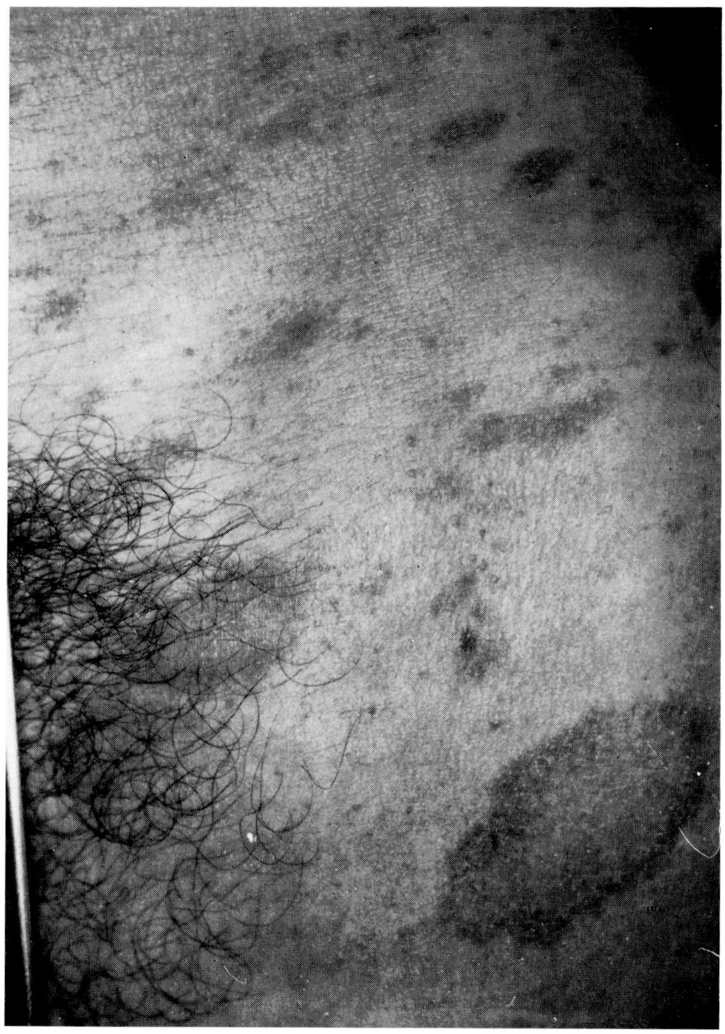

**Fig. 25-1.** Pityriasis rosea. Herald patch is larger than subsequent lesions.

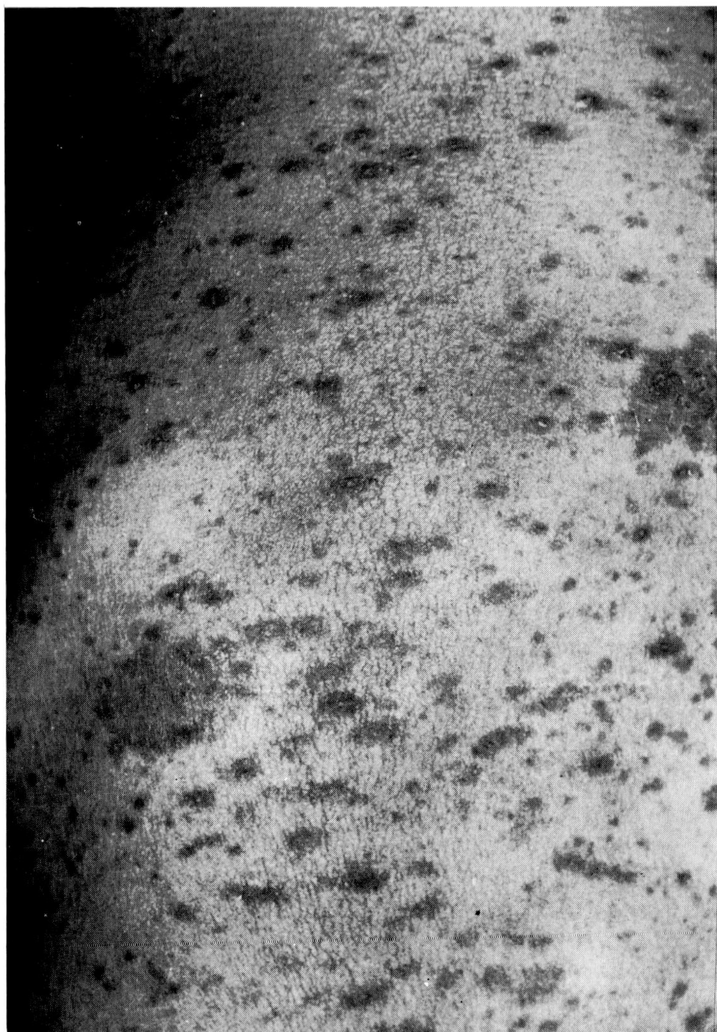

**Fig. 25-2.** Pityriasis rosea, with prominent papular lesions.

| | |
|---|---|
| Menthol | 0.25% |
| Phenol | 0.25% |
| Dermabase | 2 oz. |
| Water | to 8 oz. |

Apply three or four times daily.

| | |
|---|---|
| Trimeprazine tartrate (Panectyl) | 2.5 to 5 mg. |

Label: 1 tablet at bedtime.

Ultraviolet light exposure will hasten the course of the disease, as shown by Merchant's clever one-sided treatment with ultraviolet light. The treated side, if it desquamated, improved promptly.

## REFERENCES

Björnberg, A. and Hellgren, L.: Pityriasis rosea: a statistical, clinical, and laboratory investigation of 826 patients and matched healthy controls, Acta Derm. Venereol. **42**(suppl. 50):1, 1962.
**90 year old's familial occurrences and multiple attacks, as well as the classic cases. All are in this excellent paper.**

Merchant, M. and Hammond, R.: Controlled study of ultraviolet light for pityriasis rosea, Cutis **4**:548, 1974
**This ingenious study of one-sided ultraviolet-light therapy (successful) in 66 confirms treatment of pityriasis rosea with ultraviolet light.**

Takaki, Y., and Miyazaki, H.: Cytolytic degeneration of keratinocytes adjacent to Langerhans cells in pityriasis rosea, Acta Derm. Venereol. **56**:99, 1976.
**Finding cytolytic changes adjacent to Langerhans cells in herald plaques is of etiologic interest.**

CHAPTER 26

# Primary irritant dermatitis (hand eczema) and nummular dermatitis

## PROTECTIVE BARRIER FUNCTION OF SKIN

The barrier function of the skin prevents passage of water in or out through the stratum corneum, although there is some minimal transepidermal loss of water as a part of the insensible perspiration and the keratinization process. So little moisture is exchanged that in an environment of low humidity, the stratum corneum can lose its integrity from extreme dryness and prolonged submersion in freshwater or saltwater but has virtually no effect on the internal milieu.

The barrier, rather than being a well-defined layer at a specific depth, appears to encompass all the layers of the stratum corneum and decreases gradually as these layers are stripped away.

Gases, with the exception of carbon monoxide, pass freely through the skin.

Water-soluble substances that also have good lipid solubility penetrate the epidermis well. Highly ionized polar substances may not. The compounds that do penetrate the corneal barrier, do so promptly, but in minute amounts through the appendages—the sweat glands and hair follicles, which are breaks in the integrity of the outer layer. Slower but much more significant penetration occurs as these compounds move through the intact epidermis between and through cells.

Phenol, salicylic acid, resorcin, fat-soluble hormones, vitamins, and certain other substances can penetrate the epidermal barrier. The chief avenue of absorption of these substances (except for gases) is through damage to the stratum corneum or through the hair follicles and sebaceous glands.

The normal barriers to penetration of all substances are greatly altered and may be completely lost in certain cutaneous diseases in which the epidermis is damaged. Penetration of drugs is increased in acute contact dermatitis, for example, so that greater untoward effects as well as therapeutic benefits must be expected from topically applied medications.

The subject of vehicles for carrying medications through the skin is a complex one. The vehicle can establish only an *optimum* environment for penetration by the desired substance. There is no ideal vehicle, as the usefulness of the vehicle is proportional to the solubility of the desired medication in the vehicle as compared to its solubility in the stratum corneum. The vehicle should carry the drug but deliver it up readily to the tissue.

Paradoxically, the skin of the palms and soles, once used only for bearing weight, now in the case of the palms, is required to function as a barrier against wetness and strong toxic agents such as solvents and detergents. No part of our skin surface is less able to comply. The cells of the palms are more easily damaged by trauma, alkalis, and chemicals, contain only half the amount of water-soluble substances, become brittle on drying, and are much more permeable to water and chemicals than other parts of the skin (Montagna).

Increased hydration enhances the penetration of medications. This process is accomplished clinically by the use of plastic occlusive films over a medication, a procedure that has been shown to increase by many times the amount of drug penetrating the skin.

Dimethyl sulfoxide (DMSO) has exceptional qualities as a solvent and as a vehicle to enhance penetration into the skin. It increases the epidermal reservoir of steroids and promotes penetration of other compounds, to the degree produced by occlusion with a plastic film.

#### REFERENCE

Montagna, W., and Parakkal, P. F.: The structure and function of skin, ed. 3, New York, 1974, Academic Press, Inc., p. 63.
**A short digression on the properties and function of the stratum corneum.**

## PRIMARY IRRITANT DERMATITIS

Hand dermatitis from exposure to primary irritants is responsible for housewife's eczema and most of the industrial dermatoses. Large numbers of patients suffer from this common dermatological disorder.

### *Natural course*

Out of 107,206 persons in a general health survey over 10 years, Agrup found that there were 827 cases of hand eczema, of which almost 500 were primary irritant in origin.

Hand eczemas from entirely different causes may closely resemble one another.

Initially, the affected areas, which are most often the fingers, hands, wrists, and forearms, become erythematous and pruritic. Patches of small vesicles develop in the more acute forms of this condition. Dryness of the area, with some scaling and fissure formation, is not unusual (Fig. 26-1). Lichenification, hyperkeratosis, and fissuring and cracking, secondary to inflammation, may occur in long-standing cases.

The potentially irritating industrial soaps, detergents, and common household cleaning products most often believed to be responsible for this form of dermatitis are so frequently used that the industrial worker or housewife fails to appreciate the actual role that these irritants play in the production of dermatitis. Primary irritant chemicals, such as acids, solvents, lime, alkalis, oils, and other compounds, produce identical dermatitides. Alkalinity is a hazard to the stratum corneum.

These agents usually produce their effect slowly, and rarely is there a clear-cut, sudden onset of the dermatitis. It is always necessary to determine the extent of exposure in time and concentration of the irritant, in order to evaluate its capacity to produce a dermatitis. The appearance is not specific and may vary from simple dryness and chapping to erythema, hyperkeratosis, or the recurrent itchy vesicles of sweat retention on an altered stratum corneum.

The course of primary irritant dermatitis may be prolonged, with exacerbations and remissions dependent on the degree and times of exposure. At the onset there may be periods of complete freedom, but periods of involvement become longer and clear periods shorter, with steadily worsening signs. In allergic contact dermatitis, weekend and holiday remissions are usually quite apparent. With the slower reacting primary irritant dermatitis, however, it may take longer than a vacation period to produce a subsidence of the dermatitis. The reasons for this are poorly understood, but the phenomenon is frequently observed. This produces obvious difficulties in establishing a firm diagnosis of primary irritant dermatitis early in the disease.

The degree of inflammation varies considerably from individual to individual. This may depend on such factors as race, degree of perspiration, type of skin, preexisting disease, and family history. It is known that blacks, Orientals, and the descendants of persons from the southern European and Mediterranean areas, with easily pigmented skin, are less subject to the effect of irritants than persons with fair complexions.

Perspiration varies in pH from person to person and also in one individual, and alkalinity of sweat seems to be a predisposing factor to primary irritant dermatitis. Excessive perspiration has been recognized as a hazard and warned against as early as 1839 by writers in Germany. This is particularly true of workers handling certain solid substances that become irritants when moistened.

Another hazard is the repetitive use of water, as occurs with compulsive hand washers, or housewives who are compulsive house cleaners, and also professional dishwashers, salad makers, bartenders, dental hygienists, and nurses, who must wash their hands fre-

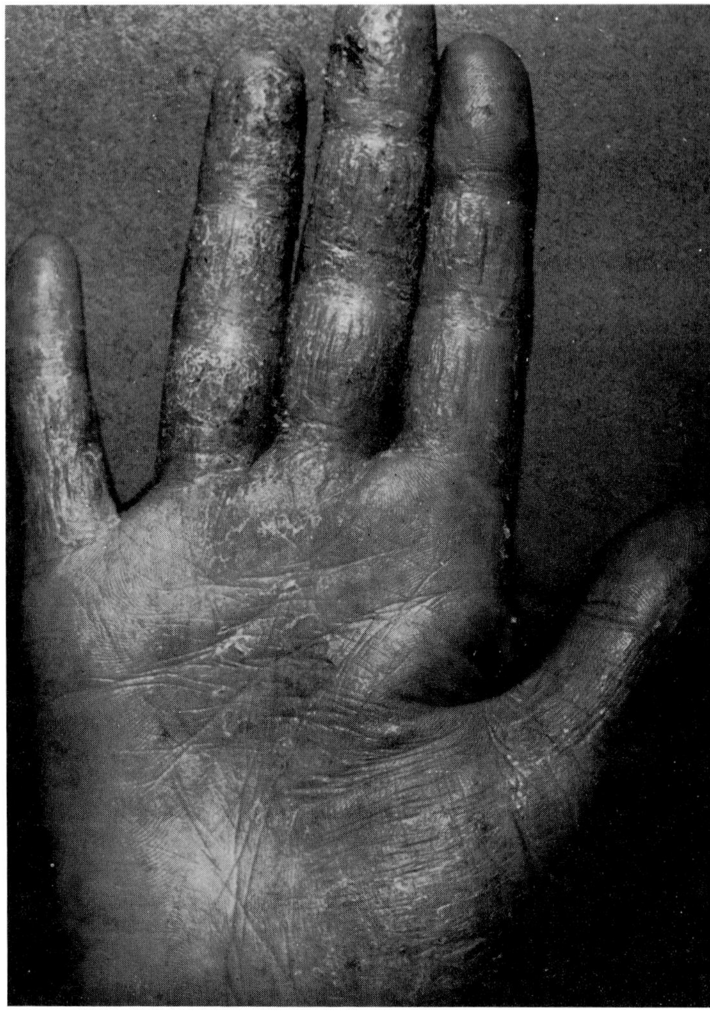

**Fig. 26-1.** Primary irritant dermatitis (housewife's eczema).

quently. However, Rietschel did demonstrate that the striking inflammation Willis observed from water immersion was not always a sequel.

Excessive moisture, either external or from perspiration, hydrates the outer stratum corneum, increases the penetration of many substances, probably compromises the barrier function of the skin, and promotes friability of the protective layer. This occurs because of loss of the water-soluble components of the epidermis that are able to bind water and maintain the integrity and pliability of the stratum corneum. This is accompanied by a drying and fissuring of the affected part. With defects in the epidermal barrier, chemicals that ordinarily are not irritants may become so (Suskind).

Atopic skin is more susceptible of primary irritation than normal skin. It is also susceptible to the development of chronic dermatitis.

Frequently a primary irritant dermatitis, particularly in the atopic individual, is complicated by secondary bacterial infection. This may not be immediately apparent, as the signs of infection may be limited to multiple small vesicle formation and minimal crusting.

Repeated episodes of irritation, from whatever cause, produce an abnormal thickening, or hyperkeratosis, which probably increases the incidence of sweat pore occlusion and sweat retention, as evidenced by the recurrent itchy vesicles seen at the site of inflammatory skin disease (inner aspect of fingers).

Not infrequently, the occurrence of sweat retention, or dyshidrosis, complicates the orderly resolution of the dermatitis. If the patient's activities encourage undue sweating or if the environmental temperatures are increased, sweat retention is more likely to occur. The sweating and heat generated by wearing of rubber gloves often play a provocative role. *However, one can counteract this aggravating factor by applying potent glucocorticoid creams on the hands before the gloves are used.*

The prognosis in industrial primary irritant dermatitis is for a prolonged course. Once the skin is thus damaged, recovery occurs *very* slowly. Burrows reports discouraging figures for complete recovery: 79% of 113 patients still required treatment 10 to 13 years later. The consensus is that housewife's eczema too is a prolonged affair.

The process of hardening is as yet poorly understood, but occurs in people repeatedly exposed to irritants or sensitizers that initially produce inflammation, which the skin learns to tolerate. Suskind believes that this is a process that involves not only the external barrier of the stratum corneum, but also the reactivity of the living epidermal cells.

A frequently seen form of primary irritant dermatitis is *contact cheilitis*, occurring from habitual lip licking and subsequent drying of the lips in children. This produces fissuring, inflammation, and often pruritus. There is usually a peripheral red halo, which is dry and scaly, on the skin around the lips. Soap, shaving creams, alcoholic aftershave lotions, and cold creams may irritate the lips in adults.

### *Differential diagnosis*

***Allergic eczematous contact dermatitis.*** The allergic eczematous type of contact dermatitis possesses a similar clinical appearance. Diagnosis is made by history and patch testing.

At least one third of patients with hand eczema show positive patch test results when tested with a battery of allergy-producing chemicals. Foods as a cause of allergic dermatitis in housewives are sadly overlooked. A group of 53 patients demonstrating dermatitis on the fingertips was patch-test positive to garlic, onion, tomato, and carrot (Sinha). Contact with certain basic food items may produce an allergic reaction. This entity must be distinguished from primary irritant contact dermatitis.

***Atopic dermatitis.*** In atopic dermatitis there is a previous personal or family history of infantile eczema, hay fever, or asthma. Other typical areas may be involved, such as the antecubital and popliteal spaces. The skin tends to be dry and sensitive.

***Psoriasis.*** Fissuring, scaling, and nail changes are often associated with psoriasis. The presence of typical psoriatic lesions on the elbows, knees, and scalp will indicate the diagnosis. Contact dermatitis of the hands may precipitate psoriasis in this site in a susceptible individual.

***Fungal infection.*** Dull erythema and some peripheral vesiculation are present in fungal infection. Skin scrapings must be obtained for culture and mycological examination.

***Lichen planus.*** This disorder may produce a uniformly thickened, red, itchy, fissuring and scaling of the palms or the soles. It can be diagnosed by the appearance of typical lesions elsewhere, or by a biopsy.

### *Treatment*

The basic treatment principle should include protection and rest of the affected hands. Strict avoidance of heat, repetitive wetting of the affected area, soap, detergents, cleaning agents, solvents, perspiration, friction, and firm pressure (grasping, twisting) is essential.

Housewives should avoid any unnecessary wetting of the hands. When rubber gloves are worn, they should be loose, put on over a layer of prescribed topical medication, and not left on any longer than absolutely necessary. Diapers and bleach-containing cloths should not be picked up with bare fingers. Contact with citrus fruit rinds or juices, certain raw vegetables, and some meats may produce irritation. These should be avoided. All strong cleansers, detergents, and most soaps must be handled with protected hands.

In the case of the industrial worker, it is best if time off the job can be arranged. In such cases the worker should be advised to rest the affected parts completely and not contribute to further aggravation of the dermatitis by engaging in any off-the-job forms of work.

If the dermatitis is acute, Burow's solution in the form of prepared tablets or powders, 1 tablet or packet to a pint of cool water, should be used for compresses three times daily in 15-minute periods, followed by the use of a potent glucocorticoid cream, gel, or ointment, such as 0.1% betamethasone valerate, 0.025% fluocinolone, or 0.05% flurandrenolone, applied every 2 hours after the compresses and under thin plastic occlusive gloves during the hours of sleep.

WARNING: *These potent glucocorticoids should be "stepped down" to hydrocortisone or its equivalent as soon as possible.* All too often they are continued by the patient to the point of skin thinning, fragility, redness, cracking, fissuring, and susceptibility to further irritation.

Vesicle formation, accelerated drying out of the skin surface, and fissuring is greatly helped by overnight occlusion with plastic gloves over the following:

| | |
|---|---|
| Propylene glycol | 60% |
| Water | 40% |

Then the glucocorticoid cream, weak or strong as the case may be, is used through the day. After one uses weaker and weaker glucocorticoids to save the hand from the severe effects of potent medications, eventually the following cream is very helpful:

| | |
|---|---|
| Urea | 10% |
| Unibase | to 60 Gm. |

Apply multiple times daily as a hand cream for dryness.

These topical medications must be carried on for longer than one would expect, and normal patterns of activity must be resumed very slowly over a period of months. *Most recurrences are attributable to lessening therapy and increasing activity too soon.*

In acute, long-continued, or extensive dermatitis, the oral use of the corticosteroids is indicated, if there are no contraindications. The dose should be sufficient to ameliorate the inflammation.

*If the treatment measures just outlined fail to bring about clinical improvement, the following possibilities* should be borne in mind.

1. There is continued exposure to an unidentified causative agent that may be an allergic sensitizer. The medication prescribed by the attending physician may be responsible for an allergic contact dermatitis.
2. There is associated sweat retention, or dyshidrosis. This complication is more likely to occur during hot humid conditions or when the patient is attempting to carry on his duties with the aid of rubber or plastic gloves worn for excessively long periods.
3. Secondary infection may be present. Ten percent of our last 50 patients with primary irritant dermatitis had significant secondary infection.
4. Primary irritation dermatitis may be responsible for worsening a preexisting *atopic* or *psoriatic* process, and the day-by-day activities of the patient may be too rigorous for his skin to tolerate.
5. Failure on the part of the patient to use the outlined treatment is responsible for continuing dermatitis.

## REFERENCES

Agrup, G.: Hand eczema and other hand dermatoses in south Sweden, Acta Derm. Venereol. **49**(suppl. 61):1-91, 1969.

**Valuable as an epidemiologic reference.**

Burrows, D.: Prognosis in industrial dermatitis, Br. J. Dermatol. **87**:145, 1972.

**A very distressing documentation of the permanence, once established, of primary irritant dermatitis.**

Björnberg, A.: Increased skin reactivity to primary irritants provoked by hand eczema, Arch. Dermatol. Forsch. **249**:389, 1974.

**An eczema of the hands provokes increased reactivity to skin even at distant sites.**

Fisher, A. A.: Hand eczema. In Contact dermatitis, ed. 2, Philadelphia, 1973, Lea & Febiger, p. 72.
**A vast experience condensed by a superb clinician.**

Holzle, E., and Plewig, G.: Effects of dermatitis stripping and steroids on morphology of corneocytes. A new bioassay, J. Invest. Dermatol. **68**:350, 1977.
**A test that measures form and size of desquamated corneocytes that may prove useful in assessing primary irritant dermatitis.**

Rietschel, R. L., and Allen, A. M.: Effects of prolonged continuous exposure of human skin to water: A reassessment, J. Invest. Dermatol. **68**:79, 1977.
**No effect from pH or soap pretreatment, and little from water.**

Sinha, S. M., Pasrieha, J. S., and Sharma, R. C.: Vegetables responsible for contact dermatitis of the hands, Arch. Dermatol. **113**:776, 1977.
**A warning of the everyday type of exposure—tomato, onion, and garlic chiefly responsible.**

Stoughton, R. B.: The influence of soap on eczematous dermatitis, Arch. Dermatol. **92**:281, 1965.
**Not a bad influence if it is a mild soap.**

Sulzberger, M. B., and Baer, R. L.: Eczema of hands. In Sulzberger, M. B., and Baer, R. L., editors: Yearbook of dermatology 1948, Chicago, 1949, Year Book Medical Publishers, Inc., p. 7.
**Disciplined observations that will always be valid.**

Suskind, R. R., and Ishikawa, M.: Effects of wetting on cutaneous vulnerability, Arch. Environ. Health **11**:538, 1965.
**More than permeability of a dead barrier. It involves the effect on living epidermal cells.**

Wilkinson, D. S.: Contact dermatitis of the hands, Trans. St. John's Hosp. Dermatol. Soc. **58**:163, 1972.
**A comprehensive review.**

## NUMMULAR DERMATITIS (NUMMULAR ECZEMA)

A common inflammatory dermatosis of unknown cause, nummular dermatitis is associated with certain external factors that precipitate and maintain the inflammation.

### *Natural course*

The disorder frequently begins in the fall and persists through the winter. It is aggravated by soap, hot water, and degreasing agents. It occurs chiefly in adults, often elderly adults, but may be seen in patients of all ages.

The lesions are erythematous, moist, and slightly crusted patches, with a distinctive round or oval appearance (Fig. 26-2). They are finely vesicular, and there may be minimal superficial mixed infection. The lesions tend to occur on the extremities, from elbow to wrist or knee to ankle, as well as on the dorsa of feet and hands. If they clear, there is a distinct chance of recurrence at the same site. They do not ordinarily spread to cover large areas, although the periphery may slowly enlarge (Plate 43).

It would appear to be an externally caused localized dermatitis, with unknown factors damaging the epidermal cells, which for some reason are more susceptible than in the normal skin. Pathogenic bacteria are found on the lesions.

### *Microscopic findings*

The appearance is that of a subacute dermatitis, with multiple small areas of intraepidermal intercellular edema and nonspecific dermal inflammation.

### *Differential diagnosis*

***Tinea corporis.*** Circular, scaling, erythematous lesions with a clearing center and vesicular border characterize tinea corporis. Skin scrapings are positive for identification of the fungus.

***Drug eruption.*** A history of recent drug ingestion and clearing with discontinuance of the medication will confirm this diagnosis.

***Atopic dermatitis.*** Often, a patchy roughly circular involvement of the extremities will be seen in atopic dermatitis. Other characteristic lesions and a history of asthma, hay fever, or dermatitis are indicative of this diagnosis.

***Stasis dermatitis.*** The erythematous, scaling and vesicular, often secondarily infected unilateral lesions resulting from venous stasis–dependent edema, must be differentiated. Hemosiderin pigment is often an accompaniment of stasis dermatitis and in early stages tends to follow veins. (See Plate 62.)

### *Treatment*

Avoidance of excessive washing, hot water, soap, and degreasing substances such as solvents is necessary.

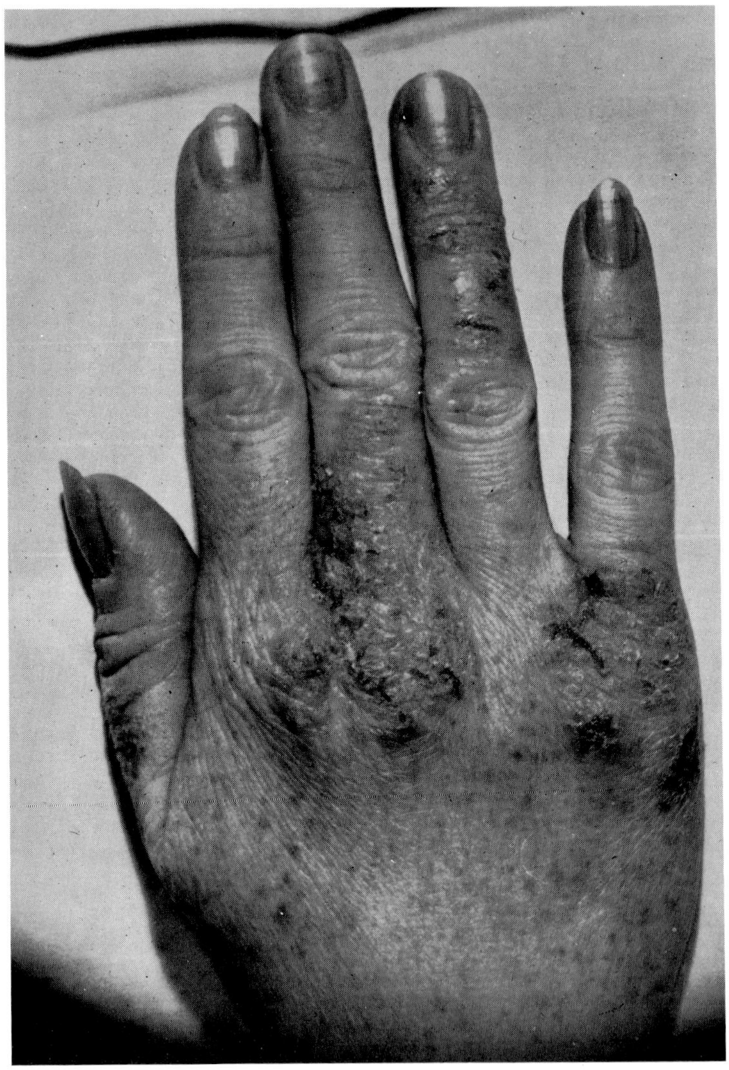

**Fig. 26-2.** Nummular dermatitis.

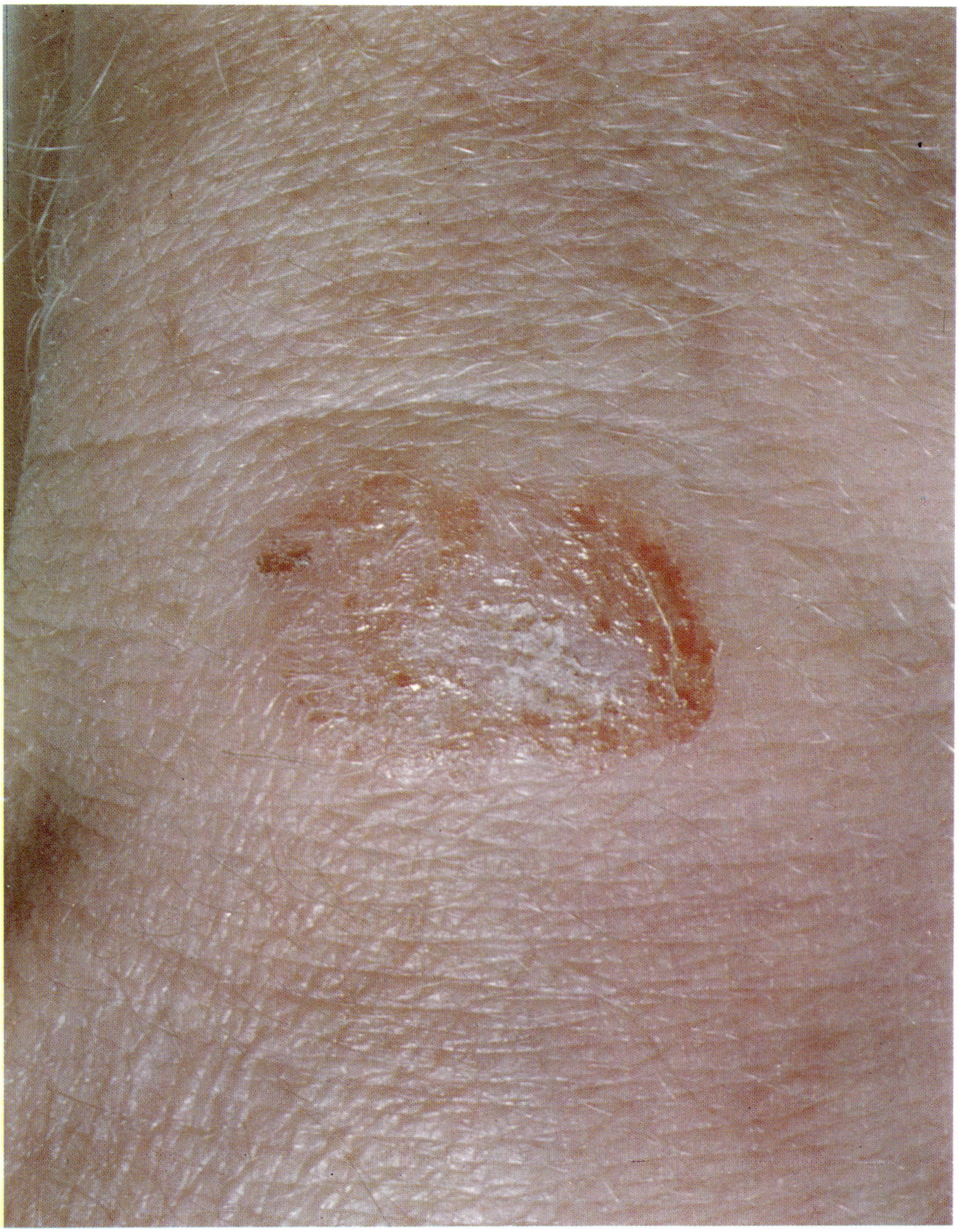

**Plate 43**

Nummular dermatitis of wrist. These lesions tend to be repetitive at the same site.

Use of proper clothing and maintenance of an environment that protects against the cold, dry, chapping effect of winter climates are indicated.

Wet compresses with prepared aluminum acetate (Buro-Sol, Domeboro), powder or tablets, 1 package or tablet to a pint of cool water, should be used three times daily for 15-minute periods. A potent glucocorticoid cream, such as 0.1% betamethasone, 0.025% fluocinolone, or 0.05% flurandrenolone, should be applied sparingly after these compresses. At first, the addition of 3% iodochlorohydroxyquin (Vioform) every 3 hours will often increase the efficacy of the cream in alleviating this disorder. Also, and perhaps they attain the same purpose, combinations of glucocorticoids and topical antibiotics are far more successful than glucocorticoids alone—betamethasone-neomycin, or hydrocortisone-neomycin combinations. Also topical antibiotic creams such as bacitracin or neosporin can be alternated with a glucocorticoid cream.

## REFERENCE

Fowle, L. P., and Rice, J. W.: Etiology of nummular eczema, Arch. Dermatol. Syphilol. **68**:69, 1953.
**Staphylococci colonize each lesion.**

CHAPTER 27

# Pruritus, including pruritus of localized areas

## STRUCTURE AND FUNCTION OF CUTANEOUS NERVES

The complicated system of reporting sensations to the brain from the multiple influences impinging on our skin is not yet understood. In addition, the motor control of cutaneous blood vessels and secretory appendages, and the relationship of intact nerves to tissue proliferation and health, are unclear. Despite this negative beginning, astonishing progress has been made in advancing knowledge of cutaneous nerve function in recent years.

First, one must emphasize the concept of the nerves as being dynamic, living, and continually mobile, not static or fixed. One needs only to see a motion picture of an advancing, palpating tip of a nerve in tissue to realize its essential participation with its neighboring cells, each of which it reacts to, and which react to it. One must realize the incredible motility of the neural cells, and the busy highway in their midst, the *axoplasm*, which carries vesicles, enzymes, particles, organisms, and macromolecules on a two-way channel up and down the nerves, separated completely from the blood or lymph. This flow approximates 5 to 10 mm. per hour. This apparently is essential for maintenance of nutrition of both the cell and the tissue it serves.

The controversy about the presence or absence of intraepidermal free nerve fibers seems to be settled by the concept of mobile nerve endings that, under certain circumstances, penetrate through basement membrane to ramify between epidermal cells (for example, psoriasis, healing wounds). This occurs under pathological and unusual conditions, and presumably when normal conditions are restored, the nerves retract. There may be some relationship to intraepidermal Merkel cells.

Identification of motor as opposed to sensory nerves, or sympathetic versus parasympathetic nerves in dermis is difficult if not impossible in many instances. The complexity of this problem can be illustrated by the observation that per square millimeter of cross-sectioned nerve, there are 10,000 myelinated and 30,000 unmyelinated fibers. A dense horizontally oriented network of wavy varying-sized fibers occurs at the papillary-reticular dermal junction. This is the first organized structure that appears in the fetal dermis. Mucocutaneous junctions and erogenous zones demonstrate coils associated with epithelial structures.

Hair follicles each retain individual sensory nerve baskets around the lower third, in hairy or smooth skin, apparently stimulated by touch. The end organs of Meissner, on the friction surfaces of palms and soles, and the Vater-Pacini corpuscles, in the deep dermis of facial planes, joints, fingers, penis, and clitoris, are all probably touch receptors.

The array of mechanoreceptors in the human skin must be able to provide for the rich complex repertoire of sensations resulting from cutaneous stimulation. This is not satisfactorily described by our present terms of touch and pressure. Present observations indicate that some 11 different receptors (Merkel, Ruffini, A-delta pacinian corpuscles and field and guard hair receptors of different types) provide different information and, depending on the way they are stimulated further, varying information still, for example, in the direction of hair movement. Some receptors are unidirectional, some are bidirectional, and some are intermediate (Horch). Some receptors have high or low threshholds, and some respond solely to a brisk tap on the skin. A unique cutaneous receptor complex, the *Haarscheibe* (hair disc), occurs very superficially and irregularly in man, is present about one per square centimeter, is related to Merkel cells, and forms a mysterious component of the touch system. Although it is identifiable, its function is unclear.

Motor nerves to the skin are sympathetic and may be cholinergic or adrenergic. A cholinergic fiber synthesizes acetylcholine, which diffuses throughout the nerve and accumulates in the terminal region. Acetylcholine esterase, the inactivator, is also formed and distributed along the fiber. Adrenergic fibers make norepinephrine to be carried in storage granules to the periphery. Individual sympathetic fibers demonstrate varicosities, which seem to be the regions of storage and release of humoral transmitters. Electron microscopic "profiles" of the axons and varicosities of nerves are best used now to identify the type of nerve and its function. The profiles reveal the type of vesicle or transmitter it is carrying in its axon. In this way, noradrenergic vesicles, cholinergic vesicles, purinergic ATP vesicles, and sensory nerve profiles are identified. The age of the biochemist is indeed upon us!

***Blood vessels.*** Arteries, arterioles, and arteriovenous shunts are constricted by sympathetic adrenergic activity. Vasodilator fibers have been recognized as well, probably operating by inhibitory sympathetic constriction, perhaps with acetylcholine. Vasodilatation can be produced by cutaneous reflex nerve action, poorly understood, or by local effects of histamine or bradykinin.

***Itch.*** Rothman believed that as the stimulus intensity is increased, itch progresses to diffuse burning pain. It is possible to separate itch from tickle and touch by a nerve block, under which circumstances it is painful. Itching can be produced by a chemical stimulus that damages cells, such as proteases, acetic acid, histamine, mustard gas, mucunain (itch powder), serotonin, and kinins. Itch may occur at the periphery of an anesthetized area in the overlap zone supplied by two segmental sensory nerves. When one is blocked, the dermoepidermal junction is the area of greatest effectiveness for producing itching. The epidermis is not necessary to its production.

***Bile salts.*** Certain bile salts produce itching (Varadi).

#### REFERENCES


Burnstock, G.: Do some nerve cells release more than one transmitter? Neurosci. **1**:239, 1976.
**Questioning the universality of the principle of limited synthesis from sensory nerves.**

Burnstock, G., and Bell, C.: Peripheral autonomic transmission. In Hubbard, J. I., editor: The vertebrate peripheral nervous system, New York, 1974, Plenum Press, p. 277
**The detailed chemistry of autonomic junctional transmission.**

Horch, K. W., Tuckett, R. P., and Burgess, P. R.: A key to the classification of cutaneous mechanoreceptors, J. Invest. Dermatol. **69**:75, 1977.
**Eleven groups, count them!**

Montagna, W., and Brookhart, J. M., editors: Cutaneous innervation and modalities of cutaneous sensibility, J. Invest. Dermatol. **69**:1, 1977.
**Special issue on cutaneous innervation.**

Rothman, S.: Pathophysiology of itch sensation. In Montagna, W., editor: Cutaneous innervation, New York, 1960, Pergamon Press, Inc.
**Careful, perceptive observations.**

Varadi, D. P.: Pruritus induced by crude bile and purified bile acids, Arch. Dermatol. **109**:678, 1974.
**The free bile acids are the villains!**


## PRURITUS

Itching is a sensation that elicits the desire to scratch. Tickle is probably a mild form of itch and is a normal sensation. Only when it reaches abnormal proportions in intensity or area or when it results from a disease does it require our attention.

It has been proposed that itching results from repetitive low-frequency stimulation of nonmyelinated C fibers, but no clear-cut definition of fibers separate from those mediating pain has emerged (Ganong). Weddell believes that itch results from a disturbance in the regular pattern of activity reaching the brain, rather than from the activation of a particular group of nerve fibers that are normally silent. The itch sensation appears to arise from nerve endings that are just beneath the epidermis and in the dermis itself. Furthermore, such stimuli as light touch, pressure, and change in temperature are all capable of initiating an intense itch sensation. Removal of the epidermis succeeds in stopping the itch sensation. However, the nerve pathways that carry sensations of itch and pain are together in the anterolateral tracts of the spinal cord, as they are both abolished by section of the spinothalamic tracts.

Shelley and others have demonstrated that the small spicules that are found on the seed pores of a plant *(Mucuna pruriens)* can produce itch when rubbed into the skin. The chemical agents responsible for the pruritus are proteolytic enzymes (mucunain) and histamine. We now know that other proteases and vasoactive polypeptides are also capable of producing pruritus. Some investigators are of the opinion that endopeptidases, which are released from epidermal cells, fungi, or bacteria, can stimulate the itch response in the superficial nerve endings during fungal and bacterial infections, atopic dermatitis, and the like. Injected trypsin also produces pruritus. The pruritus associated with hives or urticaria is largely attributable to the release of histamine. The role played by lysosome rupture and subsequent release of hydrolytic enzymes has not been clarified in relation to pruritus. It seems reasonable, however, that, along with other chemicals mentioned above, it is a significant factor.

Itching in inflamed skin can occur because prostaglandins, locally synthesized, "sensitize" nerve receptors to the pruritic effects of histamine and other mediators of inflammation. Greaves has shown that prostaglandins lower the threshold of human skin to histamine-evoked itching. Lovell has confirmed this, emphasizing that it probably applies chiefly to inflamed skin.

The existence of itching of central nervous system origin is a subject of much interest. It is seen in some nervous system diseases and psychotic states and occurs in certain central nervous system diseases of sheep, goats, and cats.

These, however, are organic diseases with demonstrable localized pathological change. The association of pruritus with psychological overtones, as has been freely discussed in the dermatological and medical literature for decades, is far less easy to assess. We describe "idiopathic" pruritus and go no further, reassured by having a word to identify it. We do not feel qualified to evaluate the ramifications of such a diagnosis in the patient's thinking. Whitlock, however, has discussed these ramifications, with the impressive methodical research, bibliographic backup, and impartiality that the reader comes to expect and enjoy in his book on psychophysiology. It is enthusiastically recommended. An ingenious electrical square-wave generator and constant-current pulse generator were used by Edwards to quantitate itch. It should be a rational approach, but the observers seem so concerned with evaluating stress and its relation to itch, a sensation we all feel, that one wonders if they will not prejudice the clinical results.

## Clinical aspects of pruritus

It is important to note a basic form of behavior of human skin in itching disorders. With the appearance of an inflammatory pruritic lesion, an area of increased excitability appears around the initial site. In this surrounding excitable area, touch, temperature change, or pressure may be interpreted as an itch. After the lesion has subsided, the area may remain hypersensitive to itch stimuli for some days (Rothman). This occurs in clinical diseases such as *insect bites* and *urticaria*, with the well-known picture of pruritus remaining in the area of a former itchy focus. Also, the tendency is for certain inflammatory pruritic disorders, such an *allergic contact dermatitis*, to produce symptoms in adjacent skin where there has been no contact with the causative agent.

In pathological states, such as *lichen simplex chronicus*, the thickening of the horny outer layer produces a pronounced effect in lowering the itch threshold, and waves of itching are easily induced by minimal stimuli. The mechanism is unexplained.

Runne and Orfanos have recently published findings that appear to confirm a long-standing clinical opinion that persistent scratching may cause neural proliferation and may thereby intensify the pruritic sensation. The unanswered question, of course, is whether the injury produced the neural proliferation, rather than the reverse. There is good evidence that nerve fibers in the epidermis only are present after injury, and the presence of multiple nerve fibers does not necessarily mean increased itch.

Three areas are most frequently affected by pruritus. These are around body orifices, which are liberally endowed with sensory nerve endings and have a greater itching excitability than normal skin. They are the areas of predilection for *pruritus ani*, *pruritus vulvae*, and *otitis externa*, three of the most common pruritic disorders. Just as these areas have a greater itching excitability than normal skin, they also have a tendency in chronic pathological states to respond to even the most transient stimulation by waves of pruritus.

We find a great variation in response to the itch stimulus from individual to individual, probably to a greater extent than any other sensation. Many factors, including the personality and bathing habits of the patient, will determine whether an itching area will be violently excoriated, rubbed gently, or ignored.

## Modifying factors in pruritus

These facts underlie the basic principles of treatment of pruritus.

AN ITCH WILL BE INTENSIFIED BY:

- Heat and warmth
- Rubbing, friction of clothing
- Wool clothing
- Perspiration
- Inactivity, relaxation (sharpens the consciousness of itch)
- Alteration of environmental temperature by heat or cold
- Inflammation of the part (external irritants, soaps, and so forth)
- Reduction of surface oily layer

AN ITCH WILL BE REDUCED BY:

- Cold and cool compresses
- Scratching (mechanism unexplained), which is best performed by moderate, firm stroking with hand or brush over a wide area
- Counterirritant or painful stimulus (for example, pin prick, pressure, pinching, slapping)
- Avoidance of overheating
- Physical or mental occupation (taking one's mind off the itch)
- Constant moderate temperature
- Reduction of inflammation
- Presence of a lubricating layer, such as sebum on the surface of the skin

## Causes of pruritus

Pruritus may result from inflammations attributable to external irritants, infections, infestations (for example, scabies), allergic reactions (for example, contact dermatitis), sweat retention (for example, miliaria), specific cutaneous disease (such as atopic dermatitis), metabolic disease (for example, diabetes mellitus, uremia), and malignancies (such as Hodgkin's disease and lymphomas), and altered physiologic states (such as pregnancy).

### REFERENCES

Arthur, R. P., and Shelley, W. B.: Nature of itching in dermatitic skin, Ann. Intern. Med. **49**:900, 1958.
**The mechanism of action of *Mucuna* itch powder and protease release as conclusions from many experiments.**

Edwards, A. E., Shellow, M. V., Wright, E. T., et al.: Pruritic skin disease, psychological stress and the itch sensation, Arch. Dermatol. **112**:339, 1976.
**There must be more to itching than stress.**

Ganong, W. F.: Review of medical physiology, ed. 6, Los Altos, Calif., 1973, Lange Medical Publications, p. 81.
**Repetitive low-frequency stimulation of C fibers.**

Greaves, M. W., and MacDonald-Gibson, W.: Itch. Role of prostaglandins, Br. Med. J. **3**:608, 1973.
**Itch response measured on the scarified forearm of volunteers from topical application**

Herndon, J. H.: Itching: the pathophysiology of pruritus, Int. J. Dermatol. **14**:465, 1975.
**A thorough review to date.**

Lowell, C. R., Burton, P. A., Duncan, E. H., et al.: Prostaglandins and pruritus, Br. J. Dermatol. **94**:274, 1976.
**A confirmation of Greaves' observations that prostaglandins potentiate histamine-induced itch.**

Rothman, S.: Pathophysiology of itch sensation. In Montagna, W., editor: Advances in biology of skin, New York, 1960, Pergamon Press, Inc., p. 189.
**Most of his conclusions and all of his observations are usable today.**

Whitlock, F. A.: Pruritus, general and localized. In Psy-

chophysiological aspects of skin disease, Philadelphia, 1976, W. B. Saunders Co., p. 110.
**Thoroughly documented discussion of causes.**

## PRURITUS ANI

Numerous and varied etiological factors will produce pruritus of the anal region.

### *Natural course*

The origin of the chronic case of pruritus ani may be any of the specific causative factors listed below; however, once the area has been made hyperexcitable, any slight movement, change of temperature, friction, or increase in perspiration can result in a wave of pruritus that demands further rubbing.

The prognosis and treatment depend on the etiology of the symptom complex. Factors that will aggravate the pruritus are excessive sweating in the area, obesity, occupations that necessitate long periods of sitting (as with executives and truck drivers), tight clothing, synthetic undergarments that will not absorb heat and perspiration, and excessive use of soap on the involved area. Frequent bowel movements, inadequate cleansing, and excessive retention of moisture must also be assessed as possible factors in each patient.

### Causes of pruritus ani

#### *Seborrheic dermatitis, psoriasis, and atopic dermatitis*

In association with one of these disorders, the onset of pruritus ani is usually insidious and may fluctuate in severity with the course of the disease.

There is perianal erythema, lichenification in long-standing cases, and involvement of the gluteal fold, often throughout its full length. There may be a painful fissure.

*Seborrheic dermatitis* may show erythema and scaling of the postauricular regions, external auditory canals, hairline of the scalp, midsternum, or navel.

Characteristic plaques of *psoriasis* may be present on the scalp, elbows, or knees. There may be pitting or ridging of the fingernails. Although not pruritic in other areas, psoriasis of the perianal area and gluteal fold may produce intense itching.

*Atopic dermatitis* may present pruritic scaling of the face, neck, and dorsum of the hands and possibly lichenification of the popliteal or antecubital fossae. There usually is a family history of asthma, hay fever, or atopic dermatitis.

***Treatment.*** See discussion of general measures of treatment for pruritus ani at the end of this section.

#### *Contact dermatitis (primary irritant and allergic types)*

The normal practices of cleansing with soap and hot water and towel drying are sufficient to cause a *primary irritation* type of contact dermatitis in susceptible individuals if frequently carried out. Also, many people will turn first to excessive use of soap at the first sign of an irritation, often worsening the situation.

The *allergic* type of contact dermatitis, on the other hand, is most frequently seen after application of local anesthetic and proprietary topical medications. *Patch tests* to identify the causative agent should be carried out after the acute phase has subsided.

Contact dermatitis of either type begins as an erythema and can progress to a weeping, oozing, erythematous acute process, sharply limited to the site of contact (Plate 44). When caused by an allergic reaction, it frequently involves the perianal area and extends onto the buttock surface. Further contact with the causative agent only causes a worsening and spread of the dermatitis. Rest and sleep become impossible, and the patient will try anything to get relief.

***Treatment.*** Whenever contact dermatitis of either type is suspected, all potential causative agents must be eliminated. See discussion of general measures, p. 446.

#### *Lichen simplex chronicus (localized neurodermatitis)*

Lichen simplex chronicus presents as a well-demarcated, lichenified patch of dermatitis, often on one side only. It is extremely pruritic and chronic. There may be excoriations. There is a distinct tendency to recurrence.

***Treatment.*** Grenz-ray therapy is helpful in stubborn cases. Triamcinolone, 5 mg./ml. in-

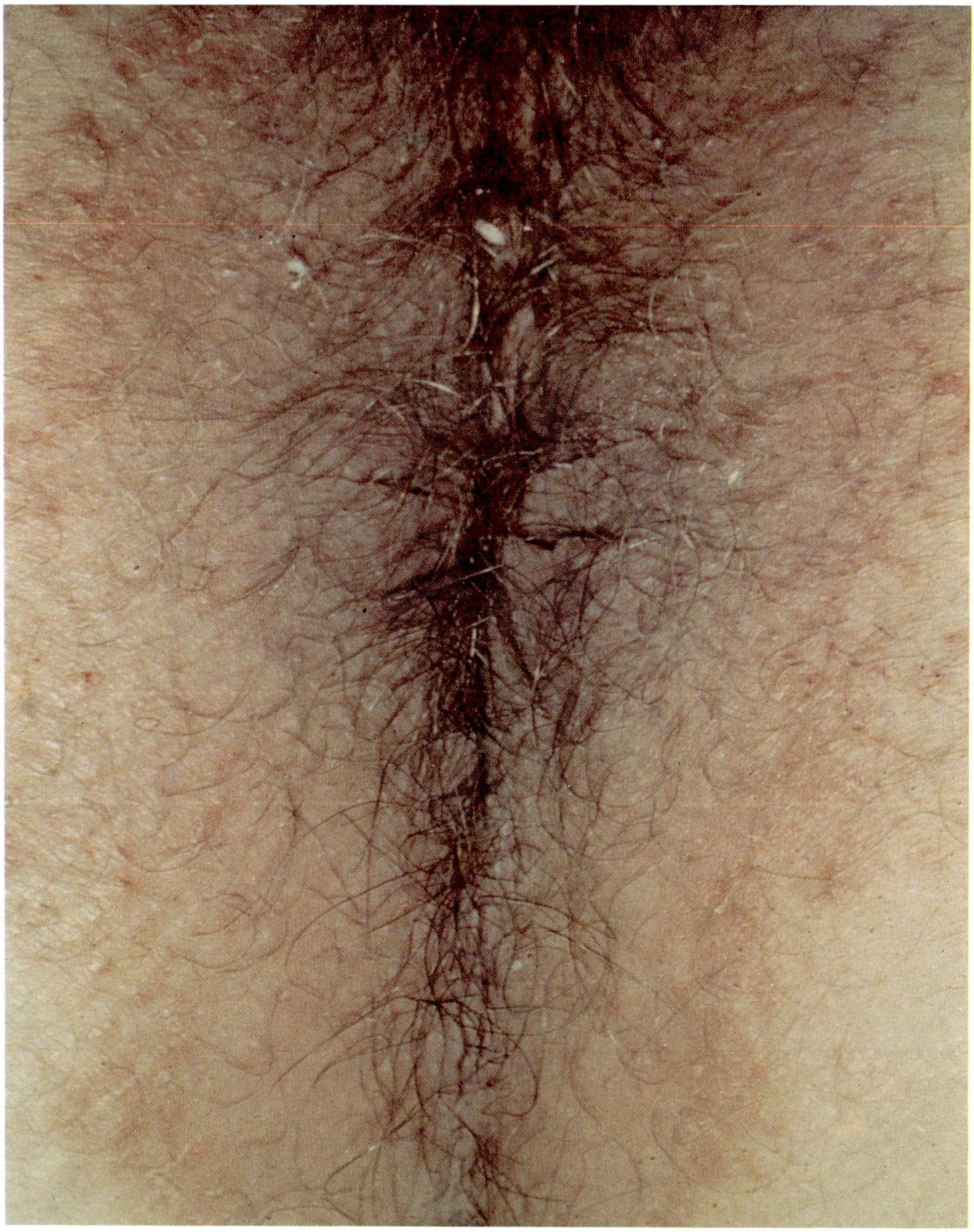

**Plate 44**

Pruritus ani (early) from allergic contact dermatitis, caused by preservatives in cream base.

jected intralesionally, is of value when other measures have failed, in protracted cases. General measures are described on p. 000.

### *Intertrigo*

Intertrigo results from the accumulation of sweat and heat in flexural areas, causing maceration, erythema, fissuring, and pruritus. It is most often seen in obese persons, in hot environments, and in association with tight clothing and excess perspiration. Identification lies in the involvement of other flexures, including the inguinal folds.

***Treatment.*** Treatment consists of the specific measures outlined at the end of this section, plus weight reduction and topical treatment of adjacent flexures and folds. Aluminum chloride salts, as in antiperspirants, function as antibacterials as well as drying agents.

### *Candidosis (moniliasis)*

Antibiotics (chiefly tetracycline) administered orally may produce pruritus ani by some mechanism other than antibacterial, allowing an overgrowth of *Candida albicans* that then involves the perianal area, resulting in erythema and pruritus. Of considerable significance is the fact that candidal pruritus ani also occurs in diabetes mellitus, where the symptoms of itching may be the first manifestation of the disease. It may spread from a primary candidal vulvovaginitis. The lesions characteristically are moist and deeply erythematous, with sharp borders, and have small pustular satellite lesions.

***Treatment.*** Treatment must include control of the primary infection with clotrimazole, miconazole, nystatin (Mycostatin) ointment, or amphotericin B (Fungizone) lotion applied topically, as well as the specific measures listed at the end of this section.

### *Fungal infection*

A dry, scaling erythema of the perianal area and gluteal walls that often has a fine vesicular border is characteristic of fungal involvement. It may be present on the inner thighs and inguinal folds of males. Microscopic examination and culture of skin scrapings will confirm the diagnosis and should be done before antifungal therapy is begun. There may be an associated involvement of toes or feet. This can so easily be missed that fungal scrapings should be performed on all nonresponsive cases of pruritus ani.

***Treatment.*** Treatment includes micronized griseofulvin, 1 Gm. daily, as well as the specific measures below. Tolnaftate, clotrimazole, miconazole, or haloprogin topically is also effective.

### *Pinworm infestation (enterobiasis)*

Pruritus caused by the presence of pinworms (*Enterobius vermicularis*) is most commonly found in children and in their families, who have contracted it from them. Most children have been infected at some time. The pruritus is most intense in the evening around bedtime and may be severe enough to be painful. Slight erythema and excoriations may be present in the perianal area and extend to the genitalia. The small white worms themselves may be seen on direct examination of the rectal canal or sometimes the stool.

A prepared cellulose tape swab rolled over the anal region (best done at night) will pick up the ova, which may be seen on microscopic examination.

***Treatment.*** See p. 339.

### *Scabies*

Scabies can cause a pruritus of the perianal area and buttocks, but this is usually submerged in the generalized pruritus accompanying the infestation.

***Treatment.*** Treatment is as for generalized scabies.

### *Warts (verruca acuminata)*

The annoying lesions of warts appear suddenly, grow rapidly, and can be very pruritic on occasion. They are very apparent on examination, tending to form soft, pedunculated, moist, lobulated lesions at the border of mucous membrane and stratified squamous epithelium. They are of viral origin.

***Treatment.*** See p. 321.

### *Gonococcal proctitis*

Fully two thirds of patients with this disorder may be asymptomatic or complain of burning or itching of the anus. Some pus is visible in the anal canal, and the mucosa is reddened and edematous. Cultures should be taken and immediately planted on Thayer-Martin media. If the test is positive, a culture from the sex partner should also be taken.

### *Hemorrhoids, anal fissure, cryptitis, papillitis, fistula in ano, and abscess*

These surgical conditions are all associated with localized anal and rectal inflammation. They are not ordinarily heralded by pruritus, despite widespread belief in the syndrome of itching piles. The act of defecation is painful, and there may be small amounts of blood or pus in the stool.

### *Carcinoma*

Rectal carcinoma has been reported to have produced no symptoms other than an initial pruritus. This bears out the fact that a digital rectal examination is a simple procedure that may allow one to make this important diagnosis early rather than late.

### *Idiopathic pruritus ani*

There remain a number of cases in which there is no association with dermatoses or disease elsewhere. Because of the nonspecificity of the clinical picture, the preceding causes of pruritus ani must be eliminated by history and dermatological examination before the patient is placed in this category. Psychogenic factors, social and emotional pressures, anxiety, concern, worry, and frustrations undoubtedly have some etiologic importance in these idiopathic cases, but these factors must be weighed as impartially as the preceding ones before one assigns them a causative role in the disease. Initially, the area shows no change but mild erythema with pruritus. As it persists, however, the erythema deepens, and thickening and lichenification of the entire area appear, with dryness and flaking of the skin. This is followed by maceration, fissuring, possibly even bleeding, and secondary infection.

The pruritus is intermittent but chronic and comes in paroxysms, particularly with the heat of bedclothes at night. Pressure of clothing, stroking, changes in temperature, and changes of position may bring on a wave of pruritus.

***Investigation.*** The following is for all forms of pruritus ani:

INITIAL

History: assessment of occupation, activities, degree of cleanliness, type and frequency of bowel habits, antibiotic therapy, oral desensitizations (for example, poison ivy), symptoms of diabetes, and general health
Digital rectal examination
General cutaneous examination
Fungal scrapings, urinalysis for glucose
Examination for pinworms

SECONDARY

As indicated from results of initial investigation.

## General treatment for pruritus ani

A methodical, rigidly enforced, but simple schedule must be established, with repeated checks of the patient to assure that the prescribed regimen is being followed. Strict adherence will show a satisfactory result in even the most persistent cases.

All irritations are to be completely eliminated, which can be achieved in part by the following rules:

1. Only minimal amounts of a mild, nonmedicated soap, used only to remove irritating residual fecal material. All soap is to be flushed or rinsed off the area after cleaning.
2. No proprietary medications applied locally
3. No tight clothing
4. No overstuffed chairs, long car rides, for at least a temporary period
5. Weight reduction, if indicated
6. Avoidance of excess perspiration

A sitz bath should be used once daily, for 10 to 15 minutes, with lukewarm water, no soap, and no rubbing. Alternatively, Burow's solution compresses using the prepared tablets or powder, 1 tablet or 1 package to 1 pint of cool water, may be applied four times daily for 10-

minute periods and allowed to dry without toweling.

Menthol, 0.5%, and 0.5% phenol added to a potent cream, for example, 0.1% betamethasone valerate, 0.025% fluocinolone, or 0.05% flurandrenolone cream are applied sparingly after the sitz bath or compresses and every 3 hours, with no excess rubbing. A less potent glucocorticoid cream must be used after the initial acute phase has been controlled. Long-term use of potent topical glucocorticoids has resulted in epidermal and dermal atrophy, telangiectasia, and striae. It may only suppress the symptoms, which can intensify on abrupt discontinuation.

Trimeprazine, 5 mg., or hydroxyzine, 25 mg., is given in the evening to encourage unbroken sleep during the time of quite severe pruritus.

Spicy foods and condiments should be avoided.

Grenz radiation may be helpful. Because pruritus ani can be a chronic or recurrent problem, the use of conventional x-ray treatment should be discouraged.

## PRURITUS VULVAE

Pruritus vulvae (Fig. 27-1), like pruritus ani, is a very common itching disorder of a friction-prone, warm, moist area generously supplied with sensory nerve endings.

### *Natural course*

A great deal is written about the sexual ramifications of this disorder (Whitlock). We find that pruritus vulvae follows the course and responds to the treatment of other orificial pruritic dermatoses. *Those cases with psychosexual associations that we have seen in our office do not have the lichenification that is a recognizable diagnostic sign of pruritus vulvae.*

Whereas the clinical findings reflect the specific cause of the disease, the course of pruritus vulvae begins with an intermittent pruritus, often occurring in episodes with asymptomatic intervening periods. With persistence, an erythema develops on the labia majora, and with long-standing cases lichenification. The pruritus becomes unremitting and worsens with tight clothing, heat and perspiration, motion, long sitting, and lying in bed at night. Unless there are particularly severe excoriations, the clinical signs are much less than the patient's complaints suggest. The process may spread along the perineum to affect the perianal region as well.

### Causes of pruritus vulvae

Many of the specific causes of pruritus vulvae are identical to those causing perianal pruritus. Overtreatment is a common outcome of initially mild irritations of this area.

### *Contact dermatitis*

The frequent use of hot water and soap and too vigorous cleansing and drying measures may lead to a persistent vulvar inflammation and pruritus from *primary irritation.* This is the most common form of contact dermatitis. It can be aggravated by the use of feminine hygiene products such as irritating deodorant sprays, douches, and heat-retaining sanitary napkins. Some women find pantyhose too occlusive and heat-retaining to be worn for long periods.

An *allergic* contact dermatitis produces labial erythema and pruritus. Weeping and vesiculation occur if it is severe from prolonged or recurrent contact with the causative agent. The area involved conforms to the site of contact with the cause (for example, the application of an ointment).

***Treatment.*** Treatment is as outlined at the end of this section, but elimination of all potential causative agents must be the first consideration.

### *Vaginal discharge*

Vaginal candidal inflammation with a vaginal discharge is very often associated with pruritus. Candidal involvement produces patchy, white lesions over the reddened inner labial mucous membrane. Moist discrete satellite lesions are seen on the perineum and in the inguinal folds. A lumpy, milky discharge is present.

*Trichomonas vaginalis* vaginitis also produces pruritus, but with somewhat fewer cutaneous changes. *Trichomonas* produces a

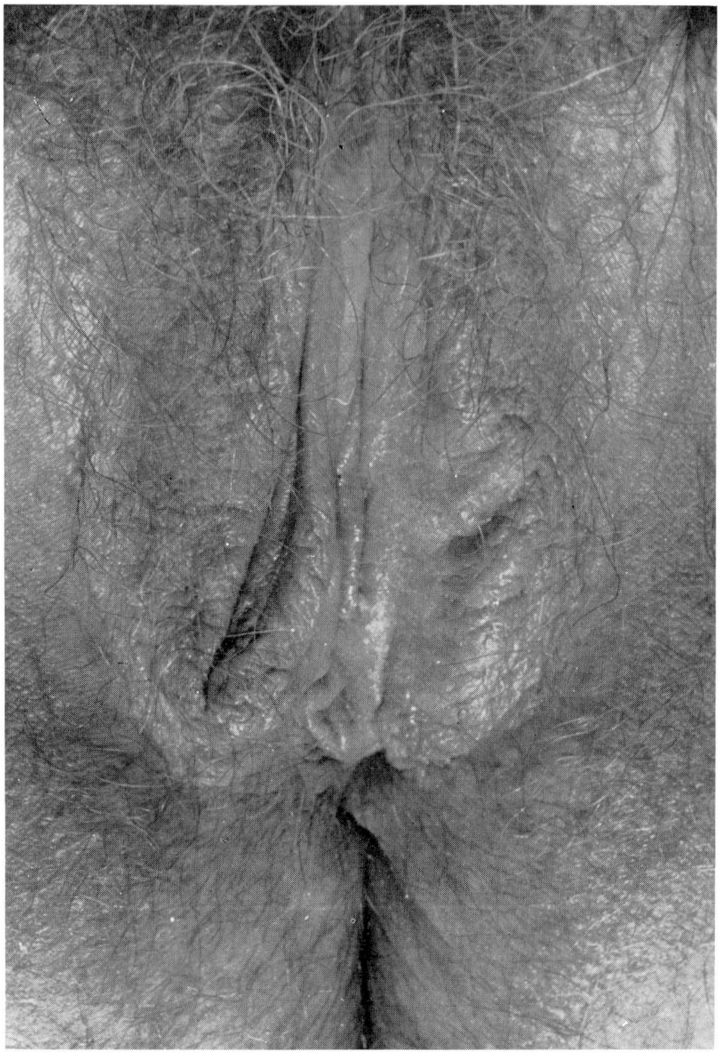

**Fig. 27-1.** Pruritus vulvae. Labia are lichenified.

frothy leukorrhea. They are frequently concomitantly present in the same patient.

The organisms may be cultured, in the case of *Candida*, or observed microscopically by the hanging-drop technique for *Trichomonas*.

***Treatment.*** For treatment of candidal inflammation, see p. 270 and 283.

*Trichomonas* infection responds to metronidazole, 250 mg., 1 tablet three times daily, plus a vaginal insert of 500 mg. nightly for 10 to 20 nights, continuing through the menstrual period. Both sexual partners should be treated simultaneously.

A thorough gynecological examination should of course be performed in all cases of vaginal discharge to determine the presence of vaginal or uterine pathological conditions.

### *Lichen simplex chronicus*

Lichen simplex chronicus usually consists of a unilateral lichenified dry plaque on one labium. The pruritus is a major, unremitting feature. There may be another similar lesion elsewhere. There are striking similarities between chronic pruritus vulvae, scrotal pruritus, and lichen simplex chronicus.

***Treatment.*** Grenz-ray therapy given in a short course, in addition to the measures described at the end of this section, is often helpful.

Glucocorticoid suspensions (for example, triamcinolone, 5 mg./ml.) may be injected intracutaneously into the lesions in resistant cases.

### *Seborrheic dermatitis*

Seborrheic dermatitis is a common condition that frequently involves the vulva and the mons pubis with a pale erythema and fine scale. It may extend posteriorly to the perianal region and include the depth of the gluteal fold (Fig. 32-4). In other areas it involves the postauricular folds, scalp, and midsternum.

***Treatment.*** Treatment is as for pruritus vulvae, with associated individual treatment of the other cutaneous areas of involvement.

### *Psoriasis*

On the mons pubis and labia, psoriasis has a sharply marginated appearance, with erythema and an overlying scale (Fig. 28-3). Where it appears in skin folds, for example, the inguinal areas and gluteal fold, it has a moist shiny surface. It is more pruritic in these areas than on other cutaneous surfaces. Confirmation of the diagnosis lies in the finding of characteristic scaling plaques elsewhere.

***Treatment.*** Grenz radiation may be given in short courses.

Tar in the form of 5% to 10% liquor carbonis detergens added to an effective glucocorticoid cream is very useful. A sample prescription is as follows:

| | |
|---|---|
| Liquor carbonis detergens | 5% |
| Hydrocortisone | 1% |
| Hydrophilic ointment | 30 Gm. |

Apply sparingly four times daily to affected areas.

Because of the heat and moisture, the area allows steroid absorption as if under occlusion, and potent steroids must be used with care.

### *Diabetes mellitus*

Diabetes mellitus may be associated with a chronic, severe, and resistant localized anogenital pruritus. This is often on the basis of a candidal infection and discharge, but such is not invariably present. The pruritus is ordinarily related to the degree of control of the diabetes. Superimposed bacterial and fungal infection must be ruled out in the presence of diabetes mellitus.

Special mention should also be made of diabetic vulvitis, which may result from irritation by heavily sugar-laden urine. However, *Candida albicans* is usually the prime offender.

***Treatment.*** Treatment consists in regulating and continuing control of the diabetes.

### *Intertrigo*

Intertrigo is most often seen in overweight patients. This condition results in a well-demarcated, erythematous, moist, pruritic dermatitis that may be virtually impossible to eliminate without weight reduction. Simple bed rest for 2 to 3 weeks for some other reason will often result in the development of an intertriginous type of pruritus of the area, probably secondary to heat, friction, perspiration, and the like.

***Treatment.*** General measures mentioned at the end of this section should be augmented by a determined weight-reduction program.

### *Senile or presenile atrophy*

Senile or presenile atrophy is usually encountered in the years after the menopause. With an atrophic vaginal mucous membrane, an irritating leukorrhea, and atrophy also present in the labial epidermis, accompanied by a chronic inflammation in the dermis, there is an intermittent and annoying pruritus.

***Treatment.*** It is difficult to assess the value of estrogens applied to these mucous membrane lesions. If used in adequate concentration, they appear to be beneficial. Systemic postmenopausal estrogen replacement therapy may also give desirable therapeutic results.

### *Urinary incontinence*

Especially in bedridden elderly females, urine contact on the vulva and perineum can produce an erythematous, irregularly pruritic dermatitis of the inguinal area and perineum.

***Treatment.*** Careful cleansing, minimal soap, and selected protective creams such as zinc oxide ointment or silicone creams with 1% hydrocortisone added are helpful.

### *Lichen sclerosus et atrophicus*

Lichen sclerosus et atrophicus is an unusual condition that is usually pruritic. It may produce itching in the early stages. It begins as white papules on the labia majora that become confluent and produce atrophic patches around the vaginal orifice (Plate 18). These then may extend to the inguinal folds or the perianal area. Atrophy and stenosis without induration of the vaginal orifice eventually may occur. Similar white patches and plaques may be present elsewhere on the cutaneous surface, usually the upper back or lateral aspect of the thighs.

***Treatment.*** Glucocorticoid compounds in maximum concentration under occlusive dressings may arrest the progress of the disease. Biopsies are important both for establishment of dysplastic or nondysplastic disease and for follow-up.

Testosterone propionate, 1% cream, has been reported to reduce itching and white patches.

### *Lichen planus*

Exceedingly severe and persistent pruritus may be associated with lichen planus, both on cutaneous surfaces generally and on the perineum and vulva. The lesions, if on the mucous membranes, form lacy gray linear patterns or white plaques. On the vulva the lesions are the characteristic papules.

***Treatment.*** Grenz-ray therapy in short courses, in addition to the general measures below, is often helpful. For resistant cases, systemic glucocorticoids give some therapeutic relief, but must be maintained.

### *Idiopathic pruritus vulvae*

Cases of pruritus vulvae that do not fit into the previous categories are, by exclusion, labeled idiopathic. The idiopathic form of pruritus vulvae begins insidiously and progresses to an increasingly severe symptom complex that interrupts the daily pattern of living and interferes with sleep at night. It is more severe around the time of the menstrual period. The vulvar area is involved first, with an erythema that may continue on to thickening, lichenification, excoriation, or secondary infection.

***Investigation.*** The following is for all forms of pruritus vulvae.

INITIAL

- History: evaluation of patient's personal proclivities toward excessive cleanliness, use of irritant deodorants or other topical preparations, history of vaginal discharge, abnormal spotting, recent antibiotic therapy, associated perianal pruritus, family history, and symptoms of diabetes.
- Pelvic examination if discharge is present
- General cutaneous examination
- Examination of vaginal discharge for *Trichomonas*, *Candida*, or bacterial infection
- Perianal swab for pinworms
- Examination of urine for glucose

SECONDARY

- Follow-up investigations in the presence of positive initial findings.

***Treatment.*** The general measures described below provide relief.

## General therapy for pruritus vulvae

There are certain basic rules for therapy of vulvar pruritus that, however, are modified for some of the specific diseases just described, as was mentioned under each entity where applicable. The patient with pruritus vulvae must be examined for diabetes mellitus, and a thorough dermatological examination of the entire skin surface must be carried out for signs of associated dermatological disease.

A methodical, quite rigid schedule must be

set up initially, and the patient should be checked to be sure that it is followed.

The following aggravating factors must be avoided:

Heat and excess perspiration
Excessive use of soap and other cleansing preparations
All potentially irritating or sensitizing sprays, ointments, and creams
Tight, occlusive pantyhose or girdles and clothing producing friction
Excessive sitting (for example, long car rides)
Rubbing and scratching
Irritating douche solutions
Sanitary pads that rub, irritate, or retain heat and perspiration

### *Treatment*

Burow's solution compresses using prepared tablets or powders, 1 to 1 pint of cool water, should be used for compresses four times daily, 15 minutes each, allowing drying in air, without rubbing.

Menthol, 0.5%, and 0.5% phenol added to a potent glucocorticoid cream, such as 0.1% betamethasone, 0.025% fluocinolone, or 0.05% flurandrenolone, are applied sparingly every 2 hours, or frequently enough to prevent pruritus. This should be maintained for a short period of time after all symptoms have subsided and then slowly discontinued. A milder topical steroid should be used in the tapering off process.

Atrophy, telangiectasia, and striae may be produced by these potent drugs in this area as elsewhere with long-term use.

Trimeprazine, 5 mg., hydroxyzine, 25 mg., or meprobamate, 400 mg., is given for nighttime sedation to encourage unbroken sleep during the time of often intense pruritus.

Grenz radiation for a short course of 3 or 4 treatments may be very helpful in otherwise unyielding cases.

#### REFERENCE

Leading article: Pruritus vulvae, Br. Med. J. **1:**17, 1973.

**A 1-page lesson in brevity with all major considerations included.**

## OTITIS EXTERNA (PRURITUS OF THE EXTERNAL EAR)

A common inflammatory condition of the external ear, resulting chiefly from trauma, moisture, and secondary bacterial colonization, otitis externa is often erroneously believed to be caused by a fungal infection.

### *Natural course*

The external auditory canal in its distal third and the skin around the meatus are the areas involved. The dermatitis demonstrates a scaling erythema that may spread to adjacent sites on the pinna, but rarely extends beyond the external ear. With increasing severity it becomes moist and oozing. Itching is the main initial sujective complaint, which is followed by pain, edema, and tenderness with persistence of the disorder.

### *Predisposing factors*

Most investigators agree that secondary to trauma and moisture, maceration is produced in the canal, with colonization by *Pseudomonas species*, *coliforms*, and *staphylococci*. Wright and Alexander have reported that the bacterial flora of the external auditory meatus, which was originally gram-positive, changes after prolonged exposure to water. Patients developed otitis externa and the bacterial flora gradually became predominantly gram-negative.

The anatomical structure of the external auditory canal, which permits poor evaporation and ventilation, predisposes to chronicity of the inflammation. The dermatitis may be aggravated and prolonged in individuals with narrow ear canals. External heat, humidity, and overzealous cleansing, as well as digging or scratching a pruritic area, are common aggravating factors. Many people are affected in tropical climates and in hot humid or wet environs, whereas in temperate zones only a few are. Swimmers are all aware of the problem. The use of irritating or sensitizing agents in this area frequently adds difficulty to the diagnosis and proper treatment. Creams and ointments or cleansing compounds are often applied with the use of cotton-tipped applicators, a habit that, in our experience, is very irritating to the canal.

Predisposition to otitis externa occurs in humid moist environments (such as in swimming), seborrheic dermatitis, atopic dermatitis, and psoriasis and may be complicated by contact dermatitis.

## Causes of otitis externa

### *Seborrheic dermatitis*

Usually seborrheic dermatitis can be found concomitantly on the scalp, postauricular regions, eyelid margins, nasolabial folds, and midsternum. It has a distinct tendency to recur.

***Treatment.*** Crusted, oozing lesions should be compressed with Burow's solution, using the prepared tablets or powders, 1 tablet or powder to a pint of cool water, for 15-minute periods three times daily.

The following topical medications are effective: a potent glucocorticoid cream such as 0.1% betamethasone, 0.025% fluocinolone, or 0.05% flurandrenolone, or, when evidence of secondary infection is present, Vioform cream with a glucocorticoid added, applied sparingly three to four times daily. Alternatively, if the external auditory canal is involved, glucocorticoid-containing eardrops can be used, but for a short time and in small quantities only. One drop is placed in the affected ear twice daily. The scalp should be shampooed twice weekly, followed by a brief application of selenium sulfide suspension (Selsun).

### *Psoriasis*

Psoriatic lesions are commonly found on the elbows, knees, scalp, or sacrum, in association with psoriasis of the external auditory canal and external ear. Psoriasis has less tendency to itch than seborrheic dermatitis. It can be a stubborn, persistent problem that is difficult to treat.

***Treatment.*** Liquor carbonis detergens, 3%, added to a glucocorticoid cream or similar tar-steroid combination, is applied four times daily.

Ultraviolet-light therapy in conventional doses should be used at least twice weekly.

Grenz radiation given in a series of divided doses is an effective method of therapy.

### *Atopic dermatitis*

A pruritic disease, atopic dermatitis occurs first in infants and children, but proceeds into adult life. There is usually a personal or family history of asthma, hay fever, or eczema. Lesions of atopic dermatitis may be present on the scalp, characterized by dryness and scaling, with pruritic involvement of the antecubital and popliteal areas.

***Treatment.*** Therapy consists of an adequate glucocorticoid cream applied sparingly every 3 hours for a temporary period and treatment of the other cutaneous manifestations of the disease. If there is considerable involvement of the auditory canal, glucocorticoid eardrops may be very helpful. One drop (no more!) is placed in each ear twice daily.

### *Allergic eczematous contact dermatitis*

An acute inflammatory dermatitis of sudden onset, allergic eczematous contact dermatitis may be superimposed on a previously existing chronic dermatitis. It spreads quickly to adjacent areas and becomes wet and oozing. The whole external ear may becomes reddened and swollen. The most common causative agents are medications applied to the ear for a previously existing condition. Hearing aids and nail polish also cause allergy here.

***Treatment.*** Therapy includes elimination of all proprietary medications and previously applied topical agents. Soap should not be used on the area.

Cool, wet compresses with Burow's solution, using the prepared tablets or powders, 1 tablet or package to 1 pint of water, or freshly prepared solution diluted 1:20, should be applied at least twice daily. Glucocorticoid cream is applied sparingly three to four times daily.

Patch tests are done to establish the causative agent after the dermatitis has subsided.

### *Lichen simplex chronicus*

Lichen simplex chronicus is usually a single, pruritic, lichenified lesion. Similar plaques may occasionally be present on the posterior aspect of the neck and about the ankles.

***Treatment.*** Glucocorticoid cream is applied sparingly at least three to four times daily, or as often as necessary to eliminate pruritus. Grenz radiation in a series of divided doses is effective.

### *Infectious eczematoid dermatitis*

An oozing, crusting, spreading erythema associated with a purulent discharge from within the ear canal occurs with infectious eczematoid dermatitis. The dermatitis first develops on the area in contact with the pus. It tends to extend to the side of the face and neck. An otitis media or a draining furuncle is the usual source of the purulent discharge.

***Treatment.*** After culture to determine the sensitivity of the organism responsible, the underlying infection is treated with the specific systemic antibiotic indicated.

Burow's solution, either freshly prepared solution diluted 1:20, or prepared tablets and powders, 1 tablet or packet to 1 pint of cool water, is used for compressing three times daily.

Antibiotic glucocorticoid-containing cream is applied after the compresses.

### *General therapy of otitis externa*

1. Eliminate potential allergens.
2. Culture for possible pathogenic bacteria.
3. Prevent trauma.
4. Eliminate itching.

All medications must be applied sparingly to avoid obstruction of the canal.

Occlusive dressings and plugs are to be avoided.

In general, a potent glucocorticoid cream such as 0.1% betamethasone, 0.025% fluocinolone, or 0.05% flurandrenolone should be used for pruritus in this area.

Medication should be maintained until well after a normal state has been attained, and then gradually discontinued. A common mistake lies in discontinuing therapy too soon. A milder concentration of cream or a nonfluorinated glucocorticoid should be substituted when the acute phase is over.

The use of home or proprietary medications must be prohibited.

Cotton-tipped applicators, hairpins, or any similar hard or sharp instrument *must not* be used in the ear canal by the patient.

The use of soap and hot water for cleansing should be discontinued.

If bacterial etiology is suspected, culture should be performed and sensitivty tests used to direct therapy. Garamycin or gentamicin topical preparations, when a topical antibiotic is essential, have largely replaced neomycin. *Pseudomonas aeruginosa* can be treated with polymyxin B or polymyxin E (colistin) topically. If *Aspergillus* is cultured in those rare cases in which it may be causative, Vioform topically has been reported to be beneficial. Gentian violet 2% in alcohol daily is a recognized treatment.

#### REFERENCES


Hoadley, A. W., and Knight, D. E.: External otitis among swimmers and non-swimmers, Arch. Environ. Health **30**:445, 1975.
**Pseudomonas, earaches, and otitis externa are more common in swimmers.**

Marples, M. H.: The ecology of the human skin, Springfield, Ill., 1965, Charles C. Thomas, Publisher, p. 701.
**A particularly well done part of this excellent book.**

Senturia, G. H.: External otitis, acute, diffuse; evaluation of therapy, Ann. Otol. Rhinol. Laryngol. **82**(suppl. 8):1-23, 1973.
**Comprehensive.**

Shelley, W. B., and Perry, E. T.: Experimental production of external otitis in man, J. Invest. Dermatol. **27**:281, 1956.
**Ingenious reproduction of the natural occurrence in three forms, allergic, irritant, and maceration.**

Wright D. N., and Alexander, J. M.: Effect of water on the bacterial flora of swimmers' ears, Arch. Otolaryngol. **99**:15, 1974.
**A very useful contribution to our understanding of a common problem.**

Wright, D. N., and Dineen, M.: A model for the study of infectious otitis externa, Arch. Otolaryngol. **95**:243, 1972.


## PRURITUS OF DRY SKIN (XEROSIS)

Three causes of pruritus of dry skin are *bath pruritus*, *senile pruritis*, and *winter itch*, all of which have a common denominator.

The clinical appearance of the skin gives evidence of dryness, with fine lines running in a pattern over the skin, and scaling. There may be transient associated erythematous patches. The legs are the most commonly involved areas. Excoriations are seldom seen.

***Bath pruritus.*** Too frequent bathing with hot water and soap removes the surface film and may not allow a replacement before the next soapy onslaught. The excitability of the cutaneous sensory nerves is increased by reduction of the surface sebum film. Pruritus then results.

***Senile pruritus.*** The sebaceous glands are reduced in number and function in old age. Cold weather and lack of humidity reduce the flow of sebum. Both tend to produce pruritus. This occurs chiefly on the legs but is often generalized.

***Winter pruritus.*** Many people, especially patients with atopic dermatitis, have dry skin and thus are particularly subject to episodes of pruritus in cold weather and with increasing age. Also, with frequent bathing and other external irritative factors such as rough or wool clothing, these individuals will experience severe and persistent pruritus. The problem is largely seasonal and is relieved by increasing environmental humidity and temperature.

### *Differential diagnosis*

Hypothyroidism may be associated with pruritus and xerosis.

Hypocalcemia attributable to hypoparathyroidism or to malabsorption can cause a generalized xerosis.

In elderly individuals one most be aware that a rising blood urea nitrogen may be associated with pruritus. Early biliary obstruction, early lymphomas, and bile salt retention can also be a cause of pruritus. (See also the following section on generalized pruritus.)

### *Investigation*

History and physical examination directed along the lines of discovering endocrine disorders, debilitating illness, and underlying lymphoma or other malignancy
Blood urea nitrogen level tests
Bilirubin and liver function tests
Serum calcium and thyroid function tests
Urinalysis for glucose; fasting or random glucose level if indicated.

### *Treatment*

Frequent baths with hot soapy water should be replaced by lukewarm short baths. Wool and rough clothing should not be worn next to the skin. Rapid and extreme temperature changes should be avoided.

The replacement of the oil film by artificial means can be attempted by the use of simple emollient preparations such as Eucerin, Lubriderm, or Nivea cream.

We have found that the addition of 10% urea to a bland vehicle such as Unibase or any of the preparations just mentioned enables the epidermis to hold water and significantly reduces dryness. This allays the pruritus very satisfactorily.

If the condition is acute, anti-inflammatory steroid therapy locally may be necessary for temporary relief. Hydrocortisone 1% to 2% may be added to the above urea-containing preparations and applied three or four times daily. Trimeprazine, 5 mg., hydroxyzine, 25 mg., or meprobamate, 400 mg. at bedtime, may be used for nighttime sedation. Some individuals obtain relief from bath oils; others have little use for them. They are worth a thorough trial (see p. 59).

## GENERALIZED PRURITUS

Generalized pruritus can signify a metabolic disorder such as diabetes mellitus, drug reaction, biliary obstruction, renal disease, dermographism, early undiscovered underlying malignancy, or pregnancy.

### Causes of generalized pruritus

#### *Diabetes mellitus*

Although anogenital or localized pruritus is the more common manifestation of diabetes mellitus, a generalized pruritus as well should lead to investigation for this disorder.

The degree of pruritus that accompanies diabetes is not related to the severity of the disease. It frequently appears early and may subside spontaneously. It is related to the degree of therapeutic control, appearing when treatment becomes inadequate. Also, increased dryness and decreased sebum production add to the pruritic tendency.

***Treatment.*** Adequate control of the diabetes eliminates pruritus. Relief is obtained by addition to the decreased lipid film of such artificial lubricants as bath oils and simple emollients.

### *Jaundice*

The pruritus associated with liver disease and jaundice may appear in the preicteric stage and may disappear even while jaundice is still present. No cutaneous lesions are visible, except for the secondary effects of rubbing and scratching. Itching occurs in approximately one fourth of patients with jaundice. It is less likely to be seen in infectious hepatitis than in other icteric disorders. Varadi has clearly shown the pruritogenic effect of purified bile acids applied to normal skin. He observed that chenodeoxycholate was mainly responsible for the pruritus. The degree of pruritus is not predictable by any of the standard laboratory tests by which liver and biliary system diseases are measured.

***Treatment.*** The pruritus can be relieved dramatically, except in complete obstructive jaundice, by the adminstration of an ion-exchange resin that sequesters the bile salts and results in their reduction in the bloodstream. Cholestyramine (Questran, Cuemid), 1 tsp. (4 gm.) of the powder in a glass of water three times a day, will relieve the itching in 5 to 10 days. Fat-soluble vitamins may be absorbed and vitamin K at least should be given prior to the cholestyramine in a twice-daily oral dose.

Relief of biliary tract obstruction surgically also produces a sudden disappearance of the pruritus.

### *Renal disease*

Chronic renal insufficiency with a rising blood level of nitrogenous wastes results in pruritus. This is most often observed in chronic pyelonephritis and prostatic obstruction. There is no direct relationship between the urea nitrogen and the intensity of the pruritus.

The number of patients on dialysis units now, because of renal failure, has produced an increase in complaints of generalized pruritus related to dialysis "run." Sometimes the pruritus may occur before, during, or after the procedure.

***Treatment.*** Relief of this uremic pruritus is successfully attained by ultraviolet phototherapy. Of the patient's minimal erythema dose, 75% is estimated by complexion and sunburn history. Treatments can be given daily as long as the erythema dose is not exceeded.

#### REFERENCE

Gilchrest, B. A., Rowe, J. W., Brown, R. S., et al.: Relief of uremic pruritus with ultraviolet phototherapy, N. Engl. J. Med. **297**:136, 1977.

**This has provided a gratifying response to simple, safe measures for an almost intolerable problem in our experience.**

### *Hodgkin's disease, mycosis fungoides, lymphoma, leukemia, and polycythemia*

Generalized itching without visible cutaneous lesions may be the first symptom of Hodgkin's disease or mycosis fungoides. After cutaneous lesions appear, many of the lymphomas are very frequently accompanied by a severe and persistent pruritus. Polycythemia rubra vera also is frequently associated with pruritus. Diagnosis may be made by cutaneous biopsy and by hematological studies.

***Treatment.*** Treatment of the pruritus is unavailing by the usual methods unless the malignant underlying process is treated by such means as radiation or cytotoxic agents, which will also relieve the pruritus. Psoralen medication, either oral or topical, and long-wave ultraviolet light has been of help in allaying this problem (see p. 474).

### *Pregnancy*

Normal pregnancy, particularly in the last trimester, may be associated with an intense generalized pruritus without visible primary cutaneous lesions. However, evidences of rubbing and scratching of the skin appear. This occurs suddenly, persists through day and night, and terminates with a normal delivery. Hepatobiliary stasis is believed to be the cause of the pruritus. Hepatosis is responsible for 70% to 80% of the cases, whereas the bulk of the balance are caused by atopic dermatitis and herpes gestationis.

### *Dermographism*

A form of pruritus that is accompanied by cutaneous lesions, dermographism is the result of an abnormal response to mechanical pressure or stroking. Wheals that normally would be the result of a blow or lash are in these cases produced after only light trauma. These are associated with itching during the transient interval of their presence, usually a few minutes to an hour or so. In some individuals this may this may occur merely from pressure of chair backs, girdles, belts, shoulder straps, and the like. It may be associated with a history of an allergic reaction to a medication (for example, penicillin) taken in the recent past.

***Treatment.*** Adequate doses of antihistaminics reduce the pruritus, although the wheals may continue.

### *Other causes of generalized pruritus*

Generalized pruritus is a well-recognized manifestation of *hypothyroidism*, whereas it occurs with less frequency in *hyperthyroidism*. *Trichinosis*, *carcinoid syndrome*, and *iron deficiency* also must be considered as causes of generalized pruritis.

Iron deficiency has been identified by Vickers as a cause of itching, and Reeves in a letter to the editor, upholds his findings and contributes two cases of his own. Lewiecki describes another case. It must be emphasized that serum iron is a better assessment of iron levels as a cause of pruritus than the hemoglobin. It should be taken at a consistent time of day for comparisons to be made.

### *Investigation of generalized pruritus*

#### INITIAL

A thorough history and physical examination is essential to rule out early systemic disease.

Laboratory studies should include the following tests:

Hemoglobin
Sedimentation rate
White blood cell count and differential
Blood urea nitrogen
Serum bilirubin
Serum iron
Sulfobromophthalein retention
Urine for glucose, and microscopic examination
Blood glucose level
Stool examination for occult blood and parasites
Biopsy of questionable lesion

#### SECONDARY

In addition, more detailed investigation should follow positive initial findings.

### *Treatment of generalized pruritus*

The only specific antipruritic agents in a case of generalized pruritus are those directed toward treatment of the underlying cause. Antipruritic measures are directed toward avoidance of irritation, reduction of inflammation, cooling, and central sedation. Antipruritic agents include (1) orally administered antihistaminics, sedatives, and tranquilizers, (2) topical medications in the form of shake lotions and creams, and (3) cool, short baths.

Although antihistaminics are of specific antipruritic value only in histamine-produced reactions, their continued wide use in other pruritic states cannot be disparaged. Sedatives and tranquilizers reduce the urgency of the pruritus and add required rest and relaxation.

It is important that antihistaminics be given in adequate doses, or up to tolerance of side effects. Sedatives and tranquilizers are to be used in adequate doses when they are necessary. Too often a therapeutic effect is hoped for with inadequate doses of these medications.

Trimeprazine in 2.5 or 5 mg. tablets, or hydroxyzine, 25 mg., two to three times daily, may cause drowsiness. Cyproheptadine, 4 mg., and methdilazine, 8 mg., are satisfactory antipruritic antihistamines. Chloral hydrate, 250 mg. two or three times a day, and diazepam, 5 to 10 mg. three times a day, are examples of sedatives and tranquilizers, respectively.

An effective shake lotion is as follows:

| | |
|---|---|
| Menthol | 0.25% |
| Phenol | 0.25% |
| Zinc oxide | 15 Gm. |
| Talc | 15 Gm. |
| Glycerin | 10 ml. |
| Alcohol | 40 ml. |
| Water | 40 ml. |

Apply with fingertips or narrow brush four times daily.

Menthol, 0.5%, and 1% hydrocortisone in hydrophilic ointment can be used twice daily over large areas. It is an effective antipruritic agent.

Cool, short baths without soap have an antipruritic effect.

### REFERENCES

Barnes, H. M., Sarkany, I., and Calnan, C. S.: Pruritus and thyrotoxicosis, Trans. St. John's Hosp. Dermatol. Soc. **60**:59, 1974.
**Supplies added emphasis to the fact that the skin often mirrors the thyroid.**

Kirby, J., Heaton, K. W., and Burton, J. L.: Pruritic effect of bile salts, Br. Med. J. **4**:693, 1974.
**Bile salts given I.V., I.M., or by mouth failed to produce itch. It takes prolonged intimate keratinocyte dihydroxy bile salt association.**

Lewiecki, E. M., and Rahman, F.: Pruritus. A manifestation of iron deficiency, J.A.M.A. **236**:2319, 1976.
**A further case report.**

Reeves, J.: Iron deficiency pruritus. Letter to the editor, J.A.M.A. **237**:1435, 1977.
**This author substantiates Vickers' observation.**

Savin, J. A.: Diseases of the skin: the management of pruritus, Br. Med. J. **4**:779, 1973.
**A practical approach to the treatment of a common, sometimes stubborn, problem.**

Schoenfield, L. J., Sjövall, J., and Perman, E.: Bile acids on skin of patients with pruritic hepatobiliary disease, Nature **213**:93, 1967.
**It was the contact with the skin that produced itching.**

Scratching the surface of the itch: Editorial, N. Engl. J. Med. **279**:715, 1968.
**Delightfully written, an editorial that produces both pleasure and pain.**

Varadi, D. P.: Pruritus induced by crude bile and purified bile acids, Arch. Dermatol. **109**:678, 1974.
**The free bile acids, deoxycholate and chenodeoxycholate are involved in the itching of jaundice.**

Vickers, C. F. H.: Iron deficiency and the skin, Br. J. Dermatol. **89**(suppl. 9):10, 1973.
**A note only, no factual data and a suggestion of the relationship of iron to pruritus.**

## LICHEN SIMPLEX CHRONICUS (LOCALIZED NEURODERMATITIS)

Lichen simplex chronicus (Plate 45) is a common pruritic disorder resulting in a localized patch of dermatitis that has a characteristic lichenification (thickening, with an exaggeration of the skin lines).

### *Natural course*

An initial sensation of itching ordinarily begins the process. It may stem from external factors such as an insect bite, the friction of a collar, or a psychogenic habit of rubbing the skin. As a result of the rubbing and scratching, a susceptible skin becomes lichenified. The slightest stimulus produces an itch sensation, and the resulting scratching and rubbing lead to further lichenification. Once established, the lesion is the source of an unremitting itch sensation.

The fully developed lesion demonstrates a sharply localized area of thickened skin, usually hyperpigmented and dry. Examination shows closely set papules interrupted by fine wrinkles. In well-developed lesions the gross appearance simulates the bark of a tree (Fig. 27-2). Lichenification may be a less prominent feature in lesions located around orifices such as the anus, vulva, and external auditory meatus. The sites of predilection are the posterior aspect of the neck (Fig. 27-3) and the extremities, but the lesion may be present anywhere on the skin surface.

The process can be diagrammatically shown as follows:

*External factors*
or
*Psychogenic stimulus*
or
*Systemic disorder that causes itching*
↓
*Itching* ⟶ *Rubbing or scratching*
↑ ↓
*Itching hyperexcitability to pruritus* ⟵ *Lichenification* (in predisposed individuals)

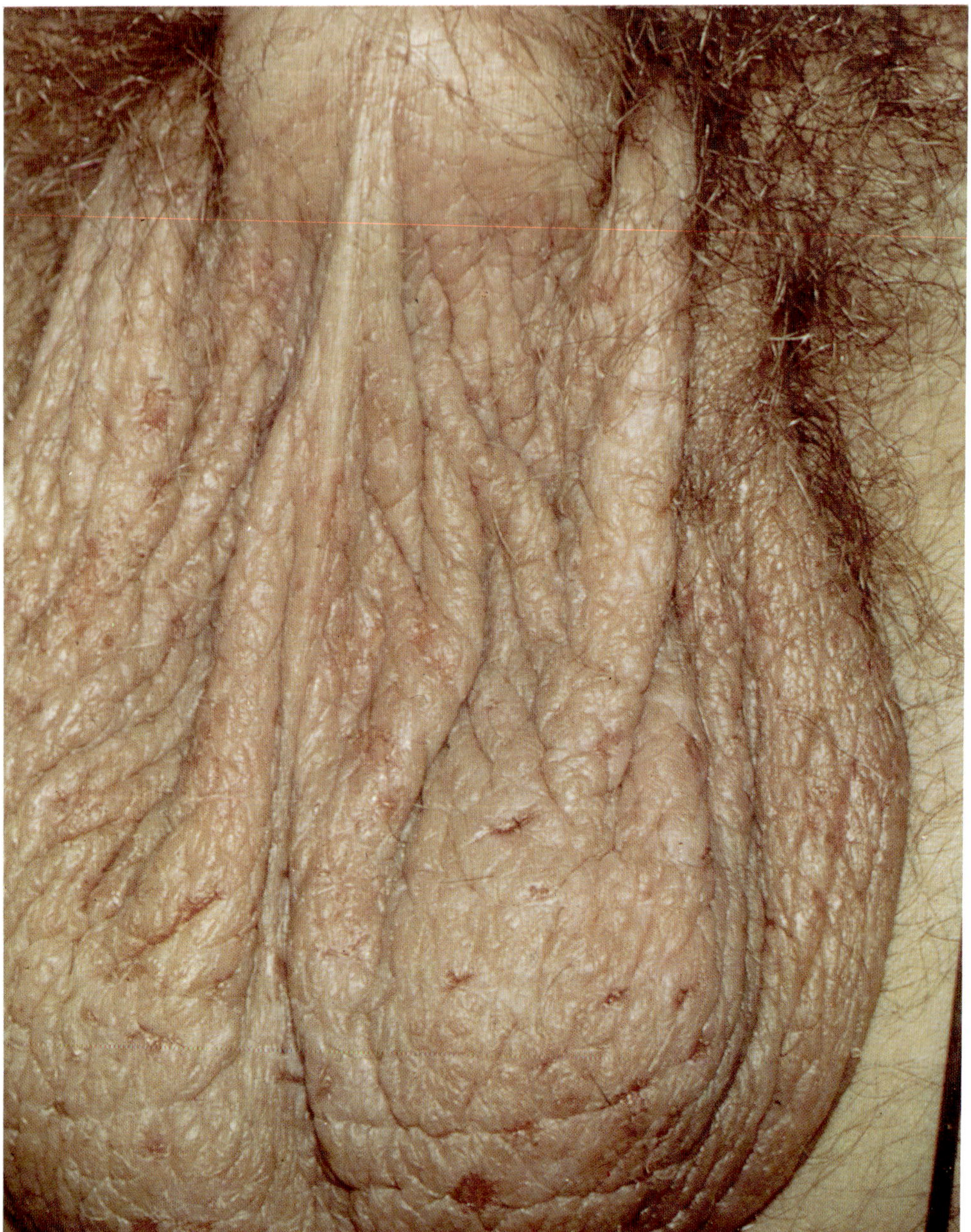

**Plate 45**

Lichen simplex chronicus of scrotum.

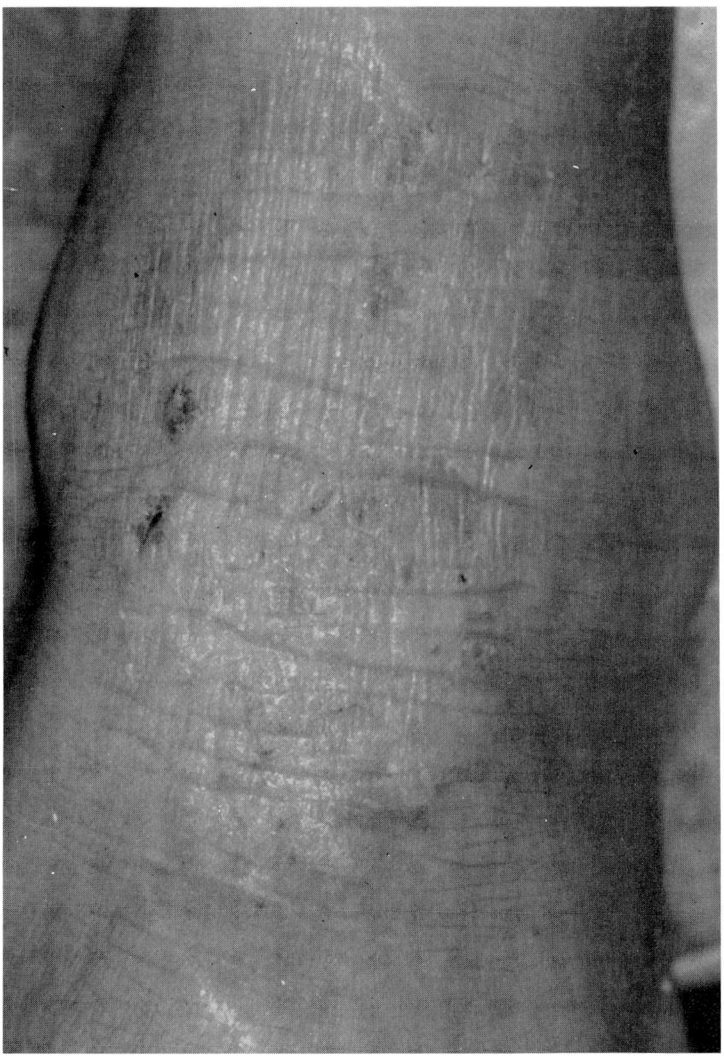

**Fig. 27-2.** Lichen simplex chronicus of ankle. Note distinctive lichenification.

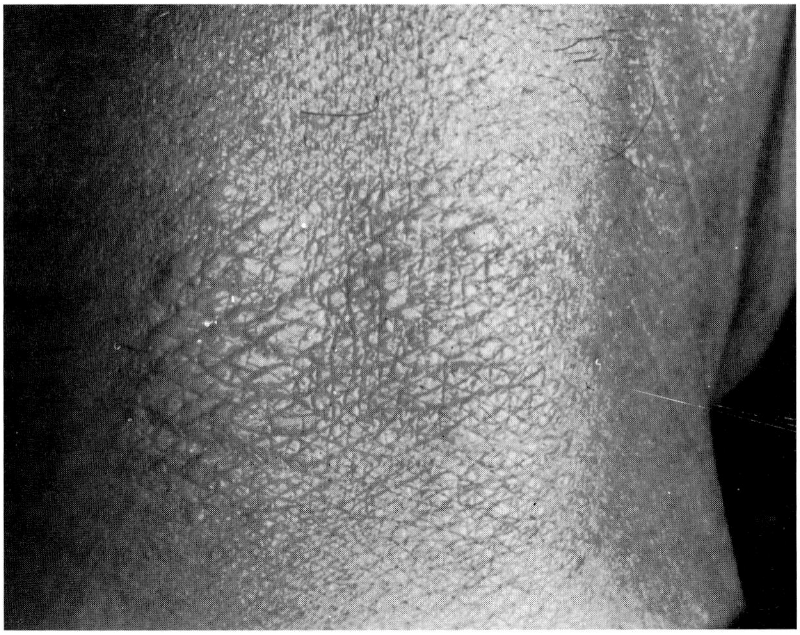

**Fig. 27-3.** Lichen simplex chronicus of back of neck, an area frequently involved in Orientals.

Marks and Wells showed increased cellular-labeling proliferation, but a slower transit time through the epidermis than normal.

If one considers that with lichenification there is decreased function or damage to epidermal sensory receptors, then the normal inflow pattern from these nerves can be considered to be less than normal. Winkelmann and Weddell (see discussion on pruritus, p. 441) have indicated that decreased input may be synonymous with itching hypersensitivity.

This disorder is three times more common in women than in men. It rarely occurs in children. For as yet unexplained reasons, it is observed seven times more often in oriental than in occidental persons.

### *Microscopic findings*

There is a hyperkeratosis and a broadening and regular elongation of the rete pegs. There is also a nonspecific inflammatory infiltrate in the dermis, chiefly perivascular.

### *Differential diagnosis*

***Atopic dermatitis.*** Atopic dermatitis usually occurs in infancy or early childhood. Bilateral diffuse lichenification may occur in long-standing cases, particularly in the antecubital and popliteal spaces. There is very frequently a personal or family history of asthma, hay fever, or eczema.

***Psoriasis*** Psoriasis is very rarely pruritic and commonly involves the elbows and knees, where erythematous plaques with a thick white scale are found.

***Stasis dermatitis.*** A thickened erythematous or hyperpigmented area on the leg is seen in stasis dermatitis. The pruritus is not severe, and examination will reveal signs of venous insufficiency.

***Contact dermatitis.*** Contact dermatitis can produce a localized area of pruritic, dry, scaling dermatitis, particularly in long-standing cases. History reveals exposure to a precipitating agent coinciding with the site of the skin surface.

***Lichen planus.*** A patch of grouped flat-topped papules resembling lichen simplex chronicus is produced by lichen planus. Evidence of lichen planus may be found in other lesions on the flexor surface of the wrists and buccal mucosa.

### *Treatment*

The patient must be firmly instructed not to rub or scratch the lesion.

A potent glucocorticoid cream, gel, or ointment, such as betamethasone valerate 0.1%, applied three times daily is the initial form of therapy. One can enhance the beneficial effect of this medication by applying it under an occlusive plastic dressing, changed daily.

An alternative effective method of therapy in stubborn cases is intralesional injection of a glucocorticoid suspension, such as triamcinolone acetonide 5 mg./ml., at weekly intervals for a total of three to four injections, the number depending on the completeness of the response (see p. 67). The total amount of the steroid should be kept below 10 mg. because of atrophy and absorption. Grenz radiation given in a short course of treatments is effective. No more than 1,000 R should be given over a 6-month period to any area.

An effective conservative approach for recalcitrant lesions on the extremities is the use of an occlusive dressing, such as a modified Unna boot (Dome-Paste Boot, Viscopaste), which reduces pruritus and also physically prevents the patient from scratching the site. This is reapplied weekly, or for longer intervals if tolerated, until the lesion clears.

#### REFERENCES

Cleveland, D. E. H.: Lichen simplex chronicus: 170 consecutive cases encountered in private practice, Arch. Dermatol. Syphilol. **33**:317, 1936.

Danto, J. L.: Incidence of lichen simplex chronicus in Orientals and Caucasians, Can. Med. Assoc. J. **75**:1029, 1956.

**Danto's follow-up substantiates Cleveland's contribution of 20 years earlier.**

Marks, R., and Wells, G. C.: Lichen simplex: morphodynamic correlates, Br. J. Dermatol. **88**:249, 1973.

**Epidermal kinetics of 16 patients with lichen simplex are compared to lichen planus and psoriasis.**

Runne U., and Orfanos, C. E.: Cutaneous neural proliferation in highly pruritic lesions of chronic prurigo, Arch. Dermatol. **113**:787, 1977.

**This work suggests that long-continued scratching is responsible for an increased number of dermal nerves, which in turn is responsible for increased itching.**

# CHAPTER 28

# Psoriasis

## CELL GROWTH

See also anatomy, p. 127, and keratinization, p. 342.

The rate of division of basal cells leads to the migration of maturing cells through the prickle and granular layers and equals the continual surface cellular desquamation. The mitotic rate follows a diurnal rhythm that is altered, among other things, by epinephrine, adrenocortical hormones, androgenic hormones, vitamin A, wounding, exercise, and the state of nutrition. Mitosis is inhibited by a tissue-specific chemical called a *chalone*, described first by Bullough, the effect of which diminishes with wounding so that a burst of epidermal mitotic activity results. Voorhees and his co-workers have also implicated cyclic adenosine-3′,5′-monophosphate (cAMP) as one, and possibly a major, mediator of epidermal cellular control.

The number of epidermal cells undergoing division at any one time under normal conditions is small, perhaps 0.1% of basal cells. The cell cycle, which is related to individual cell proliferation, is defined as *the time period separating completion of mitosis in a cell from completion of mitosis in a daughter cell.* This definition assumes an uninterrupted cycle in both cells. The phases of the cell cycle that are recognized are as follows:

- **$G_1$** From completion of mitosis to initiation of chromosomal replication: interphase.
- **S** Active nuclear DNA synthesis.
- **$G_2$** From end of chromosomal replication to cell division; resting.
- **M** Mitosis.

The time taken for an uninterrupted complete cell cycle is constant for a homogeneous cell population. Resting phases have been described as an alternative behavior to the $G_1$ phase and perhaps also for the $G_2$ phase. These are introduced as blocks by Gelfant. This is also referred to as a restriction point in the cycle. A cytoplasmic control for future cellular behavior acts at this stage. Gelfant suggests that the cell cycle in normal human epidermis is probably close to 200 hours.

Cell-cycle regulation is not well understood. There are regulators that enter cells, bind to receptors, and affect cell proliferation from within (glucocorticoids), and there are regulators that affect cell proliferation from the cell surface (chalones, cyclic nucleotides, catecholamines, HL-A antigens). Intercellular recognition and communication may also be important stimuli. Christophers postulates a relationship between epidermal cell column stacking and new cell production.

Chalones have been further purified and their inhibitory effects on cellular proliferation carefully observed. They are found to be tissue specific (epidermal chalone will not affect sebaceous gland cell growth) and cell-cycle-time specific, (epidermal chalone $G_1$ inhibits cells only at the $G_1$-S phase boundary, and $G_2$ acts to inhibit cells from entering the M phase) (Thornley et al.).

Cyclic nucleotides (cyclic AMP, cyclic GMP) control cell proliferation and perhaps differentiation. cAMP inhibits epidermal cell proliferation in the $G_2$ phase, at least, and cGMP stimulates proliferation (Voorhees).

Polyamines (spermine, spermidine, cadaverine, putrescine) provide another cell-proliferation control mechanism, widely dispersed in all living cells, that obviously goes far back in evolutionary development. They are growth stimulators that may be regulated by cAMP (Voorhees, 1977).

Epidermal growth hormone is a polypeptide only recently identified in human urine, which on topical application, stimulates growth of epithelium, with increased RNA and DNA synthesis by epidermal cells (Birnbaum).

## TRANSIT TIME THROUGH EPIDERMIS

Average time intervals for "replacement" of the epidermis, or the times taken for cells to migrate from proliferative basal cell layer to the outer cell layer of the stratum corneum are also under discussion. The age of the cells in the epidermis is crucial to an estimation of the time taken in transit from birth to death and that the age of the cells in the epidermis is dependent on the mechanism of cells that leave the bottom layer. This varies between normal, single-layer proliferative epidermis and actively dividing multiple-layer proliferative epidermis as in psoriasis (Duffill) and is of utmost importance in the calculation of the average cell transit time to the surface.

Bergstrasser and Taylor have approached the problem of determining the transit time of cells through the whole thickness of epidermis in a rather different way. They have calculated the average area of an epidermal cell of the stratum corneum and the number of cells in a column of that diameter beneath it. With a figure of 1.4 cell layers per day lost from the surface, a turnover time of 45 days for the entire epidermis is calculated.

It is obviously important to define the transit time because of its variations. Transit time may mean from mitosis to desquamation, or any portion of this, and is used differently by various writers on the subject, depending on the end point of their own investigations.

### REFERENCES

Bergstrasser, P., and Taylor, J. R.: Epidermal "turnover" time—a new examination, Br. J. Dermatol. **96**:503, 1977.
**Turnover time of 45 to 47 days—basal cell replacement of 19 days, keratinocyte transit time 14 days, corneocyte time 14 days.**

Birnbaum, J. R., Sapp, T. M., and Moore, J. B., Jr.: Effects of reserpine, epidermal growth factor and cyclic nucleotide regulators on epidermal mitosis, J. Invest. Dermatol. **66**:313, 1976.
**Assay of cell-cycle stage $G_2$ to mitosis, sensitive to agents elevating cAMP.**

Bullough, W.S.: The control of epidermal thickness, Br. J. Dermatol. **87**:187, 347, 1972.
**Chalone inhibits epidermal mitotic activity by reducing the number of actively cycling cells.**

Christophers, E., and Laurence, E. B.: Kinetics and structural organisation of the epidermis, Curr. Probl. Dermatol. **6**:87, 1976.
**The whole spectrum of cell compartments, maturation, and tissue renewal as distinct from simple cell division are considered.**

Christophers, E., Wolff, H. H., and Laurence, E. B.: The formation of epidermal cell columns, J. Invest. Dermatol. **62**:555, 1974.
**Division, speed of maturation, and division in adjacent columns of cells have an effect on individual cell mitoses.**

Duffill, M. B., Appleton, D. R., Dyson, P., et al.: The measurement of the cell cycle time in squamous epithelium using the metaphase arrest technique with vincristine, Br. J. Dermatol. **96**:493, 1977.
**Multiple layer epidermis affords different cell ages and transit times.**

Gelfant, S.: The cell cycle in psoriasis. A reappraisal, Br. J. Dermatol. **95**:577, 1976.
**Three groups of cells in the epidermis: (a) cycling, (b) noncycling blocked in $G_1$, (c) noncycling blocked in $G_2$.**

Thornley, A. L., Spargo, D. J., and Laurence, E. B.: A simple method for measuring DNA synthesis in epidermis and sebaceous glands and its application to chalone assays, Br. J. Dermatol. **97**:11, 1977.
**Effects of $G_1$ and $G_2$ chalones on strips of mouse epidermis.**

Voorhees, J. J.: Pathophysiology of psoriasis, Annu. Rev. Med. **28**:467, 1977.
**Cell surface, cyclic nucleotides, prostaglandins, and polyamines.**

Voorhees, J. J., Duell, E. A., Chambers, D. A., et al.: Regulation of cell cycles, J. Invest. Dermatol. **67**:15, 1976.
**Cyclic AMP, cyclic GMP, and pharmacologic agents affecting them.**

## CLINICAL PICTURE

Psoriasis is a very common, heritable disorder of keratin synthesis that affects more than one in a hundred individuals.

### *Natural course*

The onset of psoriasis is often insidious, asymptomatic, and initially ignored. The first lesions may consist of any of the following:

1. A diffuse scaling of the scalp that pro-

gresses to the characteristic accumulations of heavy adherent scales
2. Erythema and fine scaling of the anterior hair line and adjacent smooth skin
3. Small scaling macules arising unobtrusively on the torso or extremities
4. An erythematous patch in the perianal or perineal areas
5. Follicular papular lesions of the thighs
6. Discrete pustules of the palms or soles
7. Pitting or discoloration of the nails
8. A scaling, erythematous macule at the site of an injury
9. Discrete, guttate scaling lesions appearing simultaneously over much of the skin surface

Small scaly papules develop into patches of the characteristic deep red, thickly scaling lesions (Fig. 28-1). It begins chiefly in young adults and rarely is seen in infants or very elderly persons. Twelve to 15% of all cases begin before the age of 10.

The course of psoriasis is one of hesitating progressions with periods of inactivity and a marked tendency to regress in summer, particularly during sun exposure. Individual plaques slowly enlarge and become confluent with other plaques, covering large areas. Thick scales make the large patches dry and inflexible, and they produce deep cracks on movement. Spontaneous exacerbations, with sudden and rapid enlargement of old lesions, and the appearance of new lesions are characteristic of this unpredictable disease. Also, spontaneous remissions occur not infrequently.

Psoriasis is a disease of healthy people. Pregnancy may produce regression. Infection may produce spread and the appearance of new lesions. Anxiety, tension, worry, and emotional upset seem to be associated with an increase in pruritus and symptoms of discomfort from the lesions, but rarely with the appearance of new lesions. An interesting feature of psoriasis is the tendency of new lesions to appear at the healing sites of trauma, such as incisions, burns, and scrapes in normal skin (Koebner's phenomenon).

The lesions of psoriasis are most often found on bony prominences (knees, elbows, and sa-

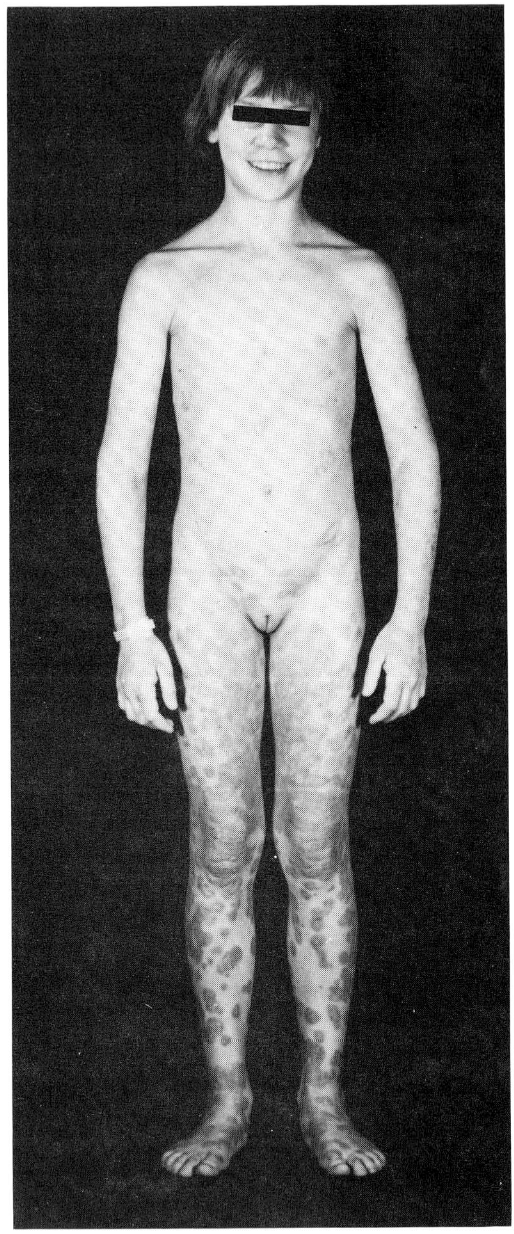

**Fig. 28-1.** Psoriasis in childhood.

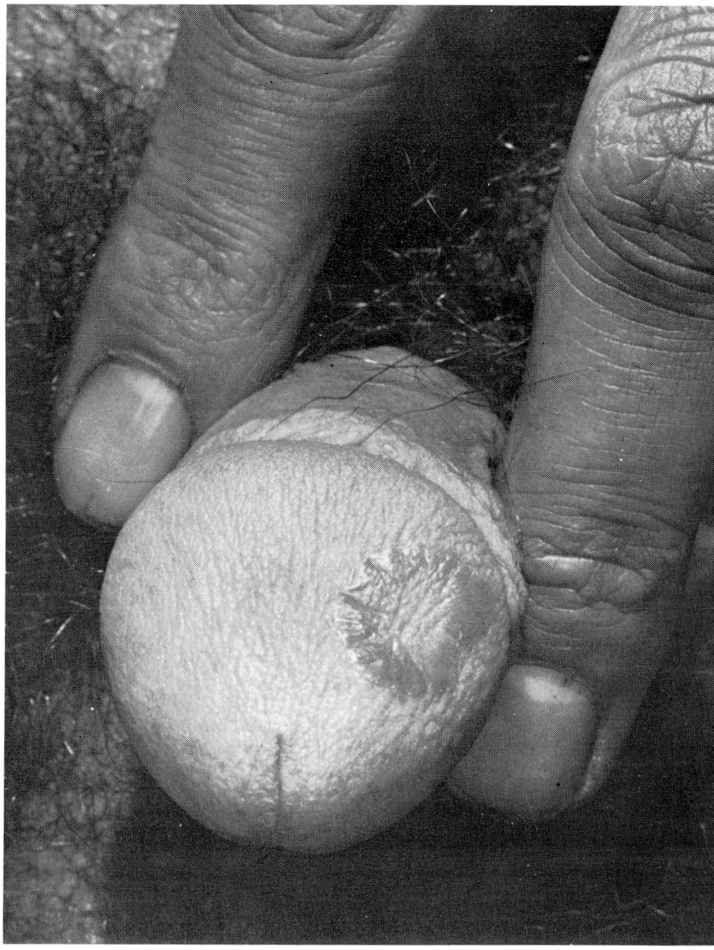

**Fig. 28-2.** Psoriasis of glans penis.

crum), scalp, external ears, genitalia and perianal area, nails, and dorsa of hands. The glans penis may show a persistent plaque (Fig. 28-2). No portion of the skin surface enjoys freedom from the disease.

The never-varying hallmark of psoriasis is the presence of a thick, silvery, overlying scale. Forcible removal of the scale reveals punctate bleeding points (Auspitz's sign). The lesion has a sharply demarcated border and a distinctive deep red color, without vesiculation, oozing, or crusting (Plate 46). Although the typical deep erythematous lesion may involve any part of the cutaneous surface, certain affected areas show distinctive features.

Lesions of the external auditory canal reveal scaling and dryness, often without erythema.

Psoriasis of the palms and soles produces vesicular and pustular pruritic lesions. Alternatively, there may be simply dryness, flaking, and fissuring.

Psoriasis of the nails is characterized by thickening, discoloration, crumbling beneath the free edge, or pitting of nails. The free edge may be elevated and separated from the nail bed.

In intertriginous areas (for example, the perianal area), smooth, shiny, erythematous lesions extend along the depth of the gluteal cleft. These, as well as vulvar lesions, may have painful fissures and are intermittently

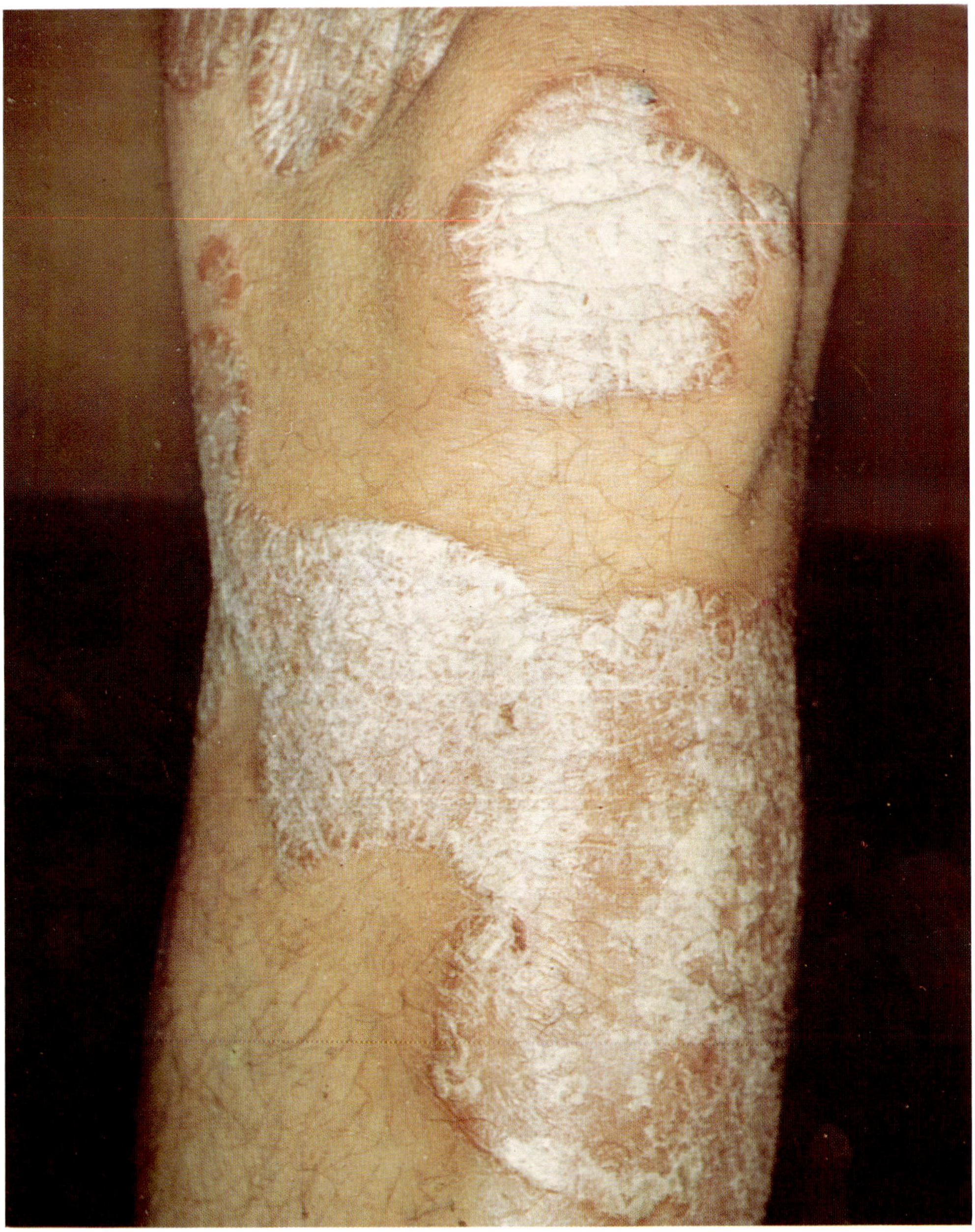

**Plate 46**
Psoriasis.

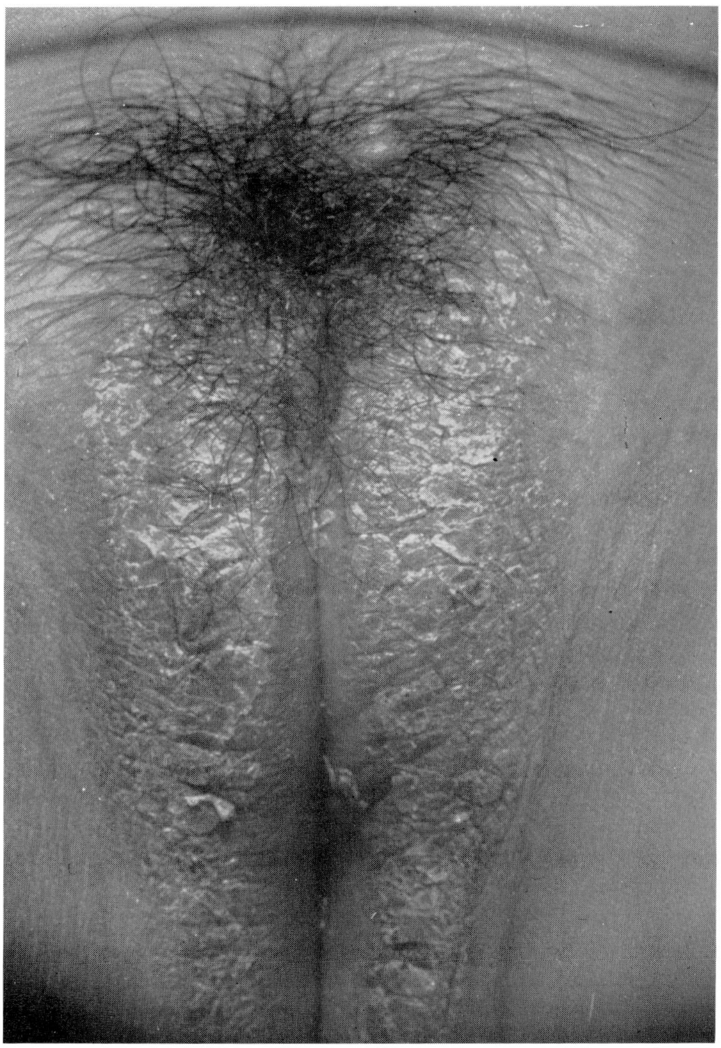

**Fig. 28-3.** Psoriasis of vulva. Pruritic.

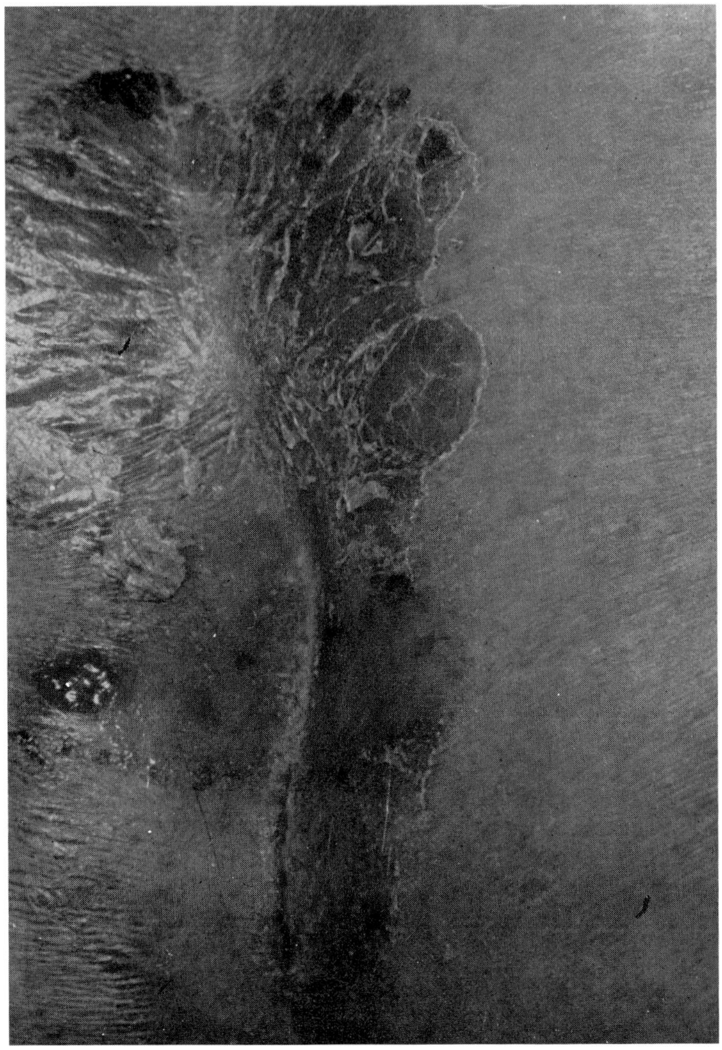

**Fig. 28-4.** Intertriginous psoriasis. Upper end of gluteal fold.

pruritic (Fig. 28-3 and 28-4). Inframammary and axillary lesions, like the foregoing, are smooth, moist, and easily fissured. Psoriatic facial lesions are often erythematous patches of the malar and paranasal areas.

*Acute guttate psoriasis* is a form of psoriasis that consists of drop-sized (guttate) lesions (Fig. 28-5) appearing suddenly over a large part of the skin surface. It may occur in association with infection, usually a streptococcal upper respiratory infection, after the infection by 1 to 3 weeks.

*Pustular psoriasis* is a chronic relapsing form of psoriasis that may involve only the palms and soles (Fig. 28-6), with pustular lesions covered by a thin scale. There may be no other characteristic psoriatic lesions elsewhere, and the differentiation from a pustular bacterial lesion may be difficult. Cultures from the psoriatic lesions are sterile. A more extensive and more dangerous form of pustular psoriasis has a generalized involvement; thousands of pustules extend over large surfaces, with the formation of lakes of pus. There are significant systemic symptoms.

*Psoriatic arthritis* occurs in a small number

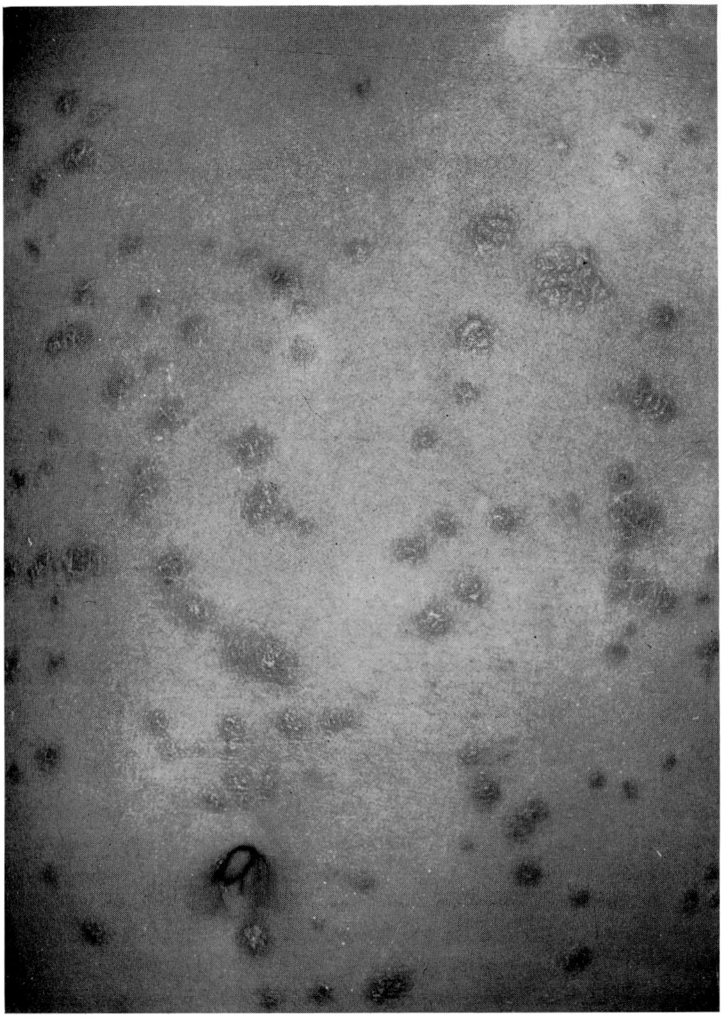

**Fig. 28-5.** Guttate psoriasis. Often seen after an upper respiratory tract infection.

of patients with psoriasis. It is an associated distinctive form of inflammatory arthritis that chiefly involves the distal small joints but can go on to attack the larger ones as well. It is usually associated with a severe psoriasis or a psoriatic erythroderma in which the nails and skin over the distal phalanges are almost invariably involved. It differs from rheumatoid arthritis in several respects. There are no subcutaneous nodules and the sheep cell agglutination test is ordinarily negative. In addition, there are consistent differences in the antiimmunoglobulin pattern of each.

*Reiter's syndrome* of arthritis, conjunctivitis, urethritis, and keratoderma blennorrhagica may be closely related to psoriasis.

*Psoriatic erythroderma* is a severe generalized exfoliative erythroderma that occurs in a small percentage of patients with psoriasis. This can occur spontaneously, but more often follows excessive irritation of existing lesions by overly aggressive therapy. Strong ointments, excessive ultraviolet radiation or sunburn, or overzealous treatment of an already spreading psoriasis can trigger a patient into an exfoliative episode. It is a serious compli-

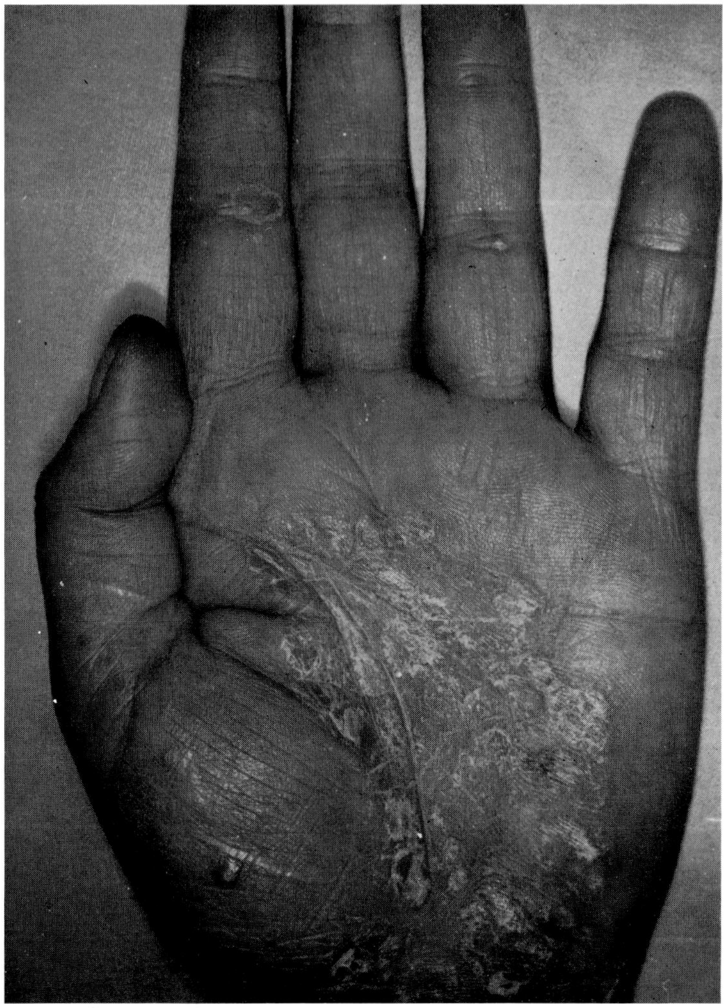

**Fig. 28-6.** Psoriasis, palmar aspect. Psoriasis of palms and soles may be pustular (see thenar eminence) or scaling.

cation of psoriasis, necessitating hospitalization and skilled management. The skin is almost totally involved, with deep erythema, massive amounts of shedding scales, and subsequent abnormalities of temperature regulation and fluid balance. The effect on the peripheral circulation can be illustrated by the fact that the increase in cardiac output in erythroderma has resulted in cardiac failure.

### *Pertinent information*

Psoriasis is essentially a proliferative aberration of the keratinizing process in association with some changes in the cutaneous vascular system. Capillaries, observed by microscopy in the living specimen, are dilated, tortuous, and elongated. There is an accelerated turnover of epidermal cells, from the basal layer through to their final imperfect cornification on the skin surface.

Normally, the transit time of cells from mitosis in the basal cell layer to the stratum corneum is approximately 26 to 28 days. After Weinstein's report on epidermal cell turnover time in 1968, there have been a number of other conflicting reports. The more recent finding of 7 days for epidermal turnover time in psoriasis appears to have more validity than the much more rapid time of 4 days as reported by Weinstein. In any event, the congestion produced by this astounding frenzy of cellular activity in a limited space conjures up vivid memories of the traffic pattern of the center of a large Italian city.

The primary lesion in psoriasis would appear to be the loss of control of epidermal cell growth, which leads to increased cell proliferation and accelerated cellular turnover. Clinically, thick scaling plaques are the result. The basic biochemical factors responsible for the loss of normal epidermal growth are not yet precisely recognized. However, recent studies by Voorhees and Mier suggest that the cyclic AMP cascade is defective because of a deficiency of cyclic nucleotides. The role of the prostaglandins has also been implicated. Most recently Beutner and others suggest an immunological mechanism that might be operative in psoriatic epidermis.

The cellular proliferation may be the result of aberrations in cellular control by epidermal chalones and the cyclic AMP system.

In the psoriatic epidermis, there seems to be an increase in intracellular structures that can release destructive enzymes. Whether these lysosomes do play a part in the abnormal keratinization in psoriasis is not yet known. The normal repair of the epidermis is disturbed after trauma, and it seems that many of the lesions of psoriasis arise after repeated minor trauma. There is a decrease in polypeptidase activity and a reduction in polypeptides. The water-binding capacity of the epidermis is lowered.

A proliferation of connective tissue in the dermis is also apparent on microscopic examination. The dermal papillae are enlarged and elongated. *Many observers believe that the psoriatic process of increased epidermal proliferation originates from a dermal stimulus.*

There is a genetic basis to psoriasis, but the mode of inheritance has not been established. In one good study, the inheritance proved to be that of an autosomal dominant with a penetrance of 60%. Farber examined the concordance rates of psoriasis for monozygotic and dizygotic twin pairs in 95 affected twin individuals. He concluded that although there is a hereditary contribution to the etiology of psoriasis, environmental factors are also important.

Psoriasis is approximately five times more frequent in persons possessing the HL-A Bw17 antigen than in persons lacking the antigen. The HL-A Bw17 antigen is associated with "hereditary" psoriasis (Jajić). HL-A B13 alone is not significantly correlated, but a sum of B13 and Bw17 antigen frequencies is statistically significant. This would be "nonhereditary" psoriasis (Jajić).

A familial incidence has been observed in as high as 80% and as low as 17% of cases. In the Indian races of North and Central America, the Canadian Eskimo, and the Japanese, the disease is a rarity.

### *Microscopic findings*

The normal keratinizing process and the progress of cells upward through the epidermis is greatly altered.

Parakeratosis with a characteristic club-shaped elongated regular acanthosis of the prickle cell layer occurs, along with thinning of that portion of the epidermal layer above the dermal papillae. Polymorphonuclear leukocytes are seen in the epidermis between epidermal cells. There are leukocyte-containing microabscesses of the epidermis (Munro's abscesses). The granular layer is diminished or absent.

Electron microscopy reveals a diminution in tonofibrils, reduction and alteration in desmosome development, enlarged intracellular spaces, and alterations in keratohyaline granules and lysosomes.

### *Differential diagnosis*

Large, dry, scaling lesions present no difficulty in diagnosis; the difficulty lies in small isolated lesions. A thorough search for other characteristic patches or involvement of knees or elbows often makes the diagnosis.

***Seborrheic dermatitis.*** Psoriasis and seborrheic dermatitis may so closely resemble one another as to be impossible to differentiate. In such cases a common name has been given to the disorder: *sebopsoriasis.* These lesions usually involve the scalp, ears, and face. Classical seborrheic dermatitis is less scaling, is more acute, may have a tendency to be moist or weeping, and is often acutely inflamed. This dermatitis has a tendency to involve the scalp, postauricular area, eyebrows, midsternum, and navel.

***Lichen simplex chronicus.*** Lichen simplex chronicus presents localized, very pruritic, thickened, unilateral, often single, chronic lesions. There is no characteristic heavy scale.

***Nummular eczema.*** Moist, coin-shaped or larger vesicular lesions that are pale and crusted, consistently pruritic, and asymmetrically placed differentiate nummular eczema from psoriasis.

***Fungal infections.*** Isolated lesions of body, face, hands, feet, or nails may all resemble psoriasis. Scrapings on three occasions with examination and culture should produce the organisms if they are present.

***Lichen planus.*** A very pruritic dermatitis, lichen planus shows flat-topped shiny lesions, not usually involving the knees or elbows. Buccal mucous membrane is usually involved with a lacy gray lesion.

***Syphilis.*** Secondary syphilis may produce the appearance of an acute guttate psoriasis. Local therapy is ineffective; history of chancre may be obtained. The serological test for syphilis is positive by the time of appearance of skin lesions.

***Pityriasis rosea.*** The history of onset of the initial herald patch followed by the generalized dermatitis is characteristic.

### *Treatment*

On the first visit the patient must be made aware of the necessity of adhering consistently to the treatment plan outlined by the physician.

A philosophy of treatment of psoriasis is best expounded as follows:

1. No therapy should produce trauma (burns or inflammation) of the skin, since this may result in new psoriatic lesions.

2. Slow, inactive, thick lesions should be treated aggressively.

3. Acute, recent, spreading lesions should be treated gently (because of the danger of precipitating a generalized psoriasis and possible erythroderma).

4. Tar and dithranol compounds should be used very cautiously in flexural and anogenital areas, if used at all, because of their irritating potential.

5. When glucocorticoids are used topically to initiate therapy and a clearing of the psoriatic process is obtained, a tar-containing preparation should be used to maintain the therapeutic effect and avoid the rebound effect seen after steroid therapy.

6. Glucocorticoids given orally should be used rarely and then only with careful consideration of the effect required of them. It is exceedingly difficult to discontinue a course of these drugs in active psoriasis, because of rapid recrudescence and rebound of the suppressed disorder.

***Topical medications.*** Ointments should be applied whenever possible after bathing has first removed the scale to allow penetration of the ointment.

A bath consisting of 2 tablespoons of a tar solution to one-half tub of water should be given for 15 minutes daily. One of the following ointments is then applied:

| | | |
|---|---|---|
| 1. | Liquor carbonis detergens | 10% |
| | Salicylic acid | 3% |
| | Hydrophilic petrolatum | q.s. |
| | Rub well into affected areas twice daily. | |
| 2. | Dithranol | 0.1%-1% |
| | Salicylic acid | 0.4% |
| | Zinc oxide ointment | q.s. |

Rub well into lesions, keeping off the normal skin and away from the eyes (may be irritating). Start with weaker concentration and slowly progress to the higher, as the response demands. Ointment stains clothing. Bandage after applying ointment once daily.

Scalp preparations include phenol-saline mixture (P & S liquid), which is quite greasy, and Pragmatar cream, either of which is massaged into the affected area of the scalp daily, and tar shampoo, which is used for cleansing the scalp thoroughly every other day.

For lesions of intertriginous areas, vulva, glans penis, and perianal region, one of the fluorinated glucocorticoid compounds (for example, 0.05% to 0.1% triamcinolone or 0.05% to 0.1% betamethasone) is most beneficial.

This is applied *sparingly* three times daily. However, the atrophy and stria-producing effect of these hormones must be monitored.

Hydrocortisone or desonide (Tridesilon) ointments only are used for psoriatic lesions of eyelids and ears, applied sparingly three times daily. Potent fluorinated glucocorticoid ointments must not be used around the eyes because of their tendency to cause an increase in intraocular pressure.

These applications must be applied regularly for some time after apparent subsidence of the lesions. *There may be a rebound of psoriatic activity after use of glucocorticoids.*

The acid radical of vitamin A (retinoic acid, tretinoin) added to a glucocorticoid, such as betamethasone valerate, has been advocated by several observers. The combination used by MacDonald and Fry involved separate but successive applications of the retinoic acid 0.1% in ointment and betamethasone valerate 0.1% ointment. A significant number of patients improved more satisfactorily than when they were treated with a glucocorticoid plus a placebo.

***Occlusive therapy.*** Triamcinolone or other fluorinated glucocorticoid cream may be applied and left on under an occlusive plastic dressing for as many hours of the 24 as possible. The area is cleansed once daily and the cream reapplied. The plastic may be held in place with articles of clothing, socks, and so forth. Use of occlusive plastic gloves is very helpful with psoriatic lesions of the hands; plastic shower caps may be used in the case of scalp lesions. The plastic covering must be completely occlusive, not allowing air to dry the area. Recurrences can be abrupt after cessation of this form of therapy.

***Intralesional injections.*** For torpid lesions, triamcinolone suspension, 5 mg./ml., may be injected intralesionally into single lesions. (See intralesional therapy, p. 473.)

***Ultraviolet therapy.*** Regular exposure to short-wave ultraviolet rays (UVB), below production of erythema or burning, is beneficial. Exposure one to three times weekly is most desirable. Gradually increasing doses, kept below erythema level, may then be instituted. With subsidence of lesions, the frequency of dose is slowly reduced and then discontinued. (See p. 474, concerning long-wave ultraviolet-light (UVA) therapy in conjuction with psoralens.)

The following two methods are useful for hospitalized patients.

***Goeckerman technique (modified).*** The photosensitizing effect of tar ointments applied in association with ultraviolet therapy is very beneficial. Although this is a messy and disagreeable method of therapy, it is acceptable in the face of stubborn, nonresponsive cases of psoriasis.

A thin layer of 1% to 5% coal tar ointment in hydrophilic petrolatum is applied and left on for some hours, preferably overnight; then, after a bath, generalized ultraviolet therapy is given in a dose allowing for the increased response attributable to the presence of tar. The patient may carry on during the day, and the procedure is repeated in the evening. This regimen is easiest when carried out in the hospital.

***Dithranol (anthralin) technique.*** This course of treatment takes approximately 15 to 20 days. The steps are as follows:

1. Tar bath of liquor carbonis detergens, 120 ml. to 80 liters of water daily.
2. Exposure to ultraviolet light by gradual increments to a level of minimum erythema. Daily treatments.
3. Dithranol paste applied to the lesions on the trunk and extremities in the following formula:

| | |
|---|---|
| Dithranol | 0.1% |
| Salicylic acid | 0.4% |
| Lassar's paste | q.s. |

   This is a simplification of Ingram's ointment. It will irritate normal skin.
4. Dusting powder applied.
5. Area covered with stockinette roll.
6. Paste removed with cotton soaked in *Arachis* oil prior to daily tar bath.

Seville has modified this somewhat forbidding formal regimen to one that is easy to follow and highly effective. We recommend it.

***Psoriasis day care centers.*** Farber of Stanford University has introduced to the United States a treatment concept similar to that established by Wilkinson at High Wycombe Hospital in the United Kingdom. The patient with severe psoriasis can undergo intensive and specialized anti-psoriatic treatment during the day and be free in the evening. Such centers are now available elsewhere in the United States and in Canada.

***PUVA therapy.*** The photochemotherapy concept for the treatment of psoriasis was first introduced by Parrish, Fitzpatrick, Tanenbaum, and Pathak in 1974. They advocated the oral administration of the photoactive drug, 8-methoxypsoralen (methoxsalen), followed by exposure to a high-intensity, long-wave ultraviolet-light system (UVA). Their 21 patients all demonstrated complete clearing of their severe generalized psoriasis. Since this initial report Wolff and Roenigk have confirmed the original favorable report of Parrish. This treatment is now available in most large centers in the Americas and Western Europe. However, we recommend that caution be exercised in the use of this new modality. A cautionary statement has been issued by the Psoriasis and Photobiology Task Force of the American Academy of Dermatology to ensure that this potentially advantageous treatment is not abused.

***X-ray therapy.*** Conventional x-ray therapy has only a minor place in modern methods of treating psoriasis. It may be used under careful supervision in the treatment of resistant nail involvement when the lesions are of sufficient importance to the patient and of sufficient severity to justify it, but only when all aspects of the therapy are carefully considered, and as a last resort. Its cumulative effect, in this modern environment of external radiation, must be taken into account in reference to the age of patient, shielding of patient, skill and experience of operator, and need of the patient for this type of therapy. Its use is largely limited to nail treatment.

***Grenz-ray therapy.*** Grenz radiation is a "soft" form of ionizing radiation with a spectrum bordering between ultraviolet rays and roentgen rays. It has no permanent effects when used correctly and has a beneficial effect on superficial psoriatic lesions. It is used chiefly for scalp lesions, perianal lesions, and genital lesions, since these are often very difficult to control by local therapy alone. It is ordinarily given in three to five treatment courses and can be repeated at 6-month intervals. It should only be used, of course, by one thoroughly familiar with both the natural history of the disease and the correct use of the modality.

***Systemic glucocorticoid therapy.*** Glucocorticoid preparations, powerful anti-inflammatory agents, will clear psoriasis when given in adequate dosage. There will be a recurrence of the disease when they are discontinued, however, and the physician must weigh this effect as well as their potential side effects against their temporary benefit in this disease. He should be thoroughly familiar with their use, which is justified only in certain carefully selected acute cases. The indications for the use of glucocorticoids must outweigh the possible undesirable results. Psoriatic erythroderma and arthritis associated with generalized psoriasis are special conditions that justify the use of glucocorticoids.

***Methotrexate.*** Methotrexate therapy has been in widespread use in North America at dermatological centers, but there is evidence that it is now being used much less, in the light of reports of deaths and liver damage attributed to its use. The drug acts to inhibit folic acid and general protein metabolism. As the proliferating epidermis is the most actively metabolizing tissue, it is inhibited to a greater extent than are other tissues.

Methotrexate is absorbed rapidly from the empty stomach and becomes bound to the plasma albumin. Its toxicity is increased by the ingestion of aspirin, sulfonamides, and sulfonamide diuretics, which displace it from the albumin binding. Methotrexate is excreted in the urine unchanged.

Methotrexate may be given at weekly intervals if routine white blood cell values and selected laboratory indices are followed. It is used intramuscularly and also orally. Therapeutic response is obtained in 10 to 12 days.

Treatment is varied according to the patient's response, with the following oral dosage schedule calculated to affect psoriatic epidermal cells and produce minimum effects on other cells: 2.5 or 5 mg. given at 8- or 12-hour intervals for 3 doses. Treatment may be repeated in a week, if laboratory parameters are not abnormal. Guidelines of methotrexate therapy for psoriasis have been published (Roenigk, Maibach, and Weinstein).

Methotrexate must not be given to females in the childbearing age who have *any possibility of pregnancy.* The patient must be under careful observation by one familiar with the course of the disease.

Other chemotherapeutic agents, including hydroxyurea, mycophenolic acid, and azarabine (triacetyl-6-azauridine) are sometimes used in selected cases or in special clinical assessment centers.

## REFERENCES


Baker, H.: Psoriasis: a review. Part I, Dermatologica **150**:16, 1975,
**The present state of our knowledge with regard to pathogenesis.**

Baker, H.: Psoriasis: a review. Part II. Dermatologica **150**:136, 1975.
**An in-depth survey of traditional as well as new topical and systemic antipsoriatic regimens.**

Beutner, E. H., Chorzelski, T.P., and Jablonska, S.: Autoimmunity in psoriasis. 1. Studies on the possible significance of the universal stratum corneum antibodies in the pathogenesis of psoriasis. In Farber, E.M., and Cox, A. J., editors: Psoriasis, Proceedings of the Second International Symposium, New York, 1977, Yorke Medical Books, p. 63.

Editorial: PUVA statement, Arch. Dermatol. **113**:1195, 1977.
**A cautionary statement.**

Farber, E. M.: Psoriasis day care centers. In Maddin, S., editor: Current dermatologic management, St. Louis, 1975, The C. V. Mosby Co. p. 44.

Farber, E. M., Nall, M. L., and Watson, W.: Natural history of psoriasis in 61 twin pairs, Arch. Dermatol. **109**:207, 1974.
**Establishes a hereditary factor.**

Farber, E. M., Pearlman, D., and Abel, E. A.: An appraisal of current systemic chemotherapy for psoriasis, Arch. Dermatol. **112**:1679, 1976.
**The most complete and objective review of the many chemotherapeutic agents advocated for use in psoriasis.**

Gelfant, S.: The cell cycle in psoriasis: a reappraisal, Br. J. Dermatol. **95**:577, 1976.
**Confirms Goodwin's work.**

Goodwin, P., Hamilton, S., and Fry, L.: Cell cycles in psoriasis, Br. J. Dermatol, **90**:517, 1974.
**Increased cell proliferation in active lesions, cell-cycle time is accelerated, but not to extent suggested by Weinstein.**

Jajić, I., Kastelan, A., and Brnobić, A.: HL-A antigens in psoriatic arthritis and psoriasis, Arch. Dermatol. **113**:1724, 1977.
**There may be two types of psoriasis, hereditary and nonhereditary.**

Jones, E. L., Epinette, W. W., and Hackney, V. C.: Treatment of psoriasis with oral mycophenolic acid, J. Invest. Dermatol. **65**:537, 1975.
**This initial report evaluates therapeutics and adverse effects in 29 patients.**

Leading article: Psoriatic arthritis: to lump or to split, Br. Med. J. **2**:491, 1976.
**Concludes that present evidence permits psoriatic arthritis to be a distinct entity.**

MacDonald, A., and Fry, L.: Retinoic acid in the treatment of psoriasis, Br. J. Dermatol. **86**:524, 1972.
**Not for everyone, but effective in some patients.**

Parrish, J. A., Fitzpatrick, T. B., Tanenbaum, L., et al.: Photochemotheraphy of psoriasis with oral methoxsalen and long-wave ultraviolet light, N. Engl. J. Med. **291**:1207, 1974.
**The original.**

Roenigk, H. H., Maibach, H. I., and Weinstein, G. D.: Use of methotrexate in psoriasis, Arch. Dermatol. **105**:363, 1972.
**Officially recognized guidelines to be followed.**

Roenigk, H. H., and Martin, J. S.: Photochemotherapy for psoriasis, Arch. Dermatol. **113**:1667, 1977.
**A review of 186 patients on PUVA.**

Seville, R. H.: Simplified dithranol treatment for psoriasis, Br. J. Dermatol. **93**:205, 1975.
**If the general practitioner sticks to this one treatment despite all the foofaraw about new methods, he will satisfactorily clear most of his psoriatic patients.**

Thomas, R. J.: Psoriasis. Case rate—HL-A antigen frequency correlation, Dermatologica **154**:23, 1977.
**Suggests that HL-A antigens B17 and B13 together with case rate in population surveyed is significant.**

Voorhees, J. J., and Marcelo, C.: Molecular mechanisms and the cyclic nucleotide cascade in psoriasis. In Farber, E. M., and Cox, A. J., editors: Psoriasis, Proceedings of the Second International Symposium, New York, 1977, Yorke Medical Books, p. 91.
**An impressive perspective.**

Weinstein, G. D., and Frost, P.: Abnormal cell proliferation in psoriasis, J. Invest. Dermatol. **50**:254, 1968.
**The forerunner of investigations into the cell cycle.**

Wolf, J. E., Jr., and Hubler, W. R., Jr.: Psoriasis, the angiogenic alternative, Arch. Dermatol. **113**:1458, 1977.
**Critical assessment of work in this field.**

Wolff, K., Fitzpatrick, T. B., Parrish, J. A., et al.: Photochemotherapy for psoriasis with orally administered methoxsalen, Arch. Dermatol. **112**:943, 1976.
**A joint, comparative study, PUVA vs UVB.**

## GENERAL REFERENCES

Farber, E. M., and Cox, A. J.: Psoriasis, Proceedings of the Second International Symposium, New York, 1977, Yorke Medical Books.
**The latest in all aspects of psoriasis.**

Maddin, S., editor: Current dermatologic management, St. Louis, 1975, The C.V. Mosby Co.
**The reader is referred to the following specific articles for the use of the therapeutic agent or technique outlined:**
McDonald, C. H.: Azarabine treatment, p. 263
Leavell, U. W., Jr.: Hydroxyurea therapy, p. 264
Weinstein, G. D.: Methotrexate treatment, p. 265
Wilkinson, D. S.: Ingram technique, p. 42

CHAPTER 29

# Psychogenic diseases (self-inflicted dermatoses)

Whitlock discusses psychogenic diseases together, without clear-cut separation, as self-inflicted dermatoses. However, we have observed that the patients involved are clearly different in the apparent psychological relationship to the cutaneous signs. To our psychiatrically naïve eyes, patients with artifactual dermatitis are malingerers or psychotic; acarophobic patients are essentially normal with, however, a selective psychologic defect in that they recognize that they suffer from a disorder that others do not, but they cannot define that defect. They cannot convince themselves their observations are invalid. Compulsive excoriators have a personality disorder that is uncompromising and rigid, but we do not believe that it actually is self-destructive as has been suggested. Trichotillomanic patients are in the bonds of a habit often more compelling than nail-biting. Children particularly are very ingenuous about it.

## FACTITIAL DERMATITIS (DERMATITIS ARTIFACTA)

Factitial dermatitis is a self-inflicted injury to the skin that is denied by the patient but is purposefully performed. The lesions are usually found on areas that are easily accessible to the fingers, for example, the forearms and face. Sensitive areas such as the genitalia, nipples, eyes, and mouth are seldom involved. The lesions develop suddenly and have variable bizarre configurations because of the great variety of agents that may be used to inflict the injury, such as scissors, acids, matches, sandpaper, hot metals, and knives. These self-inflicted lesions are produced to obtain sympathy or compensation or to escape duty. On the other hand, severe psychological illness may underlie this behavior. In some cases they are the result of hysteria.

Studies reveal that although patients with factitial dermatitis consciously produce the lesions, they are not always aware of the basic reasons for their self-destruction. Butterworth's observations on retarded children are reminiscent of some of the lesions we have seen clinically from time to time.

The lesions may be cleverly produced so as to mimic known clinical patterns of other dermatoses. This can be very confusing to the physician.

If there is difficulty in establishing a diagnosis or if this disease is suspected, the patient should be hospitalized and kept under close surveillance.

### *Treatment*

Individual lesions may be cleared by the application of an occlusive dressing, a procedure also used for diagnostic purposes. Psychiatric treatment is indicated. Unfortunately, such patients rarely accept this approach and notoriously demonstrate little or no insight into the problem. If malingering can be ruled out and superficial personality or personal problems excluded, it is of no avail and probably dangerous for anyone but a psychiatrist to try to unravel the more serious disturbances that may be present.

## DELUSION OF PARASITOSIS (ACAROPHOBIA)

In acarophobia the patient has a fixed idea that his skin is infested with bugs. There are subjective complaints of crawling and biting sensations. Frequently the patient will use the fingernails or employ tweezers to extract the imaginary parasites. To prove the existence of these creatures, the patient presents the physician with epithelial debris in jars, bottles, envelopes, and carefully wrapped facial tissue, which the patient insists contains the bugs. The patient cannot be convinced that there is no infestation. Secondary infection may develop in the excoriated areas.

This condition occurs most frequently in middle-aged and older women. A number of emotional disturbances may be responsible for delusion of parasitosis—toxic psychosis, schizophrenia, involutional depression, and paranoia. *Pellagra must be ruled out as a cause* (Aleshire).

Other fears that are similarly difficult to alter include an abnormal fear of syphilitic infection, of cancer, and of offensive body odors. These, however, are phobias rather than delusions and are more amenable to treatment.

### *Treatment*

Gould and Gragg set out a rational approach to the problem, which involves straight-forward dealing with the patient.

Delusion of parasitosis requires psychiatric therapy as early as possible in the course of the disease, after pellagra and vitamin-deficient diets have been ruled out as a cause.

It is essential that a routine search for parasites be carried out in all such patients suspected of delusion of parasitosis to avoid a dermatological discomfiture!

## COMPULSIVE EXCORIATIONS

Compulsive excoriations are self-inflicted injuries associated with an uncontrollable desire to pinch out pieces of one's skin. The patient admits to a compulsion to dig out the skin with the fingernails. This is done to remove an unsightly blemish, such as an acne papule, or to relieve an intolerable discomfort at the site. There is usually a history of a "pimple" that cannot be squeezed out, necessitating its removal with the fingernails. The early lesions consist of a crusted area, which later leaves a rather characteristic dug-out ulcer that may have a hyperpigmented border and heals with a depressed scar (Fig. 29-1, *A*). The sites of predilection are the face, arms, neck, chest, and breasts. This disorder is most frequently found in women over 30 years of age. It begins insidiously with the production of small, unobtrusive excoriations by the patient. This then develops into a chronic fixed pattern with more disfiguring lesions. The habit is almost impossible to alter.

Fisher demonstrated, with the aid of psychological testing, a uniformity of personality structure in patients afflicted with this problem. He also believed that depression played a significant part in the cause of this disorder.

### *Treatment*

The patient must be made to understand that the skin *must not* be touched by the fingernails. Encouragement and repetition of this advice with regular office visits may serve to break the habit. If distinct improvement is not apparent within a short time, psychiatric consultation should be obtained.

## TRICHOTILLOMANIA

Conscious pulling out of normally formed hair is known as trichotillomania. This syndrome may be either a benign temporary habit of no consequence or an attempt to produce a factitial dermatitis, that is, the manifestation of psychotic behavior.

Most often seen in young children, the pulling out of strands of hair seems to be associated with thumb-sucking and other similar habit patterns. It is often accomplished by twisting the strands around the fingers and semiautomatically tugging or pulling. The lesions produced are characteristic in that there are hairs of various lengths sparsely distributed over the area of alopecia. The site is rarely completely devoid of hair. The areas appear at regular intervals and tend to be in the same region of the scalp (Fig. 29-1, B). The diagnosis is usually easily made by careful observation of the child over a period of time.

When produced in adults for purposes of mimicking dermatological disease for compensation, sympathy, or other reasons, the diagnosis is made by the background facts of the case and by observing that the appearance

A

B

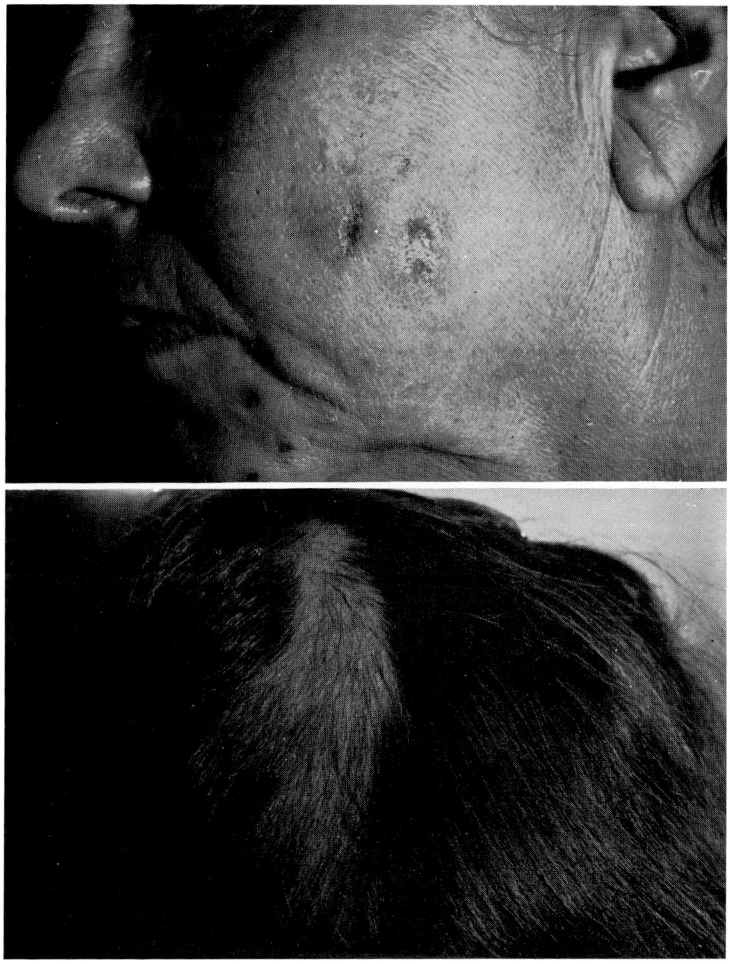

**Fig. 29-1. A,** Compulsive excoriations. **B,** Trichotillomania.

and course of the lesions do not follow the pattern of known causes of scalp alopecia. In our experience, most adults consulting us for a solution to the problem are essentially normally behaving people who find it difficult or impossible to break themselves of the habit. They find themselves perpetuating it in moments of concentration, study, or anxiety. They may be embarrased by the result, but are usually willing to discuss it freely. In one of our pediatric patients, trichotillomania was associated with a brain tumor.

Trichotillomania may be a manifestation of a psychotic disorder.

### *Differential diagnosis*

***Alopecia areata.*** In alopecia areata, usually circular areas of complete hairlessness appear suddenly on the scalp or beard and enlarge steadily. The hairs at the periphery of the lesion are often loose and easily removed.

***Tinea capitis.*** Underlying inflammation in the hairless patch occurs with tinea capitis. Skin scrapings reveal the presence of the fungus.

***Syphilis.*** After the appearance of the primary chancre, syphilis may produce an irregular, patchy, incomplete loss of scalp hair. The serological test for syphilis is positive.

### *Treatment*

Therapy consists of treating the underlying cause of trichotillomania. Close observation of the patient for a time is essential to make the correct diagnosis and also to establish a satisfactory treatment of the cause of the disorder.

Cutting the hair short may successfully curb the tendency to pull it out. In nonorganic or psychotic cases, the prognosis is entirely dependent on the ability of the patient to work out his psychological problem.

#### REFERENCES

Aleshire, I.: Delusions of parasitosis: report of successful cure with antipellagrous treatment, J.A.M.A. **155:**15, 1954.

**Nicotinic acid deficiency and its psychological effect.**

Butterworth, T. I., and Strean, L. P.: Behavior disorders of interest to the dermatologist, Arch. Dermatol. **88:**859, 1963.

**No neuroses, but patterns of purposeful "self-damage" in retarded inmates of a state school.**

Fisher, B. K.: Neurotic excoriations, Can. Med. Assoc. J. **105:**218, 1972.

**A successful endeavor to categorize this group of patients.**

Gould, W. M., and Gragg, T. M.: Delusions of parasitosis—an approach to the problem, Arch. Dermatol. **112:**1745, 1976.

**This appears to be a practical approach at least and may bear fruit.**

Ireland, P., Sapira, J. D., and Templeton, P.: Münchausen's syndrome, Am. J. Med. **43:**579, 1967.

**A form of self-mutilation that is seen chiefly by surgeons.**

Muller, S. A., and Winkelmann, R. K.: Trichotillomania: a clinico-pathologic study of 24 cases, Arch. Dermatol. **105:**535, 1972.

**A complete, instructive publication.**

Shelley, W. B.: Factitial scars. In Consultations in dermatology, Philadelphia, 1972, W. B. Saunders Co., p. 128.

**The diagnosis and management of self-inflicted injury.**

Whitlock, F. A.: Psychophysiological aspects of skin disease, Philadelphia, 1977, W. B. Saunders Co., p. 90.

**An interesting "lumping" of these four disorders, and addition of others.**

## CHAPTER 30

# Purpuras

Purpuric lesions are caused by escape of blood from a vessel into surrounding tissue. They are classed as petechiae, ecchymoses, or hematomas, in order of increasing size. They may be produced by defects of vessel wall and supporting tissue or intravascular alterations that result in blocking of blood flow and red blood cell extravasation. Most purpura-producing disorders are of such a complex nature that more than one mechanism is at fault in the production of the purpura. We include here only those forms of pupura that seem to have particular dermatological significance. Dermatologists tend to see small-lesion purpura most frequently, and this group is more likely to result from vessel wall damage or deficit, most often a vasculitis. Hematological abnormalities tend to produce large extravasations, ecchymoses, or hematomas.

Small purpuric lesions are bright red on first appearance, becoming browner with increasing age. Larger lesions are blue to black on first appearance and change through colors of green, yellow, and brown before fading (Plate 47).

## CAPILLARY WALL PURPURAS

### Vascular purpura

Purpuric lesions may arise in *normal* individuals after skin suction, quick sharp blows, anoxia, pronounced capillary dilatation, or violent muscle contraction, as in an epileptic seizure. Some women develop mild purpura at the time of the menstrual period. Ryan has noted that increased capillary fragility and permeability have been recorded in women in the fourth week of the menstrual cycle, related to progesterone levels.

### Autoerythrocyte sensitization syndrome

This is a syndrome reported by Gardner and Diamond in 1955, since which time some 50 patients have been reported with painful ecchymoses that occur on legs and thighs first and then thorax, after trauma. There has been confirmed positive skin test reactivity to their own red blood cells. They have been almost all female. There have been measurements of increased fibrinolysis during active new lesion formation. It is not a clear-cut entity but is strongly associated with emotional, neurotic, or hysterical qualities. Stigmas are compared by Whitlock. DNA autosensitivity also demonstrates tender ecchymoses. It responds to antimalarial therapy. Stocker describes two cases of psychogenic or self-inflicted purpura that may be confused.

### Orthostatic purpura

Orthostatic purpura consists of petechial to ecchymotic lesions, chiefly affecting the legs in elderly individuals after long periods of standing. There may be little evidence of venous incompetence. Tests of capillary fragility and blood clotting are normal. Brown hemosiderin pigmentation occurs slowly. Similar-appearing lesions occur in patients receiving glucocorticoid treatment and in those with Cushing's disease.

#### *Treatment*

Support of the subcutaneous tissues with elastic bandages or their equivalent is satisfactory. If venous varicosities are present, their removal will be beneficial.

### Senile purpura

Large blue-black hematomas occur without remembered cause on the dorsa of the hands, wrists, and forearms. The lesions are asymptomatic and without abnormality of the clotting mechanism. Capillary fragility may or may not be increased. The connective tissue appears to have lost some of its supporting

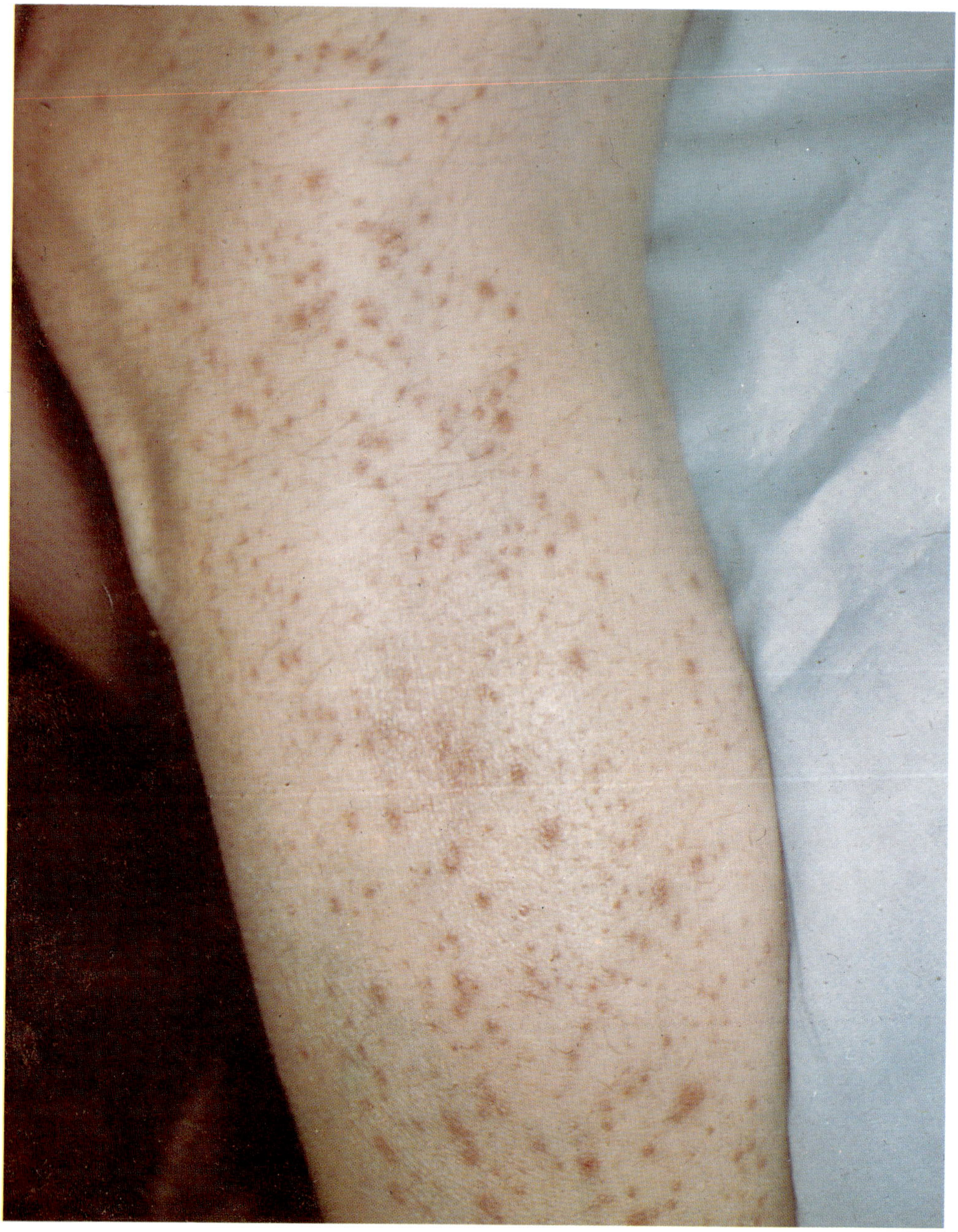

**Plate 47**

Purpura. The lesions do not blanch on pressure.

power. The disorder occurs in elderly or debilitated individuals.

***Treatment***

There is no effective treatment.

## Pigmented purpuric dermatoses (Schamberg's disease, Majocchi's purpura, pigmented purpuric disorder of Gougerot and Blum)

Pigmented purpuric dermatoses are a group of rare diseases characterized by a slightly pruritic or asymptomatic purpura of capillary origin occurring on the legs, perhaps extending to hips and forearms (Fig. 30-1).

Capillaritis is the common finding in all groups and is manifested by lymphocytes and occasional polymorphonuclear leukocytes.

The lesions are grouped, petechial, and sometimes papular, in various stages of color change from bright red to tan brown. They form annular and irregular patterns. The course tends to be chronic, with an intermittent appearance of new lesions. Capillary fragility may be increased. Clotting mechanisms are normal.

One should note here the frequent appearance of purpura in dependent areas, usually legs, of older persons, debilitated patients, and some normally ambulatory individuals, in

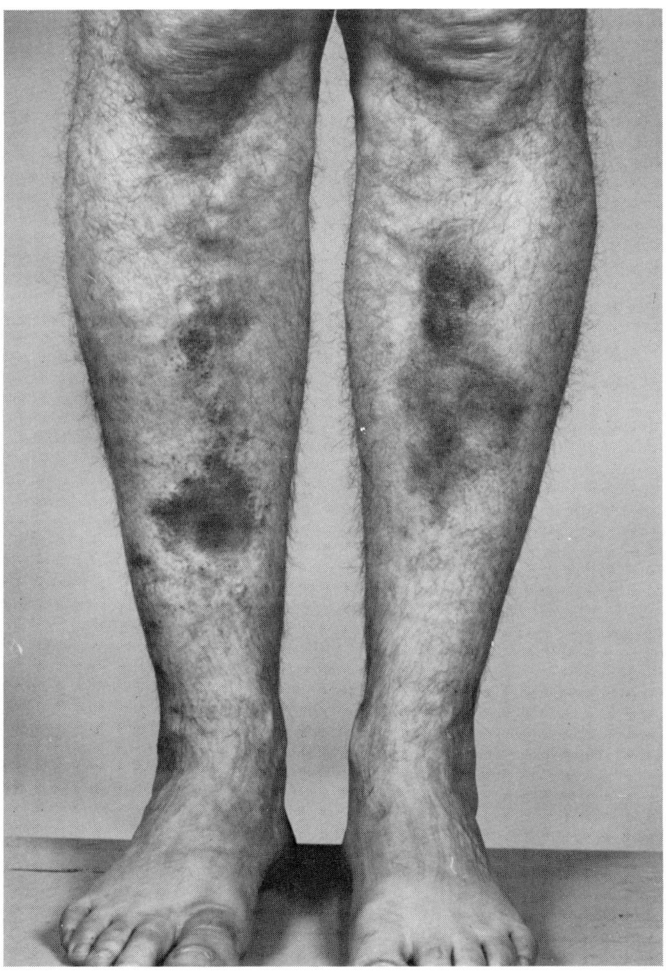

**Fig. 30-1.** Pigmented purpuric dermatosis. Coagulation mechanisms are normal.

association with inflammatory skin disorders.

### *Differential diagnosis*

Pigmented purpuric dermatoses must be distinguished from eruptions caused by drugs, specifically carbromal, but also meprobamate, sulfonamides, or barbiturates.

Other conditions that should be differentiated from pigmented purpuric dermatoses include hyperglobulinemic purpura, orthostatic purpura, and stasis dermatitis, as well as purpura caused by vasculitis of larger vessels (p. 576).

### *Treatment*

There is no effective treatment.

## Other causes of purpura attributable to capillary wall damage (nonthrombocytopenic purpura)

Drugs of many sorts cause toxic purpura in a relatively small number of patients. Drugs noted are penicillin, sulfonamides, salicylates, barbiturates, meprobamate, iodides, and quinine. Carbromal is a classic example that leaves a diagnostic clinical pattern; with other drugs, we are not so fortunate.

Infections such as meningococcemia, subacute bacterial endocarditis, viral diseases, and particularly rickettsial diseases can produce purpura.

Purpura is one of the clinical manifestations of amyloidosis, Cushing's disease, fat emboli, autoerythrocyte sensitization, and scurvy (Fig. 30-2).

Ehlers-Danlos syndrome, which includes increased cutaneous fragility, hyperelasticity of the joints and skin, and occasionally a dissecting aortic aneurysm, will produce a tendency to epistaxis, gingival bleeding, and cutaneous ecchymosis.

Hypertension, atherosclerosis, diabetes mellitus, uremia, hemochromatosis, and carcinomatosis may be associated with cutaneous purpuric eruptions.

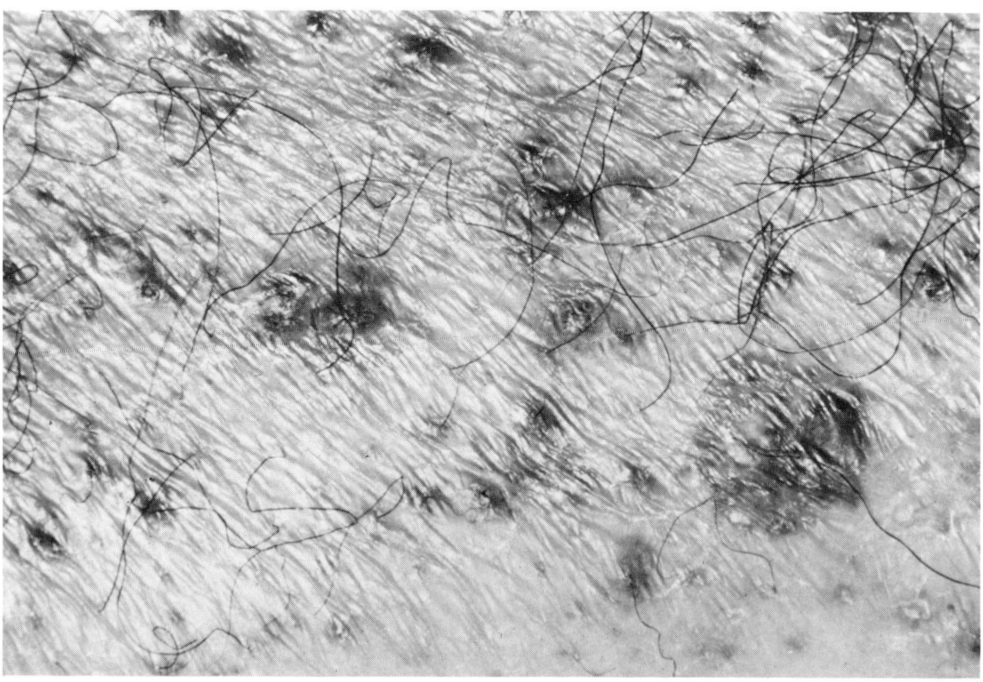

**Fig. 30-2.** Scurvy. Characteristic perifollicular distribution.

## INTRAVASCULAR PURPURAS

### Plasma coagulation defects

Hemophilia, Christmas disease, deficiency of various clotting factors, intravascular coagulation syndromes, increased fibrinolytic activity, and vitamin K deficiencies are beyond the scope of this book. These disorders generally produce more serious results of bleeding than simple purpura, although purpuric lesions may be a minor part of the clinical picture. Bleeding is ordinarily into orifices, after trauma, and is of the chronic oozing variety.

Michaelsson has reported that purpura resulted after oral provocation with azo food dyes (yellow), benzoates, and salicylates. A regimen free of these offending agents is recommended for these patients with recurring allergic vascular purpura. A diet free of natural and synthetic salicylates has been very helpful in attaining this. We have seen such patients with leg purpura cleared on this diet (Noid).

### Disseminated intravascular coagulation defect (DIC)

DIC (consumption coagulopathy) is caused by rapid intravascular coagulation leading to massive fibrin deposition. Coagulation factors are used more quickly than they can be replaced, and the blood ceases to coagulate. It occurs in a variety of life-threatening infections, complications of pregnancy, hematologic disorders, malignancy, hepatitis, postsurgery, and the like.

Cutaneous signs may be the first and often thus the most important warning manifestation. Of 36 cases described by Robboy and others, the lesions seen included petechiae, purpura, palpable purpura, hemorrhagic bullae, and acral cyanosis. In 47% of the DIC episodes, cutaneous lesions caused the patient to seek medical advice.

Fibrin thrombi were prominent in small skin vessels.

### Idiopathic thrombocytopenic purpura

With idiopathic thrombocytopenic purpura, there is a loss of platelets, because of autoimmune immunological mechanisms, and also abnormality of platelet function.

Thrombocytopenia produces purpura because of the capillary fragility associated with loss of platelets and also because of the prolonged bleeding time. The flat purpuric lesions tend to occur on the legs, arms, and buttocks. Bleeding from mucous membranes is frequent, and hematuria and profuse menses are characteristic. The disorder may be acute or chronic.

***Acute idiopathic thrombocytopenic purpura.*** Acute idiopathic thrombocytopenic purpura occurs suddenly, frequently after an upper respiratory tract infection. It is seen in children and young adults and ordinarily is self-limited, clearing within 2 months.

***Chronic idiopathic thrombocytopenic purpura.*** The chronic form occurs with a gradual onset dating back over months to years. It has a course characterized by exacerbations and remissions, although the platelet count rarely rises to normal levels. It occurs most commonly in adult females. The symptoms include purpuric lesions, hypermenorrhea, and bleeding from body orifices.

#### *Treatment*

Treatment of both acute and chronic forms of idiopathic thrombocytopenic purpura includes glucocorticoid therapy, judiciously used. Splenectomy may be necessary in treatment of the chronic form.

## DRUG-INDUCED THROMBOCYTOPENIA

Some drugs such as apronalide (Sedormid) and quinidine produce a fall in circulating platelets by allergic mechanisms; but others, such as methotrexate, nitrogen mustard, and hydroxyurea, as a result of pharmacological action. Most drugs exert their thrombocytopenic action on only certain individuals, through mechanisms that are yet unclear. Chlorothiazide, gold, barbiturates, aminopyrine, quinine, quinidine, acetazolamide, digitoxin, sulfonamides, antihistamines and paraaminosalicylic acid are some of these; hair dyes, estrogens, arsenicals, bismuth, oxytetracycline, and X rays are others.

Bacterial and viral infections, bone marrow infiltration, large hemangiomas, and splenomegaly also cause loss of platelets.

### Thrombotic thrombocytopenic purpura

A usually fatal form of rare vascular disease, thrombotic thrombocytopenic purpura includes fever, acute thrombocytopenic purpura, acute hemolytic anemia, bizarre neurological manifestations, petechiae, subcutaneous dissecting hematomas, acral cyanosis, hemorrhagic bullae, and renal abnormalities. It is significant dermatologically in that cutaneous punch biopsy can establish the diagnosis by demonstrating subendothelial fibrin deposition and hyaline thrombi of small arterioles. There is a normal coagulation profile. It has been described with systemic lupus erythematosus.

### Hypersplenism

Involvement of the spleen by infiltrates as in Gaucher's disease, Hodgkins's disease, leukemias, and lymphomas may produce thrombocytopenia and purpura. Portal hypertension, sarcoidosis, and lupus erythematosus may be similarly causative.

### Amegakaryocytic thrombocytopenia

The large category of causes of purpura known as amegakaryocytic thrombocytopenia includes chiefly agents and conditions harmful to the bone marrow. There are, however, congenital disorders and idiopathic aplastic anemias as well.

Displacement of bone marrow by leukemic cells and damage to the bone marrow by drugs and toxic agents produce the majority of these disorders. Toxic agents include ionizing radiation, cytotoxic drugs, organic solvents, arsenicals, insecticides, analeptic drugs, antithyroid drugs, chloramphenicol, barbiturates, phenothiazines, meprobamate, and many others.

## PLASMA PROTEIN ABNORMALITIES

### Collagen disorders

Purpura, as well as dysproteinemia, is a not uncommon finding in lupus erythematosus, polyarteritis nodosa, dermatomyositis, and scleroderma.

### Hypergammaglobulinemic purpura

A rare, benign, chronic disorder, hypergammaglobulinemic purpura is identified by the appearance of small, episodic, purpuric lesions over the ankles, legs, and thighs. It may be associated with joint pain and ankle edema. There is a vasculitis of the affected areas and an increase in serum gamma globulin. It occurs chiefly in women. It is a polyclonal gammopathy that may go on for 20 years or more. IgG is elevated.

### Macroglobulinemia

Waldenström's macroglobulinemia is associated with an abnormal amount of plasma proteins of very high molecular weight. There are complex clotting and bleeding disorders, as well as widespread purpuric lesions and pronounced oozing from mucous membranes. Elevated IgM and plasma cell dyscrasias are a part of this disorder. Most cases end in malignant disease.

### Multiple myeloma

Bleeding from orifices, gingival bleeding, epistaxis, and multiple purpuric cutaneous lesions are frequently seen in myeloma. Poorly defined coagulation abnormalities are also present. There is a unique monoclonal gammopathy, IgG or IgA. Diagnosis is made by bone marrow biopsy.

### Systemic amyloidosis (Fig. 6-12)

Ecchymoses and purpura of eyelids, tongue, and face are seen in systemic amyloidosis. Biopsy and immunofluorescent study of the purpuric lesion is diagnostic. Again most of these cases are now recognized to be early stages of plasma cell dyscrasia or multiple myeloma. Carpal tunnel syndrome is very common.

### Cryopathies

***Cryoglobulinemia.*** Cryoglobulins are proteins that will, on exposure to cold, precipitate and produce obstruction of small blood vessels with resultant purpuric lesions of distal aspects of extremities. They are often present in association with systemic lupus erythematosus, myeloma, Hodgkin's disease, and other systemic diseases. Some cryoglobulins are much more difficult to demonstrate (mixed type) than others (single factor).

***Cryofibrinogenemia.*** A gelatinous flocculent precipitate forms on being chilled to 4° C. This may be present in normal individuals but in limited amounts only. Larger amounts may be secondary to carcinomas, leukemia, and acute rheumatic fever. Clotting may be seen simultaneously with bleeding.

***Cold agglutinins.*** Purpura, necrosis, and gangrene of acral areas with cold sensitivity can be produced by cold agglutinins as a result of viral infections or lymphomas.

### *Investigation*

Investigation of purpura should include a thorough assessment of the patient for evidence of hepatosplenomegaly, bruising, bleeding, telangiectasia, capillary fragility, splinter hemorrhage, internal bleeding, melena, hemarthroses, or recent ill health. A thorough history of drug ingestion and precise identification of the drug are essential.

INITIAL

Blood tests including platelet count, hemoglobin, white blood cell count, differential, serum protein, and electrophoresis; platelet morphology; and bleeding time, coagulation time, clot retraction, prothrombin time

SECONDARY

Tests for partial thromboplastin time, thromboplastin generation, and fibrinolytic activity; tests for circulating anticoagulants

Recent tests for platelet function are complex and sophisticated. Tests of abnormal blood coagulation are equally complex and should be done in hematological centers.

**REFERENCES**

Gardner, F. H., and Diamond, L. K.: Autoerythrocyte sensitization: form of purpura producing painful bruising following autosensitization to red blood cells in certain women, Blood **10**:675, 1955.

**Four patients, all women, with painful bleeding into joints and organs.**

Michaëlsson, G., Pettersson, L., and Juhlin, L.: Purpura caused by food and drug additives, Arch. Dermatol. **109**:49, 1974.

**Azo food dyes, benzoates, and salicylates were responsible.**

Noid, H. E., Schulze, T. W., and Winkelmann, R. K.: Diet plan for patients with salicylate-induced urticaria, Arch. Dermatol. **109**:866, 1974.

**Also works for purpura, which is only one step more pathologically speaking.**

Robboy, S. J., Mihm, M. D., Colman, R. W., and Minna, J. D.: The skin in disseminated intravascular coagulation, Br. J. Dermatol. **88**:221, 1973.

**The cutaneous manifestations of 33 of 45 patients.**

Robboy, S. J., Minna, J. D., and Colman, R. W.: Disseminated intravascular coagulation (DIC). In Maddin, S., editor: Current dermatologic management, St. Louis, 1975, The C. V. Mosby Co., p. 134.

**Unique advice.**

Rowell, N. R.: A painful bleeding syndrome associated with increased fibrinolytic activity, Br. J. Dermatol. **91**:591, 1974.

**Spontaneous fluctuating increased fibrinolytic activity resulting in bleeding.**

Ryan, T. J.: The nerves and blood vessels. In Jarrett, A., editor: Physiology and pathophysiology of the skin, vol. 2, New York, 1973, Academic Press, Inc.

**A scholarly, imaginative sound review of these structures, their function, and selected examples of altered physiological patterns.**

Stocker, W. W.: Psychogenic purpura, Arch. Dermatol. **113**:606, 1977.

**Self-inflicted.**

Whitlock, F. A.: The autoerythrocyte sensitization syndrome: psychogenic purpura. In Psychophysiological aspects of skin disease, Philadelphia, 1976, W. B. Saunders Co., p. 100.

**Conclusion: further hematologic and psychologic investigation is necessary to explain it.**

## CHAPTER 31

# Sarcoidosis

Sarcoidosis is a granulomatous disease of unknown etiology that chiefly involves the reticuloendothelial system and can affect virtually all organs.

### *Natural course*

It may follow one of three courses: (1) resolve and disappear during the first benign stage, (2) disseminate and show multiple organ invasion during the second stage, or (3) go into the progressive stage, leading to irreversible changes and death. *The benign, completely reversible course is the most common.* Death rarely occurs from the disease. Females are more frequently affected than males. Adult North American blacks are 12 to 15 times more susceptible than are whites and have a poorer prognosis. The disease tends to be mutilating and severe in the Bantus in Africa and has curious racial and geographical variations.

An attack of *erythema nodosum* may usher in the disease, particularly in women. It is associated with bilateral hilar lymphadenopathy.

The lymph nodes are involved in most cases of sarcoidosis. A generalized, nontender lymphadenopathy is present. Bones and bone marrow are involved, with a diffuse rarefaction or circumscribed radiolucent areas apparent in the phalanges.

The lungs are most severely affected as a rule, and the radiological appearance may be out of proportion to the clinical severity. Thus an apparent extensive involvement may be accompanied by minimal symptoms. However, sarcoidosis can produce a severe, progressive, fibrosing pulmonary disease in its later stages. The increased mortality resulting from sarcoidosis is primarily attributable to pulmonary involvement.

Ocular lesions are progressive, unyielding to therapy, and present in one fourth of the cases of sarcoidosis. The eye involvement chiefly affects the lids, conjunctivae, cornea, uveal tract, and tearing apparatus. The fundus is infrequently affected. The central nervous system shows abnormalities in 5% to 15% of cases.

*Cutaneous lesions* other than erythema nodosum occur in approximately 30% of sarcoidosis cases and are generally elevated, soft and tan to purple and have raised or prominent borders. There is no characteristic distribution. They can be divided into those that appear early in the disease and those that tend to appear late. There is a predilection to lesions on the face.

Facial papular lesions may be minute and skin colored, requiring an acute observer to identify them (Fig. 31-1). Some sarcoid lesions, particularly those on the scalp, may show a distinct atrophy.

Hypopigmented lesions, described by Cornelius, are very likely to demonstrate sarcoid tubercles in these patients and should be selected for biopsy whenever possible. The reason for the decreased pigmentation is degenerative change in the melanocytes.

EARLY

- Erythema nodosum
- Papular lesions affecting the extremities and the face
- Scar sarcoid, bluish elevated lesions that occur on old scars

LATE

- Larger nodular lesions that affect the face, trunk, and legs
- Plaques that occur on the torso; lesions that appear on the forehead tend to be annular and ringed (Plate 48); persistent plaques may be associated with

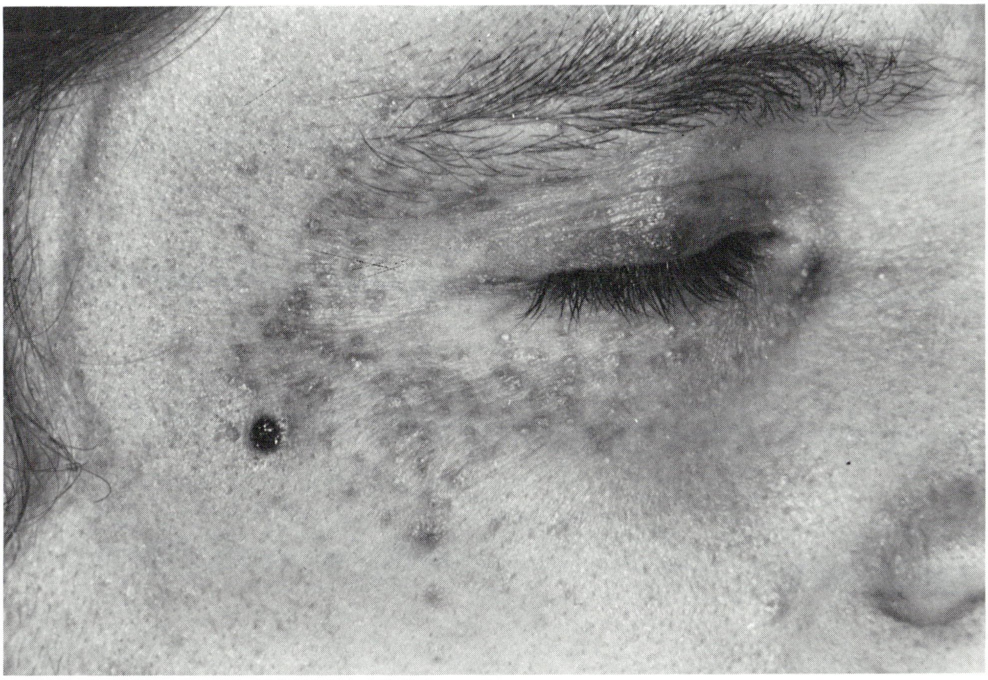

**Fig. 31-1.** Sarcoidosis. Minute discrete papular lesions.

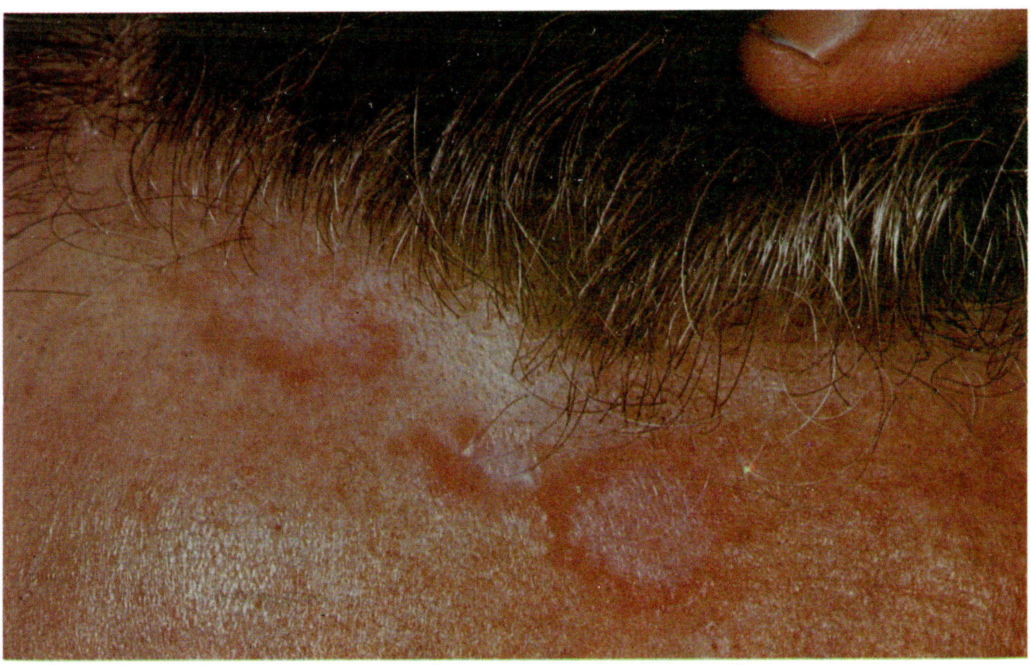

**Plate 48**

Sarcoidosis. Annular lesions with central atrophy and, significantly, depigmentation. Biopsy of depigmented lesion may provide best source for diagnosis.

pulmonary fibrosis in more than 50% of cases

There is a strong histopathological similarity to the palisading form of necrobiosis and to granuloma annulare. Very considerable overlap is present in the microscopic appearance of these diseases to the degree that one must defend their separation.

Anemia, elevated serum calcium, hypercalcemia, and increased gamma globulins are present. Most patients with sarcoidosis have functional hypoparathyroidism, on the basis of a study of 26 patients by Cushard and associates.

### *Microscopic findings*

There is a granulomatous response in which the dermis is the site of multiple tubercles made up of nodules of epithelioid cells, with few lymphocytes. There is little inflammatory reaction, no necrosis, and no sign of tuberculous caseation. The tubercles resolve slowly, if at all, and result in a fibrotic scar.

Lesions of the lungs, lymph nodes, spleen, bones, tonsils, and so forth, show an infiltration by the above epithelioid granulomas. Giant cells are present, some of which possess irregular inclusions.

### *Pertinent information*

Sarcoidosis appears to be a disease causing, or more likely a result of, a diminution of the effectiveness of the cell-mediated immune-response mechanism. Patients demonstrate an inability to develop and maintain delayed hypersensitivity. The defect in cell-mediated immunity is demonstrable by a hypo-reactivity to challenge with all topical antigens. There is decreased lymphocyte transformation to some antigens. Chemotaxis of polymorphonuclear leukocytes is impaired.

Quismorio identified IgM deposits at the dermoepidermal junction in two patients and within blood vessel walls in five patients out of a series of eight patients with active sarcoidosis. They also demonstrated IgE, IgA, and fibrin deposits in some of the lesions. Kveim test granulomas reflected similar changes to the naturally occurring lesions. It will be very important to study new lesions of sarcoidosis to assess the Ig deposits seen in recently formed granulomas and vasculitis.

The granuloma is made up of central epithelioid cells with $C_3$ and IgG(Fc) receptors. B cells are present at the periphery of the lesion. Warren suggests from his studies on chronic schistosomiasis that a modulation of cellular response to a chronic antigenic stimulus may be the basis of the sarcoid granuloma. He presents a dynamic concept of granuloma formation generally.

*It is yet undecided whether the immunological defect is constitutional or acquired because of a prior infection.*

There seems to be a considerable variation in incidence of the disease among countries. There are said to be many more undetected than known cases in North America. This has been indicated in other countries by mass radiography and other studies.

There is an as yet obscure relationship with tuberculosis. This is shown by the distinctive weak or negative reactions to tuberculin and related antigens, and in the eventual progress of the disease some patients die with tuberculosis. A rapid disappearance of sarcoid lesions may be the first sign of the onset of tuberculosis.

***Kveim test.*** Although it is diagnostic for sarcoidosis, the Kveim test must be carefully performed to extract its full significance. It is positive in over 70% of proved cases. It rarely gives false-positive results, except perhaps in recent Crohn's disease.

Heat-sterilized suspension of sarcoid tissue from human lymph nodes is injected intracutaneously into a test site. Six weeks later the site is biopsied. The presence of an epithelioid granuloma is diagnostic of sarcoidosis. The test may be negative during a clinical remission, and the tissue used for testing loses its specificity as it ages. Consequently, fresh material must be used.

### *Differential diagnosis*

Other granulomatous diseases, such as syphilis, tuberculosis, leprosy, and erythema induratum, may produce cutaneous lesions that must be differentiated from sarcoidosis. This can ordinarily be done by biopsy.

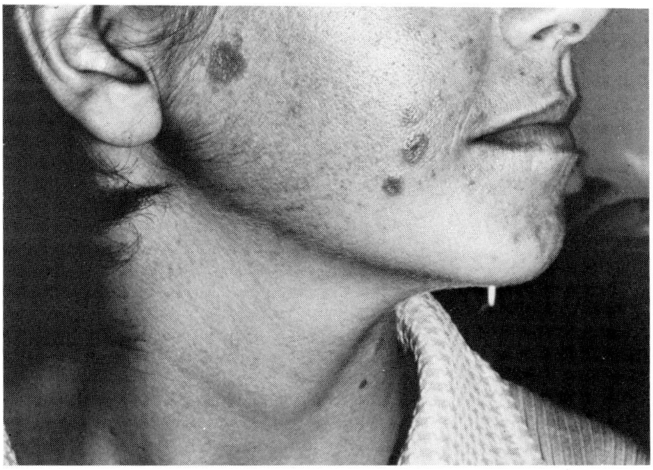

**Fig. 31-2.** Sarcoidosis. Facial, brown-red plaques.

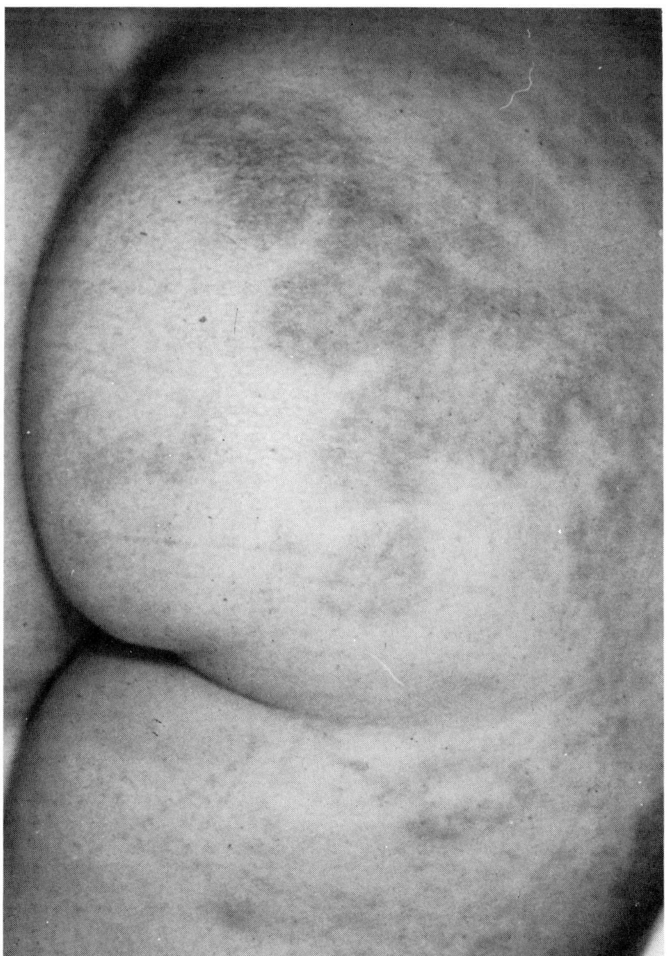

**Fig. 31-3.** Sarcoidosis. Nodular and gyrate lesions of buttocks.

Sarcoidosis lesions of the face may be confused with lupus erythematosus, syphilis, rosacea, granuloma faciale, leprosy, and polymorphous light eruption (Fig. 31-2).

Sarcoidosis lesions of the torso and extremities may be confused with lymphoma, granuloma annulare, xanthomas, necrobiosis, erythema multiforme, and syphilis (Fig. 31-3).

### *Investigation*

Cutaneous lesions are a part of the whole body involvement and serve as invitations for investigation of the total process. The following should be considered in the initial investigation:

- Physical examination, including evaluation of peripheral lymph nodes, liver and spleen, slit-lamp and ophthalmological survey, and peripheral neurological examination
- Skin biopsy (less reliable than lymph node biopsy)—if a hypopigmented lesion is available, it should be biopsied
- Chest x-ray examination for hilar adenopathy or pulmonary mottling
- X-ray examination of hands for translucent areas in phalanges, which are present in more than one half of chronic cases
- Blood studies of serum proteins for hypergammaglobulinemia
- Tests of serum and urine calcium level (elevated in less than one third of cases)
- Kveim test (fresh antigen)

### *Treatment*

Glucocorticoids seem to limit spread and progression. In more extensive cases their effect seems to be palliative only. Methotrexate and chlorambucil have been shown to be effective under some circumstances. *In sarcoidosis, treatment should be guided by one thoroughly familiar with the course and complications of the disease.*

Cutaneous sarcoidosis is often helped by local intracutaneous steriod injections, but the total course of the disease may not be altered. Individual lesions should be treated only after the stage and extent of the disease have been established.

Chloroquin orally is suggested for temporary courses in selected cases.

#### REFERENCES

Cornelius, C. E., III, Stein, K. M., Hanshaw, W. J., et al.: Hypopigmentation and sarcoidosis, Arch. Dermatol. **108**:249, 1973.
**Emphasizes the association of sarcoidosis and hypopigmentation.**

Clayton, R., Breathnach, A., Martin, B., et al.: Hypopigmented sarcoidosis in the Negro, Br. J. Dermatol. **96**:119, 1977.
**Presence of degenerated melanocytes is the reason.**

Cushard, W. G., Simon, A. B., Canterbury, J. M., et al.: Parathyroid function in sarcoidosis, N. Engl. J. Med. **286**:395, 1972.
**Calcium abnormalities elucidated.**

James, D. G.: Kveim revisited, reassessed: Editorial, N. Engl. J. Med. **292**:859, 1975.
**Positive in 968 of 1,211 patients with sarcoid with inconsequential false reactions.**

The Kveim controversy: Editorial, Lancet **2**:750, 1971.
**Doubts about the test's specificity arose.**

Kveim-Siltzbach test vindicated: Editorial, Lancet **1**:188, 1972.
**Two lots of antigen shown to be defective.**

Mitchell, D. N., Scadding, J. G., and Heard, B. E.: Sarcoidosis: histopathological definition and clinical diagnosis, J. Clin. Pathol. **30**:395, 1977.
**A good article on diagnosis.**

Quismorio, F. P., Sharma, O. P., and Chandor, S.: Immunopathological studies on the cutaneous lesions in sarcoidosis, Br. J. Dermatol. **97**:635, 1977.
**Humoral antibodies may be important in the natural course of sarcoid granulomas.**

Shelley, W. B.: On the pathogenesis of sarcoidosis, South. Med. J. **64**:988, 1971.
**A perceptive description.**

Siltzbach, L. E., editor: Seventh International Conference on Sarcoidosis and other Granulomatous Disorders, Ann. N.Y. Acad. Sci., vol. 278, 1976.
**Immunology, epidemiology, and clinical information, as well as current treatment with 15-year assessment of glucocorticoids in 250 patients. The Kveim test and other controversial matters are scrutinized.**

Siltzbach, L. E., James, D. G., Neville, E., et al.: The course and prognosis of sarcoidosis around the world, Am. J. Med. **57**:847, 1974.
**A masterful perspective.**

Tannenbaum, H., Anderson, L. G., and Rosenberg, E. H.: Diagnosis of sarcoidosis by lip biopsy of minor salivary glands, Can. Med. Assoc. J. **111**:1323, 1974.
**Diagnosis made in patients with parotid involvement by lower lip biopsy, an easy procedure.**

Umbert, P., and Winkelmann, R. K.: Granuloma annulare and sarcoidosis, Br. J. Dermatol. **97**:481,1977.
**Co-existence.**

Veien, N. K., and Brodthagen, H.: Cutaneous sarcoidosis

treated with methotrexate, Br. J. Dermatol. **97**:213, 1977.
**Skin: 12 patients of 16 cleared. Uveitis 3 of 4 cleared. No hilar changes.**

Warren, K. S.: A functional classification of granulomatous inflammation, Ann. N.Y. Acad. Sci. **278**:7, 1976.
**A dynamic concept of granulomatous inflammation.**

CHAPTER **32**

# Seborrheic dermatitis

Seborrheic dermatitis is an identification for a somewhat ill-defined, but common, chronic, recurrent, inflammatory disorder with a predilection for hair-bearing areas and facial furrows. It is of unknown etiology.

### *Natural course*

The earliest manifestation of seborrheic dermatitis is not uncommonly seen in the neonatal period as cradle cap. Here it consists of a mildly inflammatory, adherent, greasy scaling of the hair-bearing portion of the scalp.

It may also be seen in infancy as an erythematous, scaling dermatitis with poorly demarcated borders (Plate 49). It characteristically affects the scalp and diaper areas. The inflammation may spread by the appearance of new areas that become confluent with preexisting ones (Figs. 32-1 and 32-2). It is frequently pruritic.

After puberty the disease differs somewhat, particularly in the sites of predilection. The areas of most frequent involvement are the scalp, central face, external ear, postauricular region, midsternum and upper midback, and

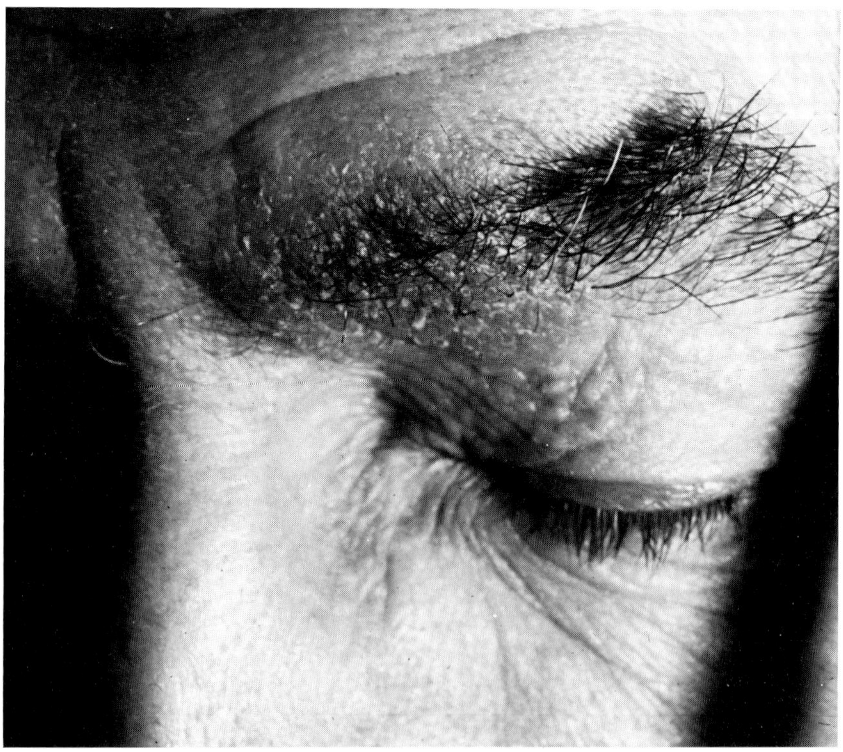

**Fig. 32-1.** Seborrheic dermatitis of eyebrow, a common site.

umbilicus and genitalia, including the hair-bearing mons pubis. In spreading, acute, or severe cases, intertriginous areas and, indeed, most of the skin surface may become affected.

Seborrheic dermatitis is a cutaneous disease of remarkable variation and exists very commonly and simply as an intermittent, mildly reddened case of scaling itchy dandruff. Few people have not had some experience with this form. It may also show evidences of secondary infection, with follicular crusts in the scalp. The hairline and adjacent hairless skin may be reddened and scaling.

A second area of common infection is the external ear, specifically the external auditory

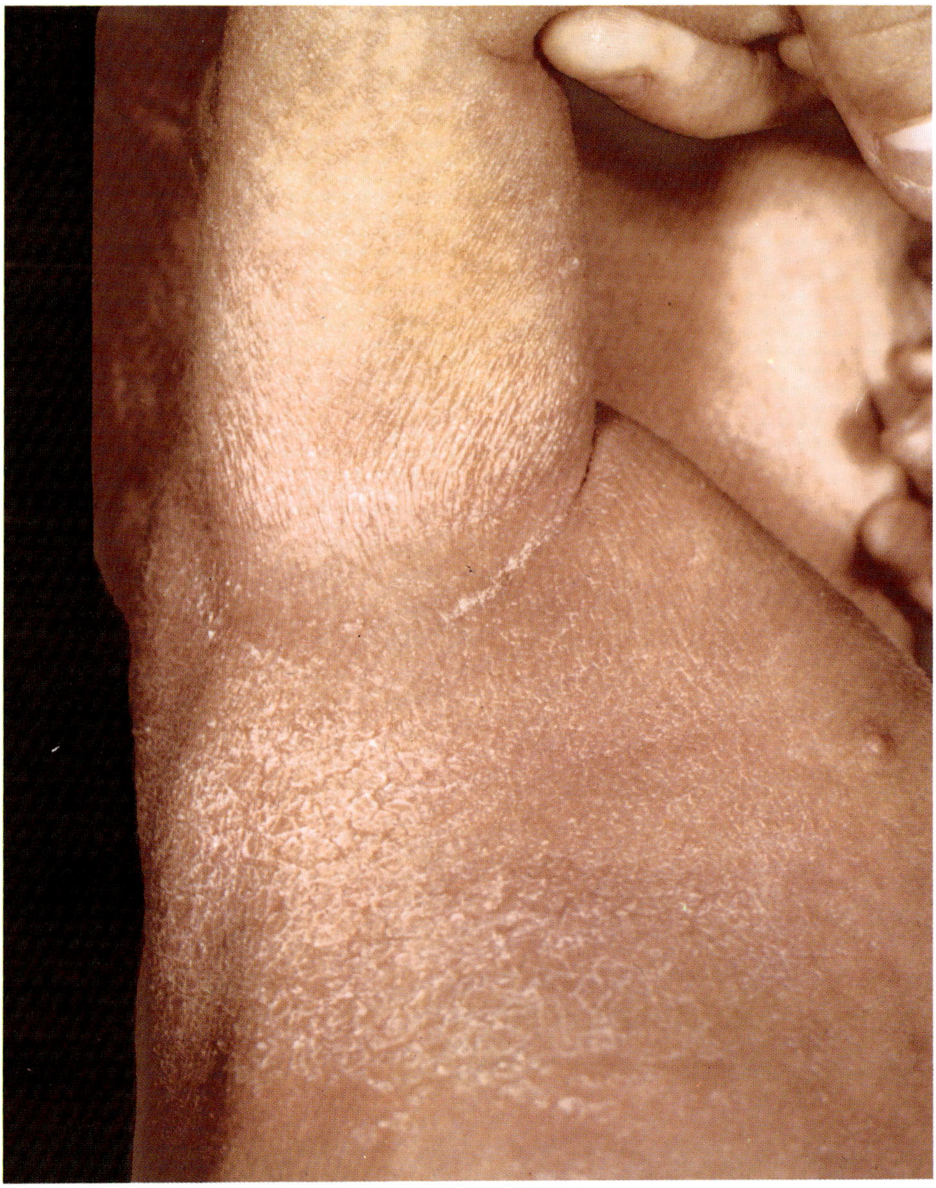

**Plate 49**

Seborrheic dermatitis in an infant.

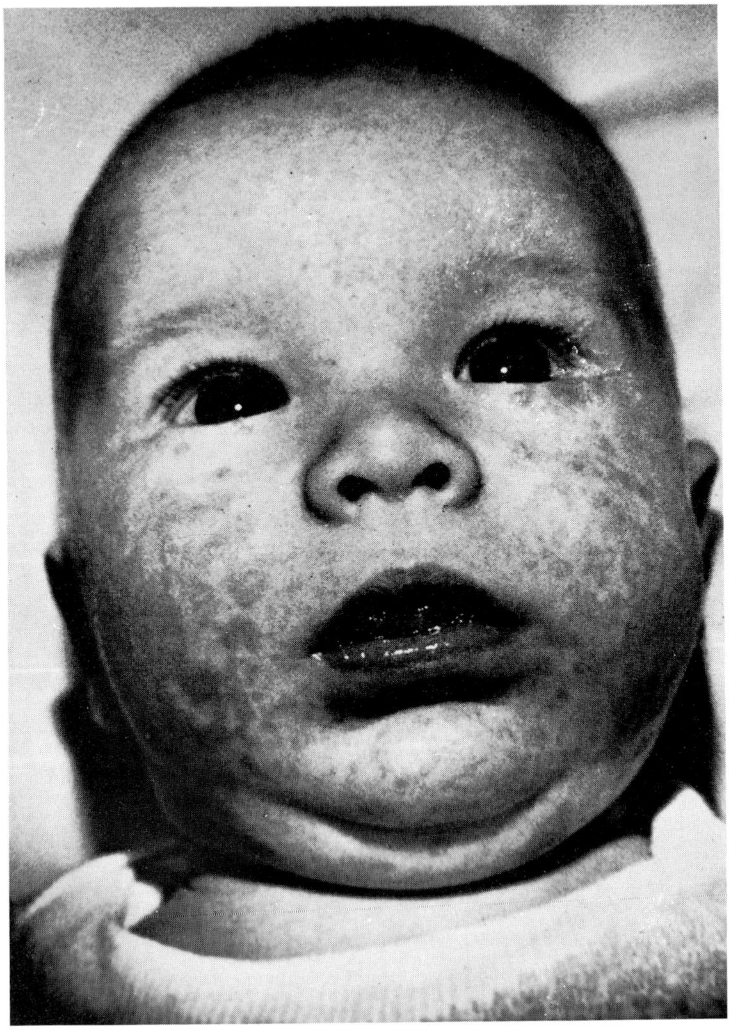

**Fig. 32-2.** Seborrheic dermatitis in infancy.

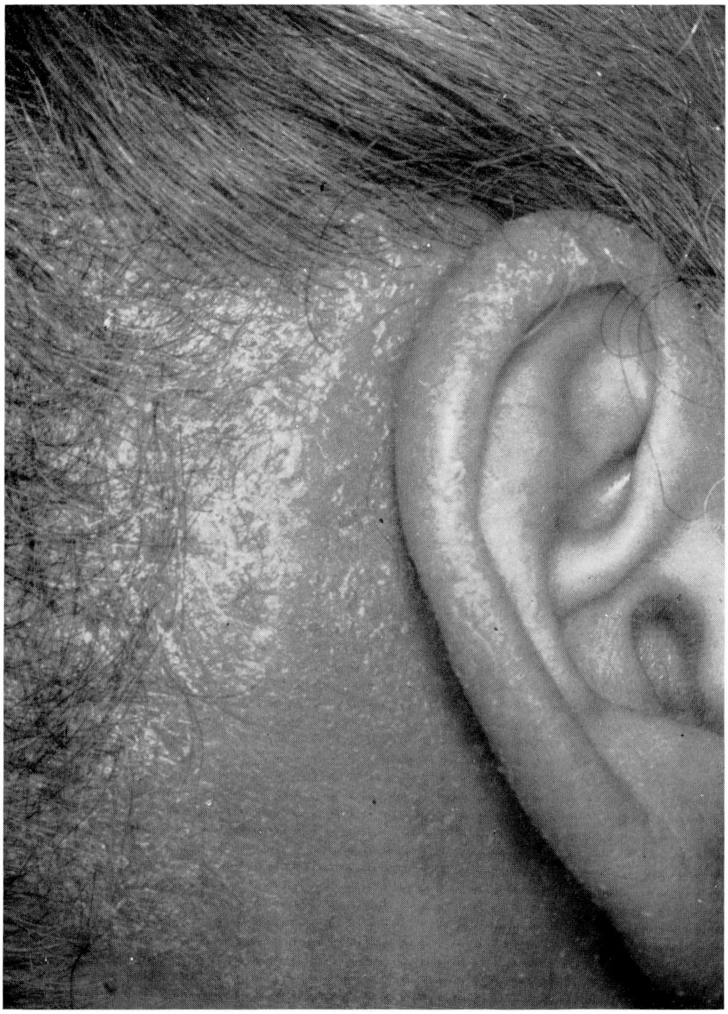

**Fig. 32-3.** Seborrheic dermatitis of postauricular area.

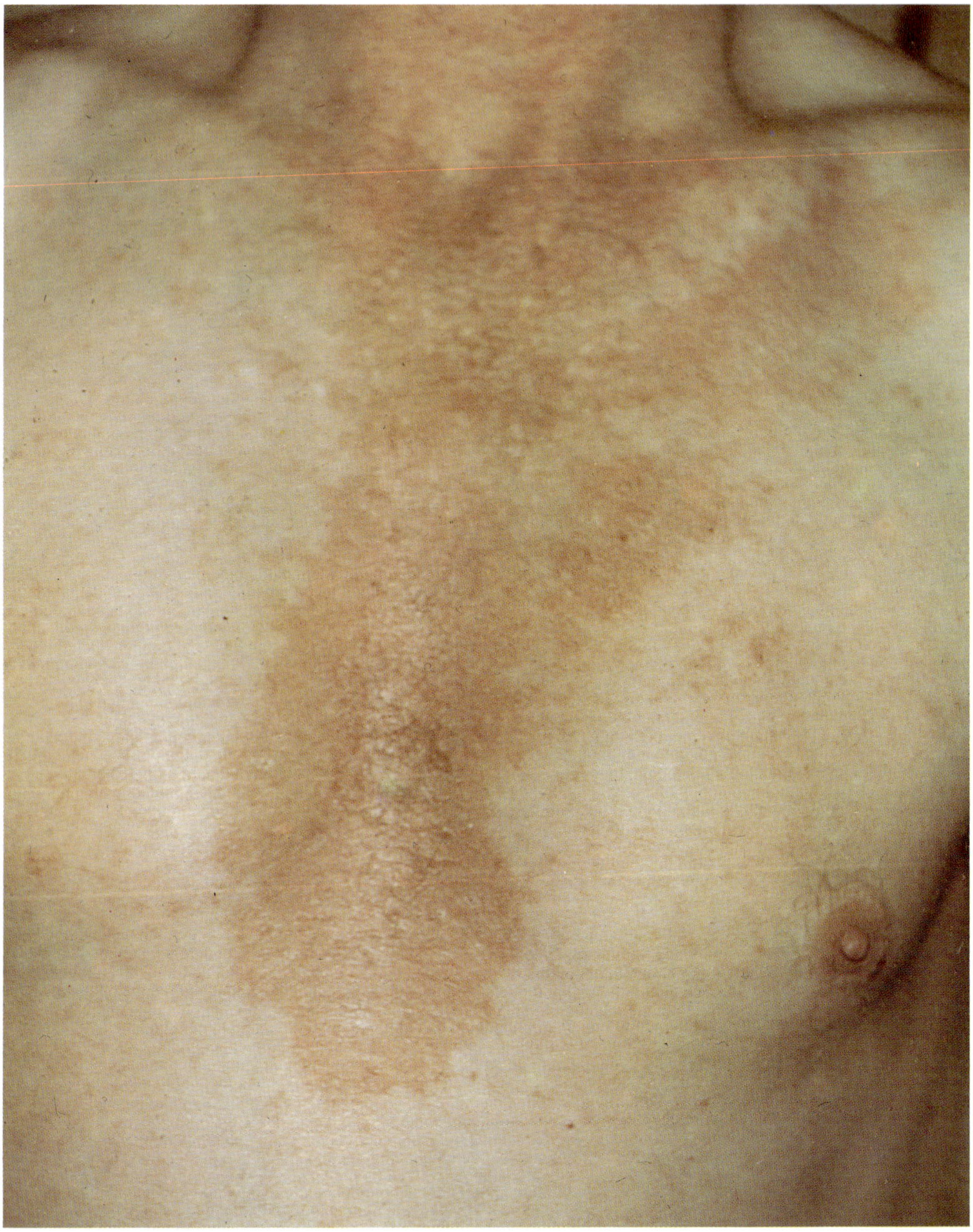

**Plate 50**

Seborrheic dermatitis.

canal and the postauricular area (Fig. 32-3). Here, again, the disease exists as an annoying persistent scaling, with episodes of crusting, weeping, and apparent secondary infection. Patchy scaling dandruff is usually associated.

Blepharitis, with a characteristic erythema and swelling of the free edge of the eyelids and an early morning crusting from overnight exudation, is common.

Other typical areas are the central midsternal area in males (Plate 50), the navel, the

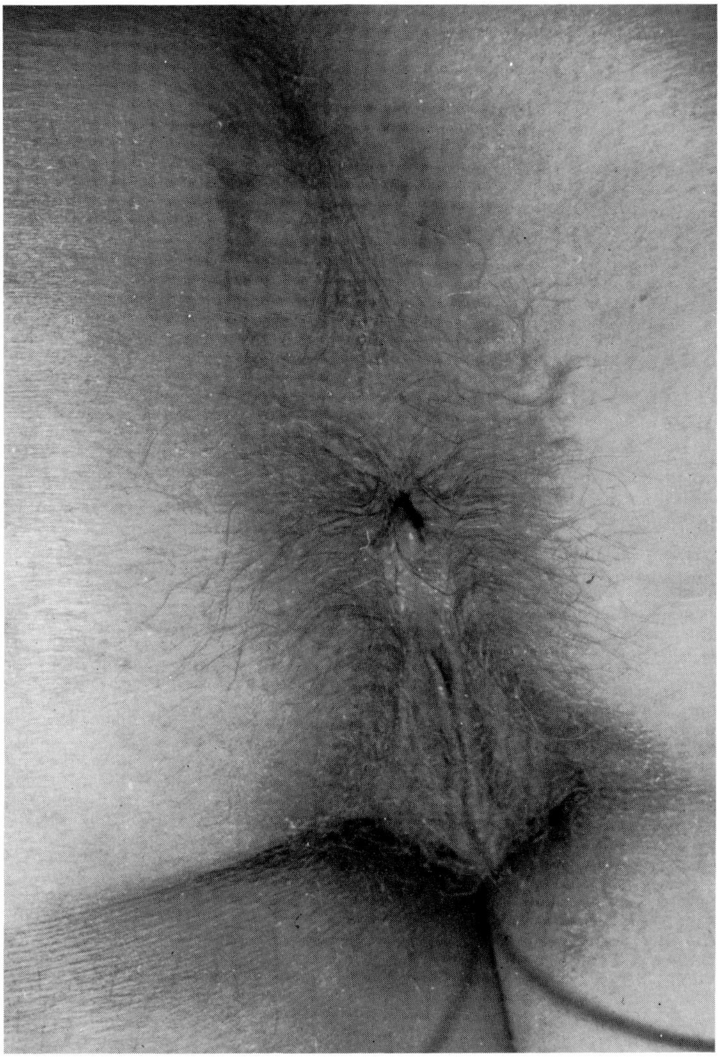

**Fig. 32-4.** Seborrheic dermatitis of gluteal cleft and perianal area.

pubis, and the perineal and perianal areas (Fig. 32-4), often with inner thigh involvement. Another affected hair-bearing area is the face, accentuated by the current popularity of beards.

The lesions are a characteristic pale erythema, with fairly sharp borders and an overlying yellowish greasy scale. They are often pruritic. In flexures the scale may not be apparent, and secondary colonization by *Candida albicans* can occur.

Seborrheic dermatitis may change rapidly from a relatively inactive disorder to a severely inflamed state, ostensibly because of secondary bacterial infection. During this acute phase new and distant areas may become affected. Oval isolated patches may appear on extremities and elsewhere. The usual appearance, however, is that of a chronic, erythematous, patchy dermatitis.

One of the common causes of pruritus ani is seborrheic dermatitis.

### *Pertinent information*

Seborrheic dermatitis is often said to occur in areas with a large number of sebaceous glands, in association with a greasy, seborrheic skin, a tendency to acne, and, later in life, to rosacea. There are persons, however, who develop seborrheic dermatitis late in life. Among these are individuals who have parkinsonism, of either the postencephalitic or the idiopathic type. These patients have excessive sebum on the skin; whether this condition is caused by increased sebaceous gland excretion or increased sweat production is not clear. In and beyond the characteristic facial and thoracic areas, these persons are much more prone to seborrheic dermatitis than are normal individuals.

Seborrheic dermatitis accompanies other neurological lesions, some in a remarkably localized manner.

There is also an unexplained association of seborrheic dermatitis with psoriasis, to which it bears many gross resemblances. Indeed, certain cases have been labeled sebopsoriasis or psoriatic seborrheic dermatitis because it is so difficult to distinguish between the two disorders. These cases are also exceedingly resistant to anti-seborrheic therapy.

Recent studies demonstrated that the increased number of scalp microorganisms (*Pityrosporon ovale*, aerobic coagulase-negative cocci, and *Corynebacterium acnes*) found in dandruff occur as a secondary event to the presence of increased nutrients. The scalp organisms play no primary role in the pathogenesis of this disease.

The areas of predilection coincide with those areas of maximum thermal sweating, which in turn are associated with an increased lipid excretion, because of the sebum-sweat surface emulsion. The pH in affected areas is strongly alkaline, which may be a factor in the etiology of the disease. It is hard to escape the view that there is some inflammatory component of the sebum, because of the increased redness in areas that tend to pool sebum.

### Microscopic findings

Microscopic findings are not specific; these include parakeratosis, some acanthosis, and intercellular edema of the epidermis. The dermis possesses a chronic inflammatory infiltrate. A recent histological study suggests that the rhythmical discharge of leukocytes and serum from the tips of engorged capillaries demonstrates a unifying feature of seborrheic dermatitis, psoriasis, and other psoriasiform states.

### Differential diagnosis

***Psoriasis.*** Psoriasis can resemble seborrheic dermatitis, particularly lesions in the scalp. However, in psoriasis the scale is thicker, the lesions are more circumscribed, and knees and elbows are involved.

***Contact dermatitis.*** Contact dermatitis can simulate seborrheic dermatitis when acute, weeping, or localized. Patch tests to detect potential causative agents produce positive reactions.

***Atopic dermatitis.*** Atopic dermatitis involves flexures and may be generalized and scaling. There is, however, a family and personal history of asthma, hay fever, and dermatitis. Atopic dermatitis in infancy can closely simulate seborrheic dermatitis.

***Tinea corporis.*** Particularly when lesions involve the inguinal or male genital areas, tinea corporis may cause localized erythema and scaling. Culture and microscopic examination of scrapings from the lesion demonstrate the fungus.

***Pityriasis rosea.*** Characteristically, pityriasis rosea begins with a herald plaque, followed in a few days by oval, uniform lesions.

***Discoid lupus erythematosus.*** The paranasal area, the eyebrows, and the upper midback, are involved, with scaling red lesions in discoid lupus erythematosus, which produce central atrophy and scarring.

### Treatment

In general, areas involved by seborrheic dermatitis are sensitive and easily irritated. All external irritants, excess heat, and excess perspiration will aggravate the disease. Rubbing and scratching will prolong the disorder and may produce infection. Frequent shampooing and the regular use of soap and warm water is the single most effective therapeutic approach.

Dandruff is controlled by use of a selenium sulfide suspension (Selsun) for frequent shampooing, after an initial cleansing shampoo to remove accumulated scale. The Selsun is left on the area for 5 minutes, then thoroughly washed away. A lotion such as 0.01% fluocinolone, 0.1% betamethasone, 0.05% beclomethasone dipropionate (Propaderm), or the equivalent in a cream base may be used, but it should be necessary only in stubborn cases.

Zinc pyrithione, 1% to 2%, in a cream base (ZP11) and in a shampoo (Head & Shoulders) has proved effective in mild cases of dandruff. Frequent shampooing is important.

Ear lesions respond to a similar glucocorticoid lotion applied three times daily. Therapy should be maintained for some time after clearing of lesions, and then the dosage should be reduced slowly. Recurrences should be treated promptly. No medication should be introduced into an ear canal by cotton-tipped applicators or other devices.

If secondary infection is present, 1% neomycin or 3% chloramphenicol (Chloromycetin) can be added for topical use.

Intertriginous lesions are most successfully alleviated by an effective glucocorticoid cream or, preferably, lotion, applied every 3 hours except at night. Slow withdrawal of medication after elimination is important.

Acute weeping lesions respond only after the exudation is dried. The use of prepackaged tablets or powders that can be dissolved in cool water to make up Burow's solution in the proper dilution is very effective. It should be used three to four times daily, and the site should be allowed to dry in the air. This is then followed by an effective glucocorticoid cream. Secondary infection characterized by crusting lesions may respond to oral antibiotics for 4 to 5 days. Tetracycline is usually the drug of choice.

If the process is severe, spreading, and uncontrollable by local therapy, then glucocorticoids orally may be used to bring the inflammation under control, after which topical medications can be applied frequently and the oral steriods slowly tapered off and discontinued. Prednisone in a dosage of 5 mg. three times daily for 2 weeks, then twice daily for 2 weeks, and so forth, may be used if there are no contraindications.

Sedatives may be necessary to ensure the necessary hours of rest at night to allow the dermatitis to subside. Meprobamate, 400 mg. at bedtime, is satisfactory.

Chronic localized lesions respond well to application of ointments such as the following:

| | |
|---|---|
| Salicylic acid | 1%-3% |
| Precipitated sulfur | 1%-5% |
| Hydrophilic ointment | 60 Gm. |

Apply sparingly twice daily.

Radiation in the form of ultraviolet-light therapy in graded increasing doses may be helpful, but often is ineffectual. Grenz-ray therapy is very beneficial. Treatment of Parkinson's disease with levodopa has been reported to improve an accompanying seborrheic dermatitis.

### REFERENCES

Hackney, V. C., and Norins, A. L.: Seborrheic dermatitis and Leiner's disease. In Maddin, S., editor: Current dermatologic management, St. Louis, 1975, The C. V. Mosby Co., p. 120.

**Treatments of choice for scalp, torso, and intertriginous areas.**

Leyden, J. J., McGinley, K. J., and Kligman, A. M.: Role of micro-organisms in dandruff, Arch. Dermatol. **112**:333, 1976.

**Another hallowed concept bites the dust.**

Seborrheic dermatitis: Editorial, Br. Med. J. **1**:436, 1973.

**A therapeutic roundup.**

Shelley, W. B.: Seborrheic dermatitis. In Consultations in dermatology, 2, Philadelphia, 1974, W. B. Saunders Co., p. 312.

**A lucid presentation on a common, often vexing problem.**

Treatment of dandruff, Med. Lett. Drugs Ther. **19**:63, 1977.

**Products containing salicylic acid and sulfur are moderately effective. Most effective: zinc pyrithione and selenium sulfide in shampoos.**

CHAPTER 33

# Sweat disorders

## SWEAT GLANDS

### Embryology

***Eccrine sweat glands.*** The eccrine sweat glands appear first on the palms and soles and arise as solid buds of epidermal cells pushing into the dermis from the crest of the ridges during the fourth intrauterine month. They become fully functional over a period of time from birth through the first year of life.

### Anatomy

***Eccrine glands.*** The eccrine glands are present almost everywhere on human skin. It has been estimated that between 2 and 5 million sweat glands are present over the surface of the body, with only the lips and parts of the genitalia being without sweat glands. They are most numerous on the sole where they approach 620 per square centimeter and are least on the arm and thigh, 120 per square centimeter. No new sweat glands develop after birth, and age does not appear to reduce their number.

These glands extend as a tube to the epidermis from the dermis or the dermal–fatty tissue border. The *duct* opens onto the surface of the palms and soles through the centers of the epidermal ridges. The epidermal *pore* opening is a well-defined orifice. It is separated from the epidermis although encased in it, surrounded by a ring of keratin, and easily blocked by superficial hydration or inflammation. Each tubule is coiled in its intraepidermal portion, then straight in its midportion, and highly coiled on itself in the deep, dermal, secretory portion, which is referred to as the basal coil (Fig. 33-1).

The *duct* is composed of two layers of cuboid cells with dark nuclei, and the secretory coil possesses dark cells with a nucleus toward the lumen and clear cells with their nucleus at the periphery. Both cells rest on a myoepithelial cell layer encased by a basal lamina that separates them from the surrounding collagen. The clear cells also reach parts of the basal lamina. Capillary loops and meshworks arising from one or more arterioles intimately enfold the coil and the duct.

### Physiology and biochemistry

*Perspiration* is of two types, sensible and insensible, a division that is obviously somewhat arbitrary. *Sensible* perspiration is eccrine in origin, visible, and produced in response to an emotional or thermal stimulus. *Insensible* perspiration emanates from the same eccrine glands, but the droplets are microscopic in size and evaporate as they reach the surface.

Insensible perspiration is also made up of that loss of body water that occurs through the intact epidermis. The two components of insensible perspiration are in continuous operation.

The chief components of sweat are water, sodium, potassium, chloride, glucose, urea, and lactate, the concentrations of which vary greatly from person to person and with the rate of perspiration.

The secretory cells of the sweat gland probably transport sodium actively into the sweat duct, rather than by a process of filtration, as occurs in the kidney (Dobson). This process, fueled by glucose metabolism as an energy source, is known as the sodium pump. Sodium is partially reabsorbed from the duct as well, a process that is under the influence of aldosterone. Sodium concentration in the sweat increases with age and is higher in an episode of rapid sweating than under basal conditions.

Eccrine sweat glands are under sympa-

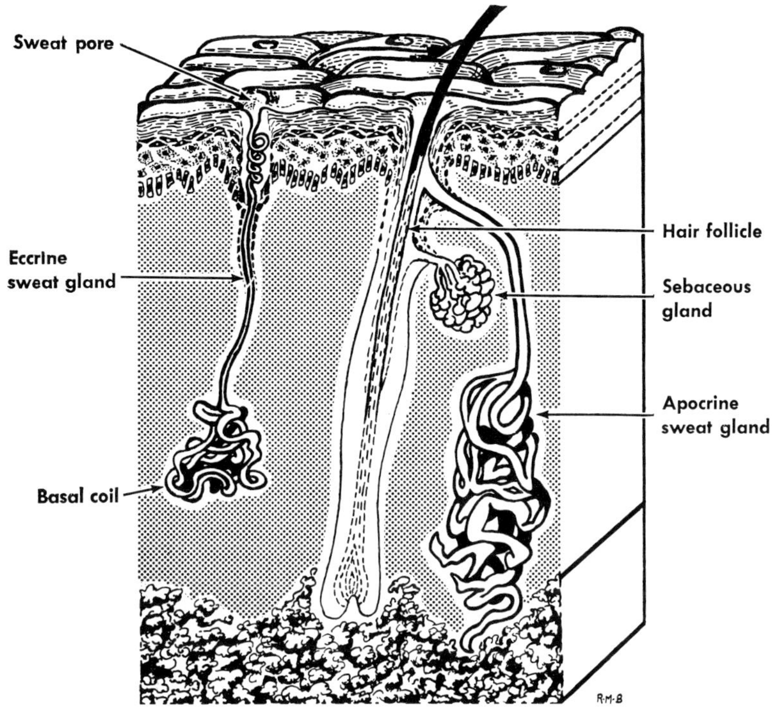


**Fig. 33-1.** Eccrine and apocrine sweat glands.

thetic control, brought into activity by the heat-regulating center in the diencephalon. The nerves coiled around the eccrine sweat glands are postganglionic sympathetic, although they release acetylcholine on stimulation. Also isolated sweat glands respond to dilute solutions of acetylcholine.

Adult males sweat one third more than do adult females, and women require a greater concentration of acetylcholine injected to initiate visible sweating. Heat augments that sweat response to acetylcholine. Epinephrine also can produce sweating and does so equally in males and females, also without alteration produced by heat.

The pH of thermal sweat, around 5.7, is more acid than that produced by exercise, around 6.4.

The palms and soles do not at first participate in this thermal response. They ordinarily produce sweat only on emotional stimulation, as do the axillae and the forehead. With more intense heating, however, the eccrine glands of palms and soles also produce sweat on thermal stimulation.

Under dry, hot conditions a man may lose 6 liters of sweat in 24 hours. A maximum sweat loss under abnormally severe conditions may produce 3.5 liter in an hour, but this cannot be sustained for long. An average figure for nonexercising individuals would be 1.5 liter in 24 hours.

With repeated exposure to heat, as in a tropical environment, acclimatization takes place. This consists of an increased rate of perspiration at a given temperature, a lowering of the temperature at which thermal sweating begins, and a more dilute perspiration, the last brought about by adrenal gland adaptation.

Antiperspirants probably act by blocking axillary eccrine gland secretion through formation of a hydroxide gel that diffuses down the eccrine duct and stops delivery of eccrine sweat to the skin surface. There is also some destruction of the integrity of the duct. The metallic aluminum salts are said to be antibacterial as well. Neomycin is a safe and effective component of deodorants, as evidenced by its use for a decade in a popular deodorant, without significant hazard. Since little axillary sweat is produced in sleep, it has been shown that it is more rational and much more effective to apply antiperspirants at bedtime to give them time to diffuse into the eccrine duct prior to the onset of perspiration in the morning. Applied in the morning when eccrine sweat begins again, much of their value is washed away (Reller and Luedders).

## HYPERHIDROSIS

Physiologically, in all individuals, emotional or "mental" factors produce sweating on the palms and soles and in the axillae. Effective stimuli include fear, excitement, pain, and mental effort. Sleep and inactivity tend to diminish this type of hyperhidrosis. Certain individuals are prone to excessive sweating in these areas so that minimal activity, mental concentration, social activity, and so forth, cause an outpouring of perspiration. The affected areas are cold, clammy, and disagreeably wet a great part of the time. The areas may visibly "drip" perspiration continuously (Fig. 33-2). In thermal hyperhidrosis, a minimal heat stimulus causes an overreaction of the sweat apparatus. This disorder commonly begins around puberty and will have a tendency to improve by the twenties.

Wolf and Maibach in studying this problem in 50 normal individuals found that although atropine blocked emotional palmar sweating,

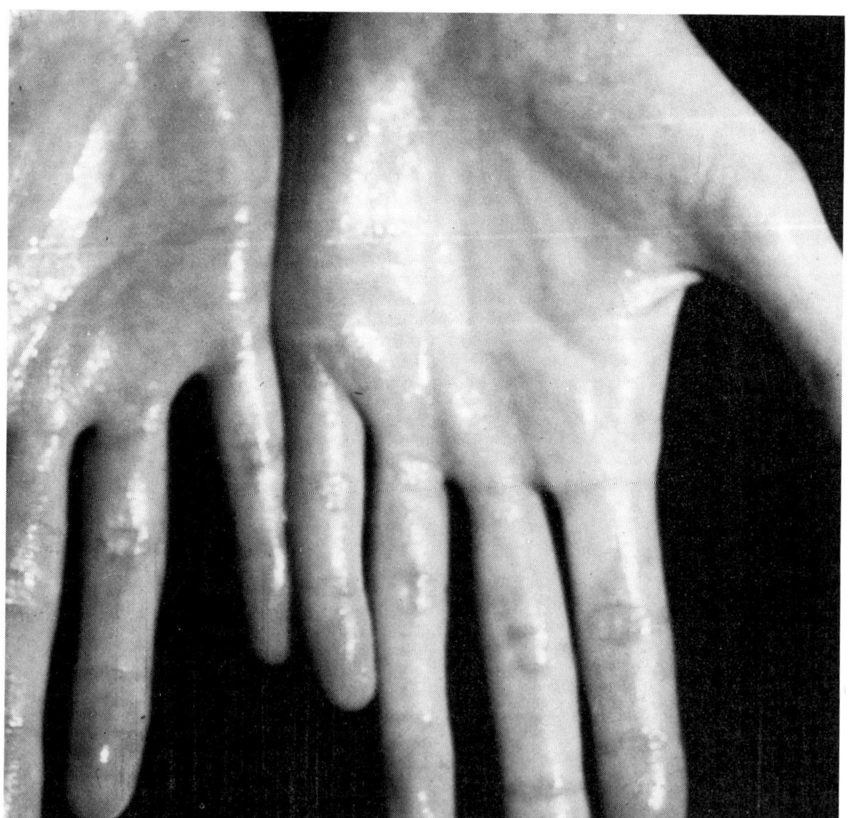

**Fig. 33-2.** Hyperhidrosis. A very real handicap, most commonly seen in teenagers and young adults.

neither it nor any other agent had any effect on spontaneous sweating.

In the axillae, any perspiration excess comes from eccrine glands.

### *Investigation*

In cases of persistent, generalized hyperhidrosis, the following systemic disorders must be ruled out: diabetes mellitus, hyperthyroidism, menopause, infections (including tuberculosis, brucellosis, and malaria), alcoholism, and generally debilitating disease. Postfebrile and postoperative patients may demonstrate intermittent hyperhidrosis.

### *Treatment*

A surprising number of patients show concern over supposedly harmful effects of reducing sweat output and must be reassured particularly if surgical removal of sweat glands is contemplated.

***Antiperspirants.*** Drysol (Person & Covey), a formulation of aluminum chloride hexahydrate in absolute alcohol, is applied to the axilla, palms, or soles at night, to be washed off the following morning. In severe cases, it can be covered with plastic overnight. One to two applications weekly suffice after it has gained control. It can, however, be irritating. Glycopyrrolate (Robinul), 2 mg. given in a dose of 2 tablets three times daily, is partially effective in controlling hyperhidrosis in selected cases.

For those individuals with severe *axillary hyperhidrosis*, surgical removal of the localized cluster of glands in the dome of the axilla gives considerable relief from the distressing disorder (Rigg).

For *plantar hyperhidrosis*, glutaraldehyde, 10% in water and buffered to pH 7.5 with bicarbonate (1.65 Gm. for a 10% solution), is applied topically two to three times weekly. It tends to discolor the area; so a weaker solution, 3% to 5%, is used for palms. After treatment is stopped, sweating recurs quickly. Regular use seems indicated. Sympathectomy is performed to produce palmar anhidrosis. It is, unfortunately, rather temporary; the excess perspiration returns. Relief may, however, be present for anywhere from 2 months to 10 years.

## SWEAT RETENTION (MILIARIA)

Obstruction of the sweat duct, either partial or complete, leads to a decrease or complete cessation of the delivery of sweat to the skin surface. The obstruction then results in the formation of a small vesicle or papule at the orifice of the sweat duct, produced by the pressure of the blocked sweat flow (Plate 51). Pressure applied by an obstructed sweat secretion has been measured at 250 mm. Hg. Sweat may then escape through the wall of the duct, dilated by pressure proximal to the obstruction, and exude into the surrounding tissue, where it sets up an inflammatory reaction. This process, referred to as *poral closure* or *sweat pore obstruction*, often follows minimal damage to the orifice of the sweat duct. The area of closure and the depth of vesicle formation reflect the depth of damage done to the duct.

*Miliaria*, or prickly heat, is a form of sweat retention. *Miliaria crystallina* is a superficial obstruction. In *miliaria rubra*, an erythematous papule is formed because of a deep obstruction and is associated with an inflammatory reaction. At times these lesions may become pustular.

Many mechanisms may act to produce the poral closure, among them the following:

1. Hyperkeratosis of the epidermis surrounding the orifice
2. Edema
3. Inflammatory processes
4. Effects of drugs

Clinically, sweat retention is seen most frequently under two circumstances: (1) after an inflammatory dermatitis, such as atopic dermatitis, and (2) after sun exposure in the spring of the year or later in the summer, in an amount excessive for the individual.

Also, the sweat obstruction may be aggravated by *increased environmental temperatures, excessively warm clothing, high humidity, prolonged bathing, febrile conditions, or excessive exercise.*

The syndrome produces an extreme and often intolerable itching, made worse by the aggravating features mentioned above.

The appearance of the lesions of the *sweat retention syndrome* is that of multiple skin-

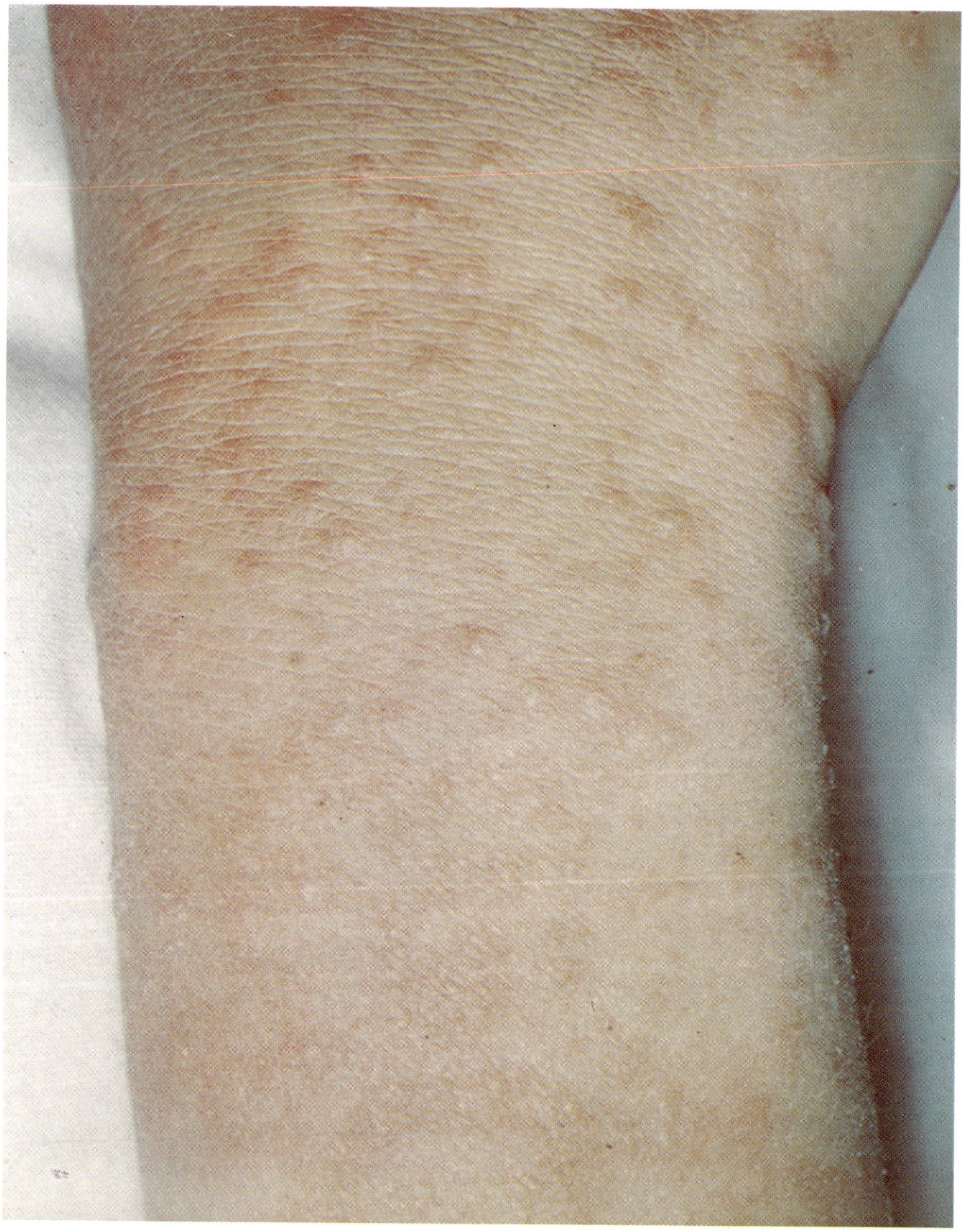

**Plate 51**

Sweat retention.

colored papules and vesicles studded over the affected area (Fig. 33-2). The deeper lesions are less well defined and may demonstrate an erythematous halo. The amount of sweat produced in the affected area is reduced. Increased heat produces a disagreeable prickling sensation leading to prolonged pruritus. Scratching this area further aggravates the condition.

A variable amount of relief is obtained by a

cool dry environment and the application of anti-inflammatory medications.

Many subsiding inflammatory dermatoses appear to undergo a relapse because of the development of a sweat retention syndrome.

### *Differential diagnosis*

***Lichen planus.*** Lichen planus shows multiple, small, papular, angular, and flat-topped pruritic lesions; however, these are not vesicular.

***Folliculitis.*** Vesicular and pustular lesions about the hair follicles are present in folliculitis, but these are usually associated with a greater degree of inflammation and infection than occurs in sweat retention.

### *Treatment*

General measures include reduction in external heat and humidity to reduce perspiration and avoidance of soap, hot water, sun exposure, and external irritants.

Cool wet compresses, using the prepared tablets or powders and 1 to 1 pint of cool water, making up a 1:20 dilution of Burow's solution, should be applied three times daily for periods of 10 minutes each. Anti-inflammatory steroids are eminently successful in reducing the inflammation. These may be topical, using a glucocorticoid preparation in a vanishing cream or lotion base. Ointments should be avoided because they tend to be occlusive.

Steroids administered orally may be necessary for a temporary period in severe or generalized cases. Sedation may be useful to reduce activity and subsequent perspiration.

Ascorbic acid, given orally, 1 Gm. daily for a 70 kg. male, has been reported by Hindson to clear the clinical effects of sweat gland obstruction and to reduce the postmiliaria fatigue known to be a factor in "prickly heat."

The topical dusting of intertriginous areas with 1% to 2% talc-containing menthol is beneficial.

#### REFERENCES

Dobson, R. L. and Sato, K.: The secretion of salt and water by the eccrine sweat gland, Arch. Dermatol. **105**:366, 1972

**Secretory cells, glycolysis, and sodium transport lucidly discussed.**

Drysol for treatment of hyperhidrosis, Med. Lett. Drugs Ther. **19**:20, 1977.

**More effective but may be more irritating.**

Ellis, H.: Hyperhidrosis and its management, Dermatol. Dig. **16**:14, 1977.

**Current surgical concepts including sympathectomy.**

Grice, K., and Verbov, J.: Sweat glands and their disorders. In Rook, A., editor: Recent advances in dermatology, ed. 4, London, 1977, Churchill Livingstone, p. 155.

**Good information, well referenced.**

Hindson, T. C., and Worsley, D. E.: The effects of administration of ascorbic acid in experimentally induced miliaria and hypohidrosis in volunteers, Br. J. Dermatol. **81**:226, 1969.

**One gram daily required.**

Hurley, H. J.: Hyperhidrosis, axillary, surgical approach and the trinary control system. In Maddin, S., editor: Current dermatologic management, ed. 2, St. Louis, 1975, The C. V. Mosby Co., p. 185.

Hurley, H. J., and Shelley, W. B.: Axillary hyperhidrosis, Br. J. Dermatol. **78**:127, 1966.

**Recommended for those who wish more detail.**

Maibach, H. I., and Prystowsky, S. D.: Glutaraldehyde (Pentanedial) allergic contact dermatitis, Arch. Dermatol. **113**:170, 1977.

**A clinically useful evaluation of glutaraldehyde.**

Montagna, W., and Parakkal, P. F.: Eccrine sweat glands. In The structure and function of skin, New York, 1974, Academic Press, Inc., p. 366.

**A tale told by experts including everything.**

Reller, H. H., and Luedders, W. L.: Pharmacologic and toxicologic effects of topically applied agents on the eccrine sweat glands. In Marzulli, F. N., and Maibach, H. I., editors: Advances in modern toxicology, vol. 4, Dermatotoxicology and pharmacology, Washington, D.C., 1977, Hemisphere Publishing Corp., p. 1.

**Pharmacologic agents and their effects, and metal salts.**

Rigg, B. M.: Axillary hyperhidrosis, Plastic Reconstr. Surg. **59**:334, 1977.

**A slightly different, but rational surgical technique.**

Wolf, J. E., and Maibach, H. I.: Palmar eccrine sweating. The role of adrenergic and cholinergic mediators, Br. J. Dermatol. **91**:439, 1974.

**A pharmacologically complex mechanism. The study includes adrenergic and cholinergic drugs, and three types of blockade.**

CHAPTER 34

# Benign tumors

## EPIDERMAL TUMORS

### Seborrheic keratosis

The common, disfiguring warty growth of seborrheic keratosis occurs most frequently after 40 years of age (Plate 52). Although the nature of seborrheic keratoses is not known, the most acceptable concept is that they are nevoid tumors. Seborrheic keratoses may vary in color from yellow to brownish or even black and have a roughened or verrucous surface. They are almost always multiple and give the appearance of being stuck on normal skin (Fig. 34-1, *A*). These lesions do not become malignant, and their chief importance is cosmetic disfigurement. The lesions are passed on from parent to offspring as a dominant trait.

Individual lesions slowly enlarge and become verrucous, dry, and fissured. When the lesions are present in intertriginous areas such as the inframammary region, they may become macerated and odorous. The sites of predilection are the back, central chest, face, and scalp. In blacks the lesions are usually smaller in size, are more numerous, and appear earlier; the condition is referred to as *dermatosis papulosa nigra*. The histopathological picture is the same as that in other varieties of seborrheic keratosis.

#### *Microscopic findings*

The two most striking features are acanthosis and hyperkeratosis. The dermal papillae are elongated, and there is a tendency for the epidermis to become invaginated. Little or no inflammation is present.

#### *Differential diagnosis*

***Pigmented nevus (mole).*** A pigmented nevus is a smooth-surfaced papule that is usually skin colored to brown and is commonly found on the face.

***Actinic (senile) keratosis.*** Actinic keratosis is a slightly elevated, dry, scaly lesion usually found on the face and dorsa of hands of susceptible people who have been exposed to an excessive amount of sunlight.

***Malignant melanoma.*** Occasionally the black-pigmented mulberry-surfaced lesion of malignant melanoma may be mistaken for a black seborrheic keratosis. Biopsy is *always* indicated in doubtful situations.

#### *Treatment*

The lesions may be removed by curettage and superficial electrodesiccation with the patient under local anesthesia. Lesions that are flat can be destroyed by the application of a carbon dioxide pencil with light to moderate pressure for 12 to 20 seconds. Scalpel surgery and the use of radiation are not justified because of the possibility of scarring and postirradiation damage that may result. Experienced use of cryotherapy with liquid nitrogen will also produce a satisfactory result.

### Actinic (senile) keratosis

Actinic keratosis is a small, unobtrusive lesion that develops on skin surfaces damaged by sunlight and may evolve into a low-grade squamous cell carcinoma. This lesion has little tendency to metastasize.

These lesions occur for the most part in persons past middle age who have a history of repeated sun exposure. Those most frequently affected are redheads and blonds, persons with fair skins, and those with a tendency to freckle rather than tan.

An actinic keratosis is a flat, skin colored to brown macular lesion with a dry, firmly at-

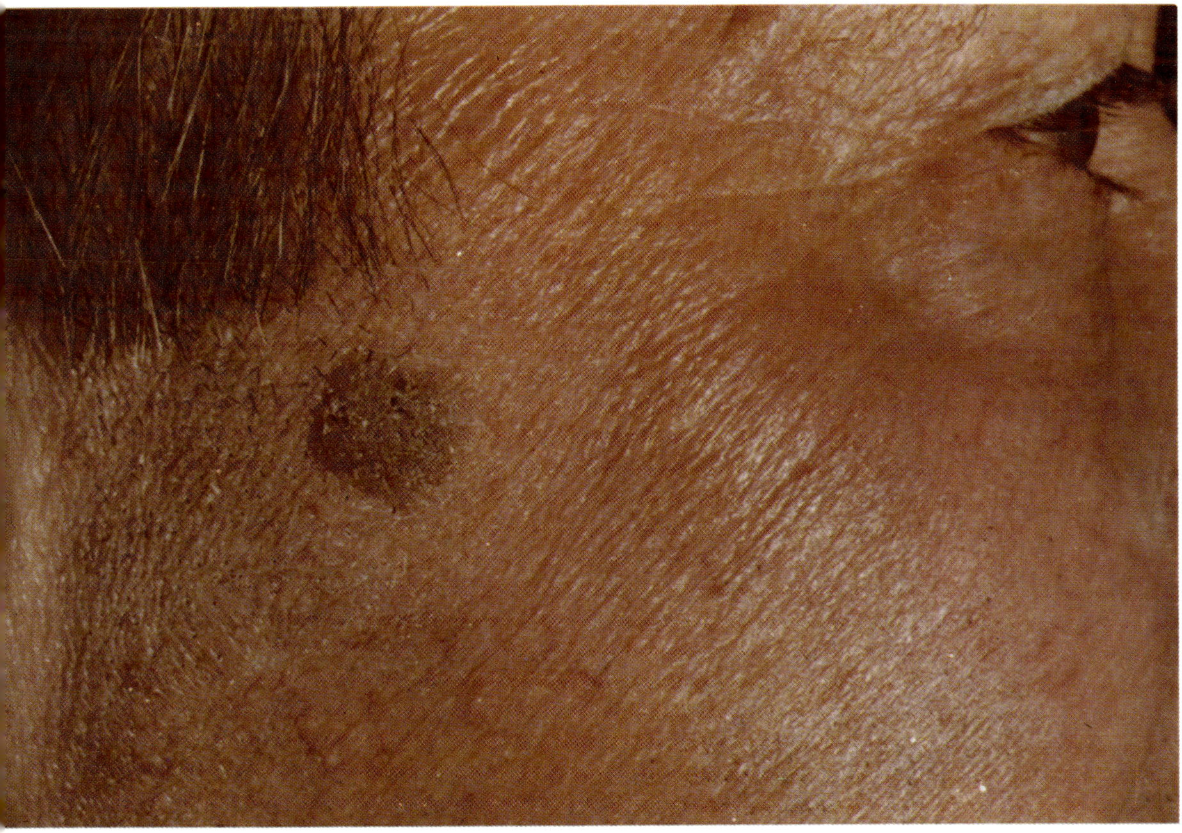

**Plate 52**

Seborrheic keratosis. This is always a benign lesion.

tached, rough scale and an underlying variable degree of erythema (Fig. 34-1, *B*). At times it may appear as a hard, dry, papular lesion. It undergoes a chronic course with repeated episodes of scaling and alternating periods of quiescence. These lesions are often just as easily felt as seen.

Usually the skin of the affected areas is dry and atrophic and shows other effects of prolonged actinic exposure. The sites of predilection are the dorsa of the hands and the forehead, ears, face, and scalp of bald-headed men. The lesions are often multiple, and after one or more lesions have appeared in sun-damaged or irradiated skin, the patient is very likely to develop further lesions. Pearse demonstrated progressive changes in surrounding skin, of which the keratosis itself is the first visible.

Actinic keratoses may occur after arsenic ingestion or inhalation of arsenic-containing sprays.

***Microscopic findings***

The microscopic findings are diagnostic, showing parakeratosis and hyperkeratosis. Areas of atrophy of the epidermis alternate with areas of acanthosis. The affected epidermal cells are sharply different from the background normally keratinizing cells, and keratinization is faulty. The deeper epithelial cells are atypical and irregular and show abnormal staining properties and increased mitotic figures. The basal cell layer is intact.

***Differential diagnosis***

***Seborrheic keratosis.*** A brown to black elevated lesion with a greasy scale that appears

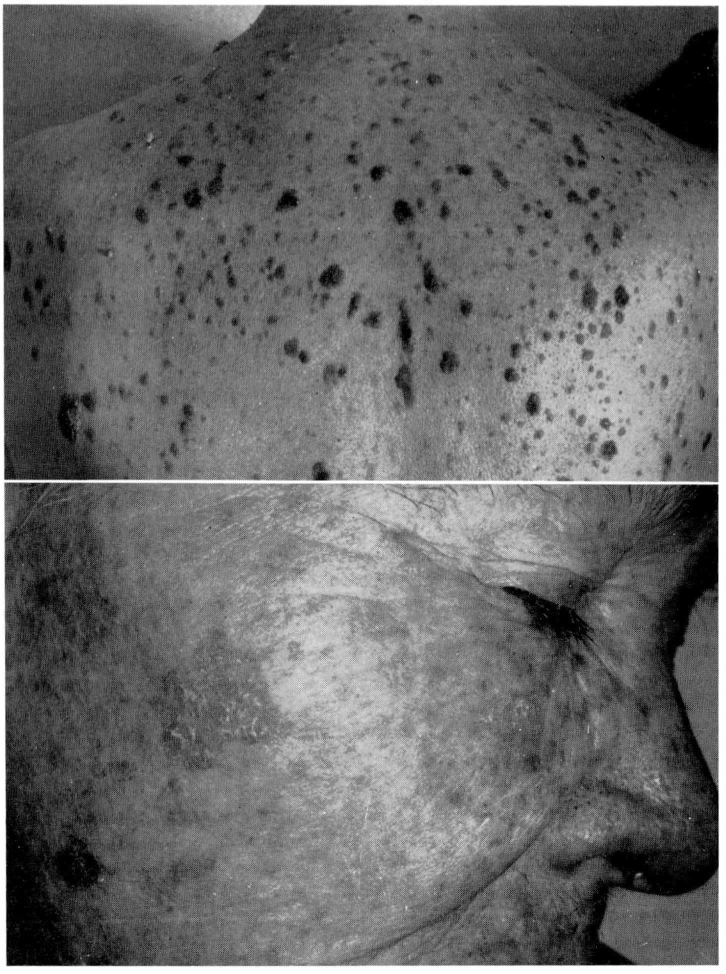


**Fig. 34-1. A,** Seborrheic keratosis. **B,** Actinic (senile) keratoses.

to be stuck on normal skin characterizes seborrheic keratosis. It is found on the back, chest, and face after middle age.

***Cutaneous horn.*** Cutaneous horn is a hard, hyperkeratotic projection found in elderly people.

### *Treatment*

Most time-honored caustic therapy has been replaced by 5-fluorouracil as a 1% solution in propylene glycol or 5% in a cream. It is used 2 times daily for 3 weeks, over normal and involved skin alike, and produces bright erythema on the actinic keratosis, often in areas unrecognized grossly as abnormal. With cessation of therapy, the scaling patch reverts to normal appearance. Normal skin is not affected. Breza and co-workers recommend the application of 5-fluorouracil followed immediately by the use of a glucocorticoid cream such as triamcinolone 0.5%. This sequential topical application reduces the brisk, sometimes alarming and unpleasant, inflammatory reaction that occurs with 5-fluorouracil. We have no evidence, however, that glucocorticoids are safe to use on potentially premalignant cells. One of us (WDS) does not believe so.

Liquid nitrogen is very effective. In the absence of sophisticated apparatus a cotton swab

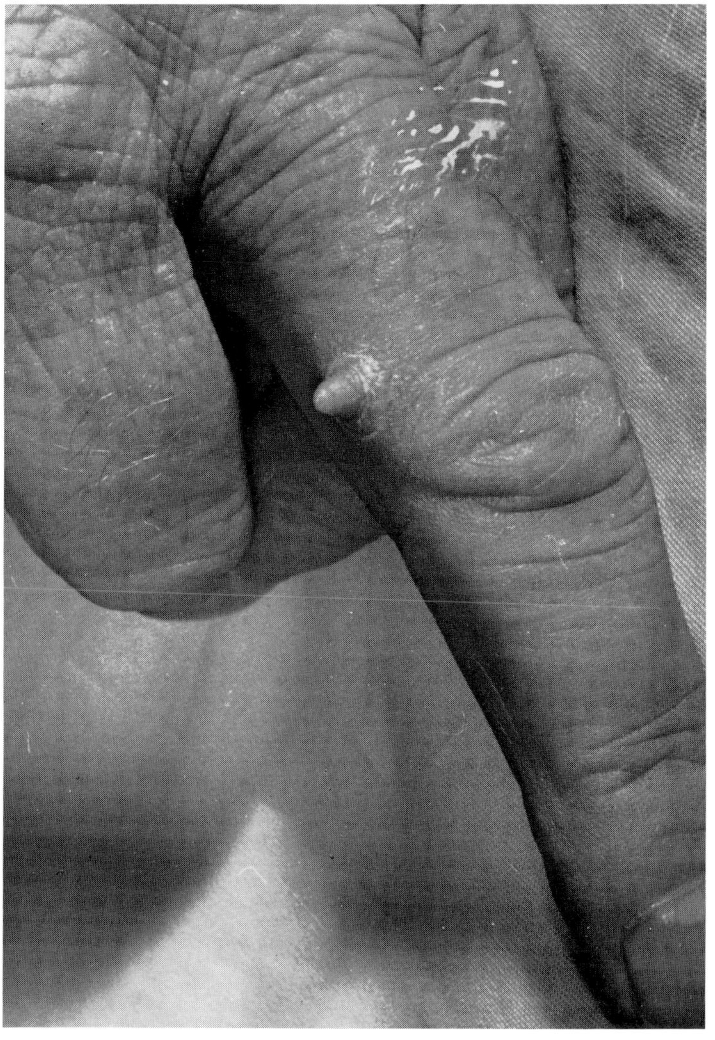

**Fig. 34-2.** Cutaneous horn.

can be used. The swab should have enough body to hold the temperature, pointed to pinpoint, and fixed in shape with hair spray. This is dipped in liquid nitrogen and applied to the actinic keratosis for 20 to 30 seconds, depending on the size and depth of the lesion. Its disadvantage is the lack of biopsy.

More extensive and recurrent lesions can be removed by curettage and electrodesiccation with the patient under local anesthesia, which tends to leave pale, superficial scars, or by liquid nitrogen applied either with a swab or the more sophisticated spray equipment. In selected patients with extensive actinic changes, dermal abrasion will remove the altered skin and reduce the number of new actinic keratoses that appear.

Prevention of actinic keratoses includes the following measures:

1. Counseling sun-susceptible persons to avoid sunlight and children prone to sunburning to protect the exposed skin
2. Advising proper clothing (for example, broad-brimmed hats and gloves)
3. Prescribing sunscreening lotions or creams (see discussion on sun-protective agents, p. 62)

Any patient who has had a senile keratosis removed should be examined at intervals for further lesions.

## Cutaneous horn

Cutaneous horn is a small, hard, keratinous projection of the epidermis (Fig. 34-2). It occurs in elderly individuals, usually on the forehead and face. If neglected, these may attain considerable length. The base of the lesion microscopically demonstrates dyskeratotic changes similar to those of an actinic keratosis and should be treated as such.

## Keratoacanthoma

A benign tumor, keratoacanthoma is easily confused with squamous cell carcinoma.

This clinical entity, which bears a striking resemblance both clinically and histopathologically to squamous cell carcinoma, may develop in single or multiple lesions. It occurs predominantly in whites. It has appeared after intense sun exposure, in association with carcinogens, at sites of trauma, and we have observed multiple lesions arising at the site of occlusive topical glucocorticoid therapy of

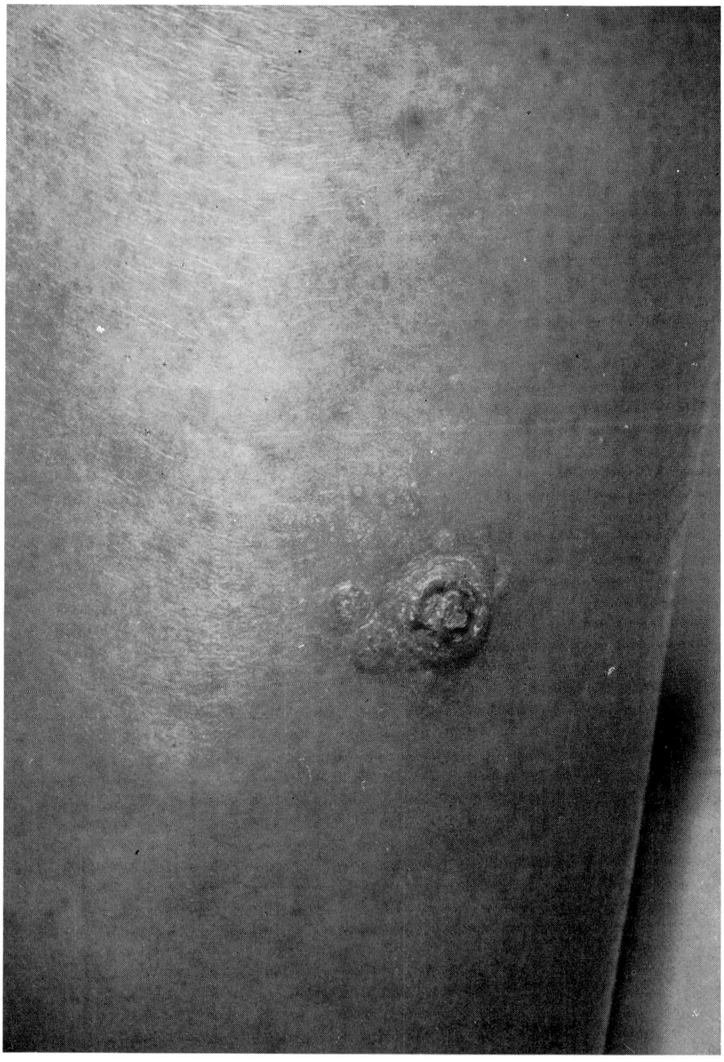

**Fig. 34-3.** Keratoacanthoma.

psoriasis on one leg. Keratoacanthoma deserves special attention because of the fact that, although it mimics squamous cell carcinoma, it runs a quite rapid but benign self-limited clinical course, averaging 17 weeks, after which it involutes completely. Lesions may persist for 3 years or more, particularly in older patients. Initially, keratoacanthoma begins as a red maculopapular lesion that becomes dome shaped, with a central keratinous plug (Fig. 34-3). The diameter seldom exceeds 2 cm. and is usually around 0.5 cm. Sites of predilection are the exposed areas—the central face, hands, and wrists—and less commonly the covered areas of the trunk. The scar that results from spontaneous involution of a keratoacanthoma tends to be pitted and to have an overhanging border.

### *Differential diagnosis*

***Squamous cell carcinoma.*** In appearance and course, squamous cell carcinoma may closely resemble keratoacanthoma, although its initial development is not usually so rapid. Biopsy must be done to differentiate between them.

***Basal cell carcinoma.*** Basal cell carcinoma has an elevated border and a slower growth rate than does keratoacanthoma.

***Cutaneous nodule.*** A dome-shaped, firm lesion, cutaneous nodule has an extremely slow growth and no central depression.

### *Treatment*

The course of treatment must be decided only after careful biopsy and consideration of size, location, and course of the individual tumor *by one experienced in the natural course of this lesion*. The biopsy should allow the pathologist to view a cross section of the whole lesion for proper assessment. The great danger lies in failing to recognize a true squamous cell carcinoma.

Choices of treatment include observation awaiting spontaneous involution, excision, curettage and electrodesiccation, adequate cryotherapy, intralesional injection of glucocorticoids, or radiotherapy. Since spontaneous involution may produce permanent scarring, early electrodesiccation and curettage after biopsy may produce the best cosmetic result.

These lesions ordinarily do not recur.

## Milium (epithelial cyst)

Milium is a pinhead-sized, asymptomatic, white, globlar lesion that is usually found in small numbers around the eyes and forehead (Fig. 34-4, *A*). It may develop spontaneously or be secondary to dermal trauma that occurs after thermal burn, incision, dermabrasion, or bullous disease.

Microscopically, it is an epidermal cyst.

### *Treatment*

Treatment consists of incising the overlying epidermis and expressing the keratinous core with a comedo extractor.

## Wen (epidermal cyst, sebaceous cyst)

Sebaceous cyst, or as the international nomenclature of disease would have it, sebaceous tumor, is a name that is almost surely here to stay. Too many nondermatologists refer to these fluctuant, painless, subepidermal tumors as sebaceous cysts to convert them all to more accurate nomenclature.

However, dermatopathologists for years have pointed out that histologically the sebaceous gland is not the cyst-forming structure and have suggested truer names for these cysts. Thus epidermal, keratinous, pilar, trichilemmal cyst, and trichochlamydocyst have been propounded, each for carefully thought-out reasons. It may be that wen, like mole, is a lay term that best encompasses a variety of growths with subtle technical differences and is a satisfactory noncommittal name for these structures.

A wen (Fig. 34-4 *B*) is a globular, tense, cystic structure, fluctuant and asymptomatic, that is attached to the skin. It is usually less than 3 cm. in diameter, but can enlarge to the size of a small orange.

The content of the cyst, which is the product of the obstructed hair follicle, is soft, yellow-white, and has a rancid odor. It is formed as a result of the continuing keratinization of the cells lining the cyst, and its exact nature depends on the level of the obstruc-

A

B

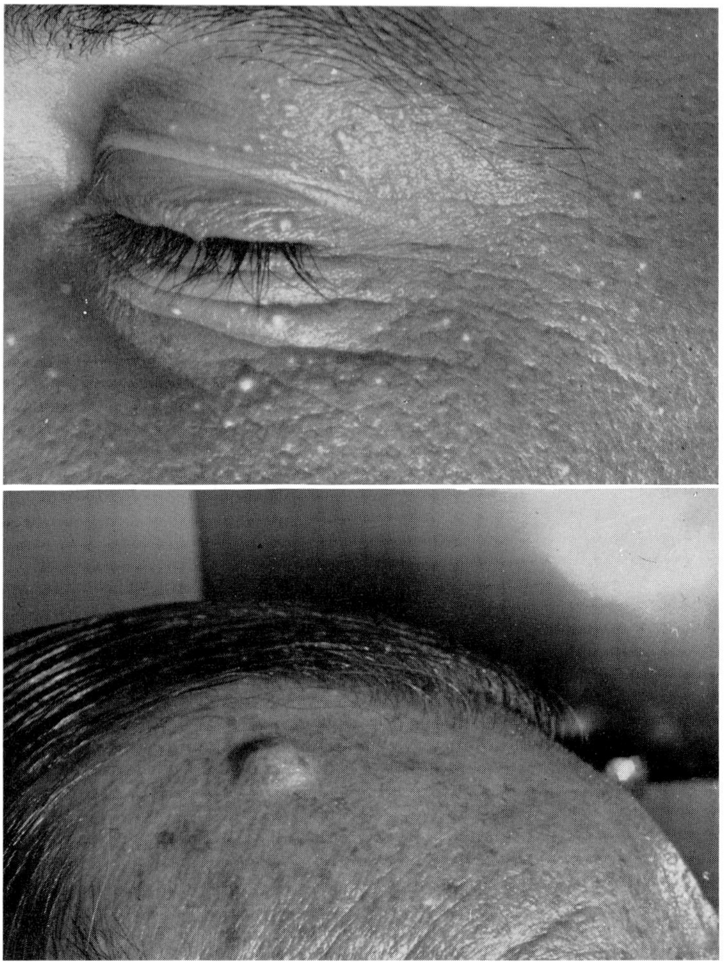

**Fig. 34-4. A,** Multiple milia. **B,** Wen (sebaceous cyst).

tion. It may arise because of the obstructing effect of acne vulgaris and seborrhea, in which case it is found chiefly on the face, neck, shoulders, and chest, regions involved by the acne process. Cysts occurring without preceding inflammation are often found on the scalp and thorax. When present on the scalp, the lesions frequently result in loss of scalp hair overlying the cyst. The tendency to develop these cysts without preceding inflammation can be inherited as an incomplete dominant trait.

Microscopically, the cyst is seen to be lined by epithelial cells that arise from the pilosebaceous follicle and continue to keratinize, and which, in comedones at least, have been shown to have an increased mitotic rate over normal epidermis. The type of keratinization observed leads to the specific delineation of the nature of the cyst.

### *Differential diagnosis*

***Steatocystoma multiplex or sebocystomatosis.*** Multiple elastic, globular, yellow-white cysts appear after puberty as an inherited trait. They occur on the axilla, thorax, and scrotum.

### *Treatment*

Treatment may be effected in several ways.

In the Kanee procedure (modified Danna

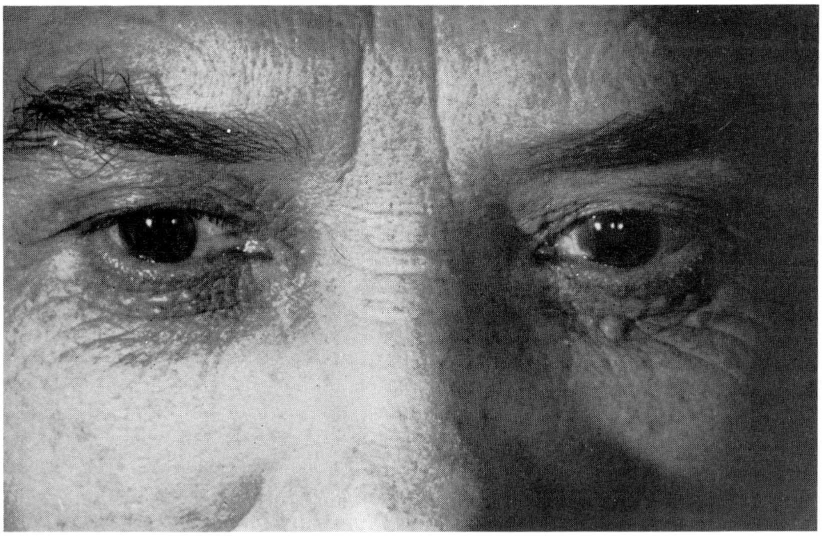

**Fig. 34-5.** Trichoepithelioma.

technique), the skin overlying the cyst is anesthetized and electrocoagulated, and the contents of the cyst are emptied. By use of forceps and manipulation, the cyst is removed from its bed and eased through the skin opening. This is a simple and effective method.

Complete surgical excision is the most effective treatment in previously inflamed lesions that will not shell out easily because of scarring. The cyst may recur if a part of the lining remains.

## Trichoepithelioma (epithelioma adenoides cysticum)

Trichoepithelioma is a firm, small, skin-colored, waxy-appearing papule that occurs symmetrically on the periorbital skin and central face (Fig. 34-5). Lesions appear in clusters beside the alae nasi, at the inner canthi, in the paranasal areas, and on the cheeks. They occasionally appear on the scalp, neck, and upper thorax. They may range in number from a few to hundreds. Trichoepithelioma is hereditary (transmitted as an intermittent dominant) and most commonly appears in females at puberty; the lesions continue to increase in numbers during adult life. It arises from the basal cells, forming small horn cysts, and may be very similar microscopically to basal cell epithelioma.

### *Treatment*

Trichoepithelioma can be treated by dermabrasion if there are large numbers of lesions or by electrodesiccation if there are only a few.

Cryotherapy carefully done, with either solid carbon dioxide or liquid nitrogen, can be used successfully to eradicate the superficial lesions.

## Tuberous sclerosis (adenoma sebaceum, Pringle's disease)

The cutaneous lesions of tuberous sclerosis, or Pringle's disease, appear in childhood and consist of small, tan-colored, telangiectatic and fibrous papules of the nose, alae nasi, cheeks, and central face. The classic triad of symptoms includes skin tumors, mental deficiency, and epilepsy. There are also subungual fibromas and thickened, soft, discrete patches of skin (shagreen patches) on the sacral area. White leaf-shaped macules recently were found in 50% of these children. Tumors and other cellular abnormalities are found in the brain, retina, heart, and kidneys.

### *Differential diagnosis*

***Flat warts.*** The plane surface nontelangiectatic appearance, and usually unilateral distribution differentiate these lesions.

***Acne vulgaris.*** The presence of comedones and inflammatory papules and pustules indicates acne vulgaris.

***Perioral dermatitis.*** This condition occurs in young adult women, and the vesicopapules are transient.

***Trichoepithelioma.*** There is a hereditary history; biopsy may be necessary to differentiate from tuberous sclerosis.

***Syringoma.*** In syringoma, there are tan to red papules, chiefly below the lower eyelid.

### *Microscopic findings*

Microscopically, the facial lesions show cellular collagen proliferation, dilation of small vessels, and abnormally stellate fibroblasts. Cerebral and retinal lesions are gliomas.

## Senile sebaceous hyperplasia (senile sebaceous adenoma)

The small, discrete, cream-colored, translucent, umbilicated papular lesions of senile sebaceous hyperplasia occur on the forehead of individuals past middle age. They are asymptomatic and consist of a hypertrophied sebaceous gland.

### *Treatment*

The lesions are treated by electrodesiccation or by cryotherapy.

# DERMAL TUMORS

## Cutaneous tag (acrochordon, squamous papilloma)

Cutaneous tag is a minute, soft, pedunculated tumor a few millimeters in length that is ordinarily skin colored but may be pigmented. The small excrescence is most frequently found around the neck, upper chest, and axillae in middle-aged women. There may be a few lesions or hundreds. The number increases with pregnancy and with the onset of the menopause. There are no subjective complaints unless the lesion is irritated. It has no clinical significance.

### *Microscopic findings*

Microscopically, cutaneous tag consists of an outpouching of loose connective tissue covered by normal epidermis.

### *Treatment*

Treatment consists of removing the lesion by electrodesiccation with the patient under local anesthesia, or by cryotherapy.

## Cutaneous nodule (dermatofibroma)

Cutaneous nodule (Fig. 34-6) is an asymptomatic, round, firm, slightly elevated lesion that may be gray to dusky red, with a yellowish tinge. It grows slowly to a size of 5 to 20 mm. and then remains stationary and asymptomatic. It is most commonly found on the extremities, especially the legs of middle-aged adults. The lesion is usually single, but may be multiple.

Recently they have been observed to appear in patients with systemic lupus erythematosus.

### *Microscopic findings*

The microscopic findings are varied. Some lesions are composed chiefly of fibroblasts (dermatofibroma), whereas others contain histiocytes as well as fibroblasts (histiocytoma). In addition, fat cells, giving the lesion a yellow color, or hemosiderin, causing a bluish color, may be present.

### *Treatment*

Usually, treatment is not necessary. The lesion may, however, be removed surgically with the patient under local anesthesia.

## Keloid (hypertrophic scar)

Keloid is a fibrous tissue tumor that is soft and pink in the early stages and then becomes firm and white. It may develop spontaneously, but most commonly it forms at the site of dermal trauma, after a thermal burn or surgical incision. We have seen a keloid develop on the presternal area as a result of acute allergic contact dermatitis from a necklace. Acne, vaccination, and hypodermic injection are also among the types of trauma that produce keloids (Fig. 34-7).

The factors that trigger this fibrous tissue proliferation are unknown. The sternum is the site of greatest predilection. Cohen and Diegelmann reintroduce Ketchum's theory that corticosteroids used in keloid therapy en-

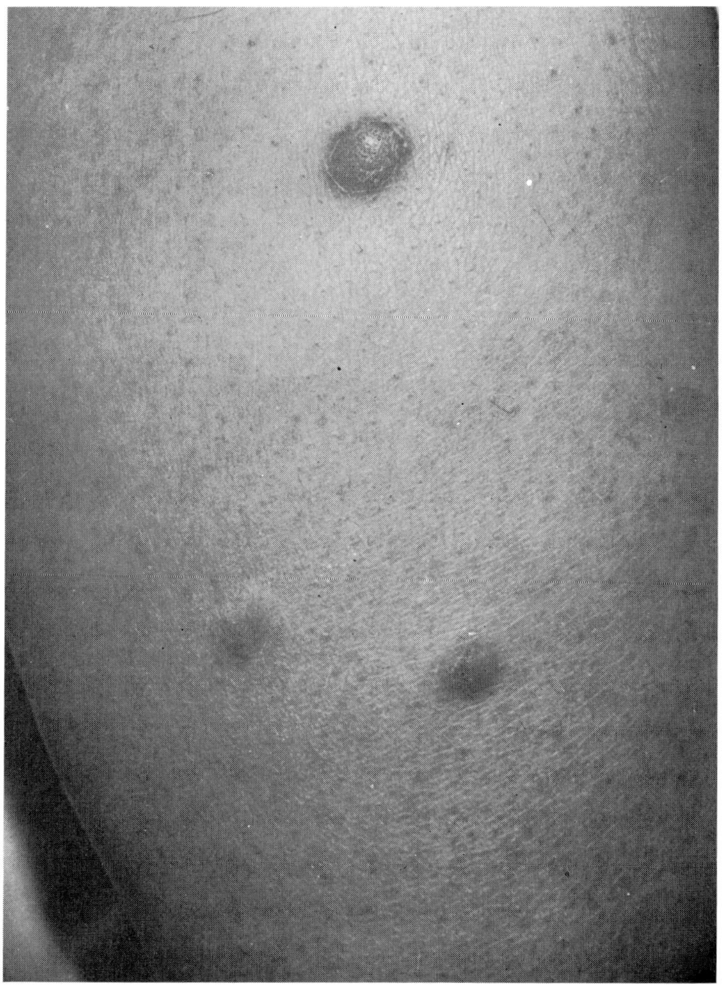

**Fig. 34-6.** Cutaneous nodule (dermatofibroma). Most common on legs.

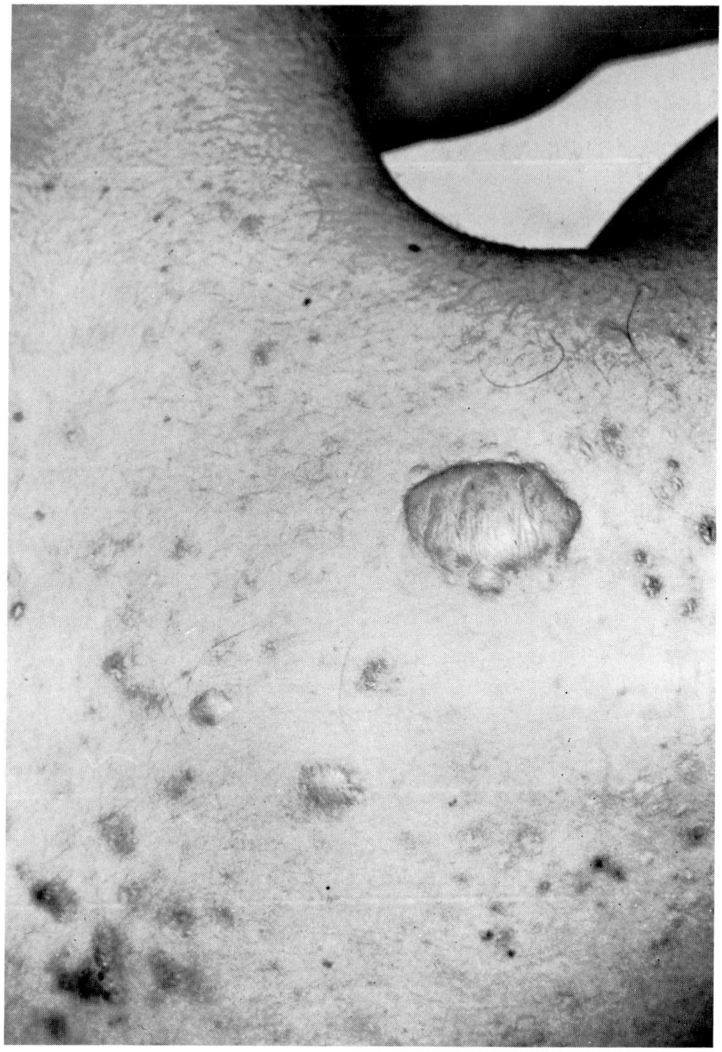

**Fig. 34-7.** Postacne keloid formation. Most eventually flatten out.

hance collagen degradation. Their investigations indicate that triamcinolone removes collagenase inhibitors. They believe that keloids may be a result of immune activity. Certain individuals are predisposed to keloid formation. This is a temporary and unpredictable tendency. It is a familial disorder occurring predominantly in children or young adults, particularly in darkskinned individuals.

Italian workers report that individuals who carry HL-A B14 or HL-A Bw16 antigens have a greater risk of developing keloids. This does not hold for hypertrophic scars.

### *Microscopic findings*

The microscopic findings consist of intertwining of collagen fibrils that become hyalinized in older keloids. Fibroblasts are present in uneven distribution and predominate in active centers.

### *Treatment*

Keloids may become worse as a result of therapy; therefore, the need for treatment must first be carefully assessed. Small keloids on the anterior chest and earlobes in young people, especially those who are darkskinned or Oriental, are *best left alone*. Time above all else gives good results.

Many, if not most, keloids will gradually soften and flatten out over a period of years, even without treatment.

Application of solid carbon dioxide to the lesion, with moderate pressure, at 2-week intervals is a safe and usually effective method of therapy. Time and pressure increase the depth of the therapeutic effect.

Liquid nitrogen, applied with a cotton-tipped applicator for a similar period of time, produces a comparable effect. It must be kept off normal skin.

Small keloids may respond to intralesional injection of triamcinolone suspension, 10 to 40 mg./ml. Ketchum discusses triamcinolone injection, pressure, and radiation as treatment forms.

Surgical excision and x-ray therapy combined appear to be an effective treatment in large keloids that demand a therapeutic attack. These modalities should be used, however, by skilled individuals familiar with the behavior of keloids. *Simple surgical excision of keloids will result in the formation of a new and larger keloid in most cases.*

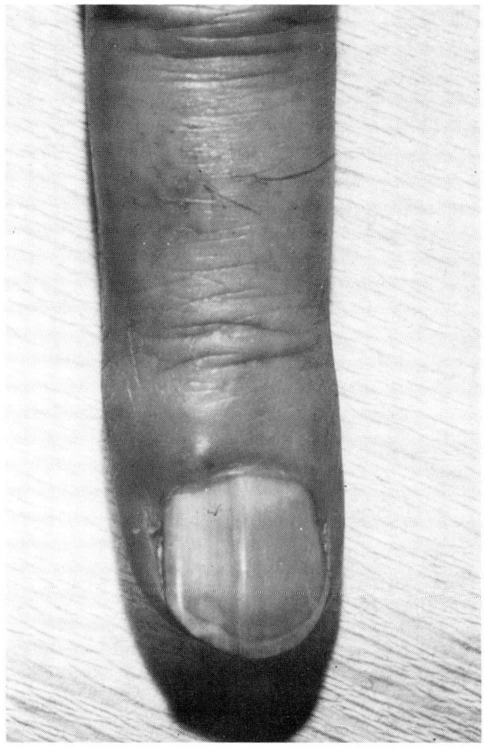

**Fig. 34-8.** Myxoid cyst. Note furrowing of nail from adjacent cyst.

## Lipoma

Lipoma is an asymptomatic, soft, compressible tumor. It is a poorly encapsulated subcutaneous collection of fat and fibrous tissue. The lesion may be a smooth swelling covered by normal skin. It may or may not be movable under the skin. It is usually single and varies greatly in size, from that of a walnut to a grapefruit. The sites of predilection are the buttocks, thighs, back, arms, and neck. Its incidence is greatest after 30 years of age.

### *Microscopic findings*

Microscopic examination shows masses of normal-appearing fat cells, some of which are in a lattice of fibrous tissue, and the tumor may or may not have a loose fibrous tissue capsule.

### *Treatment*

If the lesion interferes with function, or if cosmetic reasons warrant treatment, surgical excision is indicated. Unless carefully done, excision is likely to be incomplete, because of the indefinite borders of the lesion and its tendency to extend around muscle groups.

## Myxoid cyst (synovial cyst)

A firm, but compressible, smooth, globular tumor, myxoid cyst is found on the distal joints of the extremities, most commonly on the dorsal surface of the interphalangeal joints (Fig. 34-8). When the lesion is punctured, a glycerin-like substance is exuded. Pain or tenderness accompanies some but not all of these lesions. The cyst has been considered to have a connection with the underlying synovial cavity, but recent work suggests an alteration to the dermal connective tissue in association with a local overproduction of hyaluronic acid. This is the reason for frequent recurrence after surgery.

### *Microscopic findings*

Microscopic examination shows a cyst with a wall composed of fibrous tissue and filled with a mucinous material.

### *Treatment*

Injection of glucocorticoid compounds, for example, triamcinolone diacetate 5 mg./ml., into the cyst cavity is an effective method of therapy.

Surgical excision will usually result in a recurrence.

## Chondrodermatitis nodularis helicis

Chondrodermatitis may occur as a small, chronically tender nodule on the helix or antihelix of the external ear. It is a chronic inflammatory reaction of dermis and epidermis, with or without involvement of underlying cartilage. It may be associated with a history of trauma.

### *Treatment*

Surgical excision is the treatment of choice. Recurrences can be expected in a moderate number of cases.

## Subungual exostosis

Subungual exostosis, an essentially asymptomatic lesion, is significant chiefly for its benign nature. It may be confused with a malignant tumor of the nail bed.

It is a fibrous nodule developing on the distal phalanx of the great toe under the nail, which it pushes up and distorts (Fig. 34-9).

### *Treatment*

Removal of the nail and the tumor, with curettage of the base of the lesion, comprises the method of treatment.

## Neuroma

Neuroma is an unusual, painful, slow-growing tumor composed of bundles of nerve fibers and some connective tissue elements. It is subcutaneous, smooth, and dome shaped and is reddish or bluish in color. Injury may be a causative factor.

### *Treatment*

Treatment is by surgical excision.

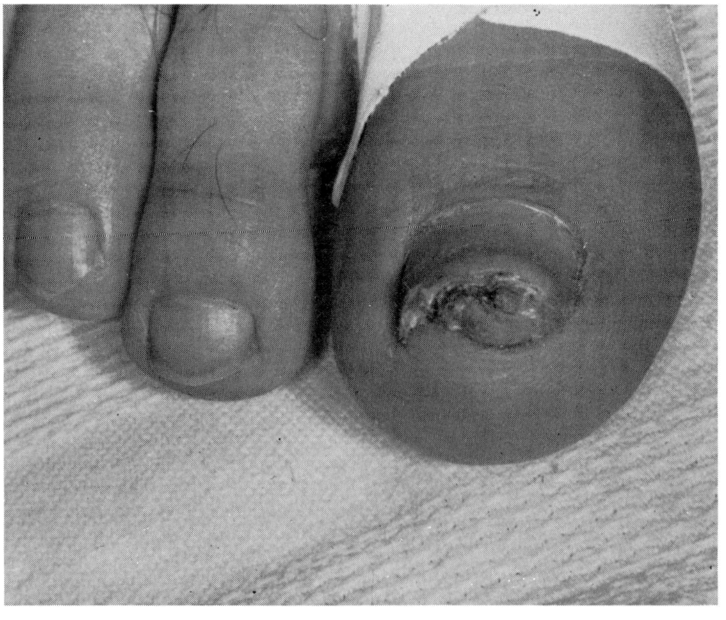

**Fig. 34-9.** Subungual exostosis.

## Neurofibromatosis (von Recklinghausen's disease)

A hereditary disorder of the nervous system, neurofibromatosis is manifested by cutaneous tumors, pigmentation, and neural tumors. It is inherited as a dominant trait and occurs once in 3,000 births.

The disease shows its first tumor formation around the time of puberty, although the pale tan to brown pigmentations have usually been present since birth or early childhood. Pregnancy may produce a rapid proliferation of tumors. Genetic counseling is important in these women. Pregnancy should not have been allowed to occur in the first place.

Pigmentation may assume various appearances. The best-known lesions are café-au-lait spots (Fig. 34-10), which are irregularly shaped, tan to brown, flat asymptomatic deposits of melanin. However, there may be multiple, very small pigmented macules, or freckling in regions such as the axilla or a portion of the thorax. Diffuse bronzing or graying may be apparent.

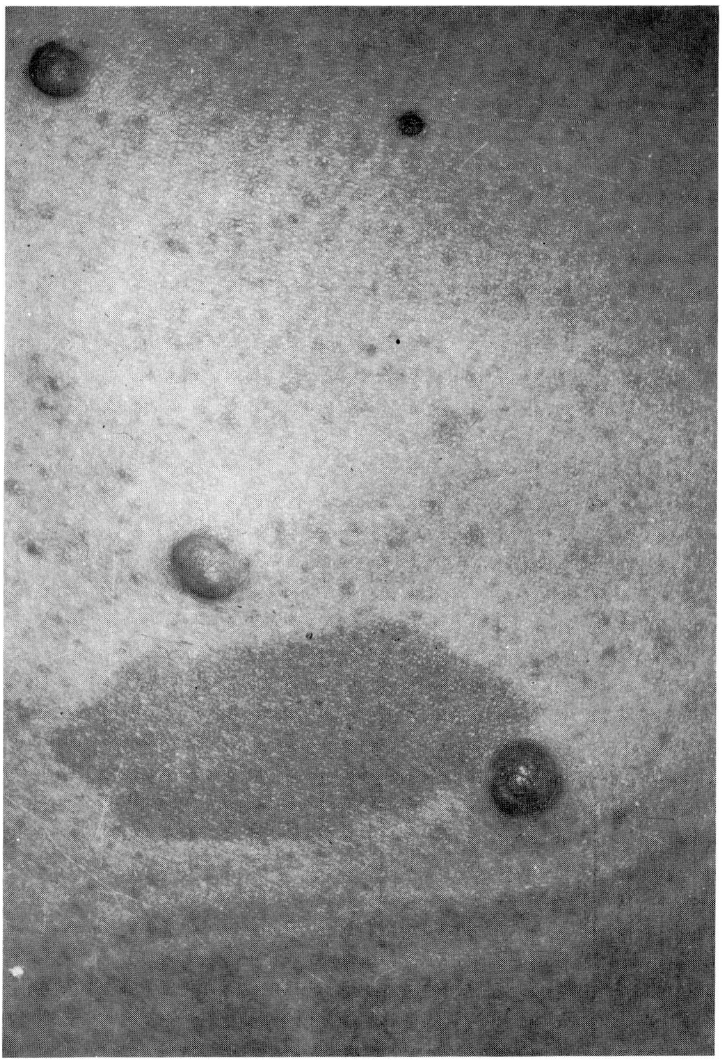

**Fig. 34-10.** Neurofibromatosis with café-au-lait spot. Tumors are soft and flaccid.

The tumors are of nerve-sheath origin and therefore may arise in the subcutaneous tissue of the oral cavity or tongue, in the walls of body cavities, or in internal organs, bones, or central nervous system, producing symptoms from local pressure as they slowly enlarge. The subcutaneous neurofibromas vary from minute lesions to large pendulous tumors. They are flesh colored, pink, blue tinted, or pigmented, with unaffected overlying skin, but have a characteristic flaccidity on palpation, like a half-deflated balloon. They occur at varying depths beneath the skin, some with only a swelling of the surface to identify them, whereas others produce pedunculated lesions.

Pressure from growing tumors may produce bone cysts, intracranial symptoms, deafness. Abnormalities of menstruation, sexual development, pituitary function, thyroid function, and mental retardation are reported.

### *Microscopic findings*

Microscopically, the pigmented lesions are composed of melanin deposition in the basal cell layer and increased numbers of melanocytes. Curiously, the pigment granules developing in the epidermal melanocytes and those delivered to the epidermal cells are very much larger than normal granules. The tumors are composed of very loose, wavy collagen, with a few nerve fibers, and frequently show a mucoid degeneration. Some deeper lesions occasionally undergo malignant degeneration to sarcomas.

### *Treatment*

Treatment consists of surgical excision of those tumors that are causing undesirable symptoms or warrant excision for cosmetic reasons. They should be completely rather than partially removed, although this may produce worrisome technical problems. Neural paralysis, pressure atrophy, and hypervascularity producing overgrowth are all problems.

## Pyogenic granuloma

A rapidly growing, small, soft, papular lesion composed of granulation tissue, pyogenic granuloma usually occurs in children, at the site of trauma. It is red, often pedunculated, and usually less than 1 cm. in diameter (Fig. 34-11). It has a smooth surface that bleeds easily and may have a superficial crust. The lesion is usually single and is most commonly found on the fingers and the face.

### *Microscopic findings*

Microscopically, the lesion consists of proliferating, newly formed capillaries in loose connective tissue.

### *Treatment*

Electrodesiccation under local anesthesia, repeated applications of a silver nitrate stick, or surgical excision may be employed in treatment. The lesion will recur if it is not completely removed.

## Glomus tumor

Glomus tumor is a small growth resulting from the proliferation of glomus cells in the glomus unit, which is a neuromuscular structure that connects an arteriole and venule of the skin, bypassing the capillary bed. It is a small, reddish-purple growth that is extremely tender to pressure and painful with cold. The pain generated is sharp, stabbing, or burning. Spontaneous pain may arise from the lesion. It is a single lesion and is most commonly found beneath the fingernails in women and on the forearm in men.

### *Microscopic findings*

Microscopic examination reveals vascular canals surrounded by a proliferation of glomus cells, which are uniform epithelioid cells with oval or globular nuclei. There is also an increase in the number of nonmyelinated nerve fibrils.

### *Treatment*

Total excision of the lesion is required. It may be difficult to anesthetize successfully. If any part remains, the glomus tumor may recur.

## Angiokeratoma of the scrotum

Angiokeratoma is a dark, purplish red firm lesion, varying from 1 mm. to 1 cm. in size.

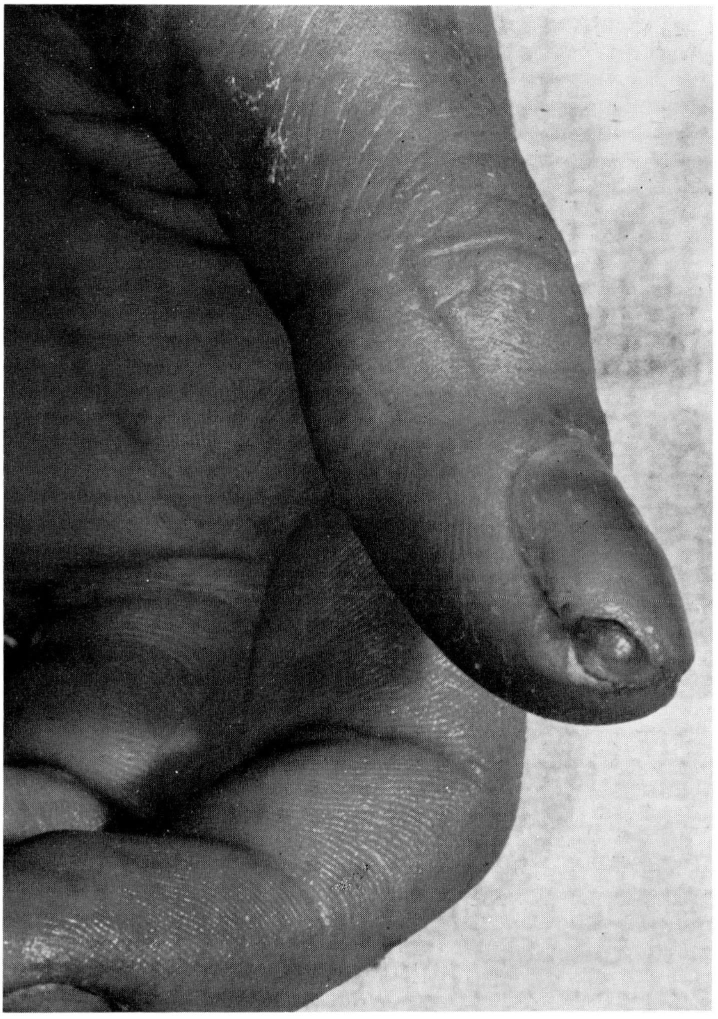

**Fig. 34-11.** Pyogenic granuloma.

The lesion is discrete and multiple, frequently occurring on the scrotum in elderly men. It is asymptomatic and has no association with other disease. There are other rare forms of angiokeratoma.

### *Microscopic findings*

Microscopically, angiokeratoma consists of dilated, thin-walled blood vessels high in the dermal papillae, some with an associated hyperkeratosis. Ectatic vessels from deeper in the dermal papillae communicate with them.

### *Treatment*

When indicated, treatment consists of electrodesiccation or cryotherapy.

## PIGMENTED NEVI (MOLES)

A nevus is a tumor arising from cells present since the embryonic period. Cells composing it are called nevus cells. These cells in adults are present in collections in the epidermis and in the dermis, having migrated to these locations during the developmental period. They may form vari-sized growths, with varying degrees of brown pigmentation, commonly referred to as moles. They are intimately associated with the pigment-producing melanocytes and are of the same neural origin. They are common to all persons, and actually most people have more than a dozen nevi (moles) somewhere on the skin. They vary from 1 or 2 mm. in size to lesions covering a large part of the body surface. They have a remarkable variation in appearance, since they may occur as flat, slightly elevated, dome-shaped, hair-bearing, smooth, or rough-surfaced lesions. Their color ranges from normal skin color through tan, gray, and dark brown to black. Their common characteristic is the possession of nevus cells, which are rounded or polygonal, pale-staining cells in the dermis, the specific location of which leads to the classification of nevi.

For some years, dermatologists have considered that selected nevi of the junctional type are most prone to develop malignant alterations and become malignant melanomas. Clarke has, after thoughtful and valuable study of the problem propounded the concept that all pigmented nevus cell nevi, regardless of type, are composed of normal melanocytes. Some 20% to 30% of malignant melanomas arise from preexisting pigmented nevi, and this can be explained statistically by the increased number of melanocytes at the site of the mole. In other words, the melanocytes in a nevus, or mole, are no more likely to become malignant than those melanocytes elsewhere in the skin. Thus, with the exception of very large inflamed or traumatized nevi, there is no reason to remove these lesions except for cosmetic purposes.

## Signs of malignant change

Signs of malignant change in a mole that demand *immediate total excision* are the following:

1. Enlargement after a long quiescent period
2. Darkening
3. Crusting
4. Bleeding
5. Inflammation
6. Ulceration
7. Appearance of satellite lesions

*There is a tendency for some of these lesions to show such changes during pregnancy, in which case they should be removed.*

## Halo nevus (Fig. 34-12)

The significance of this lesion, which consists of a central pigmented nevus surrounded by a depigmented halo, has only recently

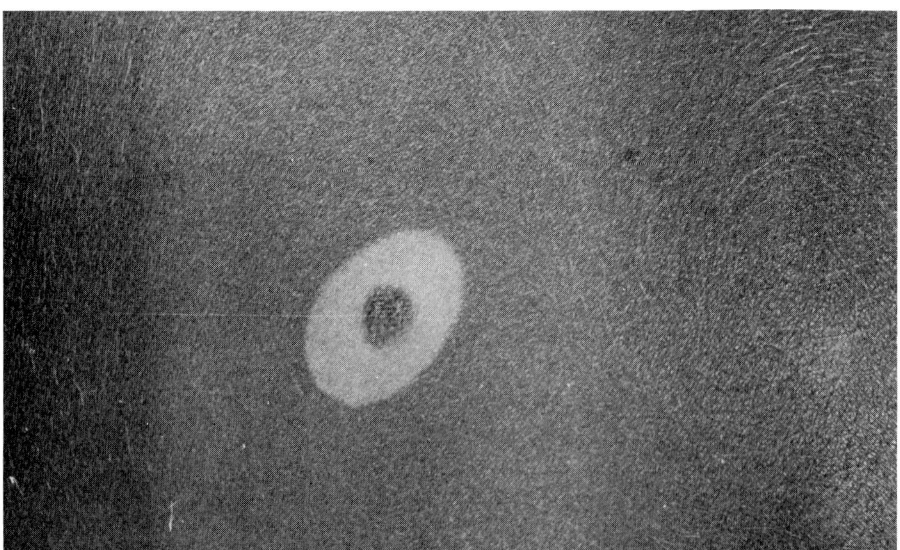

**Fig. 34-12.** Halo nevus. A significant immunological "happening."

been understood. The nevus, or mole, is the focal point of the depigmenting process, which results in destruction of the melanocytes.

*Natural course*

The pigmented mole develops a sharp, oval, or circular depigmented halo, without particular preference as to site or age of the patient. The mole may then show various and sometimes alarming morphological changes, including thickening, darkening, lightening, papule or nodule formation, inflammation, or crusting. It will subsequently disappear, and the halo usually will repigment eventually. The whole process may take years. These nevi are associated with a greater than expected incidence of vitiligo. Kopf reported one patient in whom the halo nevus developed into a malignant melanoma.

*Significance*

Copeman, Lewis, and associates postulate that this process represents an accelerated and successful rejection phase of a pigmented mole developing malignant change. They have demonstrated a circulating antibody against the cytoplasm of melanoma cells in patients with malignant melanoma *and in patients with halo nevi*. At the time of detection of the antimelanoma antibody and the development of the halo, masses of lymphocytes are

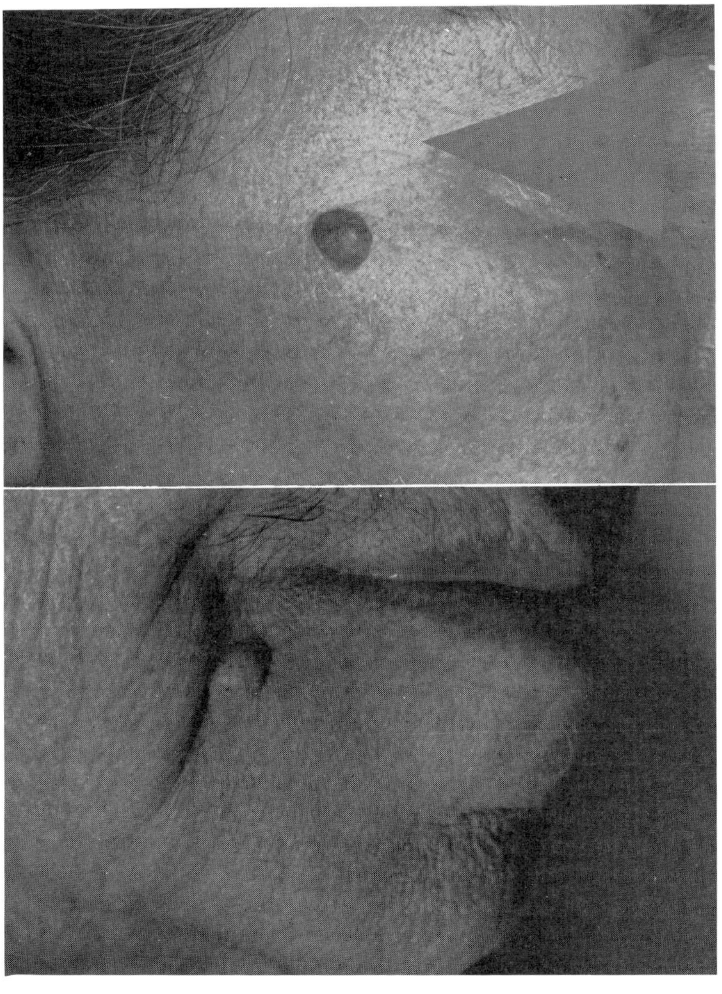

**Fig. 34-13.** Benign intradermal nevi.

seen to infiltrate the nevus. Similar areas of lightening and depigmentation occur in the lesions and in the vicinity of malignant melanoma lesions, particularly superficial spreading melanoma.

## Intradermal nevus

Nevus cells wholly in the dermis characterize a benign lesion, an intradermal nevus (Fig. 34-13). The pale, fairly uniform cells are in clusters and cords in the upper dermis and are surrounded by collagen bundles, with little or no inflammation. Most dome-shaped and hair-bearing nevi are intradermal nevi. Most intradermal nevi, however, possess some junctional nevus cell elements. This does not alter the clinical fact that these flesh-colored or pigmented, dome-shaped, and hair-bearing lesions are benign lesions that do not tend to become malignant.

### *Treatment*

No medical reason exists for removal of an unchanging intradermal nevus, and when treated it is for cosmetic reasons only. One may excise it in toto or may partially remove it by excising (shaving off) that area above the skin surface, leaving a level surface. Although this procedure does not allow a complete examination of the dermal extent of the lesion, it does allow microscopic examination of the most important area, the dermoepidermal junction, where most melanomas are identified in their earliest stages. Light electrodesiccation of the base then prevents bleeding and produces a good cosmetic result. All excised portions of any pigmented nevus must be sent for histological examination.

If hairs are present in a benign intradermal nevus, they are best removed by electrolysis before treatment of the nevus itself.

## Junction nevus

Nevus cells lining the dermoepidermal junction, usually in circumscribed nests or clusters, characterize a junction nevus, and the activity and position of these cells may provide the recommendations for removal of the lesion. Pigmented nevi of the palms, soles (Fig. 34-14), genitalia, and mucous membranes are almost always junction nevi. In addition, flat or slightly elevated dark brown or black nevi are usually junction nevi. Pigmented lesions of the mucous membranes, as well as those subject to repeated trauma, should probably be removed prophylactically. One wonders if the superficial location of these pigmented cells exposes them to more actinic damage, trauma, and other carcinogenic factors.

### *Treatment*

Removal of a junction nevus, if indicated, should be total, employing either punch biopsy or scalpel biopsy. The tissue should then be examined histologically as a routine measure.

## Compound nevus

Compound nevus is a lesion that has nevus cells both deep in the dermis and also lining the dermoepidermal junction. From the clinical appearance of the cutaneous lesion, it is not possible to predict which has junctional elements and which does not.

### *Treatment*

As with junction nevi, the compound nevus should be totally removed if any part of it is to be removed.

## Large hairy nevus

Large hairy nevus may be present from birth, is without hair for the first years of life (Fig. 34-15), and may cover as much as half the skin surface. Although it has been regarded as a benign lesion, there is now evidence that the large, hairy, extensive pigmented nevus (bathing suit nevus) should also be watched for signs of malignant change. A significant number of these lesions, between 2% and 14%, will develop into malignant melanoma. Any questionable area should be excised and sent for microscopic study.

### *Treatment*

The nevus should be observed for signs of irritation or change. As the malignant potential of melanocytes seems to bear a direct relationship to the number and perhaps superficial location of these cells, lesions such as

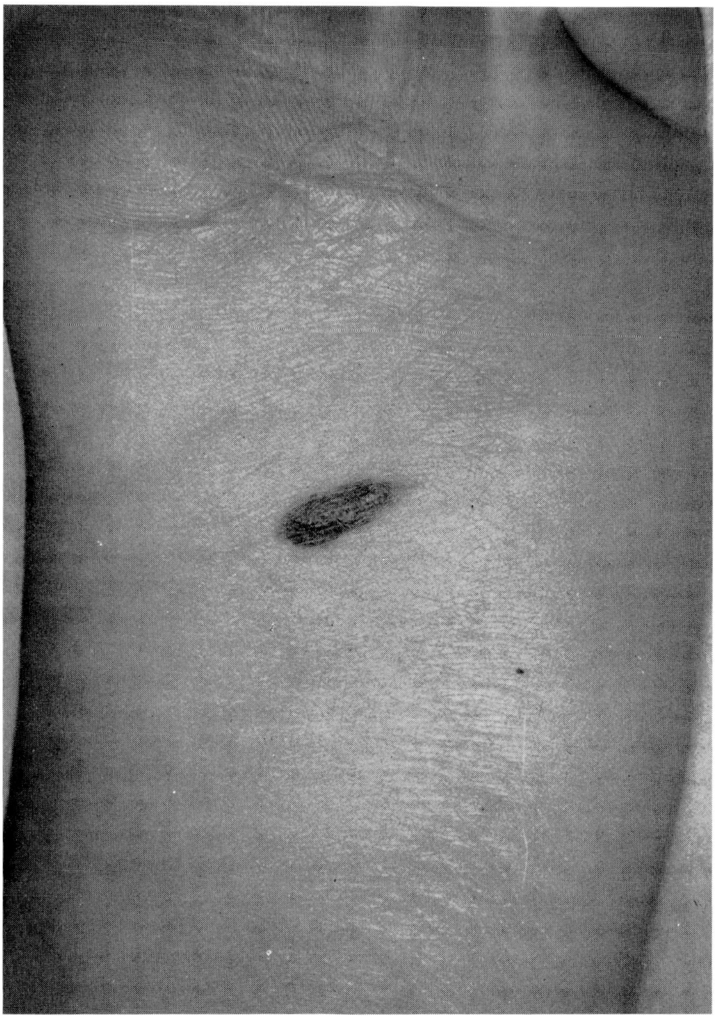

**Fig. 34-14.** Junction nevus on sole.

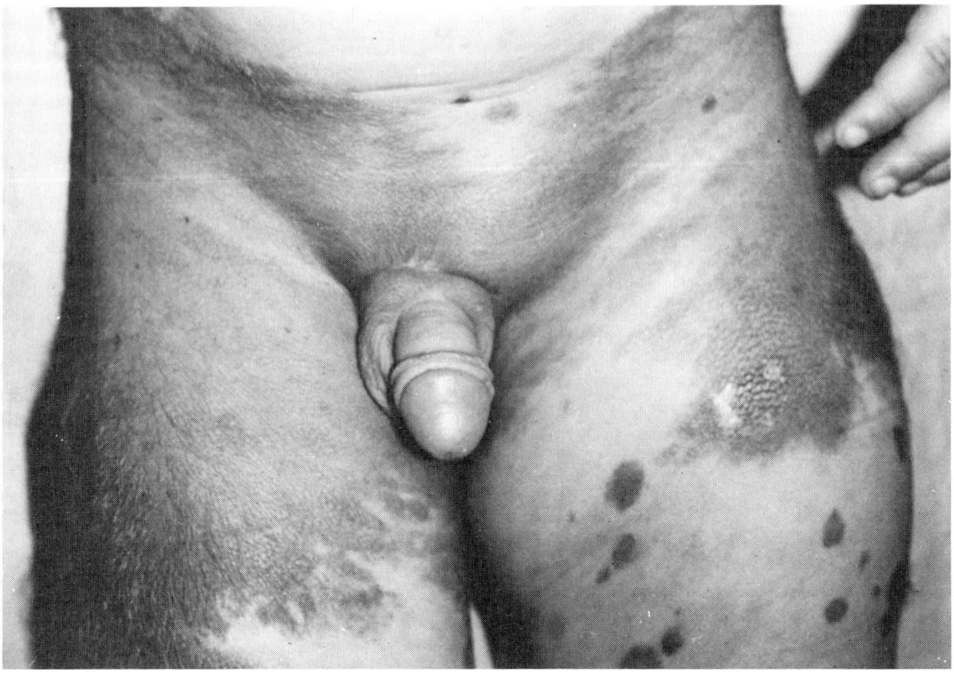

**Fig. 34-15.** Large hairy nevus, or bathing suit nevus. Must be watched for malignant changes.

these, with very large numbers of melanocytes, have a greater chance of becoming malignant. Serious consideration should be given to complete removal of the nevus and replacement by full-thickness skin grafting.

## Juvenile nevus (benign juvenile melanoma)

Juvenile nevus is a smooth, nodular or papular, lightly pigmented lesion arising before puberty. It has a predilection for the face and the lower extremities. It is a very active compound nevus, with enhanced junctional activity. It has in the past been mistaken for a malignant lesion on microscopic examination, because of its great similarity to an active adult malignant melanoma. *It is a benign lesion.* If such a lesion is biopsied, the age of the patient must be stated in the report, so that proper consideration may be given to this diagnosis by the pathologist.

### *Treatment*

Treatment consists of observation only.

## Blue nevus

This pigmented nodular lesion possesses a blue color because of the concentration of melanin and its depth below the epidermis. It occurs usually as a solitary lesion on the dorsal surface of hands, on the face, or on the buttocks. The lesion is present from birth and characteristically remains unchanged. The *nevus of Ota*, a rare pigmented lesion involving the sclera, cornea, orbital area, and retro-orbital tissues, is a variant of blue nevus.

Histologically, the melanin pigment that gives the lesion its color is within the nevus cells lying in groups and whorls in the dermis.

### *Treatment*

Because malignant change is such an extreme rarity and because the depth of the lesion makes a cosmetic defect likely, treatment is not ordinarily indicated.

## Mongolian spot

A dusky blue pigmentation, blending into surrounding normal skin and appearing chiefly in the lumbosacral area of Oriental infants, is known as a mongolian spot. It may also be seen in darkskinned races, but rarely in whites. The lesions vary in size from a centimeter to many centimeters. They are asymptomatic and disappear, for the most part, during childhood.

### *Microscopic findings*

Nests of spindle-shaped nevus cells, many of which contain melanin, are shown by microscopic examination to be lying in the mid-dermis.

### *Treatment*

Treatment is not indicated.

#### REFERENCES

Breza, T., Taylor, R., and Eaglestein, W. H.: Noninflammatory destruction of actinic keratoses by fluorouracil, Arch. Dermatol. **112**:1265, 1976.
**Recommends sequential topical application of 5-fluorouracil and triamcinolone to reduce inflammatory reaction.**

Cohen, I. K., and Diegelmann, R. L.: The biology of keloid and hypertrophic scar and the influence of corticosteroids, Clin. Plast. Surg. **4**:297,1977.
**An approach involving fibroblast growth study.**

Copeman, P. W., Lewis, M. G., Phillips, T. M., et al.: Immunological association of the halo nevus with cutaneous malignant melanoma, Br. J. Dermatol. **88**:127, 1973.
**Anti–melanoma cell cytoplasmic antibody present in resolving halo nevi.**

Epstein, E., and Epstein, E., Jr.: Skin surgery, ed. 4. Springfield, Ill., 1977, Charles C Thomas, Publisher.
**A thorough and nonpartisan description of available cutaneous surgical techniques.**

Ketchum, L. D.: Hypertrophic scars and keloids, Clin. Plast. Surg. **4**:301, 1977.
**Experienced, practical, imaginative.**

Krebs, J. A., Roenigk, H. H., Jr., Deodhar, S. D., et al: Halo nevus: Competent surveillance of potential melanoma? Cleveland Clin. Q. **43**:11, 1976.
**The prevailing opinion explained.**

Laurentaci, G., and Dioguardi, D.: HLA antigens in keloids and hypertrophic scars, Arch. Dermatol. **113**:1726, 1977.
**HL-A B14 and HL-A Bw16 carry with them an increased risk of developing keloids.**

Linares, H. A., Kischer, C. W., Dobrkovsky, M., et al.: The histiotypic organization of the hypertrophic scar in humans, J. Invest. Dermatol. **59**:323, 1972.
**A hypertrophic scar is made up of nodules or centers of highly stellate fibroblasts where the most active scarring occurs.**

Main, R. A.: Neurofibromatosis, In Maddin, S., editor: Current dermatologic management, ed. 2, St. Louis, 1975, The C. V. Mosby Co., p. 225.
**A clinically oriented presentation readily solving management problems.**

Mehregan, A. H., and Mishima, Y.: Pigmented lesions, benign and malignant. In Maddin, S., editor: Current dermatologic management., ed. 2, St. Louis, 1975, The C. V. Mosby Co., p. 244.
**Succinct, authoritative.**

Pearse, A. D., and Marks, R.: Actinic keratoses and the epidermis on which they arise, Br. J. Dermatol. **96**:45, 1977.
**Actinic keratoses occur on an already half abnormal epidermis.**

Shelley, W. B.: Keratoacanthoma, In Consultations in dermatology, 2, Philadelphia, 1974, The W. B. Saunders Co., p. 24.
**An impressive clinical presentation.**

# CHAPTER 35

# Malignant tumors

## EPIDERMAL TUMORS

### Malignant melanoma

Melanoma is the most malignant primary cutaneous tumor. It is the leading killer in dermatological disease and is increasing with an anticipated 8,000 deaths per year by 1980. Its behavior varies in each race.

#### *Natural course*

About one tenth of malignant melanomas have microscopic evidence of nevus cells present. One fourth of these patients remembers a lesion present for less than 3 years prior to the diagnosis of malignant melanoma. Clark suggests that melanomas arise from pigmented nevi and from melanocytes elsewhere in the skin in simple proportion to the numbers of melanocytes in each location. He believes that there is no basic difference in malignant potential between the melanocytes in either area.

The potential for malignancy in congenital nevi is not clear, but the large "giant" nevi, often hairy in adult life, have the greatest potential. (Fig. 34-15). Melanomas arising from 2% to 42% of these "bathing trunk" nevi have been rcported. Most of these melanomas (over half) arise in the first decade, one tenth in the next decade, and one third after that.

The change from a benign to a malignant lesion produces so few warning symptoms that it is often unobserved. The classic signs that herald the transformation are rapid change in size or color, development of inflammation, bleeding, ulceration, and appearance of pigment around the lesion. These are, however, usually signs that it is already too late.

The diagnosis of malignant melanoma from a pigmented nevus at a time when an aggressive approach will be beneficial is carefully delineated by Mihm, Clark, and Reed and includes (1) subtle changes in color, (2) loss of surface markings, and (3) irregularities in border (Plate 53).

Malignant melanomas are classified into (1) *lentigo maligna melanoma*, (2) *superficial spreading melanoma*, and (3) *nodular melanoma*. An excellent series of clinical photographs illustrating these lesions and their variations and behaviors can be found in The New England Journal of Medicine (November 8, 1973), and Dr. From's 27-picture art gallery in Modern Medicine of Canada, November 1977.

Levels of invasion of these tumors are very important in regard to surgical or radiological therapy and are directly related to survival (Clark, McGovern). Thus the initial superficial nature and knowledgeable prompt therapy of types 1 and 2 of these tumors reassures the physician of the success of his treatment.

***Lentigo maligna melanoma*** (Fig. 35-1). Lentigo maligna, or Hutchinson's freckle, is a tan macule or patch ocurring most frequently in elderly persons on the side of the face. It constitutes 12% of malignant melanomas and follows a slow, steady progression through enlargement, mottling, darkening, and eventual thickening and nodule formation. The color gradually darkens overall but, in the process, may demonstrate flecks of irregular pigmentation. The initial flat stain, which may rarely be amelanotic (pink toned) eventually forms papules and then nodules, often so unobtrusively the patient professes to be unaware of the change. Lightening of pigmentation may occur as well. This whole process takes years,

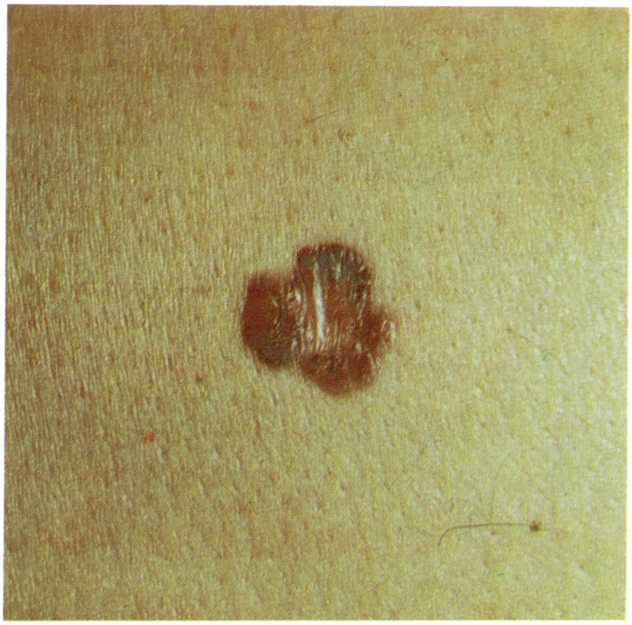

**Plate 53**

Superficial spreading melanoma. Horizontal spread and limited to epidermis at first. Note irregular, notched border.

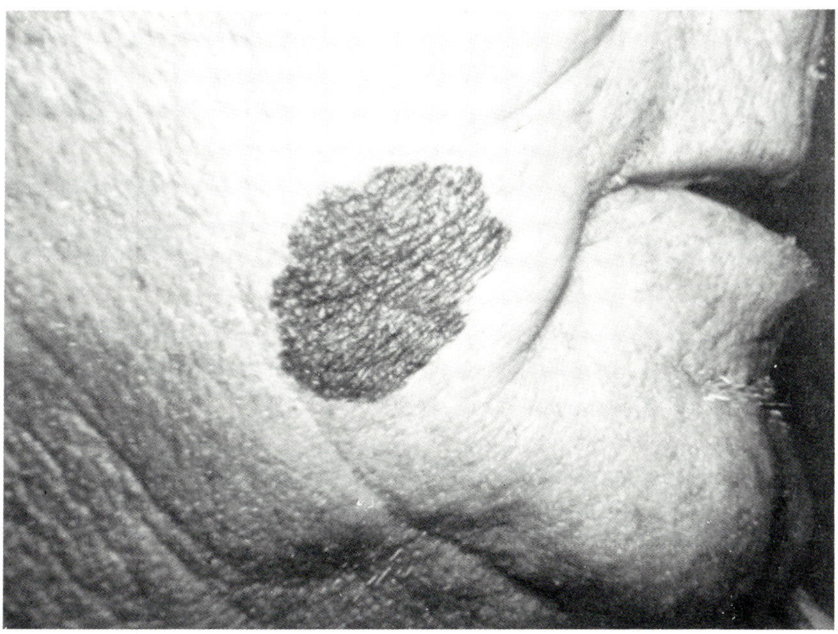

**Fig. 35-1.** Lentigo maligna melanoma. Part of a long, slow process of development into malignancy, before truly nodular changes became apparent.

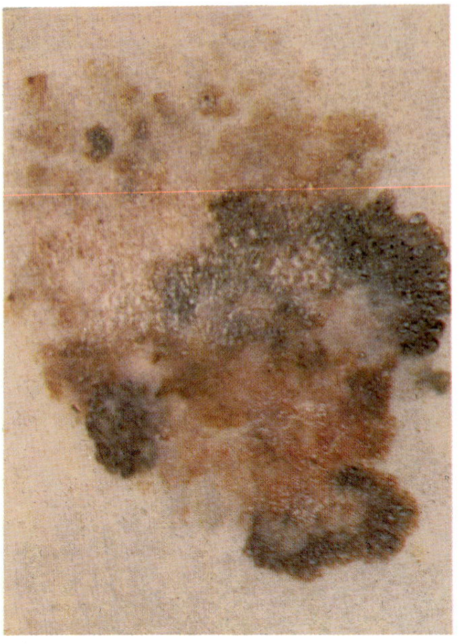

**Plate 54**

Superficial spreading melanoma—red, brown, and black with gray-white areas of regression on midback.

and not all of these lesions eventuate into invasive melanoma. This lesion is amenable to local excision, with good prognosis throughout most of its course.

***Superficial spreading melanoma.*** This lesion constitutes 55% of Clark's 208 malignant melanomas. It begins in middle age and has no predilection for specific areas of the skin. It may be flat or very slightly elevated. It has an irregularly spreading border and demonstrates a play of colors from tan to yellow and from red to dark brown or black (Plate 54). It begins as a small pigmented lesion that may, because of a blue hue in its brown-tan milieu, irregular border, smoothing out or interruption of normal skin markings, and disordered appearance, betray its malignant nature. Here, also, lightening may occur. Although this tumor is confined to the epidermis and even the superficial dermis, the prognosis with adequate local excision is excellent. With further extension downward, the prognosis worsens rapidly.

***Nodular melanoma.*** The characteristic nodular melanoma, on the other hand, is an invasive lesion. It is pigmented, round to irregular, slightly elevated, and embedded beneath the surface (Fig. 35-2) and constitutes 30% of malignant melanomas. The color usually consists of shades of gray and gray-blue on the background of brown to black. A pigmented halo is not uncommon. Amelanotic melanomas possess the gray-blue overlay despite a pink to red basic color. The surface is smooth, rounded or slightly lobulated, and rarely verrucous. The border is less irregular than with the slower growing melanomas.

### *Regional vagaries*

***Palms and soles.*** These areas are less affected in whites than tradition would indicate. The pigmented races have an increased incidence. Lesions are brown-blue-black, flat, and slightly roughened. The amelanotic lesions may be mistaken for pyogenic granulomas.

***Nail bed.*** Streaks are brown, black, blue, tan, or white, and there are split nails or ingrown nails. They have been bilateral (Mihm). Biopsy adequately.

***Exposed areas.*** The sun is the chief trigger to malignant change in the nonpigmented races. A clear relationship has been established between latitude and melanoma death rate. The tumor is unpredictable and widespread from only a minute primary lesion (Fig. 35-3). Regional lymph nodes are involved early.

A study in Australia on 400 cutaneous melanomas showed that over 80% of the lesions were 2 cm. or less. Melanomas in blacks are much more virulent than in whites, as are most skin cancers.

The incidence of the tumor is higher in females than in males and hits a peak around the menopausal years. It is very rare before puberty. Most lesions occur on the back in males, and on the lower extremities in females. Approximately 15% of these tumors appear on the head and neck. *Lentigo maligna melanoma* is an exposed area tumor for the most part. *Superficial spreading melanomas* are anywhere, but chiefly on the back, head

A

B

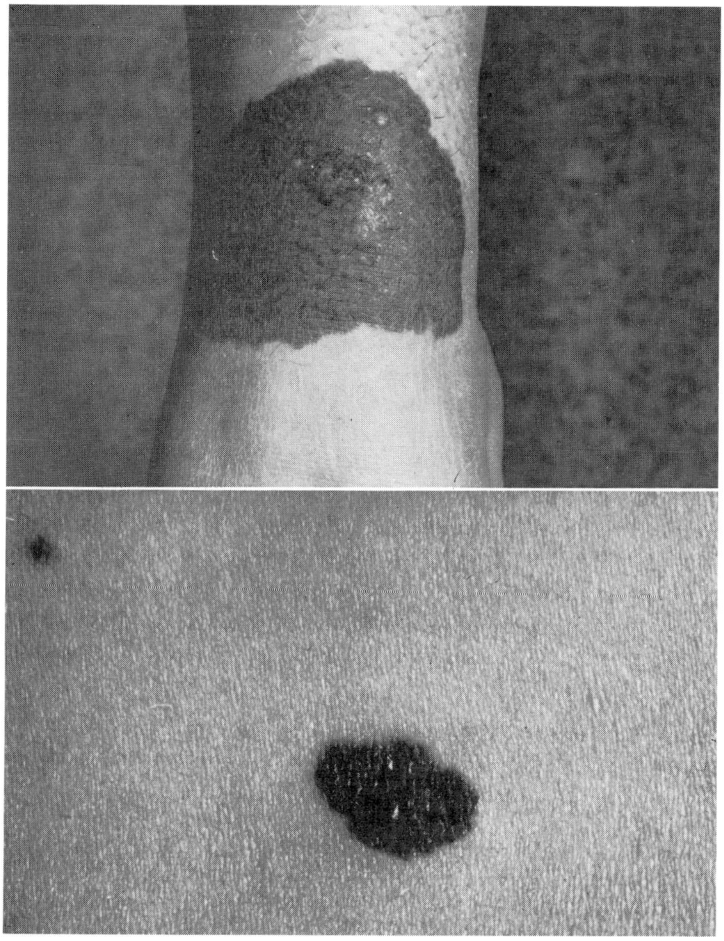

**Fig. 35-2. A,** Nodular malignant melanoma in center of congenital nevus on ankle. **B,** Nodular malignant melanoma, with blue-black color, verrucous surface, and irregular border.

and neck, leg and foot. *Nodular melanomas* are more furtive, since they appear on the sole of the foot, leg, buttocks, and scalp. Lesions on mucous membranes are uncommon but dangerous because of the delay in diagnosis. Microscopic examination indicates most mucous membrane melanomas are superficial spreading melanomas in behavior, and 50% are amelanotic.

Scalp melanomas have a particularly poor prognosis because they are first of all hidden, and the rich vascular and lymphatic drainage aids metastases.

*Statistics leave no doubt that the most significant feature for the patient's survival lies in an early diagnosis and immediate therapy.*

### *Pertinent information*

After observing homograft rejection, Thomas, as quoted by Burnet, conceived immunological surveillance as a host defense against neoplasia. This has been used more effectively in malignant melanomas than in other tumors.

For many years, evidence has been accumulated that there is a host reaction to this tumor, first measured nonspecifically by the cellular infiltrate surrounding the malignant cells and by observations of regression and

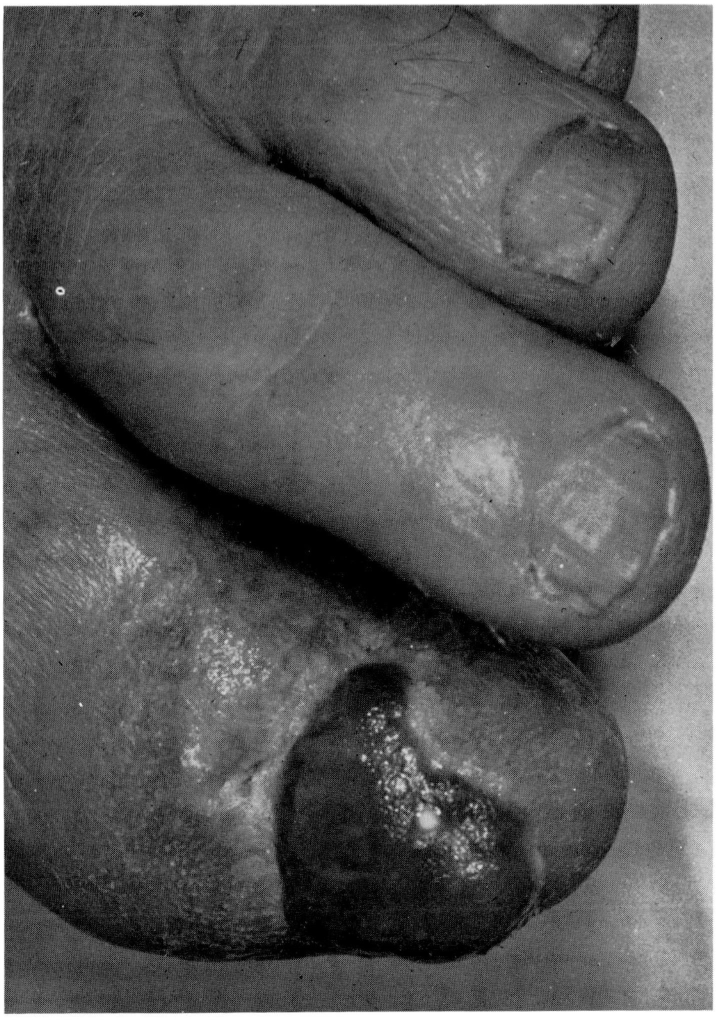

**Fig. 35-3.** Malignant melanoma. This began with minute lesion of large toe.

spontaneous disappearance of both tumor and metastases. Also, many melanomas remain localized for long periods of time before invasion. Subsequently, cytotoxic antibodies against tumor cells were identified. It was found that stimulation of the T-cell system of lymphocytes in sensitized subjects by BCG or other agents could be directed against the invading melanoma. There are thus both circulating antibodies and cell-mediated immunity used by the host against cancer that can be commandeered by a therapist and used to destroy melanoma cells. Encouraging results of this form of therapy combined with surgical resection of larger masses of tumor have been reported. Further encouragement arises from Conrad's study of 663 patients with invasive melanoma. He reported 5-year tumor-free survivals of 33 patients with metastatic melanoma.

Complications from BCG therapy include systemic BCG dissemination in an anergic individual, with granulomatous hepatitis and infection of lungs and other organs. Vaccinia virus, purified protein derivative of tuberculin (PPD), dinitrochlorobenzene (DNCB), and other nonspecific immune potentiating agents are being evaluated at present.

The following few facts in our currently incomplete knowledge emerge:

1. Immunotherapy can be a successful adjunct to chemotherapy.
2. The most favorable response occurs when the host's tumor load is reduced to the lowest possible mass by surgery.
3. Some forms of immunotherapy may block antibodies and enhance tumor growth.

### *Microscopic findings*

The level of invasion of the dermis becomes most crucial when one considers survival rates after diagnosis. Clark has divided the invasion of the tumor into six levels, each very closely allied to prognosis varying from almost 80% survival to 8% in 5 years.

***Lentigo maligna melanoma.*** There is an increased number of melanocytes in the basal cell layer, to the extreme of complete replacement by these cells. The melanocytes are pleomorphic and atypical. They extend along hair follicles and sebaceous glands for years contained within the epidermis. Initial spread is lateral through the epidermis.

***Superficial spreading melanoma.*** There are uniform, large malignant melanocytes lacking the pleomorphism of lentigo maligna melanoma. There are nests and clumps of invasive cells of a clearly malignant nature. The spread is essentially through the epidermis, although individual Pagetoid cells invade the upper dermis and the hair follicles. Initial spread is lateral through the epidermis.

***Nodular melanoma.*** Clearly malignant melanocytes arising at the dermoepidermal junction invade the dermis directly. *There is no lateral spread through the epidermis.*

Because of the extreme variation in the histological changes in these lesions, we cannot emphasize strongly enough that evaluation should be performed by an *experienced* dermatopathologist before radical therapeutic measures are undertaken. Series of melanoma statistics in the literature reveal many erroneous diagnoses in patients suspected of having had malignant melanoma (Epstein). The time saved by performing immediate extensive surgery before a careful and accurate diagnosis and assessment can be made does not justify unnecessary mutilation.

### *Differential diagnosis*

***Benign pigmented nevus.*** Present since early life, a benign pigmented nevus changes only very slowly if at all.

***Seborrheic keratosis.*** Very slowly growing and stationary, the pigmented warty lesions of seborrheic keratosis have a "stuck-on" appearance and are chiefly to be found on the chest, back, and temporal area.

***Pigmented basal cell epithelioma.*** Pigmented basal cell epithelioma is slow growing and elevated, with a distinct border. A biopsy identifies this lesion.

***Juvenile melanoma.*** A benign lesion arising before puberty, juvenile melanoma may closely resemble a malignant melanoma microscopically. It is unrelated immunologically to malignant melanoma. It occurs on the face, arms, and trunk.

### *Biopsy procedure*

Exposed or large pigmented lesions probably benign, with a possibility of malignancy, can be safely biopsied without fear of spread. The danger of a small biopsy is in missing the malignant portion.

A biopsy of a probable malignant melanoma should be total excision and microscopic examination of the whole lesion. Although it is permissible to biopsy a benign-appearing lesion, it is not recommended that such a procedure be carried out in a pigmented lesion demonstrating possible malignant transformation. The procedure of "shaving" the projecting portion of a pigmented nevus for diagnostic purposes does not permit full microscopic assessment of the dermal portion for malignant changes.

### *Treatment*

Treatment of a histopathologically proved malignant melanoma now depends on the level of invasion, the cell type, the host response, the presence of metastases, and other factors. Adequate surgical excision is the first choice for noninvading lesions. For nodular, invasive lesions and for those with clinical evidence of metastases, it still may well be the selected therapy since these are not contraindications.

Gumport and Harris of New York University recommend for treatment of localized melanoma: Wide and deep excision of primary site with 5 cm. margin when possible. No covering of excision site defects *by flaps*. This may conceal a recurrence. Should lymph nodes be removed prophylactically? Not for levels I and II or lentigo maligna melanoma. Not if primary site drained to several groups of nodes. Not in presence of serious concomitant disease, old age, or distant metastases. When nodes are involved clinically and confirmed microscopically, the survival rate falls to 10%. Treatment of metastasizing, complicated melanoma must be highly individualized.

There is no question but that immunotherapy is yet in its infancy, though some control of the disease by this means is possible. Surgical removal of the tumor burden, followed by continued chemotherapy and immunological manipulation of host response would seem to bear the greatest potential for the immediate future.

## REFERENCES

Barnes, H. M., Calnan, C. D., Sarkany, I.: Malignant melanoma: a 20 year survey, Clin. Exp. Dermatol. **1**:353, 1976.
**A very revealing survey covering 83 patients over 20 years.**

Blois, S., and Epstein, W. L.: Melanoma—value of early detection and treatment, Postgrad. Med. **61**:82, 1977.
**Data from 975 patients.**

Bodurtha, A. J., Berkelhammer, J., Kim, Y. H., et al.: A clinical, histologic and immunologic study of a case of metastatic malignant melanoma undergoing spontaneous remission, Cancer **37**:735, 1976.
**Cancer in retreat. Lymphocytotoxicity destroyed the melanoma cells.**

Burnet, F. M.: The concepts of immunological surveillance, Prog. Exp. Tumor Res. **13**:1, 1970.
**A primary mechanism for national defense against neoplasia as well as microorganisms and parasites.**

Clark, W. H., Jr., From, L., Bernardino, E. A., and Mihm, M. C.: The histogenesis and biologic behavior of primary human malignant melanoma of the skin, Cancer Res. **29**:705, 1969.
**Salutary combination of concerned clinicians and computers.**

Conrad, F. G.: Cures achieved in patients with metastatic malignant melanoma of the skin, Cancer **30**:144, 1972.
**Important factor of unpredictability can be favorable in this disease.**

Conrad, F. G.: Treatment of malignant melanoma, Arch. Surg. **104**:587, 1972.
**Twenty years of experience, 640 patients, comparing wide excision alone with lymphadenectomy. Clinically involved by lymph nodes is the deciding factor.**

Cosman, B., Heddle, S. B., and Crikelair, G. F.: The increasing incidence of melanoma, Plast. Reconstr. Surg. **57**:50, 1976.
**Increased sun exposure is again critical factor.**

Davis, N. C., Herron, J. J., and McLeod, G. R.: Malignant melanoma in Queensland: analysis of 400 skin lesions, Lancet **2**:407, 1966.
**Over 80% were 2 cm. or less, yet one half had clinically involved lymph nodes. Over two thirds were invasive (nodular).**

deGast, G. C., The, T. H., Koops, H. S., et al.: Humoral and cell-mediated immune response in patients with malignant melanoma, Cancer **36**:1289, 1975.
**Defects in lymphocyte function are related to subsequent tumor growth.**

Epstein, E., Bragg, K., and Linden, G.: Biopsy and prognosis of malignant melanoma, J.A.M.A. **208**:1369, 1969.
**559 patients with black lesions: 7.1% were malignant melanomas, 12 were proved to be such.**

From, L.: Malignant melanoma: atlas of clinical appearance and differential diagnosis, Mod. Med. Canada **32**:1423, 1977.
**A superb collection of clinical pictures.**

Gumport, S. L., and Harris M. N.: Melanoma of the skin. In Andrade, R., Gumport, S. L., Popkin, G. L., Rees, T. D., editors: Cancer of the skin, Vol. 2, Philadelphia, 1976, W. B. Saunders Co., p. 950.
**A good overview, including recommendations for specific treatment.**

Gutterman, J. U., Mavligit, G., Reed, R., et al.: Immunology and immunotherapy of human malignant melanoma: historic review and perspectives for the future, Seminars in Oncology **2**:155, 1975.
**A realistic appraisal; 227 references.**

Kaplan, E.: The risk of malignancy in large congenital nevi, Plast. Reconstr. Surg. **53**:421, 1974.
**From 2% to 42%: 60% develop within the first 10 years.**

Leading article: Treatment of malignant melanoma, Br. Med. J. **1**:306, 1973.
**A review of the presently available therapy.**

Lewis, M. G., Ikonopisov, R. L., Nairn, R. C., et al.:

Tumour-specific antibodies in human malignant melanoma and their relationship to the extent of the disease, Br. Med. J. 4:547, 1969.
**The exciting news that 80% of unselected patients with melanoma had autoantibodies if the disease was localized; if not, the antibodies had disappeared.**

McGovern, V. J.: Spontaneous regression of melanoma, Pathology 7:91, 1975.
**A look at the favorable side of this often lethal growth.**

McGovern. V. J., Mihm, M. C., Bailly, C., et al.: The classification of malignant melanoma and its histologic reporting, Cancer 32:1446, 1973.
**A classification and nomenclature in a standardized form suitable for international use.**

Mihm, M. C., Clark, W. H., and Reed, R. J.: The clinical diagnosis of malignant melanoma, Seminars in Oncology 2:105, 1975.
**Meticulous clinical detail.**

Mihm, M. C., Fitzpatrick, T. B., Brown, M. L., et al.: Early detection of primary cutaneous malignant melanoma. A color atlas, N. Engl. J. Med. 289:989, 1973.
**A duplication of authentic color of melanoma types.**

Rosenberg, E. B., Kanner, S. P., and Schwartzman, R. J.: Systemic infection following BCG therapy, Arch. Intern. Med. 134:769, 1974.
**Systemic BCG infection in an anergic individual.**

Wanebo, H. J., Woodruff, J., and Fortner, J. G.: Malignant melanoma of the extremities: a clinicopathologic study using levels of invasion (microstage), Cancer 35:666, 1975.
**There are indications that measurement by ocular micrometer may offer best criteria for estimating prognosis of tumor.**

## Basal cell epithelioma (basal cell carcinoma)

Basal cell epithelioma, a locally eroding malignancy, accounts for approximately 65% of all skin cancers.

### *Natural course*

The most common variety of basal cell epithelioma begins as a papule that enlarges peripherally. It soon develops a central depression, may become crusted, and bleeds easily. At times the central area may become necrotic and depressed, leading to ulcerations and the classical *rodent ulcer*. Close examination of the border shows that it is translucent and elevated, with a smooth shiny appearance on which fine telangiectatic vessels may be found (Fig. 35-4).

The lesion tends to be asymptomatic. In 90% of cases the lesion occurs in the area between the hairline and the upper lip, but it never occurs on the palms or soles. This lesion is usually single, but under certain circumstances more than one may be present. Occasionally one sees patients with an inherited tendency to multiple recurrent basal cell epitheliomas.

This is a locally invasive cancer that destroys underlying and adjacent tissue. After a prolonged period, cartilage and bone may be involved. It rarely, if ever, metastasizes.

Safai and Good, however, recount a remarkable provocative case with immunodeficiency and metastasizing basal and squamous cell carcinoma. They propose that there may have been a transition from one to the other.

### *Pertinent information*

Although not unequivocably confirmed as the sole cause of basal cell epitheliomas, the major factor seems to be prolonged sun exposure. The greatest natural inherent protection is pigmentation, as shown by the sharply decreased incidence in blacks and in Oriental races, in a ratio directly proportional to the degree of the pigmentation. Basal cell epithelioma may also develop at the site of excessive x-ray exposure, lupus erythematosus lesions, and thermal burns. Basal cell epithelioma occurs most frequently in blondes and redheads. The incidence is greater in males. Basal cell epitheliomas have been considered to occur most frequently in the elderly. Recently, however, the incidence has increased in the younger age group, because of greater sun exposure. Also other carcinogens are enhanced by sun exposure, for example, x radiation. Experimentally, the action spectrum between 280 and 320 nm, seems most likely the carcinogenic as well as sunburn range.

### *Variants*

There are several distinct varieties of basal cell epithelioma.

***Superficial multiple basal cell epithelioma.*** These are flat, red, scaling, macular lesions

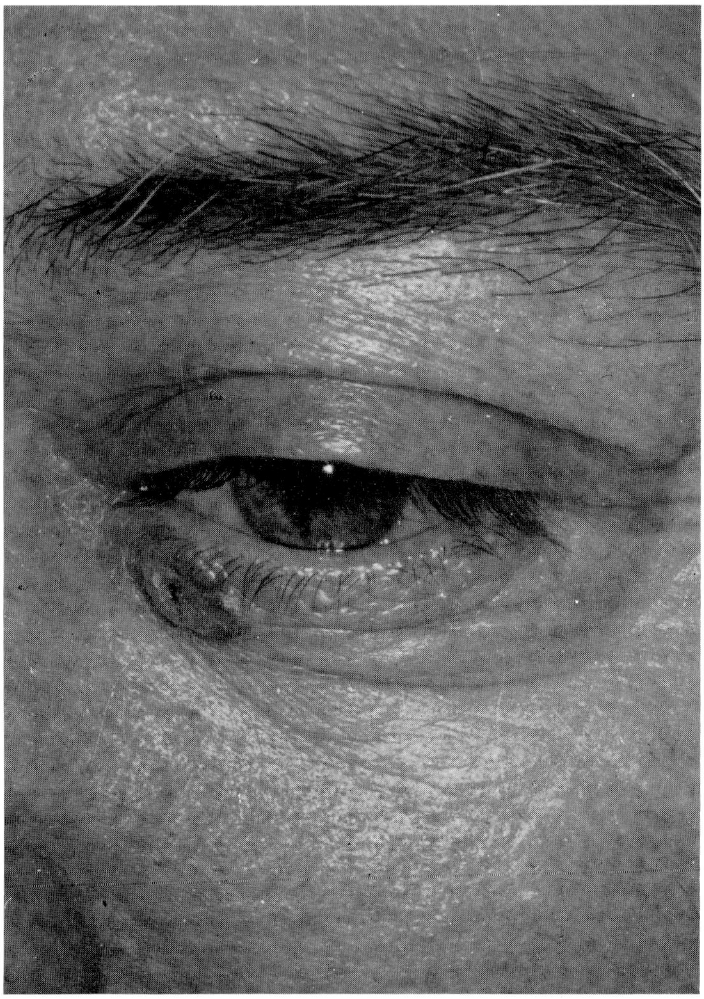

**Fig. 35-4.** Basal cell epithelioma.

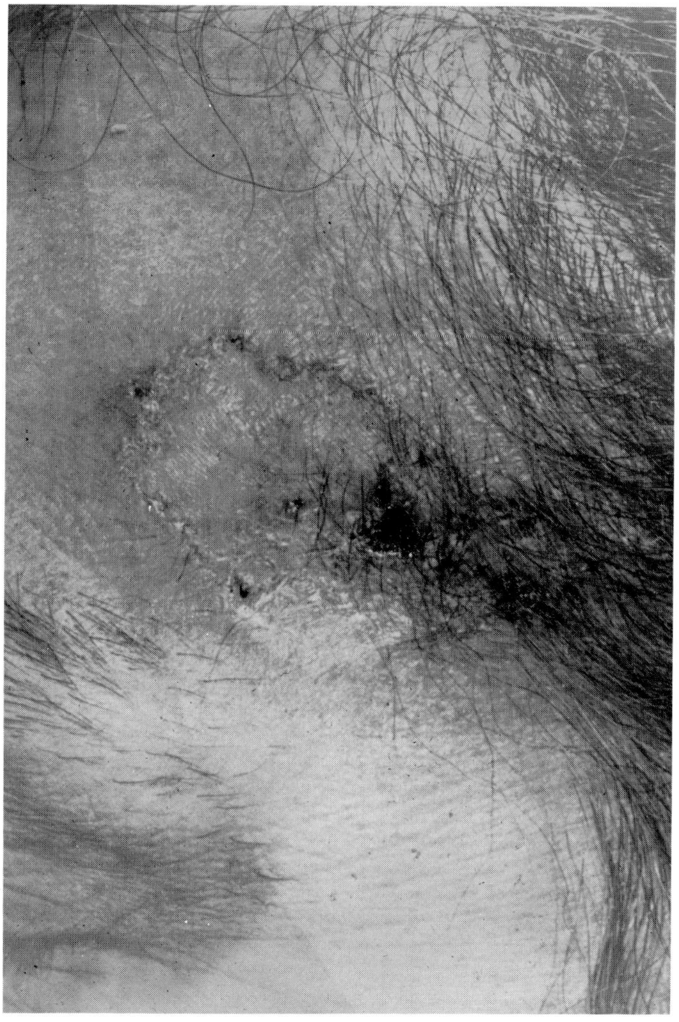

**Fig. 35-5.** Sclerosing basal cell epithelioma.

with slightly elevated borders. They occur most commonly on the *covered* portions of the body.

***Pigmented basal cell epithelioma.*** Basal cell epithelioma can be pigmented and resemble malignant melanoma. The pigment is melanin.

***Sclerosing basal cell epithelioma.*** Sclerosing basal cell epithelioma (Fig. 35-5) has the appearance of a slowly enlarging yellowish, atrophic scar with no distinct border. It is seen usually on the forehead or temples. There is a telangiectatic surface.

***Basal cell nevus syndrome.*** In basal cell nevus syndrome, multiple basal cell epitheliomas are found in all areas of the skin, associated with mandibular or maxillary cysts, frontal bosses, ectopic intracranial calcification brain tumors, and various other skeletal anomalies. Possible complications arising from the cysts include fracture, squamous cell carcinoma, and ameloblastomas, which add to the necessity to recognize the disorder (Howell).

Patients show multiple small irregularly distributed superficial discrete pits on the palms and soles.

### *Microscopic findings*

There is a projection from the epidermis into the dermis of cells having a large, dark blue–staining nucleus that gives them the appearance of basal cells. Masses of these cells are present, with an orderly arrangement of the tumor cells within the mass. There is some inflammatory infiltrate associated with the process. Various patterns of spread and extension are identified, which must be considered in the selection of optimal therapy for each lesion.

### *Differential diagnosis*

***Senile sebaceous hyperplasia.*** Yellow-white lobulated, often telangiectases-covered, papules of hypertrophic sebaceous gland. Can be mistaken for the pearly nodule of an epithelioma.

***Seborrheic keratosis.*** Seborrheic keratosis is a brown to black, elevated, warty lesion found on the back, chest, and temporal area of middle-aged to elderly individuals.

***Squamous cell carcinoma.*** Squamous cell carcinoma is usually found below the level of the upper lip and on the dorsa of the hands. Microscopic examination is essential for diagnosis.

***Actinic keratosis.*** Actinic keratosis is a flat lesion with an adherent, dry, rough scale found on exposed skin surfaces.

### *Treatment*

The effective treatment modalities to be considered are electrodesiccation and curettage, x-ray therapy, surgical excision, cryotherapy, topical chemotherapy, or chemosurgery.

The lesion must be destroyed beyond the limits of the visible border, since the epithelioma is larger than is clinically apparent. The treatment of choice is dependent on the location, size, and depth of the tumor, as well as on the expected cosmetic result. Because of the high cure rate of these lesions and the available alternative therapeutic measures, a good cosmetic result is an important consideration to the physician. Electrodesiccation and curettage is convenient, expeditious, and economical. It is well tolerated by the surrounding tissues. Its high success rate and very satisfactory cosmetic result place it as preferred therapy for these lesions. However, lesions greater than 1 cm. in diameter are ordinarily best treated by one of the other modalities. Lesions in certain locations, such as the cartilaginous corner of an ala nasi, need individual consideration of the most desirable method.

Surgical excision is equally acceptable if a good cosmetic result can be achieved. Mikhail and co-workers emphasize the rather high incidence of metastases reported in patients on whom immediate skin grafting was performed after incomplete excision of the primary tumor. If skin flaps are rotated, landmarks are lost, and the recurrence is hidden under the new tissue. X-ray therapy is also an effective method of treatment in those areas where surgery or curettage is not suitable. Treatment by any of these modalities results in a high rate of cure in uncomplicated cases, if the therapist is experienced in the natural course and behavior of these lesions. The sclerosing variety

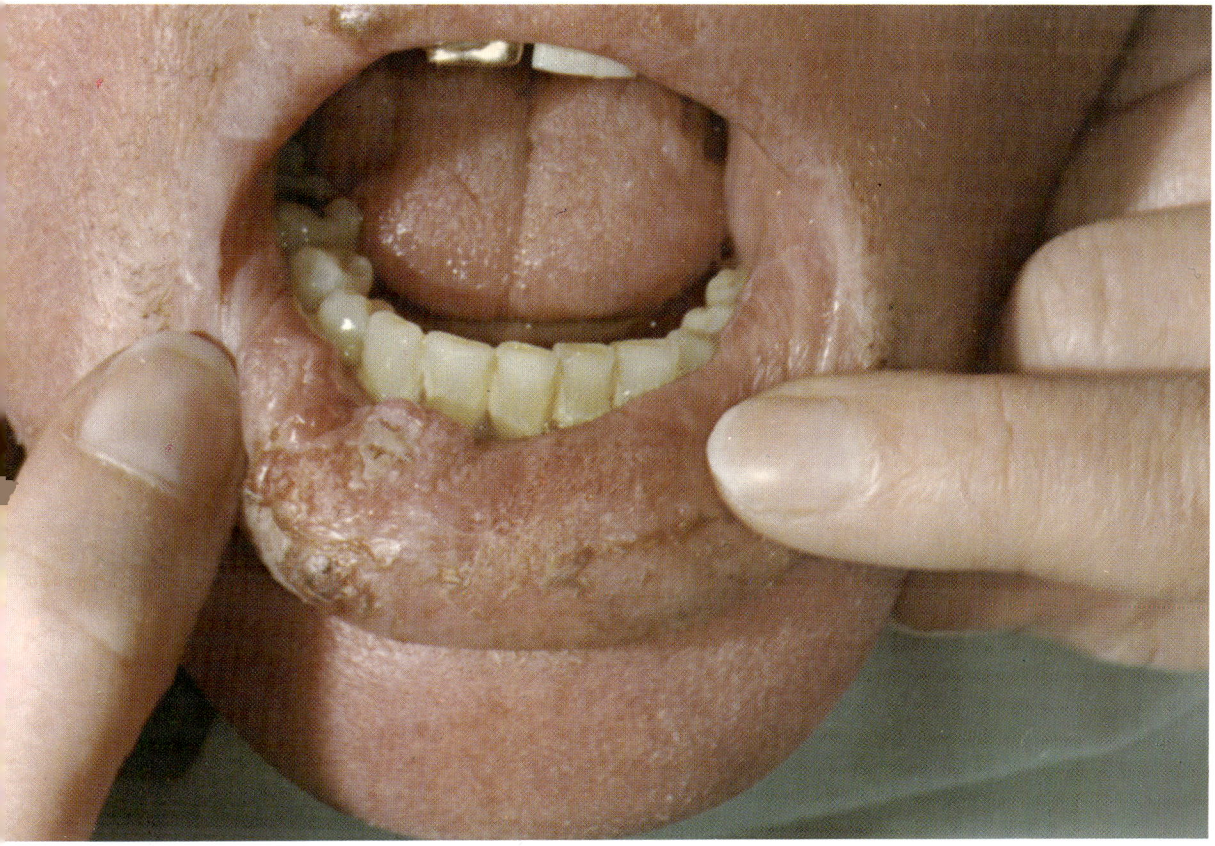

**Plate 55**

Squamous cell carcinoma.

is most satisfactorily treated by x-ray therapy or by Mohs' technique (see below).

Because recurrent epitheliomas have a high retreatment failure rate, no matter what form the retreatment takes, the initial treatment of the primary lesion must be aggressive enough to be curative. Treated patients should be checked at 6-month intervals for evidence of recurrences.

Freeman discusses the factors responsible for 53 recurrences in 2,288 skin cancers treated by various means.

Various methods of topical therapy have been tried, but have not been effective enough to replace the three time-honored methods. Mohs' technique of layer-by-layer destruction of complicated and difficult tumors under microscopic guidance is a valuable method in selected problem cases. This method now simplified and efficient has become the method of choice in sclerosing tumors, if an experienced person is available to do it (Bart). Mohs' technique, because each segment is microscopically examined, gives the best cure rate.

## Squamous cell carcinoma (epidermoid carcinoma)

Squamous cell carcinoma is a malignancy that arises on sun-exposed areas of the skin or on mucous membranes (Plate 55), invades locally, and produces metastases. It is the second most common cancer of the skin.

### *Natural course*

On the skin surface the growth usually appears as a skin-colored or reddish brown nodule, without distinguishing characteristics. It enlarges more rapidly than a basal cell epithelioma and will frequently develop necrosis with ulceration in its center. The appearance of small lesions of squamous cell carcinoma is not sufficiently distinctive for accurate diagnosis. Diagnosis must be established by biopsy. It occurs most often on the cheek and then the ear, neck and preauricular area, nose, temple, and forehead.

On mucous membranes a squamous cell carcinoma may develop from a patch of leukoplakia, appear as a fissured induration, or present as a warty growth. On the lower lip it may first appear as a persistent, scaling area that becomes thickened and later ulcerates (Fig. 35-6, *A*). In this area the lesion will infiltrate surrounding tissue and go on to metastasize more rapidly than a similar lesion of the skin. Squamous cell carcinomas arise on oral mucous membrane, resulting from the chronic irritation of pipe-smoking, dentures, or teeth, and on the glans penis in uncircumcised males.

In a series of 6,900 cases studied, Epstein recorded 2% metastases on diagnosis and a 5-year survival rate if 62% of those with squa-

A

B

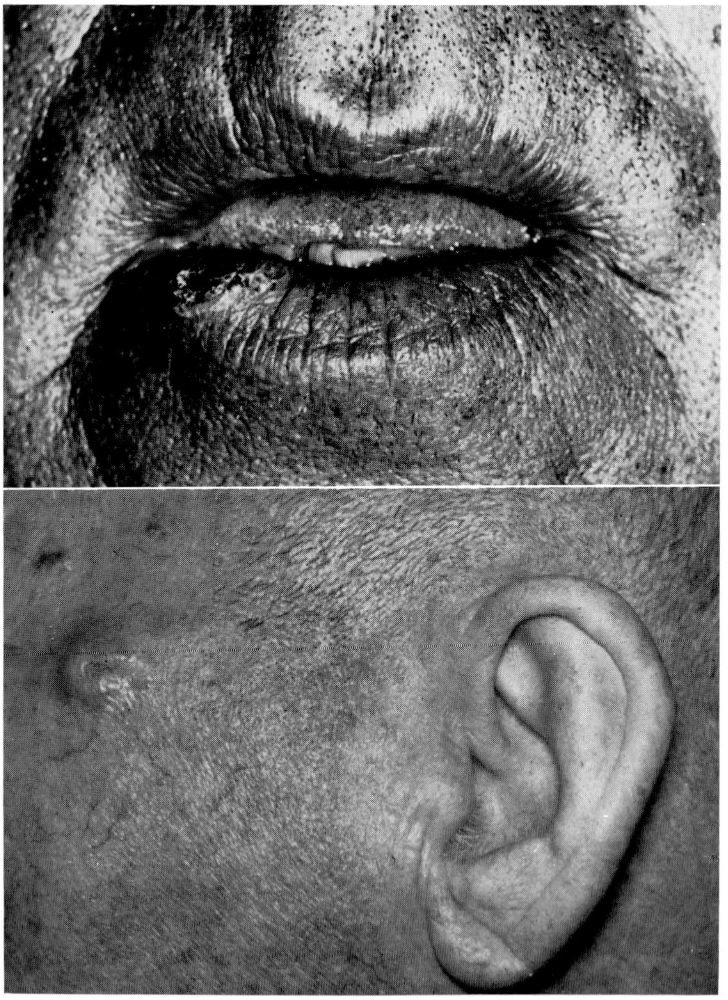

**Fig. 35-6. A,** Squamous cell carcinoma of lip. **B,** Squamous cell carcinoma in infratemporal area, one of the commonest sites for this tumor.

mous cell carcinomas. Squamous cell carcinomas are more likely to metastasize if they are located on the ears, cheeks, or temple areas, and particularly mucous membranes. Lesions of the forearms, hands, and fingers are likely to metastasize more slowly. Metastases are lymph borne, not hematogenous.

Squamous cell carcinoma occurs most frequently in males over 60 years of age, on sun-exposed areas. The face, lower lip, ears, neck, and dorsa of the hands are the sites of predilection. Ninety percent of these lesions occur on the face and ears (Fig. 35-6, *B*). A lesion appearing on the lower lip is more likely to be a squamous cell malignancy than a basal cell malignancy. On the upper lip, basal cell epitheliomas are more common. About 4% of all squamous cell carcinomas occur on the back of the hand.

Invasive squamous cell carcinomas of the glans penis, vulva, perianal area, vermilion border of lips, and ear tend to metastasize early.

### *Pertinent information*

Perhaps because of their distinctive location between environment, self, and internal milieu, a greater variety of influences seem to result in malignant changes in epidermal cells than in other cells. Of all external carcinogens, however, sun exposure is the most significant. It is the major etiological factor in the production of both squamous cell carcinoma and basal cell epithelioma of the skin. The cancerogenic rays seem to be between 290 and 320 nm. The pigment, melanin, plays a major part in protection from the development of squamous cell carcinoma. Blacks have a low incidence of this disease, although, as with other skin cancers, when it occurs in

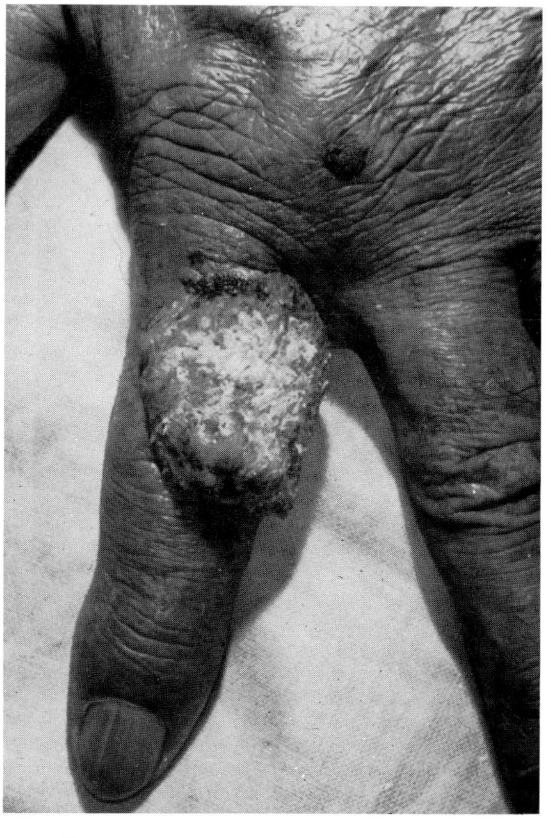

**Fig. 35-7.** Squamous cell carcinoma, secondary to x-ray exposure, low-grade malignancy.

blacks, it is very aggressive. Albinos have an exceptionally high incidence. Thus, even in northern climates, blondes and redheads are most likely to develop squamous cell carcinomas and should be warned about excess sun exposure. The incidence of skin cancer for whites doubles for each 265 miles southward toward the equator.

There are certain precancerous lesions of the skin in which squamous cell carcinoma is likely to develop. These are actinic keratosis, arsenical keratosis, cutaneous horn, leukoplakia, and xeroderma pigmentosum. Radiation (Fig. 35-7), thermal burns, chronic heat, and irritation may also damage the skin in such a way as to produce squamous cell carcinoma. These are often not related to sun exposure.

Squamous cell carcinoma, as determined in large group studies, has an association of 8% with a further internal cancer.

Epithelial malignant tumors, as well as lymphoreticular tumors, develop and proliferate more rapidly when linked with deficient or suppressed immune mechanisms. The incidence of skin carcinoma, especially squamous cell carcinomas, in renal transplant patients is greatly increased on areas of sun exposure. This deficient or suppressed immune state appears to apply to both cell-mediated (T-cell) and circulatory antibody (B-cell) mechanisms. A loss of intercellular substance, related to the epidermal cells' ability to differentiate and keratinize, normally occurs with malignant change, along with an inability to maintain the integrity of the basement membrane. This condition is reflected by an alteration in immune surveillance. There are trends toward immunotherapy in epidermal malignancies, but they are not yet well enough understood to challenge the excellent results obtained by traditional electrodesiccation, irradiation, or surgery.

### Microscopic findings

There are irregular masses and cords of squamous epithelial cells invading the dermis. Abnormal variations in the size and shape of the invading cells, deep-staining nuclei, and many mitotic figures are present. Areas of keratinization, "pearls," are seen within the masses of invading cells.

There is a wide range of biological activity of these tumors, which can be predicted by the microscopic appearance, degree of anaplasia, and so forth.

### Differential diagnosis

***Basal cell epithelioma.*** Small lesions of basal and squamous cell carcinomas may be indistinguishable one from the other. Older lesions demonstrate that basal cell epithelioma grows more slowly, is less infiltrative, has less tendency to ulcerate, and has a distinctive border. Biopsy must be performed.

***Actinic keratosis.*** Actinic keratosis also occurs on exposed areas of actinic skin damage. It is flat or only slightly elevated, with a dry scale and a tendency to bleed if scraped. It can develop into a squamous cell carcinoma.

***Seborrheic keratosis.*** Seborrheic keratosis demonstrates shades varying from tan to brown, is very slow growing, has a warty surface, and appears on normal skin. It is usually multiple and commonly found on the back and chest in older persons.

### Treatment

Anyone treating squamous cell carcinoma must be fully familiar with the natural course and the histopathology of the lesion. Where a team of cooperating specialists is available (dermatologist, radiologist, and surgeon), their services should be used. Staging of squamous cell carcinoma is helpful.

**0** In situ
**1** Confined to skin or subcutaneous tissues
  **a** Less than 2 cm.
  **b** Greater than 2 cm.
**2** **a** Invasion of deeper underlying tissue
  **b** Recurrent local disease
**3** Greater than 5 cm. with deeper invasion or metastasis to regional nodes
**4** Metastasis to distant nodes

Stages 0 and 1 can well be treated by curettage and electrodesiccation. Stage 2 and above should only be treated by experienced surgeons, radiotherapists, or Mohs' chemotherapeutists. Each lesion requires individual attention.

It is well established that retreatment of squamous cell carcinoma has a high failure rate, regardless of the form of therapy. Every lesion that recurs and is suspected of being cancer should be biopsied. Initial therapy is of paramount importance and should be sufficiently aggressive to be curative.

Recurrence of tumors may be more related to an initially aggressive tumor than to a failure or mistake in therapy (Freeman). Faced with an extremely resistant basal cell or squamous cell carcinoma, it is well to consider chemosurgery. This specialized technique permits involved tissue to be chemically treated in situ and then surgically excised and microscopically examined. The chief advantage here over other modalities is the consistent reliability of the microscopic control.

## Bowen's disease (squamous cell carcinoma in situ) (Fig. 35-8)

Bowen's disease is a slowly growing, localized, superficial variant of squamous cell carcinoma that is associated with a tendency toward the development of other malignancies.

### *Natural course*

The disease begins as a single or multiple, flat, scaling, erythematous lesion with a sharply defined border. It rarely shows induration, ulceration, or tendency to become elevated. The lesion enlarges slowly, resulting in a uniform-appearing erythematous patch of varying size, depending on its duration. It has no central pale or clearing area. There may be a superficial crust. Men and women in the 30- to 60-year age group are equally affected. On the mucous membranes, it tends to be more variable and can be thickened, white streaked, or polypoid.

The disease may occur on any area of the body, but chiefly affects unexposed areas of the trunk or mucous membranes of the mouth, vulva, or anus, thus differing from invasive squamous cell carcinoma.

Lesions of Bowen's disease may rarely progress to invasive squamous cell carcinoma,

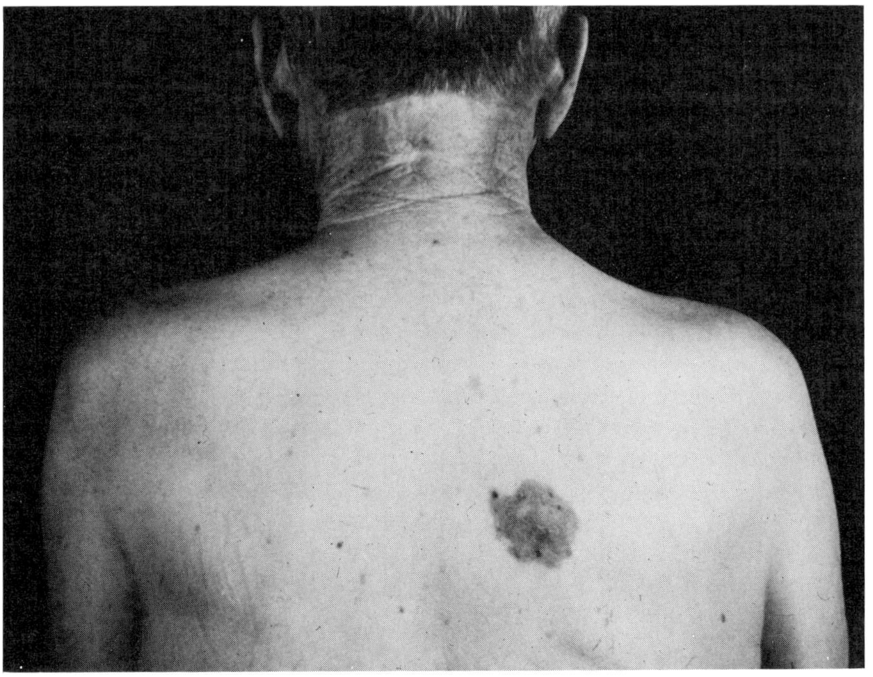

**Fig. 35-8.** Bowen's disease. Psoriasis-like patch in a characteristic location.

and biopsy specimens should be examined for signs of such change. If no invasion into the dermis has occurred, the prognosis is excellent with complete superficial removal of the lesion. If invasion is present, the situation is reversed, and the malignancy must be treated as a squamous cell carcinoma.

### *Pertinent information*

Bowen's disease occurs in individuals prone to developing other malignancies, both cutaneous and internal. Chemical analysis has shown an abnormal concentration of arsenic in these lesions, and this element is a potent carcinogen. The source of the arsenic found in these lesions is not often easily obtainable from the patient's history. The internal malignancies believed to be associated with Bowen's disease have been chiefly of the respiratory, gastrointestinal, genitourinary, or reticuloendothelial system. They have appeared several years after the diagnosis of Bowen's disease. Average age at onset is 48. The disease is most likely to occur in those with Anglo-Saxon ancestry.

### *Microscopic findings*

There is dyskeratosis within the bounds of the prickle cell layers. Cells are in complete disorientation, with atypical, hyperchromatic nuclei. Multinucleated bizarre cells and individual cell keratinization are seen. Greatly increased cell proliferation has been recorded.

### *Differential diagnosis*

***Psoriasis.*** In psoriasis there is a thick, heavy, overlying scale, with a therapeutic response to sun exposure.

***Tinea corporis.*** Sudden onset, lesions with a vesicular, actively growing border, and far more rapid growth distinguish tinea corporis from Bowen's disease.

***Superficial basal cell epithelioma.*** Superficial basal cell epithelioma can be distinguished by biopsy.

### *Treatment*

After careful biopsy and determination that the lesion is limited to the epithelium, it can be removed by curettage and electrodesiccation.

5-Fluorouracil, 5% concentration in buffered aqueous solution, applied twice daily in small areas over no more than 3 weeks, has been shown to produce excellent response with "lighting up" and subsequent clearing of previously invisible lesions.* Sometimes, in addition, occlusion under plastic helps.

Dermabrasion also produces excellent nonscarred results. X radiation is not a good choice of therapy because of poor response.

If invasion of the dermis has taken place, the lesion must be treated as an invasive squamous cell carcinoma.

The patient should be thoroughly examined for other cutaneous or internal malignancy and followed with expectation of developing such in future years.

## Erythroplasia of Queyrat (Bowen's disease of the mucous membrane)

Erythroplasia of Queyrat is a malignancy of the epithelium of mucous membranes that is microscopically similar to Bowen's disease of the cornified skin. It occurs chiefly on the glans penis, but also has been described on the buccal mucosa and on the labia minora.

The lesion is bright red, with a surface that resembles fine velvet (Plate 56). It is flat and very sharply defined. It does not ulcerate. The area slowly enlarges, and although at first it is confined to the epidermis, it will progress to an invasive squamous cell carcinoma of the penis.

There is no increased incidence of internal cancer as with Bowen's disease.

### *Microscopic findings*

Microscopically, the process is seen to be an intraepidermal carcinoma in situ. The epidermis is thickened, the basal cell layer is intact, and the prickle cells are disordered and dyskeratotic. They show the same degree of disorientation seen in Bowen's disease of the skin. With older lesions, dermal invasion is seen.

---

*Bendl, B. J.: Personal communication, 1972.

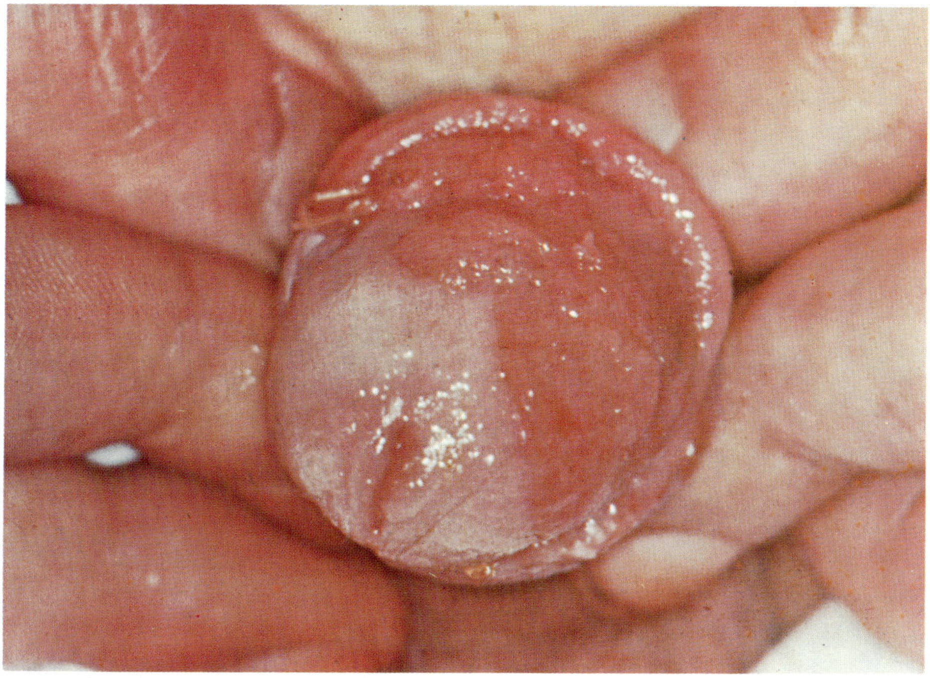

**Plate 56**

Erythroplasia of Queyrat. Features are velvety surface and sharply bordered plaque on normal mucous membrane.

### *Differential diagnosis*

***Chronic circumscribed balanitis.*** Clinically, chronic circumscribed balanitis may be impossible to distinguish from erythroplasia of Queyrat. One must perform a biopsy to make this diagnosis.

***Acute balanitis.*** An acute weeping inflammation of the glans occurring in the uncircumcised male, acute balanitis is associated with tenderness and a burning discomfort.

***Psoriasis.*** Psoriasis may present well-defined erythematous lesions of the glans. Other manifestations of psoriasis are present.

***Reiter's disease.*** Reiter's disease is a painless circular superficial erosion.

### *Treatment*

Curettage with electrodesiccation under local anesthesia is the treatment of choice. Unless all areas are adequately removed, the process will recur.

5-Fluorouracil, 1%, in propylene glycol applied twice daily, appears to be a satisfactory way of treating this disorder. In selected cases, it is reported that dinitrochlorobenzene followed by 5-fluorouracil was effective (Raaf). Careful follow-up observations should be carried out, since the long-term recurrences are not known. Radiation therapy may produce phimosis or stricture.

The patient should be kept under observation at intervals for an indefinite period, for evidence of recurrence.

#### REFERENCES

Bart, R. S., Kopf, A. W., and Gladstein, A. H.: Treatment of morphea-type basal cell carcinomas with radiation therapy, Arch. Dermatol. **113:**783, 1977.

**Contrary to what is written, x rays are effective in treatment of this type of cancer.**

Farina, A. T., Leider, M., Newall, J., et al.: Modern radiotherapy for malignant epitheliomas—a measure of last resort, Arch. Dermatol. **113:**650, 1977.

**A graphic presentation of seven cases. The clinician should never limit his therapeutic options.**

Fleming, I. D., Barnawell, J. D., Burlison, P. E., and Rankin, J. S.: Skin cancer in black patients, Cancer **35**:600, 1975.

**A picture very different from that seen in whites where sun exposure is the most important factor.**

Goette, D. K., and Carson, T. E.: Erythroplasia of Queyrat. Treatment with topical 5-fluorouracil, Cancer **38**:1498, 1976.

**Now our treatment of choice.**

Howell, J. B., and Anderson, D. E.: The nevoid basal cell carcinoma syndrome. In Andrade, R., Gumport, S. L., Popkin, G. L., and Rees, T. D., editors: Cancer of the skin, vol. 2, Philadelphia, 1976, W. B. Saunders Co., p. 883.

**A complete exposition by methodical observant authors.**

Hoxtell, E. D., Mandel, J. S., Murray, S. S., et al.: Incidence of skin carcinoma after renal transplantation, Arch. Dermatol. **113**:436, 1977.

**Significantly increased.**

Jackson, R.: Arsenic and cancer, Can. Med. Assoc. J. **113**:396, 1975.

**Seven patients that help to correlate long-term arsenic ingestion and malignant disease.**

Knox, J. M. and Joseph, L. M.: Bowen's disease and erythroplasia. In Andrade, R., Gumport, S. L., Popkin, G. L., and Rees, T. D., editors: Cancer of the skin, vol. 1, Philadelphia, 1976, W. B. Saunders Co., p. 646.

**A balanced rational consideration of the disorder.**

Kopf, A. W., Bart, R. S., Schrager, D., et al.: Curettage-electrodesiccation treatment of basal cell carcinomas, Arch. Dermatol. **113**:439, 1977.

**Confirmation of the effectiveness of the technique.**

Mikhail, G. R.: Chemosurgery in the treatment of skin cancer, Int. J. Dermatol. **14**:33, 1975.

**Well-recognized therapeutic technique limited by number of chemosurgeons.**

Mikhail, G. R., Nims, L. P., Kelly, A. P., et al.: Metastatic basal cell carcinoma, Arch. Dermatol. **113**:1261, 1977.

**Now 93 cases reported. Immediate wound closure and grafting with flaps conceal recurrences.**

Raaf, J. H., Krown, S. E., Pinsky, C. M., et al.: Treatment of Bowen's disease with topical dinitrochlorobenzene and 5-fluorouracil, Cancer **37**:1633, 1976.

**Combined local immunotherapy and topical chemotherapy may be forerunner of accepted technique.**

Safai, B., and Good, R. A.: Basal cell carcinoma with metastasis, Arch. Pathol. Lab. Med. **101**:327, 1977.

**Profound immunodeficiency, metastatic basal cell carcinoma and squamous cell carcinoma. The authors query a transition to squamous cell carcinoma as well.**

Sage, H. H., and Casson, P. R.: Squamous cell carcinoma of the scalp, face and neck. In Andrade, R., Gumport, S. L., Popking, G. L., and Rees, T. D., editors: Cancer of the skin, vol. 2, Philadelphia, 1976, W. B. Saunders Co., p. 899.

**Diagnosis, course, treatment, staging, and specific problems.**

## EXTRAEPIDERMAL TUMORS

### Paget's disease of the nipple

Paget's disease of the nipple consists of a chronic eczematous lesion from Paget's cells arising in the epidermis because of a ductal carcinoma of the underlying mammary gland.

The usual site of cutaneous Paget's disease is the nipple. Here it begins as a small, pruritic, moist, crusting patch of eczema (Plate 57). There is frequently a palpable border and a degree of induration to the lesion. The area persists, may enlarge to involve the areola and the adjacent breast, and produces symptoms, but usually it is the site of a minimal but annoying discharge. It is always unilateral. It occurs chiefly in young adult women, although it has been reported in the male.

This unusual phenomenon arises as a result

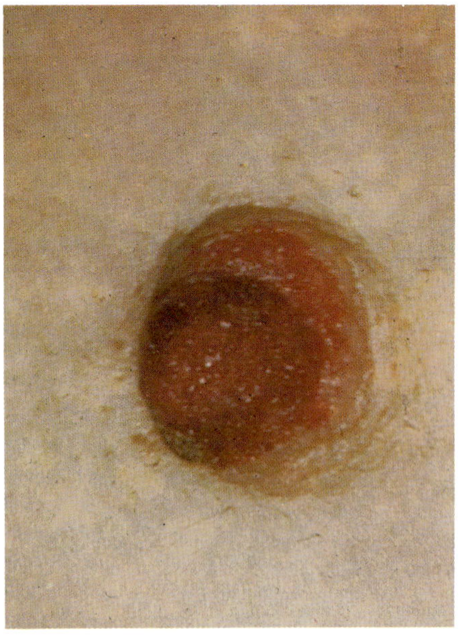

**Plate 57**

Paget's disease of nipple.

of a ductal carcinoma beginning in one of the mammary gland ducts not far from its orifice. The characteristic Paget cells that appear in the epidermis of the nipple and areola are an extension of the malignant process from the site of origin. The underlying carcinoma was noninvasive in one third of the cases studied in one series.

### *Microscopic findings*

Paget's cells are scattered through the epidermis. These are large, clear or pale-staining cells with a pale round nucleus. They have no prickles. There is an inflamatory reaction in the dermis, although Paget's cells do not invade the dermis.

There is malignancy in the mammary ducts. It remains localized for a time, but direct invasion into connective and mammary tissue occurs eventually.

### *Differential diagnosis*

Eczema of the nipple from various causes must be excluded. A chronic condition that is often bilateral, this entity consists of a localized moist patch on the nipple and areola. It responds to local glucocorticoid therapy.

*Eczema of the nipple or areola must be biopsied if it does not respond promptly to effective local therapy.*

A smear of the nipple discharge, examined for malignant cells, may give the diagnosis without biopsy. A negative result does not rule out carcinoma.

### *Treatment*

Treatment is as for carcinoma of the breast. Radical mastectomy is usually recommended.

## Extramammary Paget's disease

A change similar to Paget's disease of the nipple occurs rarely in the genital or perianal area or axilla in association with previous, simultaneous, or subsequent underlying tumors, particularly adenocarcinomas. The mean age at onset is over 62 years. Itching and burning in a reddened area followed by an oozing, verrucous surface and then vegetating lesions. The vulvar or the anogenital area is the site most often observed of this rare disease.

## Kaposi's sarcoma

Kaposi's sarcoma is a rare proliferative disorder of vascular tissue.

This disease affects all ages, but is more common in men ranging from 50 to 70 years of age. Only 6% to 19% of cases occur in women. It has been reported in several members of a family.

There is some tendency to predisposition on the basis of geographical origin, since most patients are Jewish, Russian, Polish, and North Italian. It is a more common and rather different disease in African blacks, in whom sharp differences in incidence are apparent on a geographic basis. The incidence in Indians is remarkably low. Prolonged lymphedema, trauma, and cold seem to be predisposing factors.

The lesions begin in the skin of the extremities in most cases, although some initial lesions have been reported in the gastrointestinal tract, genitalia, and internal organs. Most cutaneous lesions appear symmetrically on the hands and feet (Plate 58) and progress to involve larger areas. They are diffuse cyanotic or purpuric lesions that progress to plaques and nodules. Pitting edema, often localized below the knee, is a frequent accompaniment. Petechiae and ecchymoses are common in association with nodules in these cases and result in a hemosiderin pigmentation of the lesions. The entire cutaneous surface may become involved.

Although the skin is the primary site of the disease, it is not unusual to find visceral involvement. Nearly every organ has been reported as a site, with the gastrointestinal tract, liver, lungs, and lymph nodes the most frequently affected. In children, the peripheral lymph nodes may be generally enlarged without cutaneous involvement.

The nature of the disease is obscure. It appears to be a proliferation of the cells associated with blood vessels and lymph vessels. The prognosis is grave, with most cases proving fatal in 5 to 8 years. Remissions are seen, and some are of quite long duration. Death

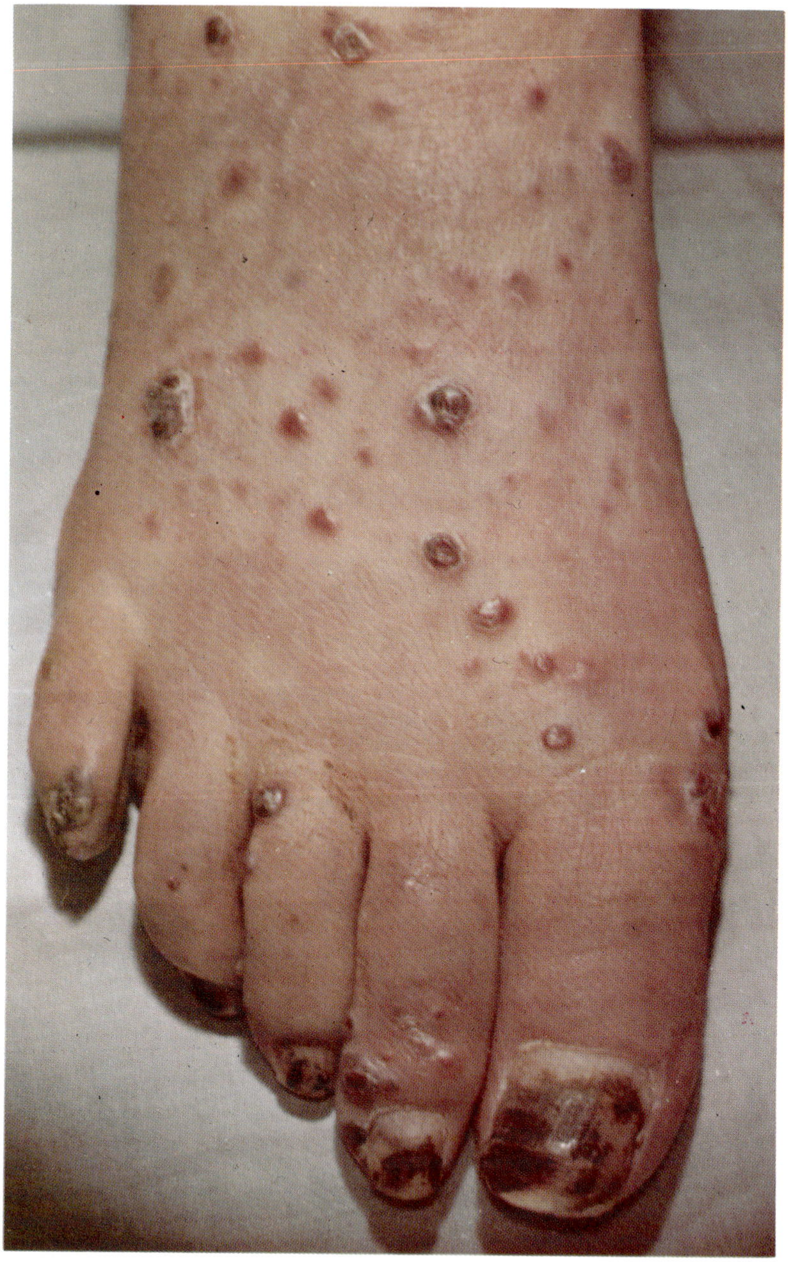

**Plate 58**

Kaposi's sarcoma.

occurs from pulmonary or gastrointestinal hemorrhage or, less often, from infection or cachexia. In Europeans, an association with lymphoma is frequent, whereas in Africans, where the disease is common and aggressive, an association with tuberculosis is frequent.

### *Microscopic findings*

The microscopic appearance of the lesions consists of a disorganized mixture of poorly formed capillaries, bundles of spindle-shaped cells, foci of hemorrhage, and fibroblastic proliferation. Malignant transformation with metastases is seen.

### *Treatment*

Tucker and Winkelmann report good results in five cases and review 18 others, treated with vinblastine. They used an impressively low dose without toxicity and with successful outcome.

Radiation therapy of a type individualized for the depth of the specific lesions treated has been the treatment of choice, although intra-arterial perfusion with nitrogen mustard, 0.4 mg./kg. of body weight into the affected limb, and other cytotoxic agents have shown a good remission. Surgery for isolated superficial nodules is acceptable in some instances.

Regression of single tumors or even disease remissions is not uncommon.

## The lymphomas

Shelley describes the clinical manifestations of the lymphomas from the vantage point of the dermatologist. He cites six cases, none with specific microscopic diagnoses initially, but all with potential clinical diagnoses.

The lymphomas comprise a group of uncommon proliferative disorders of varying degrees of malignancy that arise from lymphoid tissue. They may originate from the reticular cell or the lymphocyte. They usually develop from multiple foci, but in some instances they remain as localized tumors for prolonged periods. Current knowledge concerning etiology and consideration of infectious and epidemiological factors are thoughtfully reviewed by Aisenberg. At least some of the lymphomas are associated with a deficiency in antibody formation and hypogammaglobulinemia.

The classification of lymphomas is primarily a histological one and cannot be precise, since there are gradations between types and conversion from one type to another.

The lymphomas, excluding Hodgkin's disease, can be classified into five groups (from Aisenberg).

1. Nodular lymphoma
   a. Lymphocytic
   b. Lymphoblastic
   c. Mixed lymphocytic and reticulum cell
   d. Reticulum cell
2. Lymphocytic lymphoma
3. Lymphoblastic lymphoma
4. Reticulum cell sarcoma
5. Stem cell lymphoma

Chronic lymphocytic leukemia is most often related to lymphocytic lymphoma. Leukemia in the other types is unusual.

After being classified into these groups, patients can be staged, indicating the extent and spread of the disease. This is important for prognosis. Therapy is based on both the type of lymphoma and the stage it manifests.

As the newer concepts of origins and functions of lymphocytes are related to the clinical pictures of the malignancies of these cells, immunological classifications, including B- and T-cell malignancies and therapeutic measures most suited to each, will probably supersede this classification.

Skin manifestions of these disorders are specific or nonspecific.

***Specific lesions.*** Infiltration of the skin by the characteristic lymphoma cell produces the specific lesion, which is elevated and may be solitary or multiple. The tumor may present either as an erythematous (Plate 59) or pigmented plaque, or as a skin-colored to brown nodule (Fig. 35-9).

Microscopically, there are masses of lymphoma cells either in small or in large accumulations, trailing off into the surrounding tissue. The infiltrate has a tendency to appear uniform because one cell type predominates.

***Nonspecific lesions.*** *Generalized pruritus* is a nonspecific finding and is characteristic of lymphocytic lymphoma. Nonspecific cutaneous lesions may be macular, papular, vesic-

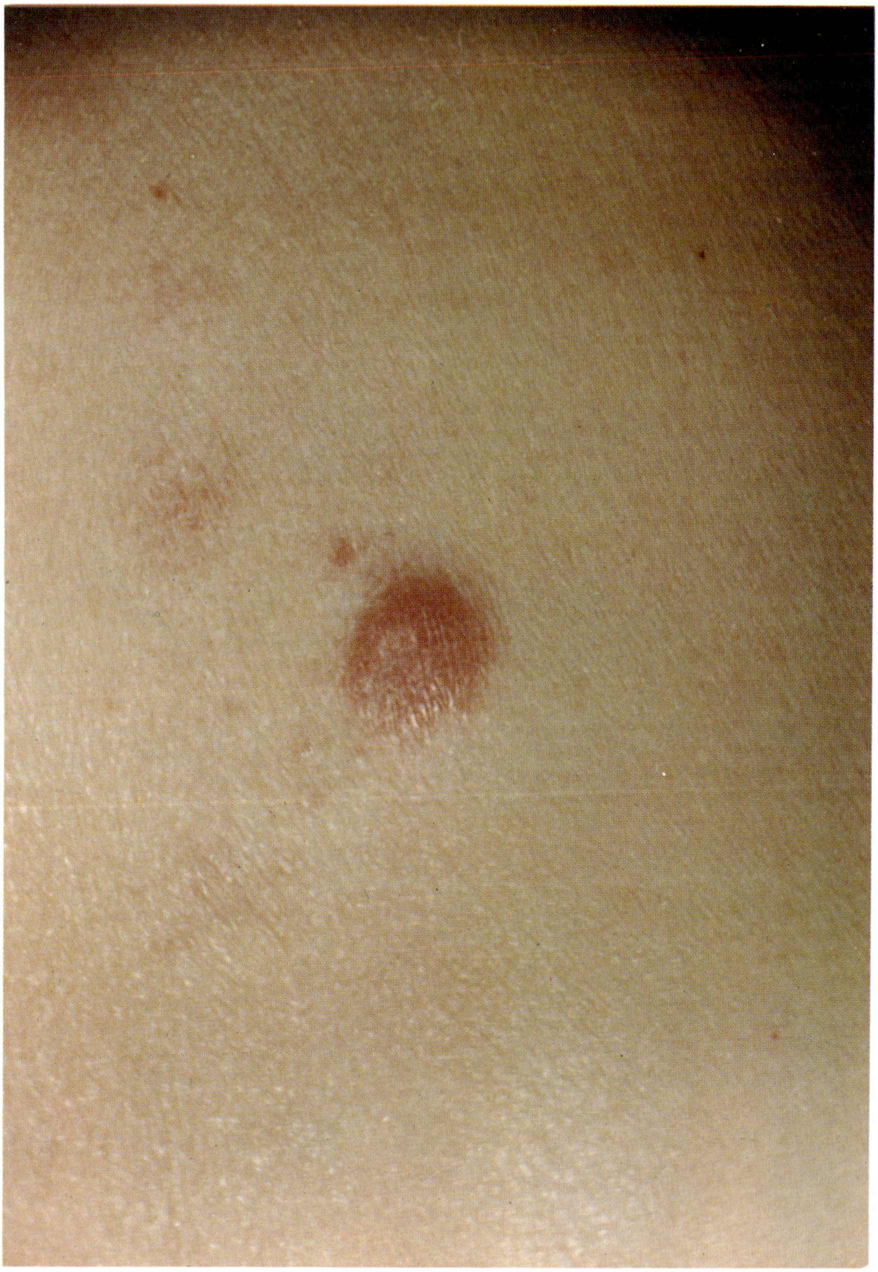

**Plate 59**

Lymphoma, skin of thorax.

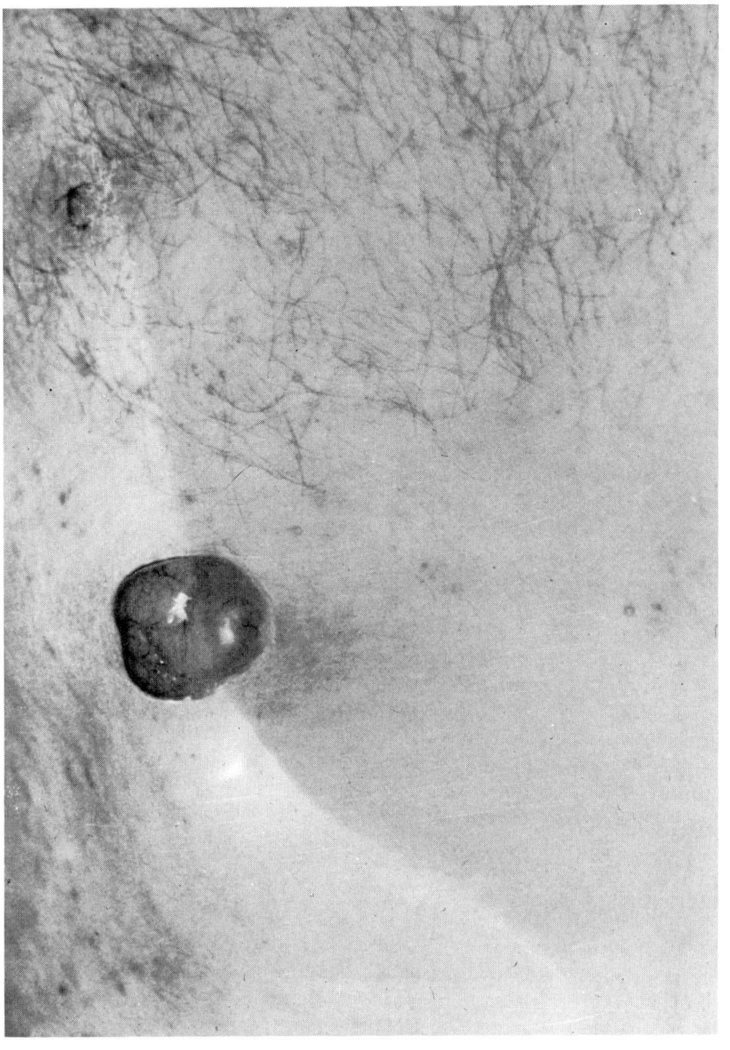

**Fig. 35-9.** Lymphocytic lymphoma of thoracic skin.

ular, or bullous. They may resemble erythema multiforme or produce an exfoliative dermatitis or erythroderma. These are attributable to the presence of the lymphoma but not to infiltration by the specific cells.

Microscopically, these lesions possess a nonspecific inflammatory infiltrate without a predominance of lymphoma cells.

### *Prognosis*

The survival rate is poor. For even the best-differentiated tumors and those most amenable to therapy, 5-year survival rates rarely exceed 50%. For lymphosarcomas and reticulum cell sarcomas, 5-year survival rates are around 25%.

Even newer therapeutic measures, sophisticated as they are, do not parallel the better results obtained with Hodgkin's disease.

### *Treatment*

The treatment of the lymphomas and related tumors should be carried out in an institution or medical center where sufficient numbers are seen for those directing the therapy to be experienced in the best therapeutic measures. Logic favors treatment centers that see a minimum of 25 to 50 new patients with lymphoma a year (Aisenberg). Changes are occurring so rapidly in the fields of immunotherapy, chemotherapy, and radiotherapy of cutaneous and deeper forms of malignancy that one method or drug is supplanted by another fairly quickly. In radiotherapy, supervoltage techniques with meticulous care in field selection and shaping are of utmost importance to prevent serious radiation sequelae and to achieve the best possible results.

The drugs used for therapy of this group of diseases can be divided into the following groups:

1. Alkylating agents. Alkylating agents are unstable compounds whose antineoplastic action is directed against the cancer cell nucleoproteins, the exact mechanism being unknown. Examples are nitrogen mustard, melphalan, chlorambucil, triethylenemelamine, cyclophosphamide, and busulfan.
2. Antimetabolites. Of the antimetabolites, the most frequently used are methotrexate, a folic acid antagonist; 6-mercaptopurine and 5-fluorouracil, purine and pyrimadine antagonists; vinca alkaloids, which arrest mitosis; procarbazine hydrochloride; and actinomycin D, an antibiotic that inactivates DNA.
3. Hormones. Glucocorticoids may produce tumor remissions but are used chiefly to allay fever, malaise, and secondary effects of the malignancy and to improve general well-being.
4. Mixed therapy. Cyclophosphamide is currently the single drug of choice for most of these tumors, but various studies on mixed chemotherapy and radiation, or a careful mixing of chemotherapeutic agents, is beneficial.

## Hodgkin's disease

The malignant disorder known as Hodgkin's disease is ordinarily classed with the lymphomas and comprises slightly more than one third of the cases of that group. It is considered separately here because the cutaneous manifestations of Hodgkin's disease are more characteristic than those of the lymphomas. Between 25% and 40% of patients with Hodgkin's disease have cutaneous manifestations, chiefly pruritus.

In Hodgkin's disease the now well-defined immune deficiency state parallels that of the thymectomized animal. T-cell function is selectively involved with depression of established delayed hypersensitivity and an inability to acquire new similar allergic responses. Clinically, this situation is demonstrated by a lack of ability to sensitize these patients to contact allergens, and in the depression of the lymphocyte transformation tests. The greater the extent of the disease, the more severe the immune deficit.

### *Natural course*

The disease occurs more than twice as frequently in males as in females. Young adults are usually affected, although persons of all ages are susceptible. The course is one of steady, fairly rapid progression to a fatal termination, usually within 3 years after the diagnosis has been made.

The first symptom may be either a severe pruritus that is unresponsive to therapy or an asymptomatic lymph node enlargement, or both. There is frequently a diffuse brownish pigmentation, most apparent in the areas of pruritus. Other nonspecific lesions include macular erythematous lesions, papules, and, at times, exfoliative dermatitis or erythroderma.

Specific lesions, which contain the characteristic cellular infiltrate, include skin-colored to brown plaques, nodules, and tumors. These are less common than the nonspecific lesions.

Lymph nodes, spleen, liver, and other organs become involved with the cellular infiltrate, with a resulting downhill course leading to death.

### *Pertinent information*

The 5-year survival rates in Hodgkin's disease have risen sharply with modern methods of radiation and chemotherapy, with reported figures of 85% to 90% in stages 1 and 2 (localized or regional disease) (Table 7). It has been

**Table 7.** Histological classification of Hodgkin's disease (Aisenberg)

| | Percent of cases | Percent of 5-year survival |
|---|---|---|
| Lymphocyte predominance | 5 | 90 |
| Nodular sclerosis | 50 | 70 |
| Mixed cellularity | 40 | 35 |
| Lymphocyte depletion | | |
| Diffuse fibrosis | 0 | 0 |
| Reticular | 5 | 35 |

established that Hodgkin's disease affects clones of lymphocytes. It spreads chiefly by contiguous lymphatics, but has hematological dissemination as well. Liver, spleen, abdominal lymph nodes, and kidneys may be affected, with no histological evidence of invasion by lymphoma cells.

Lymphangiography is used extensively to assess the location and extent of lymph node involvement.

Laparotomy has been recently employed in the initial assessment of Hodgkin's disease in order to determine accurately the extent of the disease and to self therapy.

After carrying out an epidemiologic review of Hodgkin's disease in a New York State high school, Vianna and his colleagues suggest that the disease is an infective condition with a long incubation period and transmitted by person-to-person contact.

According to Thorling and Thorling, serum copper estimates reflect the activity of Hodgkin's disease—the level rising as the disease becomes more active. It has also been observed that herpes zoster infections occur more frequently in patients with Hodgkin's disease, serum copper levels fall steadily for as long as 200 days prior to the appearance of herpes zoster.

### *Microscopic findings*

Microscopically, the cellular infiltrate is comprised of chronic inflammatory cells and cells of the lymphocytic series in various stages of maturation. There are characteristic Reed-Sternberg cells that are pathognomonic of Hodgkin's disease. These are large, atypical early cells of the lymphocytic series.

Nodular sclerosis describes a pattern of involvement that includes broad bands of collagen or the presence of shrunken "lacunar cells," which are a form of the Reed-Sternberg cell. There is a favorable outlook for successful treatment of nodular sclerosis.

### *Treatment*

The best therapeutic results have arisen from radiation therapy. Carefully planned supervoltage therapy by radiotherapists who see this disease frequently has produced the increase in survival rates noted above. Complications can include radiation pneumonitis or pericarditis, radiation-induced leukemia, or hypothyroidism.

Chemotherapy now includes quadruple drug therapy with nitrogen mustard, vincristine sulfate, prednisone, and procarbazine hydrochloride. This therapy appears to be more suited to the asymptomatic patient than to the patient with advanced symptoms. Choice of therapy should be made by an experienced clinician. Some evidence of an increase in nonlymphomatous malignancies may accompany intensive therapy of this anergic state.

## Mycosis fungoides—Sézary syndrome

A cutaneous infiltrative process of malignant T-lymphocytes, mycosis fungoides occupies a unique position in the spectrum of cutaneous diseases. It may remain localized to the skin for years before disseminating to other internal organs or structures. It has a nonleukemic and a leukemic (Sézary syndrome) phase.

### *Natural course*

Mycosis fungoides follows a pattern that progresses slowly but inexorably through three characteristic stages. The usual course takes many years.

The *exanthem or macular stage* resembles psoriasis, parapsoriasis, and Bowen's disease, with bright erythematous patches having a slight superficial scale. These patches enlarge peripherally and also tend to change their location slowly. Average duration of this stage is 10 to 12 years. Microscopic examination reveals only a nonspecific cellular reaction, and few firm diagnoses are made in this stage.

The *second stage, plaque formation,* varies from the first only by the development of specific cellular infiltration, and thus lesion elevation, adding a third dimension to the previous lesion. Average duration is less than 10 years (Plate 60).

The *third stage* is characterized by *tumor formation.* The lesions are of various sizes, ranging from 1 to many centimeters in diameter, with ulceration, necrosis, and areas of infection. Average duration is 2 to 3 years.

Pruritus is frequent in the first two stages. The chief clinical manifestations are those of increasing general discomfort and limitation of normal living habits by the extending plaques and oozing, crusting, and ulcerated surfaces that progress to universal cutaneous involvement. In the later stages, this becomes virtually intolerable. In the final stage, intercurrent infection or general debility may result in death. In some cases, only cutaneous infiltration may be demonstrable at autopsy, yet in other cases, infiltrative lesions are found in the viscera, where the lymph nodes, lungs, spleen, and the liver are most fre-

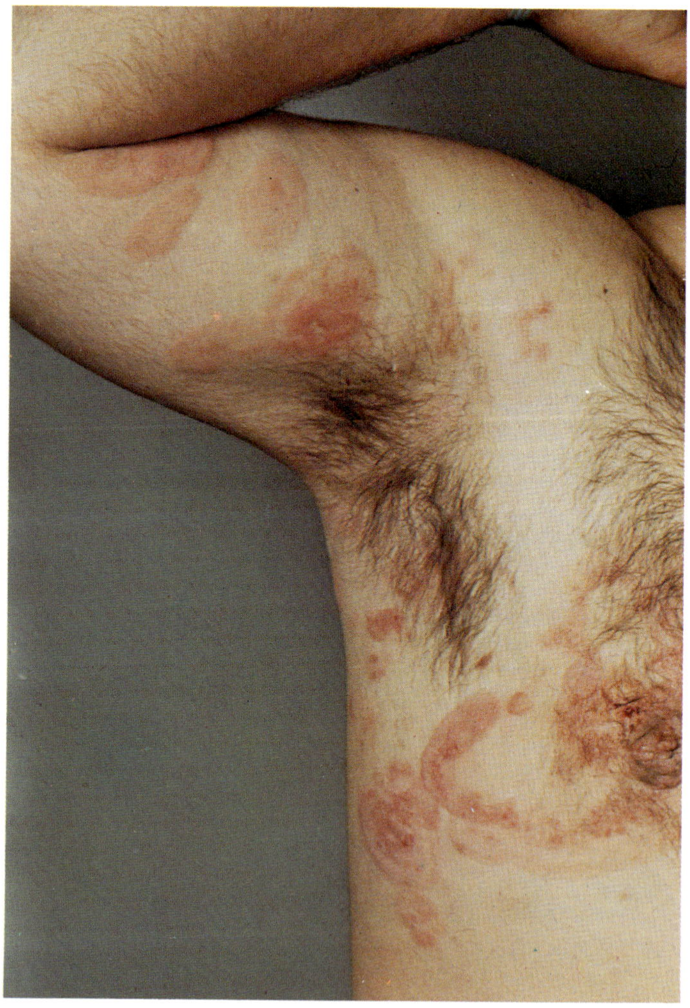

**Plate 60**

Mycosis fungoides, stage II. Crescentic plaque formation.

quently affected by the characteristic cells. Involvement of the bone marrow occurs late.

The Sézary syndrome, a part of the mycosis fungoides picture, may present as a cutaneous plaque or diffuse erythema that progresses in 1 to 5 years to an exfoliative erythroderma with atypical circulating cells, a distinct leukemic phase.

### *Pertinent information*

Mycosis fungoides is a T-cell lymphoma with a leukemic phase that remains unique from the traditional malignant lymphomas and from Hodgkin's disease (Fig. 35-10). It has been clearly demonstrated to have epidermotropism and probably begins in the skin. It has epitheliotropism and selectively invades certain organs and tissues on that basis. In its later disseminated phases it has been shown by Rappaport to invade virtually all organs and tissues, but relatively spares some, for example, bone marrow. It remembers its T-cell origins and selectively invades T-cell areas of lymphoid tissue.

The malignant cells, whose origin has been unclear until recently, are identified by cell membrane markers as T-cells (Edelson). There are other T-cell lymphomas and Lutzner suggests that they be lumped together as the "cutaneous T-cell lymphomas," because of the common epidermotropic propensity.

The Sézary syndrome, which does not occur in all cases of mycosis fungoides and which may develop de novo, is the leukemic phase of this malignancy. Atypical cells with deeply indented nuclei are circulating in numbers up to 200,000 per milliliter or more and demonstrate a similar biological behavior in all respects to that of the mycotic cells. The Sézary syndrome demonstrates an exfoliative erythroderma and a pronounced cellular immune system impairment, in contrast to mycosis fungoides, which, at least in the initial stages, has intact cellular immunity.

As the disease progresses, cellular immunity begins to fail, the number of normal T-cells falls, and dissemination may follow. Fuks believes that lymphangiography may help to demonstrate early lymph node involvement in pelvic and para-aortic nodes at this stage, and even dermatopathic nodes that may be

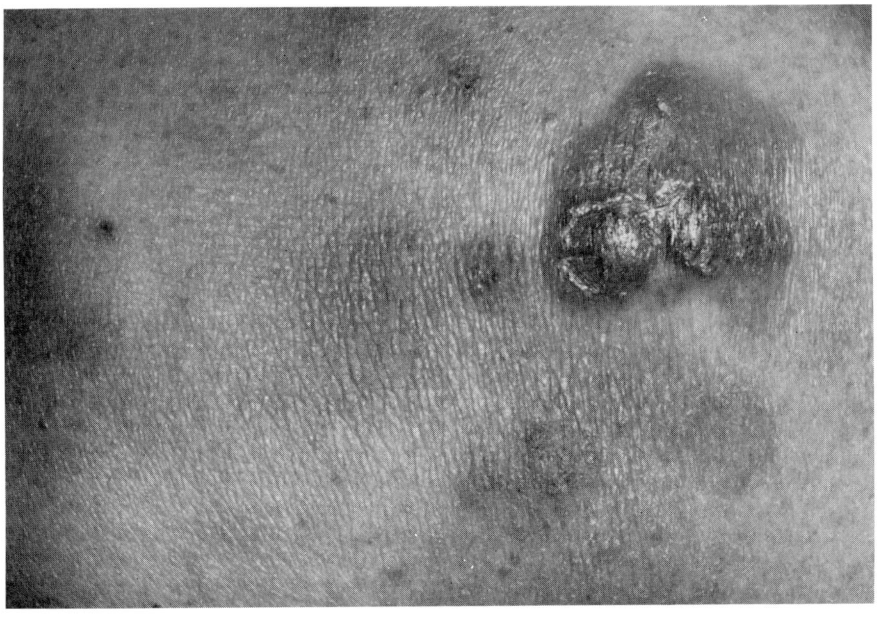

**Fig. 35-10.** Mycosis fungoides. Innocent-looking plaque with a suspicious crescentic border.

the first to attract malignant invasion. It was formerly held that mycosis fungoides changed its nature to one of the other malignant lymphomas, but it is now recognized that it retains its characteristic cellular components.

The diagnosis of mycosis fungoides is still impossible from microscopic examination in the early stages. When there are sufficient malignant cells in the upper dermis and in the epidermis, electron microscopic examination of an individual cell will identify them earlier than will light microscopy.

### *Treatment*

In the first stage, and even in some infiltrated lesions of the second stage, ultraviolet light has produced temporary remissions and served to relieve the pruritus. Psoralen therapy combined with intense ultraviolet-light exposure (PUVA) is an accepted method of therapy, as long as the tumor remains responsive. It is not known yet how long this is likely to be. Until this can be determined, current practices indicate the desirability of attacking the earliest lesions with either electron-beam therapy or nitrogen mustard administered topically. Gilchrist in 1976 and, more recently, Roenigk* and also Fitzpatrick* have reported on the beneficial response of patients with mycosis fungoides to photochemotherapy (PUVA).

Nitrogen mustard solution, 20% in water, may be used topically on infiltrated lesions, and since the medication is an active sensitizer, allergic dermatitis will usually result. Klein and Van Scott have both demonstrated beneficial effects from minute amounts of nitrogen mustard administered topically in the range of 1 part per million to sensitized patients. However, inducing specific immunological tolerance by intravenous administration prior to beginning topical nitrogen mustard therapy does not interfere with the effectiveness of the drug. Low does intravenous nitrogen mustard was used in late stages by Van Scott, with 78% remission, at least temporarily.

*Personal communications, 1978.

High-voltage electron-beam therapy, penetrating 1 cm. into the skin, achieves satisfactory remissions and has been claimed to result in cures (Fuks). Conventional, superficial x-ray therapy is good in selected cases with localized disease, but is of temporary value only. The tumor eventually becomes radioresistant.

Chemotherapy and alkylating drugs such as cyclophosphamide and chlorambucil have been shown to be effective, although resistance may develop. Antimetabolites, for example, methotrexate, can be used.

Cameron and Pauling have demonstrated that vitamin C in large daily doses is clearly helpful in prolonging life in cases of advanced cancer of various types.

## Metastases to skin

Lesions in the skin that are metastases from a distant neoplasm rarely divulge the tissue of origin by their clinical appearance. They are ordinarily firm, skin-colored, erythematous or telangiectatic nodules. They may be embedded in the skin itself or lie in the deeper subcutaneous tissue.

These are all rare lesions, but carcinoma of the breast results in more cutaneous metastases than any other tumor. These metastases may be accompanied by a erythematous inflammatory reaction of the surrounding skin. They may first appear on the scalp.

In a study of 724 records of patients with metastases to the skin, it was found that in men, cutaneous metastases developed from carcinoma of the lung and large intestine, melanomas, and carcinoma of oral cavity, kidney, and stomach, in that order of frequency. Women experienced metastases to the skin from primary tumors in the following order: breast, large intestine, melanomas, ovary, and lung.

The scalp and the abdominal wall were the most common areas for tumors that appeared as cutaneous metastases, although the numbers were few. Sources of the tumor were the large intestine, lung, stomach, ovary, and breast. Interested readers are referred to the excellent article by Brownstein and Helwig.

## Cutaneous manifestations of internal malignancy

***Gardner's syndrome.*** This is a dominantly inherited syndrome characterized by multiple sebaceous cysts present in early childhood primarily on the face and by fibromas, osteomas, and rectal polyposis. At least 40% to 50% of patients develop carcinomatous changes in the polyps, beginning at age 20.

***Peutz-Jeghers syndrome.*** Peutz-Jeghers syndrome is dominantly inherited and characterized by (1) hyperpigmented macules of the lips, oral mucosa, perioral, perinasal, and periorbital skin, and dorsal aspects of the fingers, toes, palms, and soles (the cutaneous pigmentation may fade and disappear with age, but the mucosal pigmentation persists); and (2) polyposis, chiefly of the small intestine. Carcinomatous change in the polyps is rare, but there is an increased incidence of gastric, duodenal, and colon carcinoma.

***Exposure to arsenic.*** Inorganic arsenic (Fowler's solution, processing of copper and other ores, insecticides, and electroplating) may result in a mottled hyperpigmentation primarily of the trunk, hyperkeratotic yellowish papules on the palms and soles, and multiple superficial basal cell carcinomas, often of the trunk. There is a high incidence of internal carcinoma, especially of the lung and gastrointestinal tract.

***Bowen's disease.*** This is an epidermoid carcinoma in situ, appearing clinically as a relatively flat, well-circumscribed, erythematous scaling patch that often resembles eczema. There is disagreement concerning the incidence of internal malignancy, which is as high as 80% of patients in some series. The underlying carcinoma is not specific and can be in any organ system. Arsenic may be responsible for the associated malignancies.

***Paget's disease.*** This can be either mammary or extramammary (especially perineal and axillary). Classically, it appears as a red, scaling, eczematous eruption. If it is on the areola, it is associated with duct carcinoma of the breast. Extramammary location, usually anogenital, is associated with underlying sweat gland or other carcinoma.

***Acanthosis nigricans.*** A dark brown to black, velvety thickening of axillae, groins, and sides of neck, acanthosis nigricans also occurs in obesity, endocrine disorders, and in congenital forms. The associated malignancy is commonly intra-abdominal, especially carcinoma of the gastrointestinal tract. Clinically, the benign and malignant forms cannot be differentiated. A history of adult onset in nonobese patients points toward a malignant etiology.

***Dermatomyositis.*** Dermatomyositis in adults is associated with internal malignancy in 15% to 50% of patients. It may precede (by as much as 3 years), coincide with, or follow the discovery of the tumor. It is characterized by weakness and often tenderness and pain of limb muscles. Skin changes are the following:

1. A finely scaling, nonbleeding erythema over the dorsa of interphalangeal joints as well as large joints, and an edematous erythematous eruption of butterfly distribution of the face
2. A lilac hue (heliotrope) of the eyelids
3. A diffuse violaceous, sometimes scaly eruption of exposed areas, hyperpigmented and hypopigmented macules interspersed with cutaneous atrophy
4. Raynaud's phenomenon, which may occur in adult dermatomyositis

All types of malignancies have been reported, with carcinomas of the breast and lung being reported most frequently.

***Generalized erythroderma (exfoliative dermatitis).*** Generalized erythroderma is characterized by a generalized scaling or exfoliating erythema. As a manifestation of malignancy, it most commonly occurs with lymphomas, leukemias, and mycosis fungoides. There have been a few reports of erythroderma with underlying carcinomas. Fifteen percent of patients with erythroderma have underlying malignancies.

***Acquired ichthyosis.*** This is a very dry, scaling disorder, which, when it arises abruptly in *adult life*, is a relatively specific sign of lymphoma. It has also been reported with a few cases of multiple myeloma.

***Generalized pruritus.*** Generalized pruritus is most frequent with lymphomas, especially Hodgkin's disease, and is less frequent with carcinomas, polycythemia, and leukemia.

***Bullous disorders.*** The entire gamut of blistering disorders can be associated with underlying malignancy. This includes the following:

1. Dermatitis herpetiformis—pruritic grouped vesicles on extensor surfaces, reported with choriocarcinoma, carcinomas of the ovary, uterus, prostate gland, bladder, rectum, and breast
2. Erythema multiforme—classic macules, papules, bullae, and "target" lesions that have been reported with leukemia, lymphoma, and carcinomas and in association with irradiation therapy of tumors (as a possible allergic response to necrotic tumor tissue).

***Urticaria.*** Chronic urticaria has been reported with rectal carcinoma. The association frequently mentioned with internal malignancy is perhaps exaggerated.

***Cushing's syndrome.*** Plethoric moon facies, maldistributed thoracic obesity, and striae, comprising this syndrome, have been associated with pulmonary pancreatic endocrine and gastrointestinal tumors.

***Herpes zoster.*** Both the classic zonal distribution of herpes vesicles and a disseminated form occur in increased incidence in lymphomas and leukemias, especially in Hodgkin's disease and chronic lymphocytic leukemia. It is also reported in breast cancer. It is rarely the presenting sign. The increased incidence of herpes zoster in these malignancies may be related to suppression of delayed cell-mediated hypersensitivity or abnormally depressed immunoglobulin synthesis in association with viral activation. The actual viral activation has been related to trauma in the spinal cord, such as irradiation damage from therapy and neoplastic invasion or pressure on the nerve roots.

***Purpura.*** As a manifestation of malignancy, purpura is most commonly associated with leukemias, polycythemia, and marrow metastases.

***Superficial thrombophlebitis migrans.*** Superficial thrombophlebitis migrans occurs with pancreatic and other gastrointestinal carcinomas.

***Hypertrophic osteoarthropathy.*** Hypertrophic osteoarthropathy occurs with bronchogenic carcinoma, mesothelioma, and pulmonary metastases.

***Carcinoid syndrome.*** This syndrome includes flushing, dyspnea, diarrhea, and so forth with carcinoid tumors.

## REFERENCES

Aisenberg, A. C.: Medical progress: malignant lymphoma, N. Engl. J. Med. **288**:883, 935, 1973.
**Lukes and Butler's classification with a full update on the entire subject.**

Braverman, I. M.: Skin signs of systemic disease, Philadelphia, 1970, W. B. Saunders Co.
**The major source book on this topic.**

Brownstein, M. H., and Helwig, E. B.: Patterns of cutaneous metastasis, Arch. Dermatol. **105**:862, 1972.
**724 patients with microscopic confirmation.**

Cameron, E., and Pauling, L.: Supplemental ascorbate in the supportive treatment of cancer: prolongation of survival times in terminal human cancer, Proc. Natl. Acad. Sci. **73**:2685, 1976.
**Clearly of value in prolonging survival of advanced cancer patients.**

Canellos, G. P., and DeVita, V.: Hodgkin's disease. In Maddin, S., editor: Current dermatologic management, ed. 2, St. Louis, 1975, The C. V. Mosby Co., p. 183.
**The various treatment options placed in clinical perspective.**

Edelson, F. L., Kirkpatrick, C. H., Shevach, E. M., et al.: Preferential cutaneous infiltration by neoplastic thymus-derived lymphocytes: morphologic and functional studies, Ann. Intern. Med. **80**:685, 1974.
**A remarkable attribute of some T-cells.**

Fuks, Z., and Bagshaw, M. A.: Total skin electron treatment of mycosis fungoides, Therapeut. Radiol. **100**:145, 1971.
**A plea for the earliest possible therapy.**

Fuks, Z., Bagshaw, M. A., and Farber, E. M.: Prognostic signs and the management of mycosis fungoides, Cancer **32**:1385, 1973.
**Fourteen of 132 patients disease free for 3 to 14 years. Lymphopenia described as a bad prognostic sign.**

Gilchrist, B. A., Parrish, J. A., Tannenbaum, L., et al.: Methoxsalen photochemotherapy of mycosis fungoides, Cancer **38**:683, 1976.
**Good-to-excellent control of cutaneous lesions of mycosis fungoides with methoxsalen and short-wave ultraviolet light.**

Lukes, R. J.: Criteria for involvement of lymph node,

bone marrow, spleen, and liver in Hodgkin's disease, Cancer Res. **31**:1755, 1971.
**The basis for the current classification.**

Lutzner, M., Edelson, R., Schein, P., Green, I., et al.: Cutaneous T-cell lymphomas: the Sézary syndrome, mycosis fungoides, and related disorders. NIH conference, Ann. Intern. Med. **83**:534, 1975.
**Characteristics are skin infiltrating, marrow sparing, and localization in T-cell regions of lymphoid tissue.**

Newbold, P. C. H.: Skin markers of malignancy, Arch. Dermatol. **102**:680, 1970.
**Omitting urticaria, a number of sound additives.**

Nordquist, B. C., and Kinney, J. P.: T and B cells and cell-mediated immunity in mycosis fungoides, Cancer **37**:714, 1976.
**Cell-mediated immunity falls as mycosis fungoides progresses. A patient with Sézary's syndrome had 75% null (neither B nor T) cells in the circulation. It is suggested these represent the malignant T-cells.**

Rappaport, H., and Thomas, L. B.: Mycosis fungoides. The pathology of extracutaneous involvement, Cancer **34**:1198, 1974.
**45 cases with extracutaneous infiltation of all organs is 71%.**

Shelley, W. B., and Wood M. G.: Observations on occult malignant lymphomas in the skin, Cancer **38**:1757, 1976.
**Pain was a feature in half.**

Templeton, A. C.: Kaposi's sarcoma. In Andrade, R., Gumport, S. L., Popkin, G. L., and Rees, T. D., editors: Cancer of the skin, vol. 2, Philadelphia, 1976, W. B. Saunders Co., p. 1183.
**Thorough, complete, and up to date.**

Thorling, E. B., and Thorling, K.: Serum copper in Hodgkin's disease before and after herpes zoster, Lancet **2**:1396, 1974.
**An interesting observation, without explanation at present.**

Tucker, S. B., and Winkelmann, R. K.: Treatment of Kaposi's sarcoma with vinblastine, Arch. Dermatol. **112**:958, 1976.
**Successful, particularly in progressive extensive disease.**

Van Scott, E. J., Grekin, D. A., Kalmanson, J. D., et al.: Frequent low does of intravenous mechlorethamine for late stages of mycosis fungoides lymphoma, Cancer **36**:1613, 1975.
**92 courses for 46 patients; 35% became at least clinically disease free.**

Vianna, N. J., Greenwald, P., Brady, J., et al.: Hodgkin's disease. Cases with the features of a community outbreak, Ann. Intern. Med. **77**:169, 1972.
**An extended epidemic studied at a New York State high school. Findings suggest an origin from person-to-person contact.**

Vonderheid E. C., Van Scott, E. J., Johnson, W. C., et al.: Topical chemotherapy and immunotherapy of mycosis fungoides, Arch. Dermatol. **113**:454, 1977.
**220 patients followed as the benefits and problems produced by topical application of dilute aqueous mechlorethamine.**

## CHAPTER 36

# Urticaria pigmentosa (mastocytosis)

Urticaria pigmentosa is an uncommon disorder produced by accumulations of *mast cells* in the dermis in the cutaneous form of the disease. Symptoms arising from the lesions are caused by histamine secretion from the mast cells.

### *Natural course*

Cases may have single or multiple lesions. Most single lesions disappear in a few years after an appearance at birth or in early childhood. They may be on the extremities or the torso and are round to oval, brown to red, 0.5 to 3 cm. Multiple lesions also usually begin at birth or in the first 2 years of life with small, irregular, tan to brown, poorly defined, often "blurry" macules or papules over the body, arms, and less often the face (Fig. 36-1). These are usually pruritic, and rubbing or scratching of the areas makes the lesions urticate or swell up noticeably (Fig. 36-2), a feature that is diagnostic. Bullous lesions may appear on the infant's feet or legs early in the disease. At least half of children with involvement show vesicular or bullous lesions.

Multiple lesions commencing in early childhood will usually disappear. Half will go by puberty, and the rest by degrees, but they will be faint and asymptomatic. Dermographia is present in about half of the patients at some time, on normal-appearing skin. Flushing from the secreted histamine occurs in less

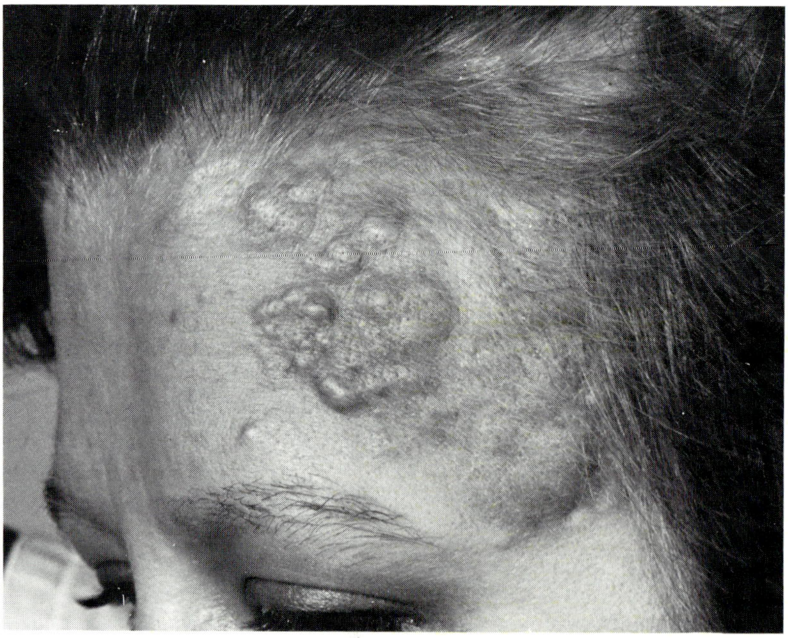

**Fig. 36-1.** Nodular mastocytosis. An unusual presentation.

than 10% of the cases and is not related to extent or number of mast cells in biopsy.

Lesions in the adult form are generally multiple, small, firm, slightly pigmented nodules that are concentrated in the inguinal area (inner thighs) and over the lateral aspect of the thorax. It may be macular, with a generalized telangiectasia that does not urticate on rubbing. It has a generally good prognosis although it does not show any tendency to clear.

Lesions that begin in adult life tend to persist. Also, adult forms of the disease are more likely to have associated lesions of the bones, liver, spleen, lymph nodes, and gastrointestinal tract, which may be progressive. Fully 40% of these patients have roentgenographically detectable bone lesions, which may be thinning, cystic changes or a form of sclerosis. Of the one fifth of adult patients that demonstrate involvement of internal organs, fully one third develop the rapidly progressive form of the disease.

The symptoms of mast cell disease may include pruritus, episodes of flushing, palpitation, cramping, abdominal pain, and sudden diarrhea. A form of facial flushing that spreads to the neck and chest is sometimes seen.

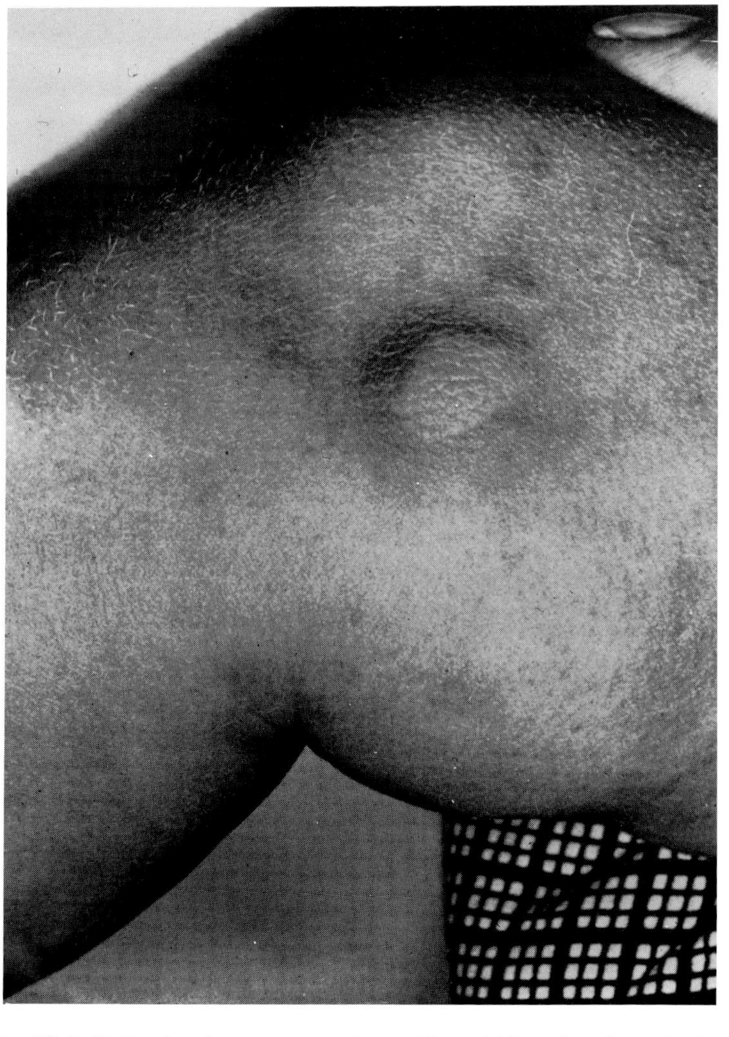

**Fig. 36-2.** Urticaria pigmentosa urticated by rubbing. A solitary lesion.

Complications that may arise because of the secretion of histamine and heparin include peptic ulcer, hemorrhagic tendencies, shock, and severe allergic reactions. Tissue infiltration and a leukemoid picture of bone marrow and blood may be present.

### *Pertinent information*

Mast cells in connective tissues are ubiquitous but often sparsely distributed. They are identified by special staining and so are not seen on routinely examined sections. Green reports their presence in epidermis in larger numbers in various inflammatory dermatoses. They are very similar but not identical to circulating basophils. They are present in the connective tissues of most organs and in pericapillary and adnexal regions of the dermis. They have large granules, which on stimulation are extruded from the cell, liberating histamine and heparin. There is a variety of chemical compounds in animal mast cells, but some disagreement exists over their presence in man. Mast cells have been shown to have high-affinity surface receptors that attach to IgE.

There is a tendency to familial occurrence in some patients.

The lesions in urticaria pigmentosa have been found to contain histamine liberated from the mast cell accumulation. This is produced by trauma such as rubbing and is responsible for the urtication. Some patients have a definite histaminuria.

Certain drugs will cause liberation of mast cell histamine, producing flushing, headaches, and symptoms in the gastrointestinal tract, and should be avoided by these patients. These drugs include *aspirin*, *polymyxin B*, *alcohol*, and the *codeine-morphine* group of alkaloids. Physical irritation such as brisk toweling should also be avoided.

### *Microscopic findings*

In the papular and nodular forms of mastocytosis, there is an accumulation of mast cells that is usually in the upper third of the dermis, but may be deeper in the modular lesions. Mast cells possess deeply basophilic granules in their cytoplasm. In the macular and diffuse forms, the mast cells are less in evidence and indeed may be difficult to identify.

The pigment is melanin.

### *Investigation*

INITIAL

- Biopsy of cutaneous lesion (with minimal manipulation to avoid degranulating the mast cells), with specific instructions to the pathologist to identify mast cells

SECONDARY

- In adult patients, investigation of systemic involvement
- Bleeding and coagulation time
- X-ray study of skeleton for areas of translucence
- Urinalysis for histamine
- Study of peripheral blood and bone marrow, if indicated, for circulating abnormal cells
- X-ray study of gastrointestinal tract

### *Treatment*

Oral antihistaminics and reserpine both have demonstrated some benefit in this distressing disease. There is, however, no effective treatment. Occasionally, the surgical excision of a solitary mastocytoma is possible. Remember that even minor surgical procedures can cause excessive histamine release in these patients, with various degrees of shock as a result. It has been recently reported that infusion of 2.5 mg. of mithramycin brought about dramatic relief of bone pain within 24 hours, but without altering anything else of the patient's symptoms.

#### REFERENCES

Caplan, R. M.: The natural course of urticaria pigmentosa, Arch. Dermatol. **87**:146, 1963.
**112 cases: an excellent background to the understanding of this disease.**

Conrad, M. E., Carpenter, J. T., Jr., Todd, J. N., III, et al.: Mithramycin in the treatment of systemic mastocytosis, Ann. Intern. Med. **83**:659, 1975.
**One dose relieved bone pain alone.**

Dennis, D. J.: The mastocytosis syndrome: clinical and biochemical studies, Ann. Intern. Med. **59**:194, 1963.
**Caused by histamine release and occurs in less than 15% of patients with mastocytosis.**

Eady, A. J. R.: The mast cells: distribution and morphology, Clin. Exp. Dermatol. **1**:313, 1976.
**What mast cells are, and more.**

Green, R. M., Cordero, A., and Winkelmann, R. K.: Epidermal mast cells, Arch. Dermatol. **113**:166, 1977.
**Increased epidermal mast cells in cutaneous inflammation, particularly in mucous membrane disorders.**

Sagher, F., and Even-Paz, Z.: Mastocytosis (urticaria pigmentosa). In Maddin, S., editor: Current dermatologic management, ed. 2, St. Louis, 1975, The C. V. Mosby Co., p. 216.
**Comprehensive coverage of the disease.**

Sahihi, T., and Esterly, N. B.: Atypical diffuse cutaneous mastocytosis, Am. J. Dis. Child. **124**:133, 1972.
**Interdicts certain drugs and unnecessary mechanical irritation.**

Warin, R. P.: Clinical aspects of mast cell disorders in man and considerations of factitious urticaria, Clin. Exp. Dermatol. **1**:323, 1976.
**A variety of mast cell–related disorders are covered.**

CHAPTER 37

# Vascular diseases: disorders of the cutaneous blood vessels

## BLOOD VESSELS

### Embryology

The epidermis contains no blood vessels. Endothelial and pericapillary cells arise from the mesoderm, developing recognizable simple channels by the tenth week of intrauterine life, which form arterioles and venules only after blood flow. By birth, the skin shows a disorderly capillary network, most prominent in skin creases. A more orderly arrangement is apparent after the first week of extrauterine life. Superficial capillary loops appear in selected areas above the general cutaneous vasculature and grow into the developing ridges of the papillary dermis to the dermoepidermal junction. A distinct horizontal vessel orientation and uniform looping papillary vessels are present in all areas of the skin by the fourteenth to seventeenth week after birth (Perera).

### Anatomy

This network of vessels in the dermis is supplied from the segmental arteries and their branches, the musculocutaneous or the direct cutaneous arteries. Arterovenous shunts are present in the fingers, toes, and palms, where they are called *glomus bodies*, and form neuromyoarteriolar structures between the arterial and the venous sides of the circulation. The role of these shunts is not clear. The area of capillary perfusion of the skin is less than that in muscle, and numerous shunts allow for lessening capillary flow still more.

Reticular patterns on the skin, "mottled skin," reflect the anatomical disposition of the dermal vessels, blood flow, and temperature. The light areas in the elliptical pattern, 2 cm. or thereabouts in diameter, correspond to the arterial system; the blue periphery of the ellipse marks the stasis zones in dilated venules.

The dermis, in its 0.5 to 2.5 mm. thickness, probably does not possess plexuses or recognizable levels of intercommunicating blood vessels, arterial and venous. There seems to be rather a general interlacing of the whole dermis with an efficient infinitely adaptable system of vessels of varying sizes. The chief attribute of this system seems to be its ability to meet any reasonable exigency by a flexible, mobile, protective outer layer often compressed and ischemic from external factors. The system is composed of arterioles and smaller vessels, rich in intercommunicating shunts between arterioles, so that there are preferential channels and multiple alternate channels at all levels.

Montagna and Parakkal suggest that two interconnected vascular areas can be recognizable in this network, the periadnexal or perifollicular baskets with their connections, and the general vascular background of the dermis.

### Physiology

Observations of the superficial capillaries and blood-flow studies indicate that the flow in individual capillaries is intermittent in a more or less rhythmic pattern. With maximal capillary dilatation, flow is slowed, and cells and fluid leak through walls. Generalized cutaneous vasodilatation produces heat loss and may initiate chills and shaking. This is seen in erythroderma.

Sympathetic stimulation, acetylcholine, and norepinephrine produce cutaneous vasoconstriction and cooling of the skin. Sweat gland activity is accompanied by kinin release and cutaneous vasodilatation. Vasoconstriction predominates and is evoked by skin cooling, noise, pain, forced breathing, or carbon dioxide inhalation. Vasodilatation appears to result from irritation of skin, noxious neural stimulation, and, in general, inhibition of sympathetic tone.

If an area of skin or an extremity has been subjected to temporary interruption of its blood supply, as occurs during sitting, lying, and so forth, that area undergoes an increased blushing when the circulation is reestablished. This mechanism is called *reactive hyperemia* and may be more prolonged after longer periods of interruption.

*Erythema* is produced by exposure to ultraviolet light, with the degree and duration being dependent on the wavelength, duration, and quantity of ultraviolet radiation. Wavelengths at 250 nm. are the most efficient erythema producers.

General body irradiation with ultraviolet light immediately causes a fall in systolic and diastolic blood pressures, sometimes lasting for several days.

Ingestion of substantial meals, particularly those high in protein content, produces cutaneous vasodilatation lasting for about 2 hours. Alcohol produces facial vasodilatation and subsequently more generalized increased blood flow without hyperemia, resulting in a pronounced heat loss over a period of time.

The normal whealing reaction of the skin is composed of three parts, referred to as the *triple response of Lewis*: (1) local vasodilatation caused by histamine or substances from damaged cells, (2) the red flare of arteriolar vasodilatation dependent on axone reflexes, and (3) localized, increased permeability independent of local innervation.

## Adaptability

It is yet to be generally appreciated that the *endothelial cell* is an active, migrating, secretory dynamic cell, rather than the static fixed structural component of the capillary we envisage (Majno). It also possesses multiple fenestrations, develops gaps between cells, and demonstrates evidence of considerable mitotic activity (Ryan). The material in the interstitial spaces is a *gel reticulum* containing mostly hyaluronic acid, which controls the degree of water imbibition and also the size of particles in the dermis, in acting as a coarse water-absorbing sponge.

The function of the cutaneous vasculature has undergone reconsideration since the days of Starling and the rigid interpretation of varying pressures at opposite capillary ends.

Ryan proposes an ever-changing balance between high volume of blood flow, slow flow, multiple channels in use, coiled papillary capillaries, cellular activity and turnover, and the opposite less exuberant situation with low volume, but faster flow, few channels, constricted capillaries, and tissue atrophy. Fibrin deposition is countered by fibrinolysis secreted by endothelium. Hypoxia and stasis result in *leaky capillaries* because of endothelial cell gaps. If fibrin is then deposited, neutrophils accumulate and *inflammation* develops because of vascular damage. Reparative responses include fibrinolysis, phagocytosis, new channels developed, and a tissue proliferation. *This is an ongoing process, and many skin diseases can be considered in this light.* Ryan (1973) has exhaustively reviewed his concept of this dynamic process, and the reader is commended to this work.

*These patterns are emphasized because it is vital to impress anyone attempting to understand the circulation of the skin with its variability, adaptability, and continued remodeling.* Both nerves and blood vessels in the dermis have been pictured as static as road maps for years. They are actually proliferating and atrophying continuously. Ryan has been chiefly responsible for introducing the idea of this dynamism. He denies the time-honored concept that the profusion of cutaneous vessels is primarily for thermoregulation and proposes that it is a feature of an active tissue continuously undergoing growth and repair.

Ryan describes cutaneous microcirculation

in terms of the *atrophy and ischemic tissue damage resulting from reduced channels and decreased blood flow, as opposed to the hypertrophy, tissue growth, and proliferation of channels that result from increased blood flow*. Coagulation, fibrin formation, fibrinolysis, telangiectasia, and their relationship to tissue growth are not understood, yet in some instances each of these processes also causes hypertrophy of the tissue they supply. Epidermis and epidermal extracts are among the most potent stimulators of new vessel growth in vitro. Added to these factors, the looseness and flexibility of skin, the presence of skin folds and creases, multitudinous episodes of ischemia from local pressure or creasing eliminate rigid concepts of blood vessel patterns within the skin.

*It must adapt infinitely, become ischemic, die a little, regrow, reform, proliferate under friction or pressure, and respond to extremes of temperature.* Despite this incredible adaptability, our concept has been for years that the chief function of the cutaneous vascular system is temperature regulation when its complexity may indeed demonstrate that its chief function is to survive while functioning protectively.

## LYMPHATICS

The lymphatic vessels terminate in the tissues as a system of blind endothelial tubes. The endothelial cells making up the walls of these tubes are shown by electron microscopy to separate readily when necessary, producing gaps through which cells, particles, and large molecules may pass into the lymphatic circulation (Courtice). A large portion of the plasma protein is continually leaking through the blood capillaries into tissue fluid and must be returned by way of the lymphatics. This large amount of high-protein tissue fluid, estimated at 100 to 200 Gm. per day in the skin is being continually returned to the vascular system through the lymph vessels. There is evidence that arterial pulsation and muscular movement is helped in maintaining lymph flow, by independent lymphatic contraction.

Cells in the efferent lymphatics of the sheep are mature lymphocytes at approximately 10,000 per milliliter; cells in the afferent channels are fewer, consisting of 10% macrophages with the rest being lymphocytes, normally 500 to 600 per milliliter in sheep (Courtice). When antigen is returned to the lymph node, processed by macrophages, the lymphocyte circulation stops, the efferent channel becomes cell free, and in 24 hours, the time for antigen processing, cell recruitment begins. This lasts for 72 hours, during which small mature lymphocytes circulate through the node. Then the doors open; transformed lymphocytes appear in large numbers in the lymphatics, to be returned to the bloodstream; and antibody is present in the lymph. Plasma cells for the most part remain in the node, manufacturing antibody.

### REFERENCES


Courtice, F. C.: Lymphatic function concepts old and new, Med. J. Aust. **1**:379, 1968

**A thorough statement of knowledge.**

de Micheli, P., and Glässer, A. H.: The effects of catecholamines and adrenoceptor blocking drugs on the canine peripheral lymph flow, Br. J. Pharmacol. **53**:499, 1975.

**Alpha-adrenergic receptors in lymphatics enable lymph flow to increase independent of blood flow or pressure.**

Majno, G., Shea, S. M., and Leventhal, M.: Endothelial contraction induced by histamine-type mediators: an electron microscopy study, J. Cell Biol. **42**:647, 1969.

**A dynamic view of cutaneous circulation.**

Montagna, W., and Parakkal, P. F.: The blood supply. In The structure and function of skin, New York, 1974, Academic Press, Inc., p. 142.

**An informed authoritative discussion on the subject from distinctive views held by the author for over a decade.**

Perera, P., Kurban, A. K., and Ryan, T. J.: The development of the cutaneous microvascular system in the newborn, Br. J. Dermatol. **82**(suppl. 5):86, 1970.

**Careful observations by capillary microscopy on 40 infants, related to function and environment.**

Ryan, T. J.: The blood vessels of the skin. In Jarrett, A., editor: The physiology and pathophysiology of the skin, vol. 2, The nerves and blood vessels, New York, 1973, Academic Press, Inc., p. 577.

**Here the reader gets the full treatment.**

Ryan, T. J.: The blood vessels of the skin, J. Invest. Dermatol. **67**:110, 1976.

**An incredibly short review of a complex concept.**

## VASCULAR TUMORS

### Hemangiomas

Hemangiomas (vascular nevi, or birthmarks) are congenital vascular lesions that appear at birth or in the neonatal period and have different patterns of behavior.

#### Superficial fading infantile hemangioma (salmon patch)

The most superficial and transient form of hemangioma is the superficial fading type. It is present on the central forehead and face in a large proportion of neonatal infants as a blotchy, irregularly shaped, salmon-colored patch. It is faint and is paler than the deeper colored port-wine stain. It fades spontaneously but slowly and disappears by the end of the second year. Interestingly enough, it continues to be apparent throughout adult life in some individuals when they flush or become angry—an important indicator of their feelings to those who know them!

#### Nevus flammeus (port-wine stain)

Nevus flammeus is a flat, capillary lesion that varies in color from red to reddish purple. This type of hemangioma is apparent at birth. The most common site is the occipital area of the scalp. Here the lesion is asymptomatic, does not enlarge, and poses no cosmetic or other problem. In other areas, however, the lesion is deeper colored, is present at birth, and does not tend to disappear with time. Unfortunately, it usually occurs on the face (Fig. 37-1, *A*). The color, which varies from light to dark reddish purple, depends on whether the superficial, middle, or deep dermal vessels are involved. This lesion persists, does not enlarge, but gradually may develop a verrucous, thickened nodular surface (Fig. 37-1, *B*). The lesions are usually unilateral and may follow the course of a cutaneous nerve.

Nevus flammeus of the central face, associated with convulsions, disturbed intelligence, hemiplegia, and ocular changes (signifying abnormal intracranial vascular channels), is referred to as *Sturge-Weber disease*.

The blood vessels composing this lesion are mature capillaries.

##### *Treatment*

Treatment is not satisfactory. A good cosmetic result may be obtained by the use of a properly selected, skin-colored, waterproof cosmetic such as Covermark, and this is almost always the most satisfactory therapy.

Some improvement may be obtained in the verrucous lesions by electrodesiccation or cryotherapy, if very carefully performed.

Goldman has carried out some interesting work using a laser technique in the treatment of cavernous and port-wine hemangiomas. The results are impressive in one case, although the course of treatment he reported took 7 years.

#### Hemangioma simplex (strawberry hemangioma)

Hemangioma simplex is a raised, red to bluish red, soft lesion with strawberry-like lobulations. It is usually present at birth but may develop shortly thereafter. It may enlarge for the first 6 to 9 months, but rarely does it increase in size after the first year. It may occur on any part of the skin surface. Despite its early enlargement, it will involute and eventually spontaneously disappear completely. Of all lesions, those involving the lips carry the least likelihood of resolving completely. *The earliest sign of involution is the appearance of linear, gray-white patches* in the center of the nevus (Plate 61). Very rarely one of these lesions will show a tendency to increase rapidly in size. The potential complication of enlargement is distortion of cosmetic areas (for example, nose, eye, and ear). Most of these enlargements return to normal, but if they do not, the condition may be best handled by plastic surgery after all activity has ceased. Consultative advice by one familiar with the course of these lesions should be sought under these circumstances.

##### *Microscopic findings*

The lesion is a capillary angioma showing cellular proliferation, often in several layers around the capillary lumen. In older lesions, fibrosis replaces the capillaries.

A

B

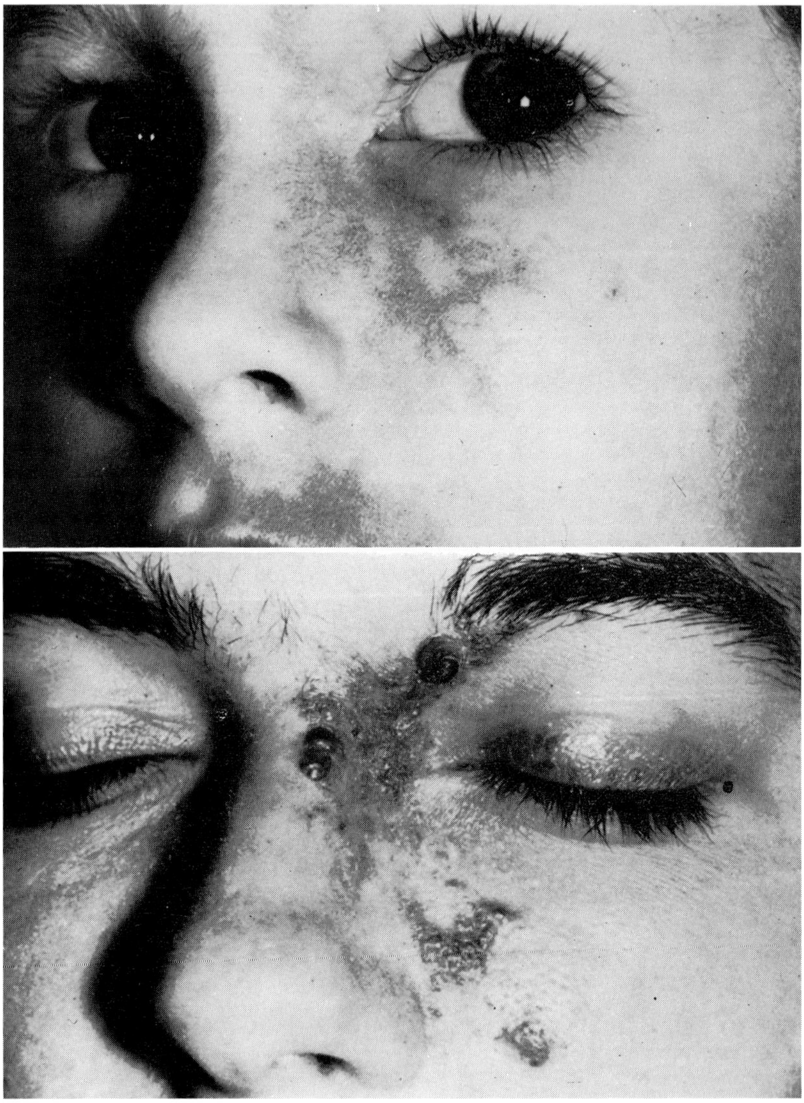

**Fig. 37-1. A,** Port-wine hemangioma in an infant. **B,** Port-wine hemangioma in adult. Note development of verrucous nodules.

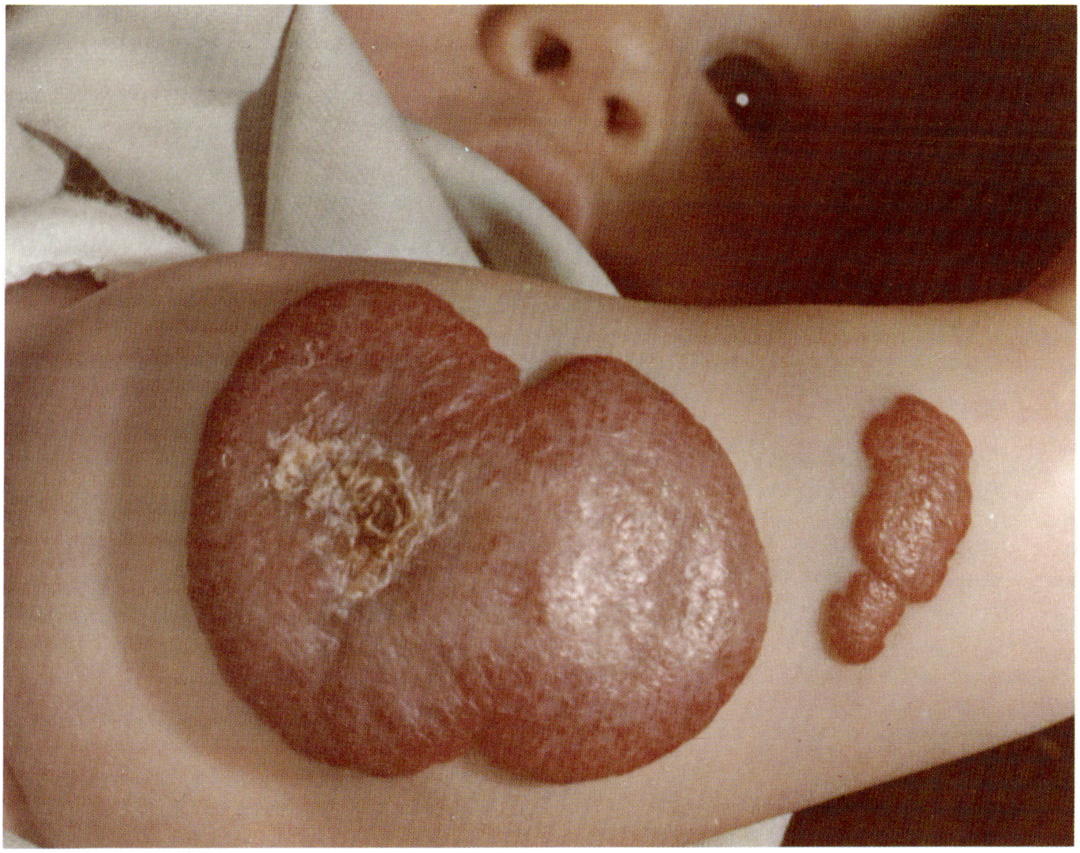

**Plate 61**

Hemangioma. Note gray patches and crusting, which are signs of resolution.

### *Treatment*

Virtually all strawberry hemangiomas involute spontaneously by the fifth year if they are left completely alone. They seldom produce scars or other residual effects. However, to gain their cooperation, parents must be reassured that this method of watchful waiting will produce the best cosmetic result.

Under certain circumstances, more aggressive therapy is indicated. These are (1) involvement of a vital structure; (2) rapid growth, with serious cosmetic sequelae; (3) mechanical orificial obstruction; (4) hemorrhage or hemorrhagic tendencies; and (5) threatened cardiovascular collapse.

When the need for intervention is present, based on the criteria listed above, early and aggressive use of prednisone may be indicated for rapidly growing strawberry type of hemangiomas. Varying schedules have been used, up to 20 mg. daily intermittently from 5 weeks to 2 years.

## Cavernous hemangioma

The cavernous type of hemangioma is a soft, rounded, compressible, reddish blue to skin-colored tumor that may occur on any part of the skin surface. Fortunately, this is the least common hemangioma. It is situated deeper in the dermis than are the other varieties. A growing body of observers believes that these also involute spontaneously. A phenomenon that must be kept in memory is the type of cavernous hemangioma that is associated with severe platelet destruction, bleeding, and the threat of death. The hemangioma rapidly increases in size.

Large "giant" hemangiomas of an extremity may set in motion the fibrinolytic system and begin a consumptive coagulopathy in the Kasabach-Merritt syndrome.

### *Microscopic findings*

The lesion consists of large vascular lakes lined by mature endothelial cells in the dermis and subcutaneous tissue.

### *Differential diagnosis*

***Lipoma.*** Lipoma is a soft, skin-colored tumor that usually appears long after infancy. It is soft, but retains its shape on pressure. It is not truly compressible and lacks the blue color of the hemangioma.

***Mongolian blue spot.*** Mongolian blue spot is dusky blue, nonvascular, and flat, is found in the lumbosacral region in Oriental and black infants, and usually disappears during childhood.

### *Treatment*

Certainly almost all of these lesions will involute spontaneously. It is not possible to determine in advance which lesion will involute and which will not. Radiation therapy in these lesions does not appear to produce any more rapid resolution than does nontreatment, and guidelines like Rowell's must be maintained. Judicious plastic surgery may offer cosmetic benefit, but this should be performed only after all possibility of involution has passed.

## Senile angioma (cherry angioma)

Senile angioma occurs chiefly on the chest and back in middle-aged and older individuals. It is 1 to 5 mm. in diameter, bright red, soft, multiple, compressible, and globular. It does not cause symptoms.

### *Treatment*

Electrocoagulation or cryotherapy is the accepted treatment.

## Nevus araneus (spider nevus) (Fig. 37-2)

Nevus araneus is a small vascular lesion with a bright red central dot that is an arteriole leading into radiating vessels around it. It is found in persons of all ages and usually is without significance. It is present in 25% to 50% of normal children. The maximum number of lesions recorded under these circumstances is 12. The spider-like lesion is found chiefly on the face and upper chest. It is induced, however, by liver damage and by pregnancy, apparently because of the higher estrogen level. Trihexyphenidyl (Artane), a drug used in treating Parkinson's disease, may produce these lesions.

### *Treatment*

Electrolysis is the preferred method of treatment. Electrodesiccation will destroy the lesion, but may produce a scar. Judicious

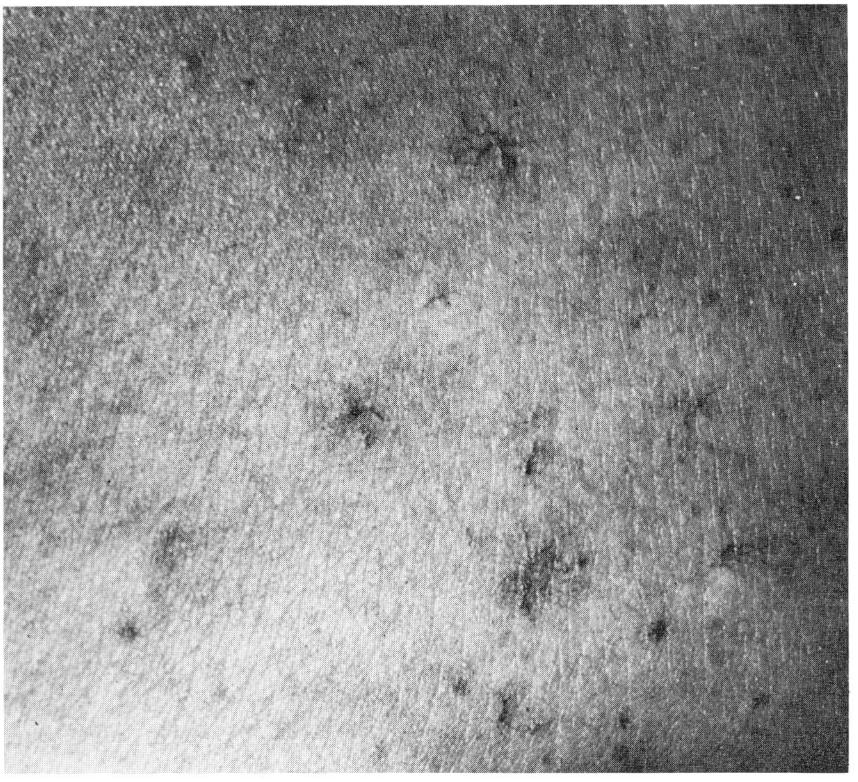

**Fig. 37-2.** Spider nevus. May occur in apparently normal individuals.

cryotherapy with liquid nitrogen may be successful.

### REFERENCES


Fost, N. C., and Esterly, N. B.: Successful treatment of juvenile hemangiomas with prednisone, J. Pediat. 72:351, 1968.

**Under critical conditions, aggressive steroid therapy is indicated. The problem is after stopping it.**

Goldman, L. and Dreffer, R.: Laser treatment of extensive mixed cavernous and port-wine stain, Arch. Dermatol. 113:504, 1977.

**Despite technical shortcomings, this may be the future approach in special cases.**

Goldwyn, R. M., and Rosoff, C. B.: Cryosurgery for large hemangiomas in adults, Plast. Reconstr. Surg. 43:605, 1969.

**Successful.**

Leopard, P. J.: Cryosurgery for facial skin lesions, Proc. Roy. Soc. Med. 68:606, 1974.

**Interesting technique of intermittent freezing of cavernous and capillary hemangiomas.**

Margileth, A. M.: Hemangiomas, lymphangiomas, and variants. In Maddin, S., editor: Current dermatologic management, ed. 2, St. Louis, 1975, The C. V. Mosby Co., p. 168.

Rowell, N. R.: A follow-up study of superficial radiotherapy for benign dermatoses: recommendations for the use of x-rays in dermatology, Br. J. Dermatol. 88:583, 1973.

**No sequelae noted in five patients given 6,400 to 12,800 rad in fractionated doses for port-wine stain. No patient should get more than 1,200 rad of conventional x rays.**

Thompson, L. R., and Holauf, H. J., Jr.: Hemangioma associated with thrombocytopenia: report of two cases and review of literature, Milit. Med. 129:652, 1964.

**Kasabach-Merritt syndrome.**


## TELANGIECTASIA

Telangiectasia results when superficial dermal capillaries and venules become visible as individual, fine, bright red lines. This is produced by persistent dilatation and is made more apparent if the epidermis, the dermis, or both become atrophic. An atrophic epidermis and dermis occur with increasing age in certain disease states and under the influence of long-term potent topical glucocorticoid therapy.

Actinic damage on the face is most prominent on the malar prominences, nose, and ears. In whites, as a result of ineffectual pigmentary protection from the sun, telangiectasia may be intense enough to give the appearance of a red face (see Fig. 19-1, *A*).

Telangiectasia is also seen over areas of atrophy-producing dermatoses such as necrobiosis lipoidica, on skin tumors such as sebaceous cysts and epitheliomas, as well as in sites of persistent vasodilation, as from longstanding rosacea and polycythemia. It may be a component of a spider nevus, which may be associated with an increased level of estrogens. This type is arterial in origin, with small radiating, telangiectatic vessels.

Telangiectasia as a component of systemic disease occurs in dermatomyositis, lupus erythematosus, scleroderma, the adult form of mastocytosis, and hereditary disorders such as ataxia telangiectasia. Primary telangiectasia occurs in *generalized essential telangiectasia*, a spreading disorder beginning on the legs of adult women, in hereditary hemorrhagic telangiectasia (see below), and in some angiomatous diseases.

### Treatment

Electrolysis is the treatment of choice for localized forms of telangiectasia. This makes use of a galvanic direct current of electricity of less than 2 milliamperes. A very fine flexible needle is inserted into the lumen of the vessel, and free hydrogen is liberated from the needle, which is wired to serve as the negative electrode. This obliterates the tiny vessel. For larger areas, an acceptable waterproof covering such as Covermark can be used with benefit.

## HEREDITARY HEMORRHAGIC TELANGIECTASIA (RENDU-OSLER-WEBER DISEASE)

In hereditary hemorrhagic telangiectasia, a rare disorder, multiple small telangiectatic lesions of the skin and mucous membrances may appear in childhood, but most commonly after puberty, and tend to increase in number throughout adult life. The disease is hereditary, with a dominant pattern of inheritance.

Symptoms are usually initiated by nosebleeds, but bleeding may occur from lesions in the mouth, pharynx, and gastro-intestinal or urogenital tracts.

Unfortunately, the more follow-up done on patients with hereditary hemorrhagic telangiectasia, the more we become aware of the appreciable percentage of these patients demonstrating neurologic symptoms, pulmonary arteriovenous fistulas, and proved cases of cerebrovascular malformation. The lesions may not appear until the patient is in the thirties.

Lesions are slightly elevated, circumscribed, red papules, 1 to 3 mm. in diameter, that blanch on pressure. They tend to occur on nasal mucous membranes first, but new lesions continue to appear on the face, pharynx, lips, hands, fingertips, and thorax. They have a definite bleeding tendency that may be difficult to control, despite their minute size. Anemia may result from continued oozing, despite a normal clotting mechanism.

### Treatment

Treatment consists of local destruction of the lesions in mild cases. Cyclic estrogen therapy has been used, resulting in a reduction in bleeding tendency in some patients. Skin grafts have been helpful.

## CUTIS MARMORATA

An intermittent bluish mottling of the skin of the extremities characterizes cutis marmorata. It reflects the distribution of the deeper venous channels and can be shown by infrared photography of normal skin. In those individuals, chiefly normal children, who are so predisposed, it is most apparent on exposure to cold. It has no significance.

## LIVEDO RETICULARIS

On examination, livedo reticularis presents a latticework of blue to red subcutaneous mottling, caused by cyanosis in small dilated vessels of the legs and arms.

Capillary microscopy and other studies indicate a variable flow through the small vessels leading to the skin and variable stasis in the most superficial capillaries.

## Idiopathic livedo reticularis

This disorder, similar to cutis marmorata, also involves the extremities but is persistent rather than episodic. It never disappears entirely. Symptoms of coldness, paresthesias, numbness, and aching of the areas may accompany the vascular mottling, which can extend to the trunk.

There are no abnormalities on microscopic examination, although occasionally superficial recurrent ulcers may appear over the affected sites on the legs, in which case a localized vasculitis may be found.

### *Treatment*

Treatment is not effective, although cold should be avoided. In some cases oral reserpine (0.25 to 0.5 mg. daily) has produced dramatic relief.

## Secondary livedo reticularis

Livedo reticularis may appear as part of a primary vascular disorder, including chilblains, rheumatoid arthritis, collagen disorders, thrombocythemia, malignancies, chronic infection, arteriosclerosis, arterial occlusion, and vasculitis, particularly periarteritis nodosa. When it occurs in a previously unaffected adult, particularly if it demonstrates an asymmetrical patchy appearance, the patient warrants further investigation.

An asymptomatic livedo reticularis has been reported in patients receiving amantadine in the treatment of parkinsonism. It is abolished by epinephrine or norepinephrine (vasoconstrictors) and accentuated by isoproterenol (vasodilator). A reticulated pigmentation has been seen as a result.

### *Treatment*

Treatment is of the primary disease.

#### REFERENCES

Champion, R. H.: Livedo reticularis, Br. J. Dermatol. **77**:167, 1965.

**Primary and secondary.**

Vollum, D. I., Parkes, J. D., and Doyle, D.: Livedo reticularis during amantadine treatment, Br. Med. J. **2**:627, 1971.

**Possibly the amantadine was responsible for the release of dopamine and other catecholamines—result, vasoconstriction.**

## ACROCYANOSIS

Acrocyanosis is a symmetrical vascular disorder that results in persistent coldness and a blue-red cyanosis of the distal aspects of the extremities. The hands are usually most affected, and in severe cases the ears and nose are also involved. Cold weather aggravates the condition, but it does not completely disappear in warm weather. Swelling and aching accompany exposure to the cold.

The disorder occurs most often in young women. It persists throughout life and is lessened by living in a warm, even climate. There are no evidences of atrophy, ulceration, or alteration in the affected skin.

There is no histopathological evidence of vascular disease, but a physiological narrowing of the arterioles and precapillaries appears to be present. Interested readers should consult Ryan's review of current knowledge regarding dermal blood flow and platelet stickiness in this and associated disorders caused by cold.

### *Treatment*

A steady, even environmental temperature should be sought, since medications are of little value to date.

#### REFERENCE

Ryan, T. J., and Copeman, P. W. M.: Microvascular pattern and blood stasis in skin disease, Br. J. Dermatol. **81**:563, 1969.

**The normal increase in blood viscosity on cooling was accentuated.**

## ERYTHROMELALGIA (ERYTHERMALGIA)

Erythromelalgia is a vascular disorder without apparent pathological alteration of the blood vessels, in which temperature elevation or exercise produces pronounced erythema and local discomfort. There is usually a critical temperature above which symptoms appear.

The disorder has been reported to precede the development of polycythemia, systemic lupus erythematosus, and rheumatoid arthritis in some patients.

It affects the feet in middle-aged men chiefly. With increased local environmental temperature, heavy or occlusive socks or footwear, and hot weather, the skin becomes very red, and rather severe burning discomfort develops. There may be associated swelling. Cooling of the feet causes the symptoms to disappear more quickly, although each episode may last only 2 to 3 hours. The cause is unknown.

### *Treatment*

Treatment is not specific, except for maintenance of an environmental temperature below that which produces symptoms. Acetylsalicylic acid in adequate doses may give relief. The patient should be examined and observed for possible underlying hematological or collagen disorder.

## VASCULITIS

Vasculitis is a rather comprehensive identification for a group of cutaneous disorders that have in common as their major feature a functional fault in the integrity of the vessel's wall. In part, this can be classified according to the size of the vessel, but this gets lost in the variety of causes. We are still classifying these disorders largely as to cause.

The disorder, as Ryan clearly states, is one of degree. The fault in the vessel wall results in either erythema, effusion, purpura, or necrosis. The process is one of "leakiness" and is very complex. Some vessels in some areas such as the nose are very prone to be affected, and others such as in the brain are very unlikely to be affected.

Vasculitis, in the definition of a cellular vascular or perivascular infiltrate, results from the leaky vessel. This is most often produced by an immune process and can be identified by various means as such.

The intravascular complement system and the fibrinogen-fibrin-fibrinolysin system are always in action and in a balanced adversary position at all times. An alteration in these factors may begin the process that leads to a mild or a fulminating cell-and-tissue destroying vasculitis.

To divide this continuum into stages or processes, or even diseases, is difficult. Ryan, in his masterful exposition of this subject, fits the pieces together to produce the blueprint for the functioning system. There are vasculitides whose effects are limited to the skin or to the skin and internal organs, whereas some may not involve the skin at all.

The diseases range in severity from extremely mild to fulminating and fatal (Winkelmann, Soter, Chumbley, Conn, Ryan).

Vasculitis producing cutaneous lesions is characterized by the following findings: (1) erythematous papules and plaques, (2) nodules, (3) purpuric or hemorrhagic papules and vesicles, and (4) pustular and necrotic lesions.

There is a previous history of drug allergy in many patients.

Lesions are most often seen on the legs, thighs, and buttocks; they occur in crops and may last for a limited time only. Some lesions will begin as erythematous papules or plaques and progress to ulceration. The ulcerated lesions heal slowly. With the severe forms, lesions are ulcerative and progressive, with more evidence of extension than of healing; with progression, other organs and systems show involvement as well. (Palmer, Sams and Winkelman, and Ditto).

### *Pertinent information*

Recent studies indicate that immunological mechanisms are at work in this group of diseases. Sufficient evidence is not available to offer a satisfactory working classification nor to clarify pathogenetic mechanisms. Such diversified diseases as streptococcal and other bacterial infections, tuberculosis, leprosy, drug reactions, serum sickness, neoplastic diseases, rheumatoid arthritis, and lupus erythematosus are all associated with cutaneous vasculitis.

Immunoglobulins IgG and less often IgM and IgD have been demonstrated by immunofluorescence in vasculitis lesions, along with consumption of complement. It is believed that immune complexes as a result of soluble circulating antigen-antibody union form a basis for the pathogenic process, and other factors including stasis, cold, epinephrine secretion, attraction and destruction of leukocytes, local cell injury, increased blood viscosity, and other findings combine to allow vascular damage. Abnormal fibrin deposition occurs, and measurements of serum fibrinolytic activity are significant in the assessment of therapy of the disease process. Fibrinolytic activity is almost absent in the skin of the lesions of vasculitis and reduced in the normal leg skin.

### *Microscopic findings*

All aspects of the vascular system may be affected, including veins, venules, capillaries, arterioles, and arteries. A biopsy should, therefore, include all these blood vessels for assessment of the process. Three types of inflammation, based on the predominant cell type, has helped to form a classification of the process of vasculitis (Copeman and Ryan): predominantly (1) polymorphonuclear, (2) lymphocytic, and (3) granulomatous cellular infiltrates are described, with classification as well of the size of the blood vessel—small dermal vessels and large subcutaneous vessels.

Other features that aid in the assessment of the type and severity of vasculitis are fragmentation of nuclei of inflammatory cells, fibrinoid deposition, hyalinization of vessel walls, degree of inflammatory change, and presence of necrosis. Immunofluorescence has helped to unravel the mechanism of some of these processes.

## Selected clinical forms of vasculitis

The following are selected examples of clinical disease in which vasculitis is the major pathological process.

***Urticaria.*** Urticaria produced by histamine may in some patients extend, become painful and bruised, and show extravasation of red blood cells. Urticaria may be associated with systemic lupus erythematosus and is a part of Schönlein-Henoch vasculitis. A variety of drugs and chemicals, including salicylates and related compounds, can produce this picture (Fig. 37-3).

***Pigmented purpuric dermatoses.*** Several clinical entities demonstrating various degrees of capillary inflammation are included in this category. They have in common small, often asymptomatic, purpuric macular lesions of the ankles and legs, spreading progressively. Some of these, notably carbromate purpura, are the result of drug sensitivity, but more often the etiology is undetermined. Males seem to be most frequently affected in most forms. The process is lymphocytic and pericapillary and results in leakage of red blood cells, with hemosiderin deposits in the dermis.

***Erythema multiforme.*** Erythematous papules, plaques, vesicles, and bullae of varying etiology reflect an underlying small-vessel lymphocytic vasculitis.

***Acute parapsoriasis.*** Acute parapsoriasis is an acute, often self-limited process of unknown etiology, affecting children more commonly than adults. The lesions are small and usually asymptomatic and comprise papules, vesicles, and small necrotic lesions that heal without permanent scars. The small vessels involved show a lymphocytic infiltrate.

***Allergic cutaneous vasculitis.*** This disorder chiefly affects the extremities, involving the skin primarily, with any of the above lesions presented by a vasculitis process. Systemic signs of fever and arthralgia, as well as renal involvement, are not uncommon, however. The process affects small blood vessels, with an acute polymorphonuclear inflammatory process in the vessel wall. It may be caused by drugs, hormones, a variety of diseases, and bacterial, viral, and fungal infection. Acute and chronic forms are seen.

***Atrophie blanche (livedo vasculitis)*** (Fig. 37-4). Atrophie blanche is a chronic recurrent atrophic vasculitis of the lower extremities particularly around the malleolar areas. It often begins with purpuric lesions that progress to thin, fragile, white, stellate, taut scars that are penetrated at their periphery by small vessels that are notable by their fragility in turn. Pain and tenderness is a feature. Small to confluent superficial slow-healing ulcers

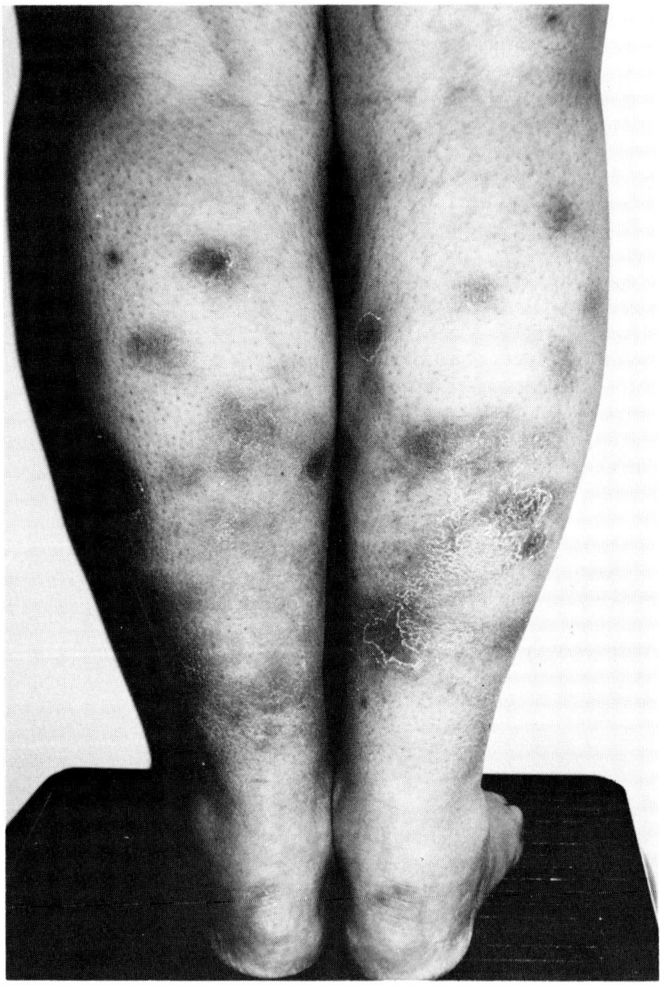

**Fig. 37-3.** Vasculitis from salicylates. These drugs can produce vasculitis as well as urticaria.

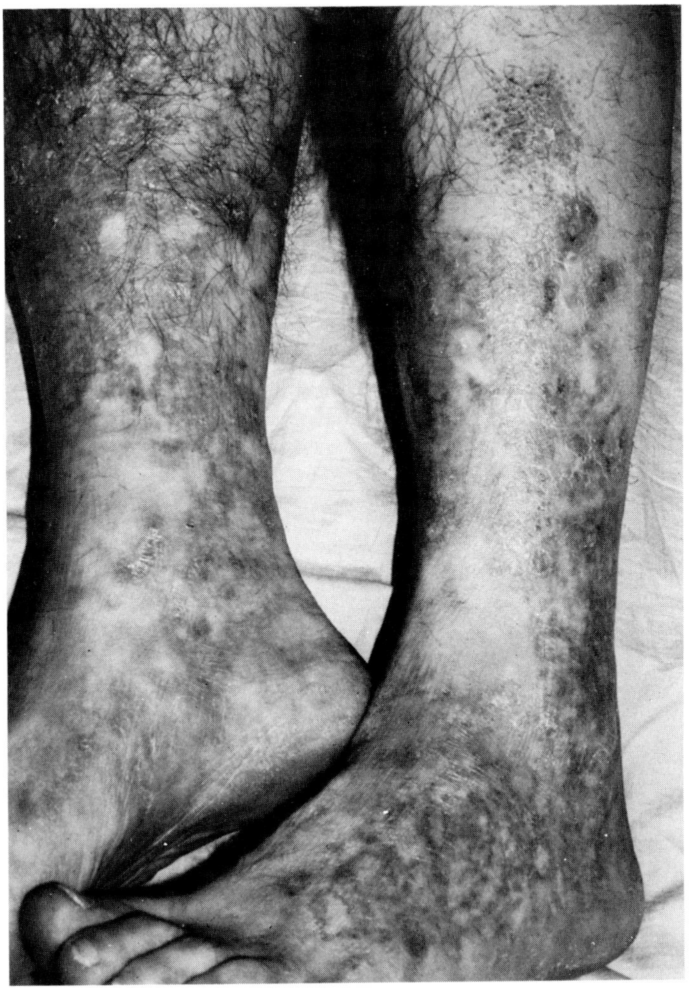

**Fig. 37-4.** *Atrophie blanche* (livedo vasculitis).

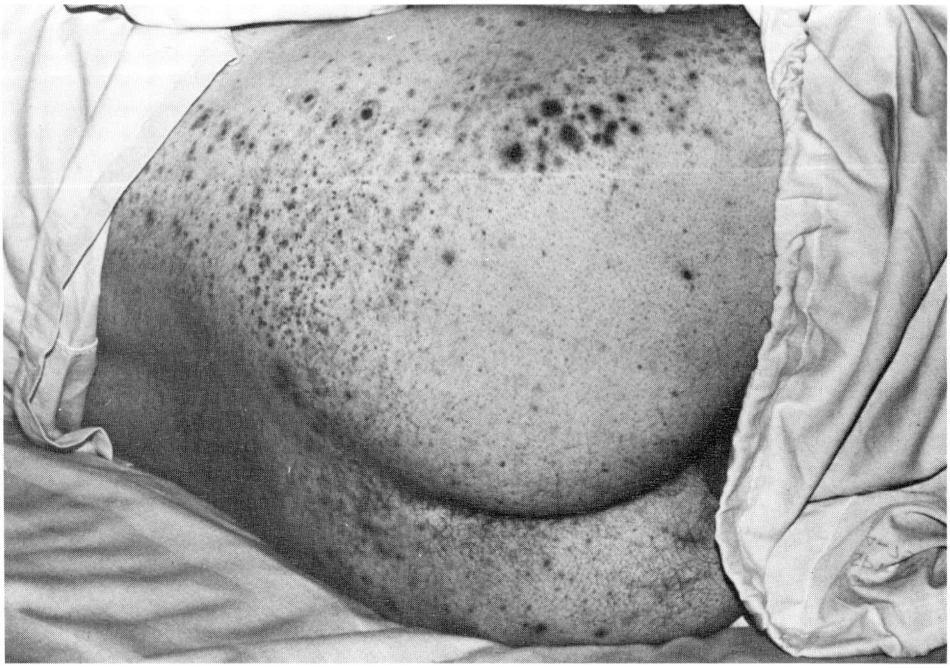

**Fig. 37-5.** Schönlein-Henoch purpura. Note ringed and multiform shapes of lesions.

are a major feature. Arterial pulses are intact, and normal skin surrounds the area. Immunoglobulins IgG, IgD, or IgM may be deposited and complement as well.

TREATMENT. The treatment of atrophie blanche has been successful by means of fibrinolytic therapy with phenformin and ethylestrenol. We can confirm the effectiveness of this therapy advocated by Ryan. However, there have been warnings about the problem of lactic acidosis and increased cardiovascular complications in diabetes from phenformin.

The drug has been recalled in Canada. It increases anaerobic glycolysis. Metformin is not an effective substitute.

***Schönlein-Henoch purpura (allergic purpura, anaphylactoid purpura)*** (Fig. 37-5). Schönlein-Henoch purpura occurs chiefly in children, although it can affect persons of any age. Some of the cases follow an upper respiratory tract infection within 3 weeks. Drugs, particularly thiazide diuretics, must be considered as possible causes. The disorder begins with fever, followed by a characteristic type of purpura, abdominal pain, localized edema, joint pain, and often renal involvement, shown by hematuria. Some characteristics of the disorder are similar to those of serum sickness; hence the name allergic or anaphylactoid purpura. There is a leukocytoclastic vasculitis of the vessels of the middermis, with fibrinoid necrosis and endothelial proliferation.

The cutaneous findings are those of irregularly shaped petechiae or ecchymoses, with inflammatory papules associated with urticaria, thus giving an unusual appearance. They are usually confined to the legs and buttocks. Localized urticarial edema is also present and is one of the prime features of the disease, appearing mostly on the hands, feet, and face.

Other characteristics that are significant include transient migratory joint pains of the lower extremities, renal lesions that may be persistent, and colicky abdominal pain.

The disease is self-limited, lasting less than 6 weeks as a rule, although longer cases are by no means unusual. Recurrences also are not uncommon. The chronic renal lesion that develops in approximately one third of cases is the most significant aspect of the disease, since this may lead to renal failure in a few instances. Renal biopsy may be necessary for evaluation. Results of the tourniquet test are negative.

Evidence from immunofluorescent techniques indicates that antigen-antibody complexes are found in both skin and kidney arterioles.

TREATMENT. Investigation for a source of infection, hematological disease, and dysproteinemias and elimination of drug allergy as a causative factor are necessary before treatment is instituted. Glucocorticoids will not significantly shorten the course of the immediate attack but may be effective in treatment of the persistent renal disorder. They may slow its progression and improve a nephrotic syndrome.

***Nodular vasculitis.*** Nodular vasculitis is characterized by painful, tender, bluish red, nodular lesions of the legs of middle-aged women. These persist for weeks to months but seldom ulcerate. There are no systemic symptoms. The process is predominantly lymphocytic, with a granulomatous component, and affects vessels larger than those in the dermis. This may be a chronic form of erythema nodosum.

***Hypersensitivity angiitis.*** A universally distributed, acute, necrotizing disease of small arteries, hypersensitivity angiitis involves most organs. A polymorphonuclear, cellular inflammation of the walls of these vessels progresses rapidly to a fatal outcome. The disease is caused by drugs and serum used as therapeutic agents.

***Wegener's granulomatosis.*** A progressive, nodular, destructive, granulomatous vasculitis that affects chiefly the midline structures of the mouth, pharynx, larynx, and trachea, as well as the lungs, kidneys, and spleen, Wegener's granulomatosis is fortunately rare, but almost always fatal.

***Polyarteritis nodosa.*** Polyarteritis nodosa is a disorder caused by widespread necrotizing inflammation of the small and medium-sized arteries throughout the body. The skin is not involved in all cases of this major multiple organ disease of the blood vessels, but when they occur, the lesions are chiefly on the legs and consist of blue-red, tender, painful nodules that may ulcerate. A primarily cutaneous variety exists, with a less grave prognosis.

### *Investigation*

Investigative tests for vasculitis should include the following:

1. Biopsy, for routine stains and immunofluorescence, for diagnosis and assessment of type and severity of vasculitis
2. Tests of hemoglobin, white blood cell count, and sedimentation rate, for estimates of systemic involvement
3. Antinuclear factor and serum proteins, rheumatoid factor, and serological test for syphilis, to determine if collagen disease is present
4. Culture and antistreptolysin titer, to detect infection
5. Microscopic urinalysis for red cells and casts
6. Serum complement, cryoglobulins
7. X-ray films of the chest, sinus tract, and teeth
8. X-ray films of the gastrointestinal tract, if indicated by symptoms
9. Determination of serum fibrinolytic activity

### *Treatment*

Rest, protection from cold, movement of legs to maintain blood flow, and treatment of hypertension are important measures. Elevation of blood pressure adds to the risk of further small-vessel damage. Obvious foci of infection should be cleared for the same reason.

Treatment of vasculitis involves obtaining a thorough history for possible sources of drug allergy, visceral or joint involvement, collagen disease, or evidence of bacterial infection. An examination is required to reveal possible sources or foci of infection. Systemic glucocorticoids appear to produce the most satisfactory therapuetic response in these disorders, although their use is fraught with controversy.

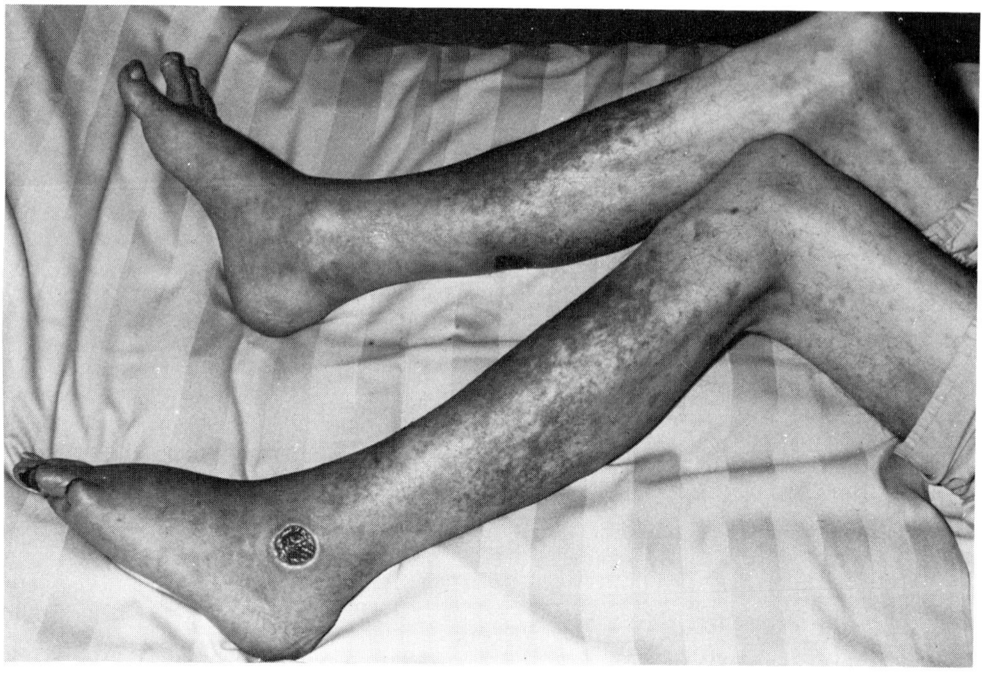

**Fig. 37-6.** Rheumatoid vasculitis and leg ulcer. A leukocytoclastic, capillary-venular microvasculitis.

They do best in deep, tender, nodular lesions and less well in superficial, painful ulcerations as in hypertensive or rheumatoid vasculitis ulcers (Fig. 37-6).

Aspirin is advocated as an anti-inflammatory agent, as it is in rheumatoid arthritis. Although it does adversely effect some urticarias, it has a fibrinolytic effect in vasculitis (Preston). Indomethacin, phenylbutazone, ibuprofen (Brufen), and iodides have been used successfully in nodular vasculitis (panniculitis) (Perry and Winkelmann) and may help in chronic erythema nodosum (Ryan).

Heparin is valuable in vasculitis when infarction, tissue death, and gangrene are possible. It is essential in some cases of disseminated intravascular coagulation and effective in myocardial infarction, pulmonary embolism, meningococcal septicemia purpura, and glomerulonephritis (Ryan). It can be used intravenously, or, as is often the case now, subcutaneously in 5,000 units at 12-hour intervals, or it has anticomplementary action and prevents platelet aggregation (Amery).

Immunosuppressives are essential in some disorders, for example, lupus erythematosus, vasculitis, and some granulomatous or malignant diseases.

Cyproheptadine, as an antiserotonin agent, may be useful in some cases of cutaneous vasculitis. The reader is referred to Ryan (1977) for a fuller consideration of therapeutic measures.

Therapy of any of these disorders requires the advice of one thoroughly familiar with the natural course and complications of the disease. Fibrinolytic therapy has been utilized, with promising results, from combinations of phenformin (DBI) and an anabolic steroid (ethylestrenol, Maxibolin) in patients with impaired fibrinolytic activity (Dodman, Cunliffe, and others).

### REFERENCES

Amery, A. H., Pergrum, G. D., Ridson, R. D., et al: Nature of hyperacute rejection in dog renal allografts and effects of heparin on the rejection process, Br. Med. J. 1:455, 1973.

**Prolongs graft survival because of its effect on platelet aggregation.**

Chumbley, L. C., Harrison, E. G., and DeRemee, P. E.: Allergic granulomatosis and angiitis (Churg-Strauss syndrome), Mayo Clin. Proc. **52**:477, 1977.
**Asthma, systemic vasculitis with nodular cutaneous involvement without renal disease.**

Coffman, J. D., and Davies, W. T.: Vasospastic diseases: a review, Prog. Cardiovasc. Dis. **18**:123, 1975.
**An inclusive review of present status of various vascular diseases.**

Conn, D. L., McDuffie, F. C., Holley, K. E., et al: Immunologic mechanisms in systemic vasculitis, Mayo Clin. Proc. **51**:511, 1976.
**Three groups, all had skin lesions; divisions made on lung or visceral involvement.**

Copeman, P. W. M., and Ryan, T. J.: The problems of classification of cutaneous angiitis with reference to histopathology and pathogenesis, Br. J. Dermatol. **82**(suppl. 5):2, 1970.
**Urticaria, the simple effusion, may be present in the most violent process.**

Dodman, B., Cunliffe, W. J., and Roberts, B. E.: Observations on tissue fibrinolytic activity in patients with cutaneous vasculitis, Br. J. Dermatol. **88**:231, 1973.
**Emphasizes the part fibrinolysis plays.**

Dodman, B., Cunliffe, W. J., and Roberts, B. E.,: Clinical and laboratory double-blind investigation on effect of fibrinolytic therapy in patients with cutaneous vasculitis, Br. Med. J. **2**:82, 1973.
**Clearly successful.**

Gilliam, J. N., Herndon, J. H., and Prystowsky, S. D.: Fibrinolytic therapy for vasculitis of atrophie blanche, Arch. Dermatol. **109**:664, 1974.
**Five patients, all responded well to phenformin and ethylestrenol.**

Mandell, F., Folkman, J., and Matsumoto, S.: Erythromelalgia, Pediatrics **59**:45, 1977.
**The clinical antithesis of Raynaud's disease. Pain is relieved by immersion in cold; unresponsive to treatment.**

Palmer, H. M., and Vedi, K. K.: Digital ischemia and malignant disease, Practitioner **213**:819, 1974.
**Further interrelation of cutaneous vessels, their coagulation-dissolution process, and disease elsewhere.**

Parish, W. E.: Cutaneous vasculitis: antigen-antibody complexes and prolonged fibrinolysis, Proc. Roy. Soc. Med. **65**:276, 1972.
**An attempt to indict bacterial infection and immunoglobulins in impaired fibrinolysis.**

Perry, H. O., and Winkelmann, R. K.: Subacute nodular migratory panniculitis, Arch. Dermatol. **89**:170, 1974.
**Iodides successful, 1.5 Gm. four times daily.**

Preston, F. E., Emmanual, I. G., Winfield, D. A., et al: Essential thrombocythemia and peripheral gangrene, Br. Med. J. **3**:549, 1974.
**Successfully treated with aspirin, which also relieved pain rapidly and predictably.**

Ryan, T. J.: Microvascular injury, Philadelphia, 1977, W. B. Saunders Co.
**The definitive source book for the world of the small blood vessels of the skin.**

Ryan, T. J.: Vasculitis, Practitioner **218**:682, 1977.
**Lucid contribution concerning a complicated disease spectrum, which includes pathophysiology, etiology, and management.**

Sams, W. M., Thorne, E. G., and Small, P.: Leukocytoclastic vasculitis, Arch. Dermatol. **112**:219, 1976.
**A new entity referring to necrotizing vasculitis of small vessels, assumed to be an immune-complex disorder.**

Sams, W. M., and Winkelmann, R. K.: Necrotizing vasculitis associated with lethal reticuloendothelial diseases, Br. J. Dermatol. **80**:555, 1968.
**The association of skin and viscera emphasized.**

Soter, N. A., Austin, K. F., and Gigli, I.: Urticaria and arthralgias as manifestations of necrotizing angiitis (vasculitis), J. Invest. Dermatol. **68**:485, 1974.
**Bringing the whole picture into focus.**

Waller, J. D., Greenberg, J. H., and Lewis C. W.: Hereditary hemorrhagic telangiectasia with cerebrovascular malformations, Arch. Dermatol. **112**:49, 1976.
**As the clinical picture continues to unfold, serious new lesions make their appearance.**

Winkelmann, R. K., and Ditto, W. B.: Cutaneous and visceral syndromes of necrotizing or "allergic" angiitis. A study of 38 cases, Medicine **43**:59, 1964
**The classic study that actually began to accumulate information.**

Winkelmann, R. K., Schroeter, A. L., and Kierland, R. R.: Clinical studies of livedoid vasculitis (segmented hyalinizing vasculitis), Mayo Clin. Proc. **49**:746, 1974.
**Nicotinic acid therapy has been gratifying, 300-500 mg. daily, and some have been helped by steroids. It is an unrelenting disease.**

## PERNIO (CHILBLAIN)

Pernio is infrequently seen on the North American continent but is common in Northern Europe. The lesions of pernio consist of symmetrical bluish red plaques and papules that may be slightly edematous; they are present over the toes and fingers, feet, legs, and face. The lesions occur after prolonged exposure to dampness and cold. Intense burning and itching occur after the exposure and are aggravated by warming. Occasionally, vesicles and bullae are formed, and the lesions may heal with pigmentation. There are acute and chronic forms.

### *Treatment*

Prevention is more successful than treatment.

Avoidance of extremes of cold and warmth, adequate covering, and protection from cold and dampness comprise the most effective therapy.

## RAYNAUD'S SYNDROME

In the vasospastic disorder known as Raynaud's syndrome, the small digital arteries of both upper and lower extremities undergo intermittent episodes of narrowing. This produces a sharply localized pallor and numbness that give way to bluish cyanosis, followed by erythema. The affected sites develop areas of cutaneous atrophy, scarring, and sclerodermatous changes in the digits. Superficial cutaneous ulcerations, which tend to heal slowly, may be seen. The disorder is symmetrical and bilateral. Cold aggravates the process. In predisposed individuals, vibratory stimuli can trigger off this disorder and lead to sclerodactyly.

Pulses are equal and palpable. Raynaud's syndrome most commonly affects young women; it may be associated with systemic lupus erythematosus and is the commonest symptom in scleroderma.

Raynaud's syndrome must be investigated to rule out *scleroderma*, *lupus erythematosus*, *rheumatoid arthritis*, *shoulder-hand syndrome*, *polycythemia*, *cold sensitivity*, *cryoglobulinemia*, *hypothyroidism*, and *drug effects* such as those from tobacco and ergot derivatives.

### *Treatment*

Treatment includes environmental temperature control to produce consistent warmth, even to moving to a warm climate. Sympatholytic and vasodilating medications may be helpful. Griseofulvin has been used in doses of 500 mg., three times a day, and is a definite benefit in mild cases. Intra-arterial reserpine is successful in some cases. Methyldopa, 1 to 2 Gm. daily, has been reported to help in some cases. Surgical sympathectomy in selected nonresponsive cases relieves symptoms, but may produce temporary benefit only.

Smoking must be discontinued.

#### REFERENCES

Blair, H. M., Headington, J. T., and Lynch, P. T.: Occupational trauma, Raynaud phenomena, and sclerodactyly, Arch. Environ. Health **28**:80, 1974.

**Vibration, cold, and genetic predisposition.**

Tindall, J. P., Whalen, P. E., and Burton, E. E.: Medical uses of intraarterial injections of reserpine, Arch. Dermatol. **110**:223, 1974.

**Appears to be helpful in some patients. A benign form of therapy.**

Varadi, D. P., and Lawrence, A. M.: Suppression of Raynaud's phenomenon by methyldopa, Arch. Intern. Med. **124**:13, 1969.

**Rational, not empirical, but side effects are bothersome.**

## ARTERIOSCLEROSIS OBLITERANS

A very common vascular obstructive disease, arteriosclerosis obliterans affects the feet and toes first, involving the upper extremities only in unusual cases. It produces slowly progressive arterial obstruction, with reduced temperature of the area, pallor on elevation, and slow return of color on dependency. The skin becomes dry, atrophic, and hairless, is easily traumatized, and heals slowly. Ulcerations are common, are usually found on areas of pressure, and are slow to heal. Infection begins easily. Diabetes mellitus predisposes to this disorder, which chiefly affects men past middle age. Peripheral pulsations are reduced or absent.

### *Treatment*

Treatment includes measures to retard the progress of the disease, or surgical correction if the process is localized.

## THROMBOANGIITIS OBLITERANS (BUERGER'S DISEASE)

Thromboangiitis obliterans is a chronic vascular disease involving both the arteries and the veins of the extremities and occurring in young men. It is characterized by pain, asymmetrical involvement, localized pallor, coolness, and edema. Pulsations are reduced in the involved extremity only. Localized areas of thrombophlebitis are present as tender erythematous nodules or plaques. Ulceration may occur. Sensitivity to tobacco is considered to be the primary cause of the disorder.

### *Treatment*

The therapeutic regimen in thromboangiitis obliterans includes interdiction of smoking, prescribed exercises, temperature control, vasodilating medications, and surgery if necessary.

## VENOUS STASIS DERMATITIS AND ULCER (HYPOSTATIC DERMATITIS CAUSED BY VENOUS INSUFFICIENCY)

Hypostatic dermatitis is a very common cutaneous problem that follows an underlying venous insufficiency. It is identified with varicose veins, with or without varicose ulcer.

### *Natural course*

One of the earliest manifestations of chronic venous insufficiency is ankle edema, usually occurring at the end of the day. After a time, patches of tan pigmentation appear on the

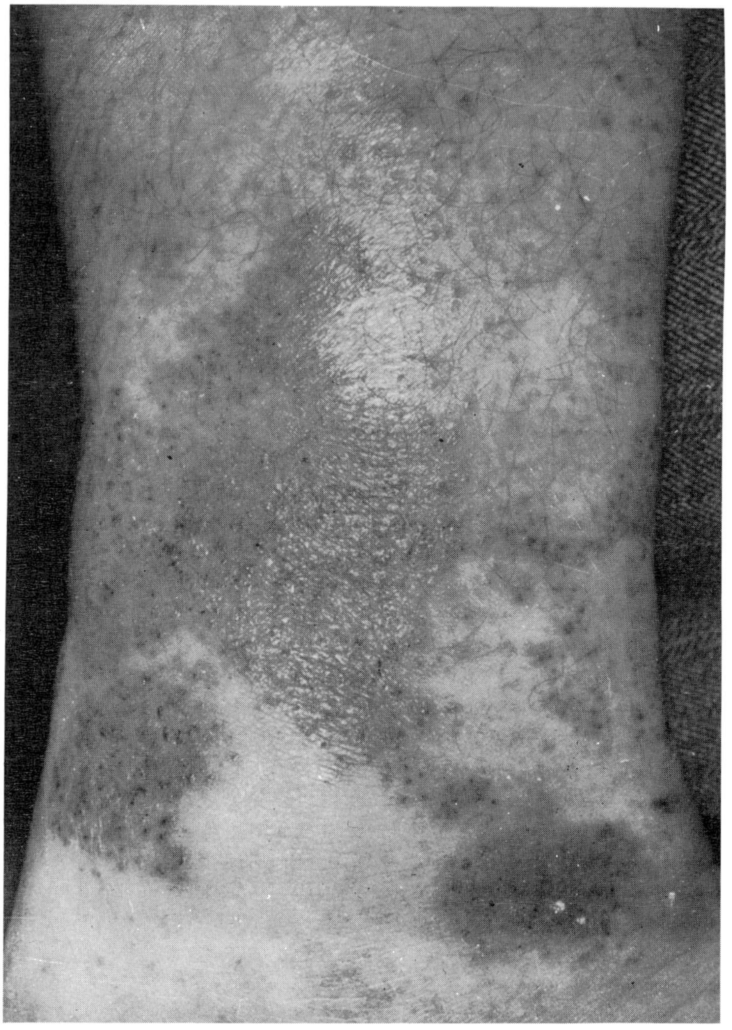

**Fig. 37-7.** Stasis dermatitis in early stage.

lower third of the leg (Fig. 37-7). This is the first evidence of the dermatitis that may follow. The pigment is hemosiderin, deposited because of extravasation of blood through capillary walls attributable to the increased venous pressure.

With continued chronic venous insufficiency, associated with edema and pruritus, a dermatitis often develops, consisting of a patchy erythema. Often, pinpoint multiple petechial lesions become visible. The area of dermatitis may be dry and scaling or oozing and vesicular. Secondary infection of excoriated areas is often seen, and progression to a more extensive involvement is to be expected. If the edema and the dermatitis persist, a characteristic subcutaneous induration may develop. The overlying skin is reddish brown in color (Fig. 37-8). The final stage is associated with atrophy and fibrous scarring of the area. At any stage of this process an ulcer may develop surprisingly quickly in the devitalized tissue. This is usually secondary to trauma and infection and is most frequent on the medial aspect, adjacent to the malleolus (Plate 62). Although some pain is usually asso-

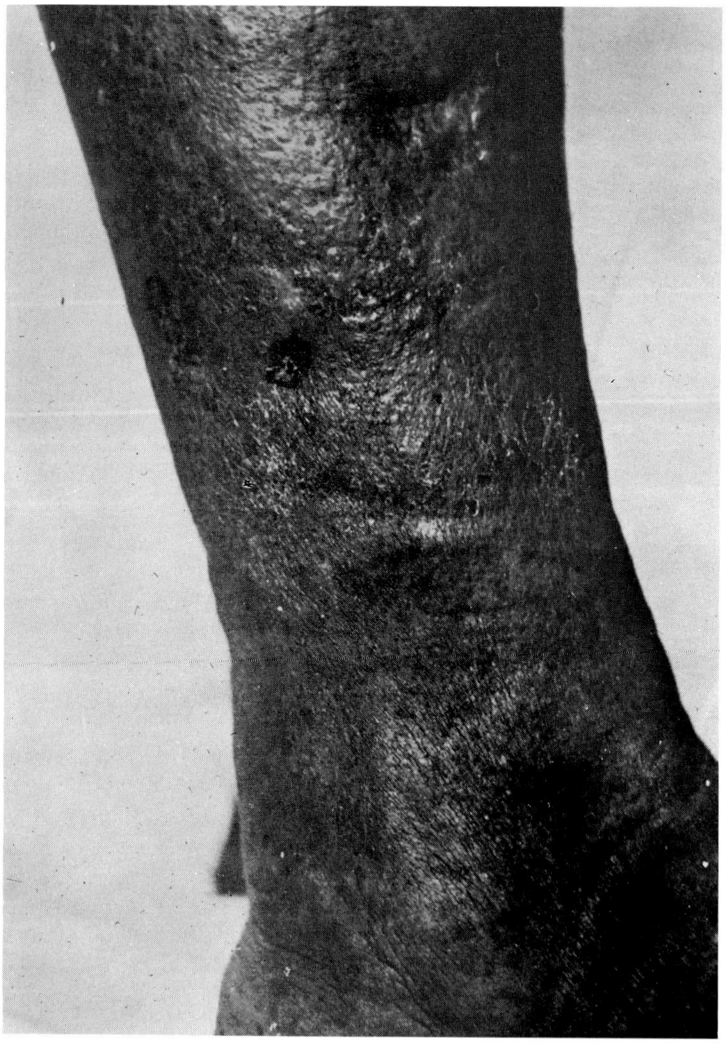

**Fig. 37-8.** Chronic pigmented stasis dermatitis with ulceration.

ciated with the ulcer, particularly on dependency, it is not the severe, sleep-destroying pain of the ischemic ulcer. Hypostatic ulcer is notoriously slow in healing, particularly with continued normal activity, and it may be infected. Usually the ulcer has a good color, unlike ulcers attributable to arteriosclerosis.

*The skin area involved with hypostatic dermatitis is peculiarly susceptible to unfavorable reactions, especially* to various topical

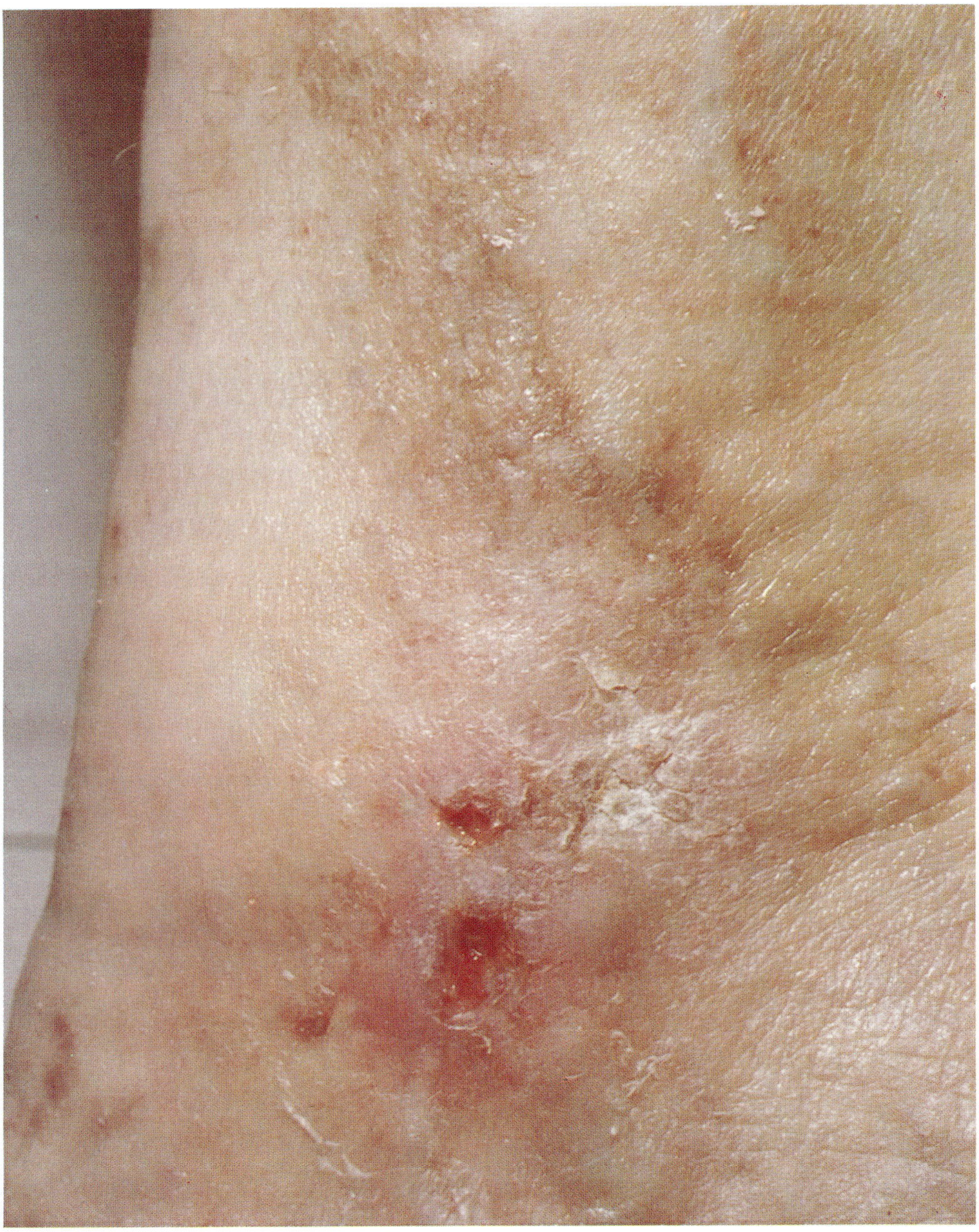

**Plate 62**

Stasis dermatitis and ulcer. Note pigmentation following course of visible veins.

medications. It is easily irritated and also appears to be easily sensitized (or made allergic) to these preparations. Therefore great care must be exercised in topical management, and bland, nonsensitizing preparations should be applied.

It has been shown that if a preparation is applied to which the patient is allergic, for example, lanolin, the leg may not show the expected acute allergic reaction, but an ulcer may simply fail to improve.

A frequent finding in hypostatic dermatitis is the concomitant development of similar pruritic patches of dermatitis at distant sites on the skin surface. These are difficult to heal if an active dermatitis remains on the ankle. If a stasis dermatitis is treated too aggressively or irritated by treatment, these distant patches of dermatitis are more likely to appear (autoeczematization).

### *Pertinent information*

The mechanism responsible for varicose veins is incompetency of the semilunar valves at the junction between the superficial (saphenous) and deep (femoral) venous systems. Normally these valves support the column of blood within the vein and thereby prevent backflow.

At least 10% of the adult population have varicose veins. A high percentage of patients with varicose veins have a familial history of this condition. Hereditary weakness in the veins and in the valves results in venous dilatation and stasis. Contributing factors usually associated with hypostatic dermatitis, varicose veins or both, include obesity, pregnancy, and thrombophlebitis. Most patients with the complete syndrome of chronic venous stasis, dermatitis, and ulcer will give a history consistent with an episode of thrombophlebitis some years previously. Long periods of standing, as required of barbers, housewives, and dentists, and conditions that lead to increased intra-abdominal pressure, such as lifting and straining, are also important factors in development of this condition.

Ryan has written a thoughtful analysis of capillary physiology at the level of the upper dermis, drawn from observations of legs of 110 patients, which is well worth perusing by students of the abnormal blood supply to the epidermis in leg disorders.

### *Microscopic findings*

Hemosiderin is present in the dermis, associated with subacute inflammation and dermal scar tissue. The arterioles and venules in the area show intimal proliferation, and there is arteriolar obliteration in ulcerated areas.

### *Differential diagnosis of edema*

Faced with the problem of a localized ankle edema, the physician must rule out congestive heart failure, renal disease, hypoproteinemia, lymphedema, arteriovenous fistula, and other less common causes of edema.

### *Differential diagnosis of dermatitis*

The differential diagnosis of the dermatitis includes several conditions with similar clinical appearance.

***Allergic eczematous contact dermatitis.*** The acutely inflamed area involved by allergic eczematous contact dermatitis conforms to the site of contact with the causative agent. This may be present to complicate a stasis dermatitis.

***Psoriasis.*** The heavy white scale with punctate bleeding points beneath is characteristic of psoriasis. The knees, elbows, and scalp are typically involved.

***Lichen planus.*** Lichen planus is manifested by hyperpigmented, chronic, pruritic scaling patches of dermatitis on the anterior surface of both lower legs. There are ordinarily other areas of involvement, with characteristic, flat-topped angular papules.

***Lichen simplex chronicus.*** Lichen simplex chronicus is a patchy, dry, lichenified, unilateral pruritic plaque.

***Fungal infection.*** A diffuse, unilateral scaling patch of erythema occurs in fungal infection. On microscopic and cultural examination, the fungus will be detected.

### *Differential diagnosis of ulcer*

The differential diagnosis of the ulcer includes similar lesions occurring with a variety of diseases.

***Arteriosclerotic ulcer.*** Pale, ischemic arteriosclerotic ulcerations appear on the foot, heel, or areas other than those adjacent to the malleolus. Pedal pulses are absent or diminished. Patients with diabetes are especially affected.

***Hypertensive ischemic ulcer.*** Hypertensive ischemic ulcers are pale, painful, and shallow; they may be of sudden onset and are usually situated laterally or posteriorly on the ankle. They have little or no granulation tissue.

***Decubitus, or pressure, ulcer.*** Decubitus ulcers occur in debilitated or bedridden individuals at points of continued pressure such as the heels.

***Ulcer occurring in anemia, arthritis, and hypersplenism.*** Leg ulcers may appear in conditions associated with splenomegaly, such as sickle-cell anemia, spherocytic anemia, and Felty's syndrome.

***Pyoderma gangrenosum.*** Concurrently with active ulcerative colitis, one may see irregular, slowly healing necrotic leg ulcers, which are often multiple, bilateral, and present mainly below the knee.

***Necrobiosis lipoidica (diabeticorum).*** The red-yellow-brown atrophic patches of this disorder seldom ulcerate, but can do so; indeed, we have seen seven or eight patches spontaneously ulcerate simultaneously.

## Some causes of leg ulcer

**CIRCULATORY**
- Venous stasis
- Arteriosclerosis
- Diabetes mellitus
- Thromboangiitis obliterans
- Hypertension
- Livedo reticularis
- Vasculitis
- Lupus erythematosus
- Periarteritis nodosa
- Raynaud's disease
- Chilblain

**HEMATOLOGICAL**
- Sickle-cell anemia
- Polycythemia
- Hemolytic anemias
- Thrombocytopenic purpura
- Hypersplenism, Felty's syndrome
- Dysproteinemias
  - Macroglobulinemia
  - Cryoglobulinemia

**BACTERIAL**
- Ecthyma
- Erythema induratum (tuberculosis)
- Syphilis (gumma)
- Diphtheria

**MYCOTIC**
- North American blastomycosis
- Sporotrichosis
- Coccidioidomycosis
- Histoplasmosis

**TRAUMATIC**
- Factitial
- Thermal
- Physical

**NEOPLASTIC**
- Squamous cell carcinoma
- Mycosis fungoides
- Malignant melanoma

### *Investigation*

The patient's history should be obtained, relative to duration, onset, previous varicosities, episodes of likely phlebitis, family history, travel, and general health.

A physical examination must be made to make certain the disorder is not a localized process. Blood pressure should be measured.

Laboratory tests should include hemoglobin, red cell morphology, blood glucose level, VDRL test, and urinalysis; culture and sensitivity of ulcer, if indicated; culture for mycobacteria and examination for fungi; and antinuclear factor, serum, or immune electrophoresis.

### *Treatment of venous insufficiency*

If the physician and patient will take adequate measures to ensure proper initial management of the acute stages of thrombophlebitis, as well as the varicose veins that are often associated with pregnancy and the immediate postpartum period, much will be done to reduce the problems that arise because of prolonged venous insufficiency. The basis of treatment of venous insufficiency is the prevention of orthostatic edema.

The following measures are suggested for those patients who, because of advanced age, previous surgical failure, pregnancy, or inoperability, should be managed in a conservative fashion:

1. Strict avoidance of standing or sitting in one position for prolonged periods of time.
2. Regular 15- to 20-minute rest periods during the day when the legs can be maintained at a level well above the heart. The foot of the bed should be raised 6 inches or more.
3. Proper instruction in the wearing of an adequate support for the limb. This can best be achieved by the careful application of an elastic bandage (3 inches wide) from the base of the toes to just below the knee. This should be applied prior to getting out of bed each morning and not removed until retiring. An individually fitted heavy elastic stocking may also be suggested. It may be necessary for the patient to wear these supports indefinitely if surgery is not feasible.
4. If obesity is a contributing factor, a proper weight-reduction diet should be instituted.

The measures just outlined should be followed throughout pregnancy and during the first 6 weeks of the postpartum period.

### *Treatment of stasis dermatitis*

Choice of therapy in stasis dermatitis, is determined by the stage of development.

*Early lesions*, which are dry and localized, respond to glucocorticoid cream applied sparingly four times daily. Elastic support, as described previously, is desirable.

*Subacute (moist) lesions* are treated with cool compresses of Burow's solution, 1:20 dilution, or the prepackaged tablets or powders, 1 to 1 pint of cool tap water. After compressing for 15 minutes three times daily and then air drying, one should apply 0.5% hydrocortisone cream or other glucocorticoid cream sparingly. Elevation of the leg for 15 to 20 minutes three times daily and elastic support (as described previously) provide additional benefit.

*Severe lesions*, or spreading and weeping dermatitis, with the appearance of distant patches of eczema, require bed rest, with the foot of the bed elevated. Burow's solution should be used for cool compresses, as for subacute lesions. Use of appropriate systemic antibiotics, determined by culture and sensitivity studies, is indicated if secondary infection is apparent. Tetracycline in a dose of 250 mg., given four times daily for 5 days, is effective in many cases. Betamethasone, 0.1%, or equivalent fluorinated steroid cream is applied sparingly after compresses. Elastic support is employed only after the acute process has subsided and the patient is allowed to become ambulatory.

With a generalized but noninfected dermatitis, temporary use of systemic oral glucocorticoids may be desirable to control the dermatitis and eliminate the distant cutaneous lesions elsewhere.

### *Treatment of varicose ulcer*

Bed rest is the most satisfactory single factor in the treatment of varicose ulcer.

*Varicose ulcer* requires culture with sensitivity studies, to determine the appropriate systemic antibiotic therapy to eliminate infection. Application of Burow's solution compresses, using the prepared powders or tablets, 1 tablet or packet to 1 pint of cool tap water, is followed by a local antibiotic such as neomycin or tetracycline powder. The leg may be covered with a commercially available gelatin—zinc oxide paste (modified Unna's boot) bandage, allowing for some shrinkage when dry. This is replaced at weekly intervals at first and then gradually at longer intervals as the ulcer heals and the patient's comfort allows.

Debrisan powder has been promoted as a method of speeding exudate and bacteria removal from wound surfaces. It is applied daily under dressing and has a strong rational background for its use. Clinical trial will help us to determine its usefulness. The beads of dextran absorb some compounds and attract others. It seems to have little value in dry, arid ulcer beds.

Zinc sulfate, 220 mg. three times a day, in capsule or tablet form for 1 or 2 months, appears to be beneficial if serum zinc levels are below normal. Goolamali and Comaish have suggested that a more critical set of studies should be carried out on the effect of zinc supplement on leg ulcer healing. The reports are in conflict, and more studies are necessary.

Pinch grafting of slowly healing ulcers has in our experience been very useful. This can be done in the hospital with a brief stay and saves much time otherwise spent languishing in bed waiting for the ulcer to heal.

Surgical intervention is called for in carefully selected cases. Active dermatitis and secondary infection must be controlled prior to any operative procedure. The earlier the chronic venous insufficiency of the limb is corrected, the more satisfactory the operative result.

*Experienced* surgical consultation is desirable to ascertain the degree of improvement to expect from venous stripping or other operative procedures. If improved venous return can be expected, then the stasis dermatitis and threat of future ulcer formation will be lessened, and surgery is recommended. Without surgery, once stasis is apparent, lifelong maintenance of an elastic support is usually necessary to avoid the development of more severe dermatitis and perhaps ulceration. These complications are far more satisfactorily prevented than treated.

### REFERENCES

Ellis, H.: Hypostatic dermatitis and leg ulcer (varicose eczema and ulcer). In Maddin, S., editor: Current dermatologic management, ed. 2, St. Louis, 1975, The C. V. Mosby Co., p. 118

Goolamali, S. K., and Comaish, S.: Zinc and the skin, Int. J. Dermatol. **14**:182, 1975.
**Reports conflict on efficacy of oral zinc in cutaneous healing, suggesting that further studies are required.**

Leading article: Venous ulcers, Lancet **1**:522, 1977.
**Responsible mechanisms covered and current treatment.**

Peachey, R. D. G.: Leg ulcers. In Rook, A. editor: Recent advances in dermatology, IV, London, 1977, Churchill Livingstone, P. 199.
**Superb.**

Roenigk, H. H., and Young, J. R.: Leg ulcers. Medical and surgical management, Hagerstown, Md., 1975, Harper & Row, Publishers.
**Well illustrated, practical, basic science emphasis, treatment oriented.**

Samitz, M. H., and Dana, A. S.: Cutaneous lesions of the lower extremities, Philadelphia, 1971, J. B. Lippincott Co., P. 154.
**A pictorial feast.**

Smith, J. D., Holder, W. R., and Smith, E. B.: Pinch grafts for cutaneous ulcers, South. Med. J. **64**:1166, 1971.
**An excellent description of a time-honored technique that should have wider application.**

# Index



Numbers in italics refer to pages with illustrations.

**D**

**F**

**I**